Evaluation of Adult Gerontology Health for the APN Practitioner

NUR 580

Division of Nursing

Keuka College

JONES & BARTLETT
LEARNING

World Headquarters
Jones & Bartlett Learning
5 Wall Street
Burlington, MA 01803
978-443-5000
info@jblearning.com
www.jblearning.com

Jones & Bartlett Learning books and products are available through most bookstores and online booksellers. To contact Jones & Bartlett Learning directly, call 800-832-0034, fax 978-443-8000, or visit our website, www.jblearning.com.

This book is produced through PUBLISH – a custom publishing service offered by Jones & Bartlett Learning. For more information on PUBLISH, contact us at 800-832-0034 or visit our website at www.jblearning.com.

Disclaimer
This publication is sold with the understanding that the publisher is not engaged in rendering medical, legal, accounting, or other professional services. If medical, legal, accounting, or other professional service advice is required, the service of a competent professional should be sought. The authors, editor, and publisher have designed this publication to provide accurate information with regard to the subject matter covered. However, they are not responsible for errors, omissions, or for any outcomes related to the use of the contents of this publication and make no guarantee and assume no responsibility or liability for the use of the products and procedures described, or the correctness, sufficiency, or completeness of stated information, opinions, or recommendations. Treatments and side effects described in this publication are not applicable to all people; required dosages and experienced side effects will vary among individuals. Drugs and medical devices discussed herein are controlled by the Food and Drug Administration (FDA) and may have limited availability for use only in research studies or clinical trials. Research, clinical practice, and government regulations often change accepted standards. When consideration is being given to the use of any drug in the clinical setting, the health care provider or reader is responsible for determining FDA status of the drug, reading the package insert, and reviewing prescribing information for the most current recommendations on dose, precautions, and contraindications and for determining the appropriate usage for the product. This is especially important in the case of drugs that are new or seldom used. Any references in this publication to procedures to be employed when rendering emergency care to the sick and injured are provided solely as a general guide; other or additional safety measures might be required under particular circumstances. This publication is not intended as a statement of the standards of care required in any particular situation; circumstances and the physical conditions of patients can vary widely from one emergency to another. This publication is not intended in any way to advise emergency personnel concerning their legal authority to perform the activities or procedures discussed. Such local determination should be made only with the aid of legal counsel. Some images in this publication feature models; these models do not necessarily endorse, represent, or participate in the activities represented in the images.

Cover Image: © Andres Rodriguez/Fotolia.com

6048
Printed in the United States of America
22 21 20 19 18   10 9 8 7 6 5 4

Contents

What Is a Nurse Practitioner?

Individuals who have never experienced the care of a nurse practitioner (NP)—whether they are physicians, reporters, lawmakers, bureaucrats, lobbyists, or new patients—often request clarification about just who NPs are and what they do.

It is their combination of the skills of both a physician and a nurse that seems to confuse people. Yet it is that combination of skills that makes an NP unique.

Definition of Nurse Practitioner

The term *nurse practitioner* has been given a variety of definitions.

- According to a state NP organization, "Nurse practitioners are registered professional nurses who are prepared, through advanced graduate education and clinical training, to provide a range of health services, including the diagnosis and management of common as well as complex medical conditions to individuals of all ages."[1]
- According to a national NP organization, "NPs are quickly becoming the health partner of choice for millions of Americans. As clinicians that blend clinical expertise in diagnosing and treating health conditions with an added emphasis on disease prevention and health management, NPs bring a comprehensive perspective to health care."[2]
- A board of nursing defines an NP as follows: "A nurse practitioner (NP) is an RN [registered nurse] who has earned a separate license as an NP through additional education and experience in a distinct specialty area of practice. Nurse practitioners may diagnose, treat, and prescribe for a patient's condition that falls within their specialty areas of practice. This is done in collaboration with a licensed physician qualified in the specialty involved and in accordance with an approved written practice agreement and protocols. Nurse practitioners are autonomous and do not practice under the supervision of the collaborating physician."[3]
- According to federal law, "Nurse practitioner means a nurse practitioner who performs such services as such individual is legally authorized to perform (in the state in which the individual performs such services) in accordance with state laws and who meets such training, education, and experience required as the Secretary has prescribed in regulations" [42 U.S.C.A. § 1395x(aa)(5)(A)].
- In California state law, "nurse practitioner means a registered nurse who possesses additional preparation and skills in physical diagnosis, psych-social assessment, and

management of health-illness needs in primary health care and who has been prepared in a program conforming to board standards as specified in Section 1484" [Cal. Code Regs. tit. 16, § 1480(a)].

For state-by-state definitions of the term *nurse practitioner*, see **Appendix A**.

An NP, by Any Other Name . . .

Other designations sometimes given to NPs include physician extender, mid-level practitioner, nonphysician practitioner, and advanced practice nurse. For a state-by-state listing of official terms for NPs, see **Appendix B**.

Physician Extender

The term *physician extender* is used by physicians' associations and publications aimed at the physician market and usually refers collectively to NPs, clinical nurse specialists, nurse anesthetists, nurse midwives, and physician assistants.

Mid-Level Practitioner

The term *mid-level practitioner* is used by some physician groups, some states, and the federal government in the Code of Federal Regulation sections dealing with Drug Enforcement Administration (DEA) registration. The DEA defines a mid-level practitioner as follows:

> The term mid-level practitioner means an individual practitioner other than a physician, dentist, veterinarian, or podiatrist, who is licensed, registered, or otherwise permitted by the United States or the jurisdiction in which he/she practices to dispense controlled dangerous substances in the course of professional practice. Examples of mid-level practitioners include, but are not limited to, healthcare providers such as nurse practitioners, nurse midwives, nurse anesthetists, clinical nurse specialists, and physician assistants who are authorized to dispense controlled substances by the state in which they practice.
>
> *Citation:* 21 C.F.R. § 1300.01(b).

Some state laws provide a definition of mid-level practitioner. For example, in Minnesota, "'Mid-level practitioner' means a nurse practitioner, nurse midwife, nurse anesthetist, advanced clinical nurse specialist, or physician assistant" [Minn. Stat. § 144.1501(f)].

Nonphysician Practitioner

The term *nonphysician practitioner* is used by the Centers for Medicare & Medicaid Services and Medicare administrative contractors. Here is the definition from one administrator's website[4]:

> For Medicare purposes, the term nonphysician practitioner (NPP) includes:
>
> - Nurse practitioner or clinical nurse specialist, as those terms are defined in section 1861(aa)(5) of the Social Security Act, who is working in collaboration with the physician in accordance with State law
> - Certified nurse-midwife, as defined in section 1861(gg) of the Social Security Act, as authorized by State law

- A physician assistant, as defined in section 1861(aa)(5) of the Social Security Act, under the supervision of the physician

Advanced Practice Nurse

Advanced practice nurse is an umbrella term used by some states and some nursing associations to cover, collectively, NPs, clinical nurse specialists, nurse midwives, and nurse anesthetists. NPs differ from other advanced practice nurses in that they offer a wider range of services to a wider portion of the population. Other advanced practice nurses compare with NPs in the following ways:

- *Nurse anesthetist*: Narrow range of services (preoperative assessment, administration of anesthesia, management of postanesthesia recovery) to a narrow base of patients (people having anesthesia).
- *Clinical nurse specialist*: Medium range of services (consultation, research, education, administration, coordination of care, case management, direct care within the definition of a registered nurse) to a narrow patient base (people under the care of a medical specialist).
- *Certified nurse midwife*: Narrow range of services (well-women gynecologic care, management of pregnancy and childbirth, antepartum and postpartum care) to a medium-sized base of patients (childbearing women).
- *Nurse practitioner*: Wide range of services (evaluation, diagnosis, treatment, education, risk assessment, health promotion, case management, coordination of care, counseling) to a wide base of patients, depending upon area of certification; a family nurse practitioner can have a patient base of any age, gender, or problem.

Services Provided by NPs

NPs may perform any service authorized by a state nurse practice act. Some nurse practice acts are so broad as to allow any service agreed upon by an NP and collaborating physician. Generally, NP services include:

- Obtaining medical histories and performing physical examinations
- Diagnosing and treating health problems
- Ordering and interpreting laboratory tests and X-rays
- Prescribing medications and other treatments
- Providing prenatal care and family planning services
- Providing well-child care and immunizations
- Providing gynecologic examinations and Pap smears
- Providing education about health risks, illness prevention, and health maintenance
- Providing counseling regarding the need for compliance with a diagnostic and/or treatment plan, course of illness, side effects of treatment, and/or prognosis
- Coordinating care and case management

Typically, an NP has the following duties and responsibilities:

- Conducts comprehensive medical and social history of individuals, including those who are healthy and those with acute illnesses and chronic diseases

- Conducts physical examination of individuals, either comprehensive or problem focused
- Orders, performs, and interprets laboratory tests for screening and for diagnosing
- Prescribes medications
- Performs therapeutic or corrective measures, including urgent care
- Refers individuals to appropriate specialist nurses, physicians, or other healthcare providers
- Makes independent decisions regarding management and treatment of medical problems identified
- Performs various invasive/clinical procedures such as suturing, biopsy of skin lesions, and endometrial biopsy, depending upon education, training, patient needs, and written agreement with physician collaborator
- Prescribes and orders appropriate diet and other forms of treatment, such as physical therapy
- Provides information, instruction, and counseling on health maintenance, health promotion, social problems, illness prevention, illness management, and medication use
- Evaluates the effectiveness of instruction and counseling and provides additional instruction and counseling as necessary
- Initiates and participates in research studies and projects
- Teaches groups of clients about health-related topics
- Provides outreach health education services in the community
- Serves as preceptor for medical, nursing, NP, or physician assistant students
- Accepts after-hours calls and handles after-hours problems on a rotating schedule
- Participates in development of pertinent health education materials
- Participates in development of clinical practice guidelines
- Initiates and maintains follow-up of noncompliant patients
- Makes client home visits and provides care in the home as necessary
- Makes hospital visits and follows hospital care of established patients
- Consults with other healthcare providers about established clients who have been admitted to hospital, home care, rehabilitation, or nursing homes
- Corresponds with insurers, employers, government agencies, and other healthcare providers about established clients as necessary
- Manages care of clients; develops plan of treatment and/or follow-up and monitors progress, determines when referral to another provider is necessary, makes necessary arrangements for further care, determines when hospital admission or emergency room visit is necessary, and determines when illness is resolved
- Assesses social/economic factors for each client and tailors care to those factors
- Manages care of clients in a way that balances quality and cost
- Tracks outcome of interventions and alters interventions to achieve optimum results
- Obtains informed consent from clients as appropriate and necessary
- Maintains familiarity with community resources and connects clients with appropriate resources
- Contracts with clients regarding provider responsibilities and client responsibilities
- Supervises and teaches registered nurses and nonlicensed healthcare workers

- Participates in community programs and health fairs, school programs, and workplace programs
- Represents the practice or the profession as an NP before local and state governing bodies, agencies, and private businesses as needed

Preparation and License Requirements

All NPs are registered nurses (RNs) with education beyond the basic requirements for RN licensure. Most NPs have master's degrees, and some have doctorates. Master's degrees for NPs are required by law in 34 states. NPs without master's degrees have completed a program that meets requirements of state law.

State-required qualifications vary widely. For example, in Alaska, NPs must have completed a 1-year academic course, have an RN license, be certified by a national certifying agency, and have 30 hours of continuing education every 2 years. In Pennsylvania, NPs must have an RN license, a master's degree, certification by a national organization, must provide evidence of continuing competence in medical diagnosis and therapeutics, and must have 30 hours of continuing education per year and 45 hours of advanced pharmacology. Federal law defers to state law regarding NP qualifications (42 C.F.R. § 440.166).

In 45 states, NPs are required by state law to take and pass a national certification exam. A state requirement that an NP be nationally certified leads to a requirement of master's education because the certifying agencies of adult and pediatric NPs require a master's degree to sit for the certification examination.

Initials

Among the initials used to designate NPs are CRNP (certified registered nurse practitioner); ANP-C (adult nurse practitioner–certified); CPNP (certified pediatric nurse practitioner); CGNP (certified geriatric nurse practitioner); RN, CS (registered nurse, certified specialist); ARNP (advanced registered nurse practitioner); and APRN (advanced practice registered nurse).

Areas of Practice

NPs may be certified in the following areas:

- Adult primary care
- Family primary care
- Geriatric primary care
- Neonatal care
- Obstetrics and gynecology
- Pediatric primary care
- Pediatric acute care
- Acute care
- Primary care of school-aged children

- Family planning
- Emergency health care
- Maternal child health
- Mental health/psychiatric care
- Critical care
- Oncology
- Palliative care
- Rehabilitation
- Community health
- Occupational health

Not all categories are recognized in all states.

According to the APRN Consensus Model (2008):

> APRNs are educated in one of the four roles and in at least one of six population foci: family/individual across the lifespan, adult-gerontology, neonatal, pediatrics, women's health/gender-related or psych/mental health.[5]

Legal History of NPs

Before the emergence of advanced practice nurses, the legal scope of nurses' practice excluded the diagnosis and treatment of medical problems. Nurses carried out physicians' orders. In the mid-1970s, some state nurse practice acts were amended to include "nursing diagnoses" in the scope of nursing practice. A nursing diagnosis "limits the diagnostic process to those diagnoses that represent human responses to actual or potential health problems that are within the legal scope of nursing practice."[6]

When a physician shortage arose in the 1960s, it became evident that the shortage and the limitations on nurses' making medical diagnoses were restricting access to health care for people in medically underserved areas. Certain nurses and physicians joined forces to solve the problem. One answer was the NP.

The first NP educational program was a joint effort between Henry K. Silver, a pediatrician, and Loretta C. Ford, then a nursing professor, at the University of Colorado in 1965. Their project was one of many efforts to deal with a physician shortage. The first NPs began practicing in the late 1960s.

As the concept was envisioned, NPs would make not only nursing diagnoses but also medical diagnoses. Further, they would treat patients with medical therapeutics, ordering pharmacotherapeutics and other treatments. It became necessary to broaden the legal scope of nursing practice.

As soon as NPs began to emerge from the training programs, a body of law emerged governing NP licensure and scope of practice. Idaho was the first state to revise its regulations to allow diagnosis and treatment by nurses.

By the mid-1970s, state legislators began to consider proposed laws regarding prescriptive authority for NPs. In some states, the prescriptive authority was granted through the regulatory process; in others, it was granted through the legislative process. By 2006, NPs had achieved some degree of prescriptive privileges in all states and the District of Columbia.

The main legal goal of NPs for 30 years was achieved. The next legal hurdle became evident with the enrollment of a large percentage of the population into managed-care plans. While NPs had the authority to bill for services to patients covered by Medicare and Medicaid, they were not necessarily credentialed as providers by the managed-care plans. So, NPs met with executives at managed-care organizations and attempted to persuade them to allow NPs to be "primary care providers" for the plans. As of 2013, that had been achieved, for the most part, in most states. The next legal hurdle is achieving the legal authority to medically manage patients within an NP's scope of practice, without mandated physician collaboration. While NPs in some states may practice without a collaborative practice agreement with a physician, the majority of states still require some form of physician involvement in NP practice.

Demographics

There are over 157,000 NPs in the United States, according to the American Academy of Nurse Practitioners.[2]

NPs in Primary Care

The concept of the NP emerged from a need for more primary care providers in underserved areas of the nation. While many NPs work in specialty and acute care settings, many provide primary care.

Because health plans designate certain generalist physicians—pediatricians, internists, and family practitioners—as primary care providers (PCPs) for groups of patients, it is important for NPs to be included in the definition of PCP. It is also important for NPs to be included as providers who can be a "medical home" for a patient.

Definition of Primary Care

The following are definitions of primary care.

According to a national health policy think tank, the National Academy of Sciences' Institute of Medicine,

- "Primary care is the provision of integrated, accessible healthcare services by clinicians who are accountable for addressing a large majority of personal healthcare needs, developing a sustained partnership with patients, and practicing in the context of family and community."[7]

A nurse practice act written by a state agency defines primary health care as:

- "that which occurs when a consumer makes contact with a healthcare provider who assumes responsibility and accountability for the continuity of health care regardless of the presence or absence of disease" [CAL. CODE REGS. tit. 16 § 1480(b)].

A state legislature's definition is:

- "the health care which clients receive at the first point of contact with the healthcare system and [that] is continuous and comprehensive. Primary health care includes health promotion, prevention of disease and disability, health maintenance, rehabilitation, identification of health problems, management of health problems, and referral" [Code Me. R. § 02 380 008(G)].

Finally, here is a definition provided by the American Academy of Family Physicians:

- "Primary care is that care provided by physicians specifically trained for and skilled in comprehensive first contact and continuing care for persons with any undiagnosed sign, symptom, or health concern (the 'undifferentiated' patient) not limited by problem origin (biological, behavioral, or social), organ system, gender, or diagnosis. Primary care includes health promotion, disease prevention, health maintenance, counseling, patient education, diagnosis, and treatment of acute and chronic illnesses in a variety of healthcare settings (e.g., office, inpatient, critical care, long-term care, home care, day care, etc.). Primary care is performed and managed by a personal physician, utilizing other health professionals, consultation and/or referral as appropriate."[8] The American Academy of Family Physicians has five definitions of primary care. One of them acknowledges that providers other than physicians provide primary care.

Primary care itself is not controversial. Who performs primary care is somewhat controversial. Who receives reimbursement for primary care is very controversial.

Legal Authority of NPs to Be Primary Care Providers

Some state laws specifically authorize NPs to be PCPs; that is, to be designated as the individual responsible for the primary care of a patient enrolled in a managed-care plan.

An example of one such law is Maryland's, which provides that "... each member [of a health maintenance organization] shall have an opportunity to select a primary physician or a certified nurse practitioner from among those available to the health maintenance organization...." (Md Health-General Code Ann. § 19-705.1).

In Maryland, a clause in the state law governing health maintenance organizations had been construed as prohibiting anyone other than a physician from being a PCP. Maryland NPs went to the legislature asking for a change in that law. In 2003, the change was made, and the language cited here was enacted.

In some states, no law prohibits an NP from being designated as a PCP.

NPs as Team Members in Secondary and Tertiary Care

Whereas the role of NP was originally contemplated to be in primary care, more and more NPs are working for specialists and in hospitals. For those NPs, state law on scope of practice and reimbursement and federal law on reimbursement are most relevant.

NP Versus Physician Assistant: What Is the Difference?

While NPs and physician assistants (PAs) may function very similarly and may, in some states, be interchangeable in terms of job description, there are differences between them in legal definition, scope of practice, licensure, and independence of practice. PAs practice medicine under the supervision of a physician, never independently, as far as the law is concerned. PAs are true physician extenders. NPs practice under their own licenses and in some states may practice independent of physician involvement. NPs may be physician extenders or practice independently, depending upon state law.

Definition and Scope of Practice of PAs, Compared with NPs

By definition, a PA is a healthcare provider who practices medicine with physician supervision. NPs define themselves as nurses with a broadened scope of practice and do not define themselves as physician-supervised professionals.

PAs include in descriptions of their duties taking medical histories, performing physical examinations, ordering and interpreting laboratory tests, diagnosing and treating illnesses, assisting at surgery, prescribing and/or dispensing medication, and counseling patients.[9] NPs would include all of these activities in their scope of practice, with the exception of assisting in surgery. While some NPs assist in surgery under practice agreements with physicians, it is not so common an activity that it is universally included in the scope of practice of NPs. NPs usually include special attention to healthcare maintenance and illness prevention in their statements of scope of practice. The nurse practice act of at least one state, Oregon, includes hospital admission in the scope of NP practice.

The scope of a PA's practice corresponds with a supervising physician's practice, with the understanding that the supervising physician will handle the more complicated medical cases. PAs are authorized to prescribe medications in all 50 states, the District of Columbia, and Guam.[9]

Physician Involvement with PA Practice

PAs acknowledge their status as physician extenders. According to the American Academy of Physician Assistants, "By design, physicians and PAs work together as a team, and all PAs practice medicine with physician supervision."[9]

The *Guidelines for Physician/Physician Assistant Practice*,[10] adopted by the American Medical Association House of Delegates in 1995, state the following:

1. The physician is responsible for managing the health care of patients in all practice settings.
2. Healthcare services delivered by physicians and PAs must be within the scope of each practitioner's authorized practice as defined by state law.
3. The physician is ultimately responsible for coordinating and managing the care of patients and, with the appropriate input of the PA, ensuring the quality of health care provided to patients.
4. The physician is responsible for the supervision of the PA in all settings.
5. The role of the PA in the delivery of health care should be defined through mutually agreed-upon guidelines that are developed by the physician and the PA and based on the physician's delegatory style.

6. The physician must be available for consultation with the PA at all times, either in person or through telecommunication system or other means.
7. The extent of the involvement by the PA in the assessment and implementation of treatment will depend on the complexity and acuity of the patient's condition and the training and experience and preparation of the PA as adjudged by the physician.
8. Patients should be made clearly aware at all times whether they are being cared for by a physician or a PA.
9. The physician and PA together should review all delegated patient services on a regular basis, as well as the mutually agreed-upon guidelines for practice.
10. The physician is responsible for clarifying and familiarizing the PA with his or her supervising methods and style of delegating patient care.

Demographics

As of June 2013, there were approximately 86,500 individuals in clinical practice as PAs.[9]

Education

PAs are educated in programs that use the medical model and are designed to complement physician training. The American Academy of Physician Assistants describes PA education in the following way: PA education includes instruction in core sciences including anatomy, physiology, biochemistry, pharmacology, physical diagnosis, pathophysiology, microbiology, clinical laboratory science, behavioral science, and medical ethics. PAs also complete more than 2000 hours of clinical rotations, with an emphasis on primary care in ambulatory clinics, physician offices, and acute or long-term care facilities. Rotations include family medicine, internal medicine, obstetrics and gynecology, pediatrics, general surgery, emergency medicine, and psychiatry.[9]

Licensure Requirements

According to the American Academy of Physician Assistants, "Before PAs can practice, they must apply for and obtain authorization from the state. In most states and DC, this authorization process is called 'licensure,' but in one state (OH) it is called 'registration.'"[9] For licensure, PAs must graduate from an accredited PA program and pass a national certifying examination.

Certification Requirements

To maintain national certification, PAs must log 100 hours of continuing medical education (CME) every 2 years. CME requirements to maintain state authorization to practice vary from state to state. PAs sit for recertification every 6 years. See **Table 1** for a comparison of PAs, NPs, and physicians according to basic and continuing education.

History of PAs

As with NPs, the birth of the concept of PAs came after a physician shortage was recognized in the mid-1960s. Dr. Eugene Stead of Duke University Medical Center established the first PA program, using already trained Navy corpsmen. He based his program on a fast-track training program for physicians during World War II.

Table 1						Nurse Practitioners' Education, License, and Certification Contrasted with That of Other Primary Care Providers

Health Professional	Years of College	Undergraduate Degree or Other Education	Graduate Degree	License	Continuing Education (Minimum)	Certification (Renewal)
Nurse practitioner	2–4	AA, BS, or RN diploma	Master's degree or doctorate required in 32 states	Yes (RN plus specific area of NP certica-tion)	75 hours/ 5 years	Yes, every 5 years
Physician assistant	2–4	BS or certificate	Not required, but the major-ity of PA programs are master's-level programs	Yes	100 hours/ 2 years	Yes, every 6 years
Primary care physician	4	BA/BS	Doctor of medicine or osteopathy required in all states	Yes (MD or DO)	50 hours/ year	Optional

Abbreviations: AA, associate of arts degree; BA, bachelor of arts degree; BS, bachelor of science degree; DO, doctor of osteopathic medicine; MD, doctor of medicine; RN, registered nurse.

Source: Data from the American Nurses Credentialing Center, American Academy of Physician Assistants and American Academy of Family Physicians.

NP Versus Physician: What Is the Difference?

NPs differ from physicians in definition, scope of practice, and education.

Definition and Scope of Practice of Physicians

A physician is a provider of medical care according to the laws of the individual states. An example of state law defining the practice of medicine is New Jersey's statute:

> The phrase "the practice of medicine or surgery" and the phrase "the practice of medicine and surgery" shall include the practice of any branch of medicine and/ or surgery and any method of treatment of human ailment, disease, pain, injury, deformity, mental or physical condition, and the term "physician and surgeon" or "physician or surgeon" shall be deemed to include practitioners in any branch of medicine and/or surgery or method of treatment of human ailment, disease,

pain, injury, deformity, mental or physical condition. Within the meaning of this act, except as herein otherwise specifically provided, and except for the purposes of the exemptions hereinafter contained in Sections 45:9-14.1 to 45:9-14.10, inclusive, the practice of medicine and/or surgery shall be deemed to include the inter alia, the practice of osteopathy…

Citation: N.J. Stat. Ann. § 45:9-5.1.

Educational Requirements of Physicians

Physicians have 4 years of medical education. See Table 1 for a comparison of NPs, physicians, and PAs on requirements for basic education, continuing education, licensure, and certification.

NP Versus Registered Nurse: What Is the Difference?

NPs and RNs differ in definition, scope of practice, education, and physician supervision.

Definition of RN

The legal definition of an RN is provided by the laws of the states. Michigan, for example, defines nursing and registered nurse as follows:

The "practice of nursing" means the systematic application of substantial specialized knowledge and skill derived from the biological, physical, and behavioral sciences, to the care, treatment, counsel, and health teaching of individuals who are experiencing changes in the normal health processes or who require assistance in the maintenance of health and the prevention or management of illness, injury, or disability. . . ."Registered professional nurse" or "RN" means an individual licensed under this article to engage in the practice of nursing which scope of practice includes the teaching, direction, and supervision of less skilled personnel in the performance of delegated nursing activities.

Citation: Mich. Comp. Laws § 333.17201.

Scope of Practice of RNs

Nursing typically includes a variety of acts, described under state law. The nursing acts described here are taken from the law of North Dakota:

The performance of acts utilizing specialized knowledge, skills, and abilities for people in a variety of settings. The term includes the following acts, which may not be deemed to include acts of medical diagnosis or treatment or the practice of medicine as defined in Chapter 43–17.

    a. The maintenance of health and prevention of illness
    b. Diagnosing human responses to actual or potential health problems
    c. Providing supportive and restorative care and nursing treatment, medication administration, health counseling and teaching, case finding and

referral of persons who are ill, injured, or experiencing changes in the
normal health processes

d. Administration, teaching, supervision, delegation, and evaluation of
health and nursing practices

e. Collaboration with other healthcare professionals in the implementation
of the total healthcare regimen and execution of the healthcare regimen prescribed by a healthcare practitioner licensed to order healthcare
regimens

Citation: N.D. Cent. Code § 43-12.1-02(5).

Education of RNs

An RN has 2–4 years of college education and may have a master's degree, a doctorate
degree, or other advanced training over and above the basic education.

Supervision of RNs

Supervision is generally not mandated by law for those activities within the scope of nursing
practice. To provide medical care, such as administering prescription medication, an RN
needs an order from a healthcare provider authorized by law to give orders or prescribe
medication.

NP Versus Clincial Nurse Specialist: What Is the Difference?

While NPs and clinical nurse specialists (CNSs) both are advanced practice nurses, they
focus on different forms of patient care. While NPs manage patients in offices, nursing
facilities, homes, and hospitals, CNSs traditionally have worked in hospitals, as resources
for other clinicians. Psychiatric/mental health CNSs traditionally have performed direct
patient care, as therapists. In the past 10 years, programs for psych/mental health NPs have
emerged, so now, both NPs and CNSs manage patients with psychiatric diagnoses. The
distinction between CNSs and NPs is important to advanced practice nurses, but probably
not so important to those who are not in the field.

Definition and Scope of Practice of CNSs

The definition and scope of practice of a clinical nurse specialist (CNS) are specified by
state law. For example, Maine law defines the scope of practice of a CNS as follows:

The certified clinical nurse specialist applies research-based knowledge, skills,
and experience to intervene in human responses to complex health and illness
problems. The certified clinical nurse specialist (1) provides case management
skills to coordinate comprehensive health services and ensure continuity of care,
(2) evaluates client progress in attaining expected outcomes, (3) consults with
other healthcare providers to influence care of clients, effect change in symptoms, and enhance the ability of others to provide health care, (4) performs
additional functions specific to the specialty areas. In addition to the above, the

certified psychiatric clinical nurse specialist may independently assess, diagnose, and therapeutically intervene in complex mental health problems using psychotherapy and other interventions.

Citation: CODE ME. R. § 02 380 Chapter 8.

Education of CNSs

CNSs have, at minimum, a master's degree in nursing and may have a doctorate degree.

Physician Supervision of CNSs

CNSs have no requirement for physician supervision unless they have prescriptive authority, in which case there often are collaboration or supervision requirements specified by state law. See **Table 2** for a comparison of NPs, CNSs, and other types of advanced practice nurses in terms of education and licensure.

Where Do Nurse Practitioners Practice?

NPs practice in health maintenance organizations, independent or collaborative private practices, hospitals and affiliated clinics, emergency departments, family planning clinics, college health services, school clinics, convenient care clinics, employee health clinics, nursing and long-term care facilities, homeless shelters, hospices, and home-based care services.

Notes

1. Nurse Practitioner Association of Maryland. (2009). Media packet. Retrieved from http://www.npamonline.org/associations/9774/files/NPAM%20Media%20packet.10.2009.pdf
2. American Association of Nurse Practitioners. (n.d.). What's an np? Retrieved from http://www.aanp.org/all-about-nps/what-is-an-np
3. New York State Education Department Office of the Professions. (2013, September 24). Nursing. Retrieved from http://www.op.nysed.gov/prof/nurse
4. Palmetto GBA Medicare. (2013, October 8). Who qualifies as a non-physician practitioner (NPP)? Retrieved from http://www.palmettogba.com/palmetto/providers.nsf/DocsCat/Providers~Jurisdiction%2011%20Home%20Health%20and%20Hospice~Resources~FAQs~Home%20Health~8GKMQC6571?open&navmenu=Resources%7C%7C
5. National Council of State Boards of Nursing. (2008, July 7). The consensus model for APRN regulation, licensure, accreditation, certification, and education. Retrieved from https://www.ncsbn.org/4213.htm
6. Smith, C. M., & Maurer, F. A. (1995). *Community health nursing: Theory and practice*. Philadelphia, PA: W. B. Saunders.
7. Institute of Medicine. (1996). Primary care: American's health in a new era. Washington, DC: IOM Division of Healthcare Services.
8. American Academy of Family Physicians. (n.d.). Primary care. Retrieved from http://www.aafp.org/about/policies/all/primary-care.html
9. American Academy of Physician Assistants. (n.d.). What is a PA? Retrieved from http://www.aapa.org/the_pa_profession/what_is_a_pa.aspx
10. American Medical Association. (1995, June). Guidelines for physician/physician assistant practice. Retrieved from http://www.aapa.org/uploadedFiles/content/The_PA_Profession/Federal_and_State_Affairs/Resource_Items/AMA-Guidelines.pdf

Table	2	Nurse Practitioners' Educational and Professional Credentials Contrasted with Those of Other Advanced Practice Nurses						
Type of APN	Years of College	Years of Training	Undergraduate Degree	Graduate Degree	License	Continuing Education	Renewal of Certification
Nurse anesthetist	4	2	BA/BS	Master's degree	Yes, RN plus nurse anesthetist	40 hours/2 years	Yes, as CRNA by NPCRNA
Nurse midwife	4	2	BA/BS	Master's degree or doctorate	Yes, RN plus nurse midwife	20 hours/5 years with other recertification options available	Yes, as nurse midwife by AMCB
Nurse psychotherapist	4	2, plus 100 hours of supervised practice	BA/BS	Master's degree	Yes, RN plus nurse psychotherapist	75 hours/5 years	Yes, as CNS by ANCC
Nurse practitioner	4	2	BA/BS	Master's degree or doctorate required in 32 states	Yes, RN plus nurse practitioner	Varies with certifying body; 75 hours/5 years (ANCC)	Yes, as NP by ANCC, PNCB, or NCC

Abbreviations: APN, advanced practice nurse; AMCB, American Midwifery Certification Board; ANCC, American Nurses Credentialing Center; BA, bachelor of arts degree; BS, bachelor of science degree; CRNA, certified registered nurse anesthetist; NBCRNA, National Board of Certification and Recertification of Nurse Anesthetists; NCC, National Certification Corporation; PNCB, Pediatric Nursing Certification Board; RN, registered nurse.

Source: Data from the American Nurses Credentialing Center, American Association of Nurse Anesthetists, and American College of Nurse Midwives websites.

State-by-State Definitions of Nurse Practitioner

State-by-state definitions of nurse practitioner, including citation of code section:

Alabama

Advanced practice nurse. A registered nurse that has gained additional knowledge and skills through successful completion of an organized program of nursing education that prepares nurses for advanced practice roles and has been certified by the Board of Nursing to engage in the practice of advanced practice nursing.

Citation: ALA. CODE § 34-21-81(3).

Practice as a certified registered nurse practitioner (CRNP) means the performance of nursing skills by a registered nurse who has demonstrated by certification that he or she has advanced knowledge and skills in the delivery of nursing services within a health care system that provides for consultation, collaborative management, or referral as indicated by the health status of the client.

Citation: ALA. CODE § 34-21-81(4a).

Alaska

"Advanced nurse practitioner" means a registered nurse authorized to practice in the state who, because of specialized education and experience, is certified to perform acts of medical diagnosis and the prescription and dispensing of medical, therapeutic, or corrective measures under regulations adopted by the Board of Nursing.

Citation: ALASKA STAT. § 08.68.850.

Arizona

"Registered nurse practitioner" means a registered nurse who:

a. Is certified by the board.
b. Has completed a nurse practitioner education program approved or recognized by the board and educational requirements prescribed by the board by rule.
c. If applying for certification after July 1, 2004, holds national certification as a nurse practitioner from a national certifying body recognized by the board.
d. Has an expanded scope of practice within a specialty area that includes:
    i. Assessing clients, synthesizing and analyzing data, and understanding and applying principles of health care at an advanced level.
    ii. Managing the physical and psychosocial health status of clients.
    iii. Analyzing multiple sources of data, identifying alternative possibilities as to the nature of a healthcare problem and selecting, implementing and evaluating appropriate treatment.
    iv. Making independent decisions in solving complex client care problems.
    v. Diagnosing, performing diagnostic and therapeutic procedures, and prescribing, administering and dispensing therapeutic measures, including legend drugs, medical devices, and controlled substances within the scope of registered nurse practitioner practice on meeting the requirements established by the board.
    vi. Recognizing the limits of the nurse's knowledge and experience and planning for situations beyond the nurse's knowledge, educational preparation and expertise by consulting with or referring clients to other healthcare providers when appropriate.
    vii. Delegating to a medical assistant pursuant to § 32-1456.
    viii. Performing additional acts that require education and training as prescribed by the board and that are recognized by the nursing profession as proper to be performed by a nurse practitioner.

Citation: Ariz. Rev. Stat. Ann. § 32-1601(19).

Arkansas

(1)(a) Any person holding a license to practice as a registered nurse and possessing the educational qualifications required under subsection (b) of this section to be licensed as a registered nurse practitioner may, upon application and payment of necessary fees to the Arkansas State Board of Nursing, be licensed as a registered nurse practitioner and have the right to use the title of "registered nurse practitioner" and the abbreviation "RNP."

2. No other person shall assume such a title or use such an abbreviation or any other words, letters, signs, or devices to indicate that the person using them is a registered nurse practitioner.

b. In order to be licensed as a registered nurse practitioner, a registered nurse must hold a certificate or academic degree evidencing successful completion of the educational program of an accredited school of nursing or other nationally recognized accredited program recognized by the board as meeting the requirements of a nurse practitioner program…

Citation: Ark. Code Ann. § 17-87-303.

California

The Legislature finds that various and conflicting definitions of the nurse practitioner are being created by state agencies and private organizations within California. The Legislature also finds that the public is harmed by conflicting usage of the title of nurse practitioner and lack of correspondence between use of the title and qualifications of the registered nurse using the title. Therefore, the Legislature finds the public interest served by the determination of the legitimate use of the title "nurse practitioner" by registered nurses.

Citation: Cal. Bus. & Prof. Code § 2834.

"Nurse practitioner" means a registered nurse who possesses additional preparation and skills in physical diagnosis, psycho-social assessment, and management of health-illness needs in primary health care, and who has been prepared in a program conforming to board standards as specified in Section 1484.

Citation: Cal. Code Regs. tit. 16, § 1480(a).

Colorado

"Practice of advanced practice nurse" means an expanded scope of professional nursing in a scope, role, and population focus approved by the board, with or without compensation or personal profit, and includes the practice of professional nursing.

Citation: Colo. Rev. Stat. Ann. § 12-38-103-8.5a.

The board shall establish the advanced practice registry and shall require that a nurse applying for registration identify his or her role and population focus. The board shall establish reasonable criteria for designation of specific role and population foci based on currently accepted professional standards. A nurse who is included in the advanced practice registry has the right to use the title "advanced practice nurse" or, if authorized by the board, to use the title "certified nurse midwife", "clinical nurse specialist", "certified registered nurse anesthetist", or "nurse practitioner". These titles may be abbreviated as "A.P.N.", "C.N.M.", "C.N.S.", "C.R.N.A.", or "N.P.", respectively. It is unlawful for any person to use any of the titles or abbreviations listed in this subsection (3) unless included in the registry and authorized by the board to do so.

Citation: COLO. REV. STAT. ANN. § 12-38-111.5(3).

Connecticut

Advanced nursing practice is defined as the performance of advanced level nursing practice activities which, by virtue of post-basic specialized education and experience, are appropriate to and may be performed by an advanced practice registered nurse.

Citation: CONN. GEN. STAT. ANN. § 20-87a (West).

Delaware

"Advanced practice nurse" means an individual whose education and certification meet criteria established by the Board of Nursing who is currently licensed as a registered nurse and has a master's degree or a postbasic program certificate in a clinical nursing specialty with national certification. When no national certification at the advanced level exists, a master's degree in a clinical nursing specialty will qualify an individual for advanced practice nurse licensure. "Advanced practice nurse" shall include, but not be limited to, nurse practitioners, certified registered nurse anesthetists, certified nurse midwives, or clinical nurse specialists. Advanced practice nursing is the application of nursing principles, including those described in subsection (o) of this section, at an advanced level and includes:

a. For those advanced practice nurses who do not perform independent acts of diagnosis or prescription, the authority as granted within the scope of practice rules and regulations promulgated by the Board of Nursing; and

b. For those advanced practice nurses performing independent acts of diagnosis and/or prescription with the collaboration of a licensed physician, dentist, podiatrist, or licensed Delaware health care delivery system without written guidelines or protocols and within the scope of practice as defined in the rules and regulations promulgated by the Joint Practice Committee and approved by the Board of Medical Licensure and Discipline.

Citation: DEL. CODE ANN. tit. 24, § 1902 (b)(1).

District of Columbia

"Practice of advanced practice registered nursing" means the performance of advanced-level nursing actions, with or without compensation, by a licensed registered nurse with advanced education, knowledge, skills, and scope of practice who has been certified to perform such actions by a national certifying body acceptable to the Board of Nursing. The practice of advanced practice registered nursing includes:

A. Advanced assessment;
B. Medical diagnosis;
C. Prescribing;
D. Selecting, administering, and dispensing therapeutic measures;
E. Treating alterations of the health status; and
F. Carrying out other functions identified in Subchapter VI of this chapter and in accordance with procedures required by this chapter.

Citation: D.C. STAT. § 3-1201.02 (02).

Florida

"Advanced registered nurse practitioner" means any person licensed in this state to practice professional nursing and certified in advanced or specialized nursing practice, including certified registered nurse anesthetists, certified nurse midwives, and nurse practitioners.

Citation: FLA. STAT. ANN. § 464.003(3).

Georgia

"Advanced nursing practice" means practice by a registered professional nurse who meets those educational, practice, certification requirements, or any combination of such requirements, as specified by the board and includes certified nurse midwives, nurse practitioners, certified registered nurse anesthetists, clinical nurse specialists in psychiatric/mental health, and others recognized by the board.

Citation: GA. CODE ANN. § 43-26-3(1).

a. A nurse practitioner is a registered professional nurse who is recognized by the Board to engage in advanced practice registered nursing.
b. The nurse practitioner practices in a manner consistent with Chapter 410-13 of the Georgia Board of Nursing Rules and Regulations.

Citation: GA. COMP. R. & REGS. § r. 410-12-.03(1).

Hawaii

"Advanced practice registered nurse" means a registered nurse who has met the qualifications for advanced practice registered nurse set forth in this chapter and through rules of the board, which shall include educational requirements.

Citation: Haw. Rev. Stat. § 457-2.

"Advanced practice registered nurse (APRN)" means a registered nurse licensed to practice in this State who has met the qualifications set forth in Chapter 457, HRS, and this subchapter, who, because of advanced education and specialized training, is authorized to assess, screen, diagnose, order, utilize, or perform medical, therapeutic, preventive or corrective measures.

Citation: Haw. Admin. § 16-89-2.

Idaho

"Advanced practice registered nurse" means a registered nurse licensed in this state who has gained additional specialized knowledge, skills and experience through a program of study recognized or defined by the board. An advanced practice registered nurse is authorized to perform advanced nursing practice, which may include the prescribing, administering and dispensing of therapeutic pharmacologic agents, as defined by board rules. An advanced practice registered nurse shall perform only those acts as provided by the board and for which the individual is educationally prepared.

Citation: Idaho Code § 54-1402(1).

Illinois

a. Advanced practice nursing by certified nurse practitioners, certified nurse anesthetists, certified nurse midwives, or clinical nurse specialists is based on knowledge and skills acquired throughout an advanced practice nurse's nursing education, training, and experience.
b. Practice as an advanced practice nurse means a scope of nursing practice, with or without compensation, and includes the registered nurse scope of practice.
c. The scope of practice of an advanced practice nurse includes, but is not limited to, each of the following:
    1. Advanced nursing patient assessment and diagnosis.
    2. Ordering diagnostic and therapeutic tests and procedures, performing those tests and procedures when using health care equipment, and interpreting and using the results of diagnostic and therapeutic tests

and procedures ordered by the advanced practice nurse or another health care professional.

3. Ordering treatments, ordering or applying appropriate medical devices, and using nursing medical, therapeutic, and corrective measures to treat illness and improve health status.
4. Providing palliative and end-of-life care.
5. Providing advanced counseling, patient education, health education, and patient advocacy.
6. Prescriptive authority as defined in Section 65-40 of this Act.
7. Delegating selected nursing activities or tasks to a licensed practical nurse, a registered nurse, or other personnel.

Citation: Ill. Comp. Stat. § 65/65-30.

Indiana

"Advanced practice nurse" means (1) a nurse practitioner; (2) a nurse midwife; or (3) a clinical nurse specialist; who is a registered nurse qualified to practice nursing in a specialty role based upon the additional knowledge and skill gained through a formal organized program of study and clinical expertise, or the equivalent as determined by the board, which does not limit but extends or expands the function of the nurse, which may be initiated by the client or provider in settings that shall include hospital outpatient clinics and health maintenance organizations.

Citation: Ind. Code Ann. § 25-23-1-1(b).

Iowa

"Advanced registered nurse practitioner (ARNP)" means a nurse with current licensure as a registered nurse in Iowa or who is licensed in another state and recognized for licensure in this state pursuant to the nurse licensure compact contained in 2000 Iowa Acts, House File 2105, section 8, and is also registered in Iowa to practice in an advanced role. The ARNP is prepared for an advanced role by virtue of additional knowledge and skills gained through a formal advanced practice education program of nursing in a specialty area approved by the board. In the advanced role, the nurse practices nursing assessment, intervention, and management within the boundaries of the nurse-client relationship. Advanced nursing practice occurs in a variety of settings, within an interdisciplinary health care team, which provide for consultation, collaborative management, or referral. The ARNP may perform selected medically delegated functions when a collaborative practice agreement exists.

Citation: Iowa Admin. Code § r. 655-6.1(152).

"Certified nurse practitioner" is an ARNP educated in the discipline of nursing who has advanced knowledge of nursing, physical and psychosocial assessment, appropriate interventions and management of health care, and who possesses evidence of current certification by a national professional nursing certifying body approved by the board.

Citation: Iowa Admin. Code § r. 655-6.1(152).

Kansas

"Advanced practice registered nurse" or "APRN" means a professional nurse who holds a license from the board to function as a professional nurse in an advanced role, and this advanced role shall be defined by rules and regulations adopted by the board in accordance with the KSA 65-1130 and amendments thereto.

Citation: Kan. Stat. Ann. § 65-1113(g).

Kentucky

"Advanced practice registered nurse" means a certified nurse practitioner, certified nurse anesthetist, certified nurse midwife, or clinical nurse specialist, who is licensed to engage in advance practice registered nursing pursuant to KRS 314.042 and certified in at least one (1) population focus.

Citation: Ky. Rev. Stat. Ann. § 314.011(7).

Louisiana

"Advanced practice registered nurse" or "APRN" means a licensed registered nurse who is certified by a nationally recognized certifying body, such as the American Nurses Credentialing Center, as having an advanced nursing specialty as described in this Part and who meets the criteria for an advanced practice registered nurse as established by the board. In the absence of the availability of a national certification examination in a selected clinical area, the board may establish commensurate requirements. An advanced practice registered nurse shall include, but not be limited to, the following:

a. Certified nurse midwife or "CNM"
b. Certified registered nurse anesthetist or "CRNA"
c. Clinical nurse specialist or "CNS"
d. Nurse practitioner or "NP"

Citation: La. Rev. Stat. Ann. § 37:913 (1).

Maine

"Advanced practice registered nursing" (A.P.R.N.) means the practice of a registered professional nurse who, on the basis of specialized education and experience, is authorized under these rules to deliver expanded professional health care.

"Certified nurse practitioner" (C.N.P.) means a registered professional nurse who has received post-graduate education designed to prepare the nurse for advanced practice registered nursing in a specialty area in nursing that has a defined scope of practice and has been certified in the clinical specialty by a national certifying organization acceptable to the Board.

Citation: CODE ME. R. § 02 380 008(1).

Maryland

"Nurse practitioner" means a registered nurse who by reason of certification under these regulations may engage in the activities authorized by these regulations.

Citation: MD. REGS. CODE. § 10.27.07.01.B(4).

Massachusetts

Nurse authorized to practice in the expanded role means a nurse with:

a. current licensure as a registered nurse in the Commonwealth;
b. advanced nursing knowledge and clinical skills acquired through an appropriate nursing education program, as described in 244 CMR 4.13 or, until April 15, 1993, as acquired through appropriate education and clinical experience, or their equivalent, as described in 244 CMR 4.14 and
c. current certification in a specific practice area as described in 244 CMR 4.13.

Citation: 244 MASS. ADMIN. CODE § 4.05.

Michigan

The board of nursing may issue a specialty certification to a registered professional nurse who has advanced training beyond that required for initial licensure and who has demonstrated competency through examination or other evaluative processes and who practices in one of the following health profession specialty fields: nurse midwifery, nurse anesthetist, or nurse practitioner.

Citation: MICH. COMP. LAWS § 333.17210.

"Certified nurse practitioner" means an individual licensed as a registered professional nurse under part 172 who has been issued a specialty certification as a nurse practitioner by the board of nursing under Section 17210.

Citation: MICH. COMP. LAWS § 333.2701(c).

Minnesota

"Advanced practice registered nurse," abbreviated APRN, means an individual licensed as a registered nurse by the board and certified by a national nurse certification organization acceptable to the board to practice as a clinical nurse specialist, nurse anesthetist, nurse-midwife, or nurse practitioner.

Citation: MINN. STAT. § 148.171(3).

Mississippi

An "advanced practice registered nurse" is a person who is licensed or holds the privilege to practice under this article and who is certified in advanced practice registered nurse or specialized nursing practice and includes certified nurse midwives, certified registered nurse anesthetists and certified nurse practitioners.

Citation: MISS. NURSING PRACTICE LAW §73-15-5(11).

Missouri

"Advanced practice registered nurse," a nurse who has education beyond the basic nursing education and is certified by a nationally recognized professional organization as a certified nurse practitioner, certified nurse midwife, certified registered nurse anesthetist, or a certified clinical nurse specialist. The board shall promulgate rules specifying which nationally recognized professional organization certifications are to be reorganized for the purposes of this section. Advanced practice nurses and only such individuals may use the title "Advanced Practice Registered Nurse" and the abbreviation "APRN."

Citation: MO. REV STAT. § 335.016(2).

Montana

1. Nurse practitioner (NP) practice means the independent and/or collaborative management of primary and/or acute health care of individuals, families, and communities including:
   a. assessing the health status of individuals and families using methods appropriate to the client population and area of practice such as health history taking, physical examination, and assessing developmental health problems.
   b. instituting and facilitating continuity of health care to clients, including:
      i. ordering durable medical equipment, treatments and modalities, and diagnostic tests;
      ii. receiving and interpreting results of diagnostic procedures;
      iii. making medical and nursing diagnoses; and
      iv. working with clients to promote their understanding of and compliance with therapeutic regimens.
   c. promoting wellness and disease prevention programs;
   d. referring clients to a physician or other healthcare provider, when appropriate;

e. providing instruction and counseling to individuals, families, and groups in the areas of health promotion and maintenance, including involving such persons in planning for their health care; and

f. working in collaboration with other health care providers and agencies to provide and, where appropriate, coordinate services to individuals and families.

2. Every licensed NP shall abide by the practice standards and guidelines established by an NP national professional organization as identified by the NP.

Citation: MONT. CODE ANN. 24.159.1470.

Nebraska

Nurse practitioner means a registered nurse certified as described in Section 38-2317 and licensed under the Advanced Practice Registered Nurse Practice Act to practice as a nurse practitioner.

Citation: NEB. REV. STAT. § 38-2312.

Nevada

"Advanced practice registered nurse" means a registered professional nurse who has specialized skill, knowledge and experience obtained from an organized formal program of training and who is authorized in special conditions as defined by NAC 632.255 to 632.295, inclusive, to provide designated services in addition to those which a registered nurse is authorized to perform.

Citation: NEV. ADMIN. CODE § 632.020.

New Hampshire

"Advanced practice registered nurse" or "APRN" means a registered nurse currently licensed by the board under RSA 326-B:18.

Citation: N.H. REV. STAT. ANN. § 326-B:2.I.

New Jersey

"Advanced practice nurse" means a person who holds a certification in accordance with section 8 or 9 of P.L. 1991, c.377 (C.45:11-47 or 45.11-48).

Citation: N.J. STAT. ANN. § 45:11-23.d.

Whenever the titles or designations "nurse practitioner," "clinical nurse specialist," or "nurse practitioner/clinical nurse specialist" occur or any reference is made thereto in any law, contract or document, the same shall be deemed to mean or refer to the title or designation "advanced practice nurse."

Citation: N.J. STAT. ANN. § 45:11-46.c.

New Mexico

"Certified nurse practitioner" means a registered nurse who is licensed by the board for advanced practice as a certified registered nurse practitioner and whose name and pertinent information are entered on the list of certified registered nurse practitioners maintained by the board.

Citation: N.M. Stat. Ann. § 61-3-3.E.

New York

The practice of registered professional nursing by a nurse practitioner, certified under section six thousand nine hundred ten of this article, may include the diagnosis of illness and physical conditions and the performance of therapeutic and corrective measures within a specialty area of practice, in collaboration with a licensed physician qualified to collaborate in the specialty involved, provided such services are performed in accordance with a written practice agreement and written practice protocols.

Citation: N.Y. Educ. Law, Art. 139 § 6902.3(a).

North Carolina

"Advanced Practice Registered Nurse (APRN)" means a nurse practitioner, nurse anesthetist, nurse-midwife or clinical nurse specialist.

Citation: N.C. Admin. Code tit. 21, r. § 36.0120(5).

"Nurse Practitioner" or "NP" means a currently licensed registered nurse approved to perform medical acts consistent with the nurse's area of nurse practitioner academic educational preparation and national certification under an agreement with a licensed physician for ongoing supervision, consultation, collaboration and evaluation of the medical acts performed. Such medical acts are in addition to those nursing acts performed by virtue of registered nurse (RN) licensure. The NP is held accountable under the RN license for those nursing acts that he or she may perform.

Citation: N.C. Admin. Code tit. 21, r. § 36.0801.

North Dakota

"Advanced practice registered nurse" means an individual who holds a current license to practice in this state as an advanced practice registered nurse within one of the roles of certified nurse practitioner, certified registered nurse anesthetist, certified nurse midwife, or certified clinical nurse specialist, and who functions in one of the population foci as approved by the board.

Citation: N.D. Cent. Code § 43-12.1-02(1).

Ohio

(J) "Certified nurse practitioner" means a registered nurse who holds a valid certificate of authority issued under this chapter that authorizes the practice of nursing as a certified nurse practitioner in accordance with Section 4723.43 of the Revised Code and rules adopted by the board of nursing.

(O) "Advanced practice registered nurse" means a certified registered nurse anesthetist, clinical nurse specialist, certified nurse-midwife, or certified nurse practitioner.

Citation: OHIO REV. CODE ANN. § 4723.01.

Oklahoma

"Advanced practice nurse" means a licensed registered nurse:

a. who has completed an advanced practice registered nursing education program for one of four recognized advanced practice registered roles,
b. who has passed a national certification examination recognized by the Board that measures the advanced practice registered nurse role and specialty competencies and who maintains recertification in the role and specialty through a national certification program,
c. who has acquired advanced clinical knowledge and skills in preparation for providing both direct and indirect care to patients; however, the defining factor for all Advanced Practice Registered Nurses is that a significant component of the education and practice focuses on direct care of individuals,
d. whose practice builds on the competencies of Registered Nurses by demonstrating a greater depth and breadth of knowledge, a greater synthesis of data, and increased complexity of skills and interventions,
e. who has obtained a license as an Advanced Practice Registered Nurse in one of the following roles: Certified Registered Nurse Anesthetist, Certified Nurse-Midwife, Clinical Nurse Specialist, or Certified Nurse Practitioner.

Citation: OKLA. STAT. ANN., § 59-567.3.5.

Oregon

"Nurse practitioner" (NP) means an advanced practice registered nurse who is certified by the Board to independently assume responsibility and accountability for the care of clients. The title nurse practitioner and population foci of practice shall not be used unless the individual is certified by the Board.

Citation: OR. ADMIN. § R. 851-050-0000(21).

Pennsylvania

Certified Registered Nurse Practitioner —A professional nurse licensed in this Commonwealth who is certified by the Board in a specialty and who, while functioning in the expanded role as a professional nurse, performs acts of medical diagnosis or prescription of medical therapeutic or corrective measures in collaboration with a physician licensed to practice in this Commonwealth and in accordance with the act and this subchapter. Nothing in this subchapter is to be deemed to limit or prohibit a professional nurse from engaging in those activities which constitute the practice of professional nursing as defined in section 2 of the act (63 P. S. § 212).

Citation: 49 Pa. Code § 21.251.

Rhode Island

"Certified registered nurse practitioner" is an advanced practice nurse utilizing independent knowledge of physical assessment and management of health care and illnesses. The practice includes prescriptive privileges. The practice includes collaboration with other licensed healthcare professionals including, but not limited to, physicians, pharmacists, podiatrists, dentists, and nurses.

Citation: R.I. Gen. Laws § 5-34-3(3).

South Carolina

"Nurse Practitioner" or "NP" means a registered nurse who has completed an advanced formal education program at the master's level acceptable to the board, and who demonstrates advanced knowledge and skill in assessment and management of physical and psychosocial health, illness status of persons, families, and groups. Nurse practitioners who perform delegated medical acts must have a supervising physician or dentist who is readily available for consultation and shall operate within the approved written protocols.

Citation: 2 S.C. Code Ann. § 40-33-20(41).

South Dakota

"Nurse practitioner," a provider duly authorized under this chapter to practice the specialty of nurse practitioner as defined in 36-9A-12.

Citation: S.D. Codified Laws § 36-9A-1(5).

Tennessee

"Advanced practice nurse" means a registered nurse with a master's degree or higher in a nursing specialty and national specialty certification as a nurse practitioner, nurse anesthetist, nurse midwife, or clinical nurse specialist.

Citation: TENN. CODE ANN. § 63-7-126(a).

Texas

Advanced practice nurse—A registered nurse approved by the board to practice as an advanced practice nurse based on completing an advanced educational program acceptable to the board. The term includes a nurse practitioner, nurse-midwife, nurse anesthetist, and a clinical nurse specialist. The advanced practice nurse is prepared to practice in an expanded role to provide health care to individuals, families, and/or groups in a variety of settings including but not limited to homes, hospitals, institutions, offices, industry, schools, community agencies, public and private clinics, and private practice. The advanced practice nurse acts independently and/or in collaboration with other health care professionals in the delivery of health care services.

Citation: 22 TEX. ADMIN. CODE § 222.1(3).

Utah

"Practice of advanced practice registered nursing" means the practice of nursing within the generally recognized scope and standards of advanced practice registered nursing as defined by rule and consistent with professionally recognized preparation and education standards of an advanced practice registered nurse by a person licensed under this chapter as an advanced practice registered nurse. Advanced practice nursing includes:

a. maintenance and promotion of health and prevention of disease;
b. diagnosis, treatment, correction, consultation, or referral for common health problems; and
c. prescription or administration of prescription drugs or devices, including:
   i. local anesthesia;
   ii. Schedule IV-V controlled substances; and
   iii. Schedule II-III controlled substances in accordance with a consultation and referral plan.

Citation: UTAH CODE ANN. § 58-31b-102(13).

Vermont

"Advanced practice registered nurse" or "APRN" means a licensed registered nurse authorized to practice in this state who, because of specialized education and experience, is endorsed to perform acts of medical diagnosis and to prescribe medical, therapeutic, or corrective measures under administrative rules adopted by the board.

Citation: Vt. Stat. Ann. tit. 26, § 1572(4).

Virginia

"Nurse practitioner" means a registered nurse who has met the requirements for licensure as a nurse practitioner as stated in 18 VAC 90-30.

Citation: 18 Va. Code Ann. § 90-40-10.

Washington

1. A licensed advanced registered nurse practitioner (ARNP) is a registered nurse prepared in a formal educational program to assume primary responsibility for continuous and comprehensive management of a broad range of patient care, concerns, and problems.
2. The ARNP is prepared and qualified to assume primary responsibility and accountability for the care of patients.
3. ARNP practice is grounded in nursing and incorporates the use of independent judgment as well as collaborative interaction with other health care professionals when indicated in the assessment and management of wellness and health conditions as appropriate to the ARNP's area of practice and certification.
4. The ARNP functions within his or her scope of practice according to the commission approved certification program and standards of care developed by professional organizations.

Citation: Wash. Admin. Code § 246-840-300(1-4).

West Virginia

"Nurse practitioner" means a registered nurse qualified by virtue of his or her education and credentials and approved by the West Virginia Board of Examiners for registered professional nurses to practice as an advanced practice nurse independently or in a collaborative relationship with a physician.

Citation: W. Va. Code § 9-4B-1(c).

"Advanced nurse practitioner" means a registered nurse with substantial theoretical knowledge in a specialized area of nursing practice and proficient clinical utilization of the knowledge in implementing the nursing process, and who has met the further requirements of title 19, legislative rules for West Virginia board of examiners for registered professional nurses, series 7, who has mutually agreed upon association in writing with a physician and has been selected by or assigned to the person and has primary responsibility for treatment and care of the person.

Citation: W. Va. Code § 16-30-3(c).

Wisconsin

"Nurse practitioner" means a registered nurse licensed under Ch. 441 or in a party state, as defined in § 441.50(2)(j), whose practice of professional nursing under § 441.001(4) includes performance of delegated medical services under the supervision of a physician, dentist, or podiatrist.

Citation: Wis. Stat. § 255.06(d).

Wyoming

"Advanced practice registered nurse (APRN)" means a nurse who:

A. May prescribe, administer, dispense, or provide nonprescriptive and prescriptive medications including prepackaged medications, except schedule I drugs as defined in W.S. 35-7-1013 and 34-7-1014;

B. Has responsibility for the direct care and management of patients and clients in relation to their human needs, disease states and therapeutic and technological interventions;

C. Has a master's degree in nursing, or an advanced practice registered nurse specialty or has completed an accredited advanced practice registered nurse educational program prior to January 1, 1999; and

D. Has completed an advanced program of study in a specialty area in an accredited nursing program, has taken and passed a national certification examination in the same area and has been granted recognition by the board to practice as an APRN.

Citation: Wyo. Stat. Ann. § 33-21-120(a)(i).

State-by-State Titles for Nurse Practitioners

ALABAMA: Certified Registered Nurse Practitioner (CRNP)

ALASKA: Advanced Nurse Practitioner (ANP)

ARIZONA: Registered Nurse Practitioner (RNP)

ARKANSAS: Advanced or Registered Nurse Practitioner (RNP)

CALIFORNIA: Nurse Practitioner (NP)

COLORADO: Nurse Practitioner (NP) or Advanced Practice Nurse (APN)

CONNECTICUT: Advanced Practice Registered Nurse (APRN) or Certified Nurse Practitioner (CNP)

DELAWARE: Advanced Practice Nurse (APN), Nurse Practitioner (NP), or Advanced Registered Nurse Practitioner (ARNP)

DISTRICT OF COLUMBIA: Advanced Practice Registered Nurse (APRN)

FLORIDA: Advanced Registered Nurse Practitioner (ARNP)

GEORGIA: Advanced Practice Registered Nurse (APRN) or Nurse Practitioner (NP)

HAWAII: Advanced Practice Registered Nurse (APRN)

IDAHO: Advanced Practice Registered Nurse (APRN)

ILLINOIS: Advanced Practice Nurse (APN)

INDIANA: Advanced Practice Nurse (APN) or Nurse Practitioner (NP)

IOWA: Advanced Registered Nurse Practitioner (ARNP) or Certified Nurse Practitioner (CNP)

KANSAS: Advanced Practice Registered Nurse (APRN)

KENTUCKY: Advanced Practice Registered Nurse (APRN)

LOUISIANA: Advanced Practice Registered Nurse (APRN)

MAINE: Advanced Practice Registered Nurse (APRN) or Certified Nurse Practitioner (CNP)

MARYLAND: Certified Registered Nurse Practitioner (CRNP)

MASSACHUSETTS: Nurse Practitioner (NP)

MICHIGAN: Certified Nurse Practitioner (CNP)

MINNESOTA: Advanced Practice Registered Nurse Practitioner (APRN) or Nurse Practitioner (NP)

MISSISSIPPI: Advanced Practice Registered Nurse (APRN)

MISSOURI: Advanced Practice Registered Nurse (APRN)

MONTANA: Advanced Practice Registered Nurse (APRN) or Nurse Practitioner (NP)

NEBRASKA: Nurse Practitioner (NP)

NEVADA: Advanced Practice Registered Nurse (APRN)

NEW HAMPSHIRE: Advanced Practice Registered Nurse (APRN)

NEW JERSEY: Advanced Practice Nurse (APN)

NEW MEXICO: Certified Nurse Practitioner (CNP)

NEW YORK: Nurse Practitioner (NP)

NORTH CAROLINA: Advanced Practice Registered Nurse (APRN) or Nurse Practitioner (NP)

NORTH DAKOTA: Advanced Practice Registered Nurse (APRN) or Nurse Practitioner (NP)

OHIO: Certified Nurse Practitioner (CNP) or Advanced Practice Registered Nurse (APRN)

OKLAHOMA: Advanced Practice Nurse (APN) or Advanced Registered Nurse Practitioner (ARNP)

OREGON: Nurse Practitioner (NP)

PENNSYLVANIA: Certified Registered Nurse Practitioner (CRNP)

RHODE ISLAND: Certified Registered Nurse Practitioner (RNP)

SOUTH CAROLINA: Nurse Practitioner (NP)

SOUTH DAKOTA: Nurse Practitioner (NP)

TENNESSEE: Advanced Practice Nurse (APN) or Certified Nurse Practitioner (CNP)

TEXAS: Advanced Practice Nurse (APN)

UTAH: Advanced Practice Registered Nurse (APRN)

VERMONT: Advanced Practice Registered Nurse (APRN)

VIRGINIA: Nurse Practitioner (NP)

WASHINGTON: Advanced Registered Nurse Practitioner (ARNP)

WEST VIRGINIA: Advanced Nurse Practitioner (ANP) or Nurse Practitioner (NP)

WISCONSIN: Nurse Practitioner (NP)

WYOMING: Advanced Practice Registered Nurse (APRN)

The Employed Nurse Practitioner

The majority of nurse practitioners (NPs) are employed by others, rather than self-employed. The advantages of employment by others are:

- A built-in collaborative agreement, in states where these are required
- No struggles for reimbursement from third-party payers, who may balk at paying NPs directly but are comfortable reimbursing physician practices that employ NPs

What Rights Does an Employed NP Have?

At Will Employment

In most states, employment is "at will." This means that employment continues at the will of both parties. Put another way, either party may terminate for any reason at any time. Unless an employee has a contract for a specified term of employment, an employee has no legal right to a job. Likewise, an employee may also end employment at any time, barring a contract for a specified term. The only protections for an employee are those offered by the equal opportunity and disability laws; that is, an employee cannot be terminated solely on the basis of age, national origin, gender, race, religion, or disability.

An NP who is employed but has no contract must negotiate terms of employment on a piecemeal basis, relying on their ability to reach agreement with the employing party as issues arise. If an employer changes the pay scale or work responsibilities for the better, the NP benefits. However, if the employer reduces the pay scale or unreasonably increases responsibilities, the NP has no recourse but to keep working under the new conditions or to leave.

Employment by Contract

Many NPs seeking employment are offered employment contracts. An employment contract is a written agreement under which the employee and employer agree on the terms and conditions of their working relationship.

Employment contracts can be complex and lengthy, and they require careful analysis. The following is a list of some of the issues often addressed in an employment contract:

- Scope of services to be performed
- Compensation

- Duration of employment
- How the agreement can be altered or updated
- Responsibility for maintaining credentials
- Terms of on-call responsibilities
- Benefits
- Time off and expenses for continuing education
- Vacation time
- Number of office hours per week
- Restriction on competition
- Bonuses
- Reasons for termination
- Assistance with continuing education

Some issues that often are not addressed but can be dealt with in an employment contract include the following:

- Extent of support service to be offered to the NP
- Expectations regarding the number of patients seen per day
- Expectations regarding nonclinical (administrative) work to be done by the NP
- Listing of the NP on the door, in directories, and in advertisements
- Use of the NP's name when the office telephone is answered
- On-call responsibilities and backup
- Release to the NP of the NP's quality performance as measured by health plan auditors

An employment agreement can include anything the parties wish to address. Often, agreements are written by attorneys for the practice and therefore are oriented to the needs of the employer. NPs should retain their own attorney to review any proposed contract and respond with counterproposals when the contract language does not mesh with their needs.

Does an NP Need a Contract?

Many NPs practiced for many years without employment contracts. In the past, an employer called to offer a job, and the employer and employee then negotiated a salary, benefits, and the hours of employment. The arrangement was typically sealed with a handshake. Details were worked out as issues arose, but NPs sometimes were unhappy with how they were handled.

Contracts have certain advantages over this informal employment arrangement. First, contract negotiation forces parties to discuss issues. When the parties agree to terms, there is a document that records the agreement and can be referred to as necessary to refresh memories about the details of the agreement. In most cases, an employment agreement is protective to both the employer and the employee.

For an employee, a contract ensures some degree of job security. In most states, unless there is a written contract defining the duration of employment, employment is "at will." As discussed, this means that either party may terminate the employment without cause at any time. For example, a practice that hires an NP and then loses a lucrative patient care contract can terminate an NP who is employed "at will" with no severance pay, even though the NP is not at fault. "At will" employees are often surprised to learn that they have no legal right to their jobs. An NP who has a contract, however, has an agreement for work for the duration of the contract, unless a clause in the contract states otherwise. An employer who wants to end the employment of the NP must wait until the contract terminates or attempt to settle the matter with the NP, possibly by offering severance terms.

For an employer, an employment agreement can afford protection against competition. An employer wants to avoid a situation where a departing NP who has built a patient following takes patients to their next position. An employer can restrict a departing NP from competing with a practice by including a restrictive covenant (discussed shortly) in the employment agreement.

A multitude of issues that affect lifestyle and workstyle can arise among coworker healthcare providers. An employment contract can delineate the expectations of employer and employee before problems arise. A contract also can specify problem-solving procedures.

Three Difficult Clauses

Three clauses commonly found in employment agreements offered by medical practices to NPs are especially difficult for NPs to interpret and can have profound effects on an NP's life. These clauses address restrictive covenants, bonus formulas, and termination clauses. These clauses often bring NPs to attorneys for advice. *Restrictive covenants* require an NP to promise, up front, not to compete with an employer when the present employment ends. *Bonus formulas* specify conditions under which an employer rewards an NP for superior performance. *Termination clauses* specify that an employer may end the agreement, without cause, with 30 days notice.

Restrictive Covenants

A restrictive covenant is a promise not to compete. Specifically, a restrictive covenant is a clause that restricts an employee from practicing within a set number of miles from an employer's business for a set period of time after the employee leaves the employer's business.

Many employers insist on restrictive covenants. An employer wants to avoid a situation where a departing NP who has built a patient following takes patients to their next position, often a neighboring practice.

Restrictive covenants are legal in many states and enforceable as long as they are reasonable. If a former employee challenges the validity of a restrictive covenant by taking the matter to court, a judge will determine whether it is reasonable. A judge will balance the needs of the employer against the harm to the employee. A judge will decide whether the geographic restriction and the time restriction are appropriate to accomplish the employer's needs, but no more. Further, a judge will consider whether there is any potential injury to the public if a restrictive covenant is enforced.

A judge will analyze the past court decisions in the state and compare the facts of those cases with the current case. Such facts include the size of the city or town the practice is in, the severity of the geographic and time restrictions in the clause, what the practice is like, the availability of other healthcare providers, and what the employment climate is like for healthcare providers.

Judges have found restrictive covenants unreasonable when the restraint is greater than necessary to protect the legitimate business interests of the employer. Judges also have found restrictive covenants unreasonable when the restraint is not greater than necessary to protect the business interests but the employer's need for protection is outweighed by the hardship to the employee. Occasionally, judges have found restrictive covenants to be unreasonable when there is neither excessive restraint nor excessive hardship but there is a likely injury to the public. For example, a covenant restricting an oral surgeon from practicing in a particular city for 3 years after termination from a practice was found to be unreasonable. The restraint was greater than necessary. However, a covenant restricting a veterinarian from practicing in a different city for 3 years after termination was found to be reasonable. In that case, the restraint was not greater than necessary. In yet another case, a covenant restricting a physician from practicing in a rural town for 3 years after termination was found to be unreasonable. In that case, there was a potential injury to the public. The injury to the public was a potential shortage of physicians if one of the two town physicians could no longer practice there. The difference in outcome in these three cases can be reconciled only by comparing the factual details of the cases. A decision that one clause was reasonable while a seemingly identical clause was unreasonable was due to differences in profession, practice, city, availability of other providers, and many other factors.

When negotiating the terms of a restrictive covenant, an NP needs to consider the circumstances of the job offer, the severity of the restriction, the potential hardship imposed on them by the covenant, the availability of healthcare providers in the area, and the availability of other practice opportunities.

In agreeing to a restrictive covenant, an NP is giving up something of value—the ability to take any other NP job that is offered to them. However, if an NP refuses to sign a reasonable restrictive covenant their employer may suspect they are looking to start a competing practice nearby. The best practice for restrictive covenants is to negotiate one the NP can live with, one that seems reasonable for all concerned under the particular circumstances of the practice and the NP. **Exhibit 1** provides examples of restrictive covenants with comments about their degree of reasonableness.

Bonus Formulas

Some employers offer NPs the opportunity for bonuses. The criteria for bonuses vary greatly. The two most important are that both employer and employee understand the formula and that it be consistent with good patient care.

The most common problem with bonus formulas is vague language. If a formula is vague, it is sure to be interpreted in different ways by different individuals. This can result in disagreements and disappointments at distribution time.

> **Exhibit 1** Restrictive Covenants
>
> Restrictive covenants are enforceable if they balance:
> - The employer's need for protection
> - Hardship to the employee
> - Likelihood of injury to the public
>
> **Example 1:** "Upon termination of employment for any reason, NP agrees not to practice in any location within 25 miles of any present or future office of this practice for a period of 5 years."
>
> **Analysis:** Accomplishes employer's need for protection but may be broader than necessary to accomplish employer's need and may put excessive hardship on employee to find alternative work 25 miles away.
>
> **Example 2:** "Upon termination of employment for any reason, NP agrees not to practice in any location within 1 mile of the Jones Road office of this practice for a period of 1 year."
>
> **Analysis:** Not a hardship on employee but may not accomplish employer's need for protection, as patients may be willing to travel 1 mile to see the NP.

Productivity-Based Formulas

Many formulas are based on the number of patient visits per year. This makes good business sense under a fee-for-service system of reimbursement. If a practice is at least half fee-for-service, patient visit–based formulas can be a reasonable choice. Tracking patient visits is uncomplicated and is not usually susceptible to vagueness. Generally, an NP who sees large numbers of patients is a productive employee who deserves a bonus.

Bonus formulas based on numbers of patient visits make less sense when reimbursement to the practice is capitated. Under a capitated system of reimbursement, a practice is paid a set fee per patient per month, regardless of the number of patient visits. Under capitated reimbursement, the ultimate goal is not a high number of visits from each patient but good patient care in as few visits as possible. Under capitated reimbursement, bonuses should be given to those providers who demonstrate high-quality care as evidenced by some documented quality measurement tool. Numbers of patient visits should not be relevant when a practice's patients are capitated. Employers have to be careful not to give providers bonuses for withholding care. Aside from the moral and ethical problems involved, there are federal laws that prohibit healthcare providers from profiting by delivering inadequate or inappropriate care.

Many practices have a mix of fee arrangements with patients and payers. Employer and employee should plan for such mixes when devising a bonus formula. A bonus formula should fit the practice's payer mix.

Quality-Based Bonuses

When more than half of patients are covered by some form of managed-care plan, NP performance can be rewarded on the basis of meeting or exceeding quality standards set by the health plan. For example, bonuses could be awarded when the percentage of patients who have met health maintenance criteria—such as childhood immunizations or mammograms for women over 50—exceeds 80%. Or bonuses could be awarded if emergency department visits declined in the past year.

While performance measures are more difficult to track than patient visits, they are more suited to managed care. Some health plans supply performance data to practices, and these data can be used to determine bonuses.

To track this kind of performance data and apportion bonuses based on performance, patients and primary care providers have to be paired. NPs need to have their own panels of patients and be designated as the primary care provider for that panel. Otherwise NP–physician teams have to work together and share bonuses.

Profit-Based Formulas

Some employers share profits with NPs. This can be satisfying to both employer and employee as long as the method for determining profits is clear.

NPs should be aware that there are accounting methods that can maximize or minimize profits and that profit is a word that has modifiers, such as *gross* and *net*, that can mean the difference between a bonus and no bonus. NPs who agree to profit-based formulas should negotiate for the right to audit financial records. NPs should also negotiate for a dispute-resolution process.

Patient Satisfaction–Based Formulas

Bonus formulas are one of the most controversial aspects of provider relationships. Many practices struggle with this issue. One approach taken by employers is to implement a bonus formula with the understanding that it can be altered and improved upon each year.

See **Exhibit** 2 for some examples of bonus formulas that have been offered to NPs.

Termination Without Cause

Typically, the termination section of an employment agreement will list events that are a basis for termination of the employee "with cause." These events often include conviction of a felony, loss of license, loss of hospital privileges, and gross negligence that compromises patient safety.

Exhibit **2** Examples of Bonus Formulas for NPs' Contracts

- Up to 15% of base salary: 5% if practice is profitable, 5% based on meeting a threshold of patient visits, and 5% based on patient satisfaction, staff satisfaction, and citizenship
- The product of "collected billings" multiplied by "total employee billings" divided by "total practice billings," with a cap
- A figure determined by a committee, based on meeting criteria for (1) financial performance; (2) quality of medical services determined by outcomes, medical appropriateness, and extent of health promotion services provided; and (3) level of patient satisfaction

---

Exhibit 3 Examples of Termination Clauses

A Termination-with-Cause Clause

The employer may terminate this agreement at the sole discretion of the employer, by written notice to the NP upon the occurrence of any of the following:

a. The NP dies or becomes disabled. . . .
b. The NP loses his or her professional license. . . .
c. The NP is limited or restricted by any governmental authority having jurisdiction over the NP to the extent that the NP cannot render the required professional services. . . .

A Termination-Without-Cause Clause (*Not Recommended for NPs*)

The employer may terminate this agreement at any time, for any reason, after thirty (30) days notice to NP.

In addition to termination-with-cause provisions, some employment agreements include a termination-without-cause clause, which states that an employer can terminate an employee at any time, without cause, with 30 days notice (see examples in **Exhibit 3**).

A termination-without-cause clause effectively defeats one of the purposes of a contract for an employee. An employee who can be terminated at any time for any reason or for no reason not only has no job security but also will think twice about pressing for performance of any of the other provisions in the employment agreement. For example, an NP may believe that a bonus was due, while the employer may believe that no bonus was due. If the NP protests too much, an employer can simply terminate the NP. If, on the other hand, an NP can be terminated only "for cause," the NP will feel freer to be assertive about ensuring that the other provisions of the contract are fulfilled.

There are reasons to agree to a "termination-without-cause" clause, however. If an NP cannot commit to a full year's employment, it may be best to agree to the "without-cause" clause. Most employers will not agree to delete a "without-cause" clause unless the employee also gives up the right to leave with just 30 days notice.

How to Negotiate a Reasonable Agreement

Preparing to Negotiate

NPs who have worked for years without contracts are now being offered them. NPs who are currently working without contracts, who foresee an offer in the future, and who want to negotiate a satisfying contract will lay the groundwork a year in advance.

First, an NP should be able to state clearly what he or she has contributed to the practice in the past year and have supporting data. Specifically, the NP should have at hand the total number of patient visits and the dollars billed and received as a result of those visits. If an NP does administrative work, he or she should make a list of administrative projects and determine the dollar worth of the projects to the practice. The NP can contrast the revenues they have brought in with the expenses related to their practice, including salary, benefits, and continuing education. If there are patient satisfaction surveys or quality-of-care data that support the NP, the NP should have those data at hand. While new NPs will not have the option of collecting data in preparation for negotiating first contracts, they should find out everything they can about the practice with which they plan to negotiate. Once employed, new NPs should begin to collect data for future contract negotiations.

First, an NP needs to make the following assessments about his or her speed and comfort level:

- How many patients can I see per hour, day, month, and year?
- How much physician consultation time will I need: a 10-minute consultation on every patient, a 5-minute consultation once a day, or a 5-minute consultation once a year?

Second, an NP should gather basic information on how the practice gets its revenues. The NP should know which insurers pay for NP services and how much they pay. If the payer mix is likely to change in the coming year, the NP must be ready to explain how their value to the practice will continue to increase in the coming year. The NP can propose ways in which the practice can increase its efficiency and revenues in the coming year and offer to help implement plans. An NP embarking on a salary negotiation needs to gather the following data from their employer:

- What is the most frequently billed CPT (procedural) code for the practice? What amount does the practice bill and receive, on average, for that CPT code?
- What percentage of practice income goes to cover practice expenses? If the employer will not reveal that information, the NP can ask how many providers share practice overhead expenses. A solo practitioner pays 43% of their income for office expenses, whereas a practice of 10 to 24 doctors pays 23.5% of their income for office expenses. Determine the appropriate rate to deduct for practice expenses.
- What is the collection rate for the practice? Remember, 90% is good.

Third, the NP should decide which terms of employment are essential and which can be given up. He or she should ask for everything they want but be ready to back down on nonessential terms.

Fourth, the NP must anticipate any drawbacks that an employer might raise in negotiations and prepare to defend or minimize those drawbacks.

Negotiating

Generally, it is best to negotiate individually rather than as a member of a group. For a variety of reasons, some NPs will be more valuable than others to an employer. A more valuable NP should get better offers. On the other hand, some employers have a standard NP offer and will not deviate for an individual NP. In that case, NPs need to negotiate as a group.

Whether negotiating individually or as a group, an NP should read a proposed contract carefully, note areas that are confusing, and get clarification. They should remember that everything is negotiable. While a contract may look intimidating, it was typed on a word processor and can be changed.

NPs should seek legal counsel to review any proposed contract.

Getting Help: What To Look for in a Lawyer

Negotiating is best done by the NP employee, but contract review is best done by an attorney. An attorney who is familiar with NP contracts and business issues is a good first choice. A second choice is an attorney who reviews contracts of other healthcare providers, physicians in particular.

NPs should avoid attorneys who need to research the law regarding NPs. One NP spent $1500 for her attorney to research the law on NPs, only to find that she knew the answers to the questions he was looking up.

Attorneys charge between $150 and $1000 an hour. Many will negotiate a flat fee for reviewing a contract. It is prudent to spend $400 for review of a contract that is worth between $80,000 and $140,000 per year to an NP. If an attorney finds vague wording that needs to be made more specific, the investment in the attorney will be repaid in the long run.

Understanding Business

If an employer has a well-run, profitable practice to which an NP contributes significantly, the NP should expect to be rewarded well under an employment agreement. If a practice is losing money, no NP will be able to negotiate a satisfying agreement, no matter how excellent they are.

NPs are clinicians by nature, not businesspeople. However, all types of clinicians are increasingly finding that they need to understand more about the business of health care. An NP who understands the financial base for a practice is in a better position to negotiate a satisfactory employment agreement than an NP who knows only the clinical side of practice. An employer will respect an NP who approaches negotiations with attention to both business principles and patient care concerns.

Negotiating Salary

New NPs are notorious for asking only two questions of a new employer: (1) What does the position pay? and (2) What are the benefits?

Four methods of payment are currently being used to pay employed NPs:

1. Straight salary
2. Percentage of net receipts
3. Base salary plus percentage
4. Hourly rate

In a straight salary arrangement, an NP is paid a set amount to perform according to a job description. In a percentage salary arrangement, an NP is paid the amount the NP bills minus accounts receivable, minus the NP's portion of practice expenses (which includes the expense of physician consultation). In a base salary plus percentage arrangement, an NP is guaranteed a set salary but can make additional salary if he or she generates practice income over some set amount. NPs working on an hourly basis are paid only for the hours worked.

Straight salary and hourly are more commonly encountered arrangements than percentage or set salary plus percentage. The advantage of percentage-based salaries is the opportunity for productive NPs to have some control over their earnings. The disadvantage is that the method sets up fellow providers in a practice as competitors for patients.

No matter what arrangement an NP chooses, it is wise to focus on hard figures that document an NP's monetary contribution to a practice and the costs of the NP to the practice.

NPs bring in income on a fee-for-service basis or a per-member-per-month basis. Calculating an NP's share of income for a fee-for-service practice is done by multiplying the number of visits by the collected fee per visit. When a practice's patients are capitated, an NP's share of income is calculated by multiplying the number of patients on an NP's panel by the per-member-per-month fee coming into the practice.

The cost of maintaining an NP is calculated by adding together practice expenses and the cost of physician consultation. Practice expenses can be estimated or calculated for a particular practice. For a solo practice, expenses can be 40–50% of the income. For a large practice, expenses are lower, 20–30% of income. Practice expenses include rent, salaries, taxes and benefits of support staff, taxes and benefits of NPs, supplies, laboratory expenses, depreciation, car, continuing education, and insurance (malpractice, workers' compensation, and premises insurance).

An NP who needs a great deal of physician consultation should expect to compensate their employer physicians for their time. An NP who needs little consultation should command a higher salary because he or she needs little of a physician's time. Until NPs no longer need a physician on written agreement, all NPs should expect to pay something for physician consultation. Experienced NPs often pay physician employers/consultants 10–15% of their net income brought to the practice.

Most employers will want a percentage of an NP's earnings as profit. An experienced NP who needs little consultation from an employer physician might consider his or her contribution to profit to be the 10–15% of net income paid for consultation, as noted in the earlier paragraph. A newer NP should expect to contribute 10–15% of net earnings to an employer as profit in addition to 15–25% of net earnings for physician consultation.

To project an appropriate salary for a particular NP, follow these steps:

1. Calculate income to the practice based on NP billings.
2. Subtract 10% for unpaid bills.
3. Subtract:
   a. The calculated figure for practice expenses (20–50% of earnings).
   b. The cost of physician consultation (10–20% of net earnings).
   c. A percentage for employer profit.

Fee-for-Service Practices. For example, an NP who sees 15 patients per day at $70 per patient visit, on average, brings in $1050 per day. Allowing 1 week off for continuing education, 1 week off for illness, and 4 weeks off for vacation, this NP will bring in $241,500 a year, potentially. However, not all bills are paid. With a 90% collection rate—a reasonable collection rate for an efficient practice—this NP actually will bring in $217,350 per year. An NP who sees 24 patients per day will bring in $1680 per day, or $386,400 per year in accounts receivable. With a 90% collection rate, this NP will bring $347,760 to the practice.

Deducting 40% of the NP's gross generated income for overhead expenses (rent, benefits, continuing education, supplies, malpractice, lab expenses, and depreciation of equipment) leaves $130,410 for the 15-patient-per-day NP and $208,656 for the 24-patient-per-day

NP. Further deducting 15% of that figure to pay a physician for consultation services leaves $110,848 in salary for the 15-patient-per-day NP and $177,357 in salary for the 24-patient-per-day NP. Deducting 10% for employer profit leaves $99,763 in salary for the 15-patient-per-day NP and $159,621 for the 24-patient-per-day NP. Note that some practices are compensated more than $70 per visit, on average, and some less. Some practices have a collections rate that is less than 90%. Note also that some practices will be able to justify 50% of generated income for practice expenses and some practices will want more than 10% profit. Ultimately the employer gets to make the final decision about these percentages. The NP's options are to accept, negotiate something better, or to find other employment.

Capitated Practices. In a fully capitated practice, an NP who has a panel of 1000 patients at an average fee per member per month of $10 will bring in $120,000 annually. There should be a 100% collection rate under a capitated system of reimbursement.

Applying 40% to overhead leaves $72,000 for the NP salary, and paying 15% for physician consultation and 10% for employer profit leaves $55,080 for the NP salary. An NP with a larger panel will make more.

The New NP. A newly graduated NP without experience may be able to see only 10 patients a day, with four or five 10-minute physician consultations per day, for the first 6 months. Plugging in the figures from the earlier examples, the NP will bill 2400 visits per year (2 weeks vacation for the new grad) at $70 per visit to total $168,000 in accounts receivable. With a 90% collection rate, the new NP will bring in $151,200.

Deducting 40% for practice expenses brings the net income to $90,720. Because a new NP often requires significant consultation time with a physician (or experienced NP), an additional 25% ($22,680) is deducted for payment for consultation, bringing the NP salary down to $68,040. With a contribution to employer profit, this new NP's appropriate salary is down to $61,236.

After 6 months, when the same NP becomes more comfortable and more efficient, the income numbers should double and consultation requirements should decrease, so that the appropriate salary will more closely approximate the salary of the 15-patient-per-day NP and eventually the 24-patient-per-day NP in the previous examples. Many employers start a new NP at a salary significantly higher than $61,236, expecting that low productivity in the first 6 months will be balanced by high productivity in the second 6 months.

There are experienced NPs who see more than 15 patients per day at CPT code level 99213 (established patient, mid-level visit) or higher who are not making the salary supported by the previous calculations. There are numerous reasons for this. First, the practice may expect more than 10% profit. Many employers expect to make a profit equal to an employee's salary. Second, the NP may have higher expenses than normal. Third, the collections rate may be lower than 90%.

Are These Projections Accurate? One could argue about whether the percentages used in the given examples are correct. In fact, some practices have poor rates of collections, some practices have higher overhead expenses, and some physicians want more payment for consultation. Some employers want more profit than projected here. However, an NP should not be subsidizing a poorly run practice and need not agree to overcompensate a physician or employer. Many practices receive more than $70 per NP visit on average. In these practices, an NP's salary should be proportionately higher.

Reported Median NP Salaries. Comparing these calculated NP salaries with some of the recently reported median salaries for NP salaries is an interesting exercise. Some medical groups use the Medical Group Management Association's (MGMA) median salary data. The median salary for a NP in 2012 was $91,000, according to the MGMA. Advance for Nurse Practitioners reported in its 2012 salary survey that the median NP salary for 2011 was $90,583.

NPs should keep in mind that salary averages are based on surveys. There is no way of knowing whether the respondents are representative of NPs. NPs who believe they are worthy of higher salaries than surveys suggest should present all of the reasons why they deserve the figure they are seeking.

As in all negotiating, there are three things to remember:

1. One who does not ask will not receive.
2. One who does not deserve will not receive.
3. Even when one asks and deserves, one will need to do some selling to get what one wants.

Negotiating Benefits

There are three yardsticks by which to evaluate a benefits package:

1. What benefits does the NP need?
2. What is reasonable?
3. What are other NPs getting?

Only the first two count. It should not matter to either the NP or the employer what others are getting, only what the NP needs, wants, or deserves and what the employer can afford and is willing to cover.

An NP in the late stages of job interviewing should ask a prospective employer the following questions:

- What benefits usually are offered?
- Does the employer pay for continuing education?
- Is time away for continuing education paid time?
- What is the retirement plan?
- What are the basics of the health plan? Is dental included? Is vision coverage included?
- If calls are required, are a cellular telephone, beeper, and car allowance included?
- What vacation time is being offered?
- How is sick time handled?
- Is malpractice insurance paid by the employer? If so, will a separate attorney for the NP be covered? Is the policy occurrence or claims made?
- Are relocation expenses paid?
- Is there a sign-on bonus?
- Are expenses of travel for the interview to be paid?

- Does the employer pay for professional dues? If so, how much?
- Does the employer pay for reference books and subscriptions to professional journals? If so, how much?
- Are there any tuition reimbursement benefits for NPs or for dependents?
- Is there a short- or long-term disability insurance benefit?
- If travel to various sites is necessary, are automobile expenses reimbursed?

Negotiating a Working Environment

Of course, many nonmonetary aspects of an NP's working life affect job satisfaction. An NP contemplating a new job is advised to spend some time thinking about and perhaps listing both the aspects of former jobs that have been most satisfying and most frustrating. Then the NP can briefly summarize the best and the worst of former jobs with the prospective employer and try to maximize the positive in the new position. Here are some appropriate questions:

- Is on-call time required? If so, how are calls shared? What backup will an NP have if consultation is needed for a call?
- What kind of and how many support staff will the practice provide?
- What will support staff do for the NP? What will support staff expect the NP to do for them?
- To whom will the NP report about medical issues? Administrative issues? Payment issues?
- What continuous quality improvement methods does the practice use?
- If the NP finds some aspect of practice organization that he or she would like to change, what is the process be for making suggestions?
- Is the NP expected to build a panel of patients or cover for overbookings of the other providers, or both?

Interviewing

A physician or administrator who is interested in hiring an NP may have significant, little, or no experience working with NPs. Therefore, NPs should be prepared to define NP scope of practice, list state requirements for collaboration or supervision, if any, and identify the sources of reimbursement for NP services.

In an interview for employment as an NP, a candidate should be prepared to answer the following questions:

- Why should I hire an NP?
- Why should I hire you?
- How many patients are you used to seeing in a day?
- Do you have a DEA [Drug Enforcement Administration] number?
- How independently are you used to practicing?
- What can you bring to the practice?
- What is your greatest job strength? Weakness?

- What can an NP legally do in this state?
- What do you want to be doing in 5 years? In 10 years?
- Does working evenings and/or weekends bother you?

Responsibilities of an NP Employee

Whether or not an NP has a contract, an NP has certain ethical responsibilities to their employer. These responsibilities include the following:

- Add to the good will an employer has built in the community by promoting the practice to the public
- Protect the employer's "trade secrets," such as patient mailing lists
- Provide one's best customer service to patients of the employer
- Remain unimpaired by alcohol or drugs
- Maintain one's credentials, knowledge of standard of care, and continuing education
- Maintain patient confidentiality

Employer's Evaluation of the NP's Performance

Some employers evaluate NP performance in highly structured ways—number of patients seen per month or quarter, income generated, detailed evaluation tools—and others use either no measure or very subjective measures.

An NP is advised to ask, in the interview stages, about the employer's expectations for productivity, measures of quality, and other performance measures. If an NP knows how their work will be evaluated, he or she has a better chance of meeting expectations. If there are no set methods of evaluation, an NP may want to offer to develop some standards.

Malpractice Insurance

The best malpractice policy for an NP is an occurrence policy, for at least $1 million per claim and $3 million aggregate, which covers the expense of an attorney for the NP as an individual. If an NP must purchase an individual policy to obtain this coverage, the NP should do so.

Collaborative Practice Agreements

In states where a collaborative agreement is required by law, the NP, the physician, or both are legally responsible for drafting and filing the agreement with the appropriate agency. The most prudent process for drafting a collaborative agreement is as follows:

- Collect information.
    1. *Review the state law regarding NP scope of practice.* Questions to be answered are: Must the practice agreement be approved by the board of nursing and/or board of medicine

prior to beginning practice? Are there qualifications for the collaborating physician? Are there limitations on the collaborating physician (such as a limit on the number of NPs who may collaborate with the physician)? Is the practice agreement required solely for prescriptive authority or for any form of advanced practice?

2. *Determine the functions that the NP will supply to the proposed collaborative practice.* Will there be in-hospital care? Suturing? Surgical assistance? Prescription of controlled substances? Nursing home practice?

3. *Determine whether the physician collaborator's area of specialty matches the NP's.* Interview the physician collaborator, much as you would conduct a job interview, and check references. Ask whether there are any current or past malpractice cases against the physician or practice. Ask whether there has been any loss of hospital privileges or loss of Medicare participation.

- Draft an agreement for the collaborator's review. Often, the board of nursing will have sample written agreements upon which an NP can base the draft.
- Finalize and submit the agreement. Sometimes the board of nursing will return an agreement with a request for more information. If so, simply redraft and resubmit.

An example of a practice agreement is given in **Appendix A**. A sample employment agreement is provided in **Appendix B**.

Sample Nurse Practitioner Collaborative Practice Agreement from the Indiana Board of Nursing

TEMPLATE

Collaborative Practice Agreement for Advanced Practice Nurses Requesting Prescriptive Authority

Rule 848 IAC 5-1-1—Initial Authority to Prescribe Legend Drugs

1. **Complete names, home and business addresses, zip codes, and telephone numbers of the licensed practitioner and the advanced practice nurse.**

Licensed Practitioner:	Advanced Practice Nurse:
Licensed practitioner name and license number	Advanced practice nurse name and license number
Street address of home	Street address of home
City, state, and zipcode of home	City, state, and zipcode of home
Home phone number	Home phone number
Business street address	Business street address
City, state, and zipcode of business	City, state, and zipcode of business
Business phone number	Business phone number

2. **List of all locations where prescriptive authority is authorized by this agreement.**
   Business street address
   City, state, and zipcode of business
   Business phone number

3. **List all specialty or board certifications of the licensed practitioner and the advanced practice nurse.**
   Licensed practitioner is certified as a _____ with a practice specialty in _____. The advanced practice nurse is a nurse practitioner, clinical nurse specialist, certified nurse midwife, etc., with a specialized certification as a family nurse practitioner, etc.

4. **Briefly describe the specific manner of collaboration between the licensed practitioner and advance practice nurse.** Specifically, how they will work together, how they will share practice trends and responsibilities, how they maintain geographic proximity, and how they will provide coverage during an absence, incapacity, infirmity, or emergency by the licensed practitioner.

How they will work together:
The licensed practitioner and advanced practice nurse shall collaborate on a continual basis, etc.

How they will share practice trends and responsibilities:
The advanced practice nurse shall make rounds at the request of the licensed practitioner and consult with the license practitioner as needed, etc.

How they maintain geographic proximity:
The licensed practitioner will maintain a physical presence within a reasonable geographic proximity to the advanced practice nurse's practice location.

How they will provide coverage during absence, incapacity, infirmity, or emergency by the license practitioner:
In the case of the absence, incapacity, or unavailability of the licensed practitioner, coverage and consultation will be coordinated and maintained by another licensed practitioner as arranged in advance by the licensed practitioner and the advanced practice nurse.

5. **Provide a description of limitations, if any, the licensed practitioner has placed on the advanced practice nurse's prescriptive authority.**
There are no additional limitations on the advanced practice nurse or there are the following limitations on the advanced practice nurse, etc.

6. **Provide a description of the time and manner of the licensed practitioner's review of the advanced practice nurse's prescribing practices.** *Specifically, the description should include provisions that the advanced practice nurse must submit documentation of prescribing practices to the licensed practitioner within seven (7) days. Documentation of prescribing practices shall include, but not be limited to, at least a five percent (5%) random sampling of the charts and medications prescribed for patients.*
The advanced practice nurse must submit documentation of the advance practice nurse's prescribing practices within seven (7) days to the licensed practitioner for review. The documentation of prescribing practices shall include at least a 5% random sampling of the charts and medications prescribed for patients.

7. **Provide a list of all other written practice agreements of the licensed practitioner and advanced practice nurse.**
There are no other practice agreements or list all other practice agreements, etc.

8. **Provide the duration of the written practice agreement between the licensed practitioner and advanced practice nurse.**

Either party may terminate this practice agreement without cause at any time, effective immediately upon notice to the other party, etc.

_____
Signature of licensed practitioner

_____
Signature of advanced practice nurse

_____
Date

_____
Date

Sample Employment Agreement

Note: The following contract is suited for a particular NP and a particular medical practice. Other NPs and practices may need different or additional provisions. NPs and employers each should seek the counsel of an attorney for drafting a contract suitable to the needs of the particular parties.

Employment Agreement

THIS PROFESSIONAL SERVICES EMPLOYMENT AGREEMENT (the Agreement) made this _____day of _____, 2013, by and between Jones Medical Clinic, a professional corporation in the State of Georgia, hereinafter referred to as "the Corporation," and Jane Doe, MS, CRNP, an individual, hereinafter referred to as "the Nurse Practitioner."

Recitals

The Corporation is a professional association formed in Georgia and engaged in the practice of medicine. The services rendered by and on behalf of the Corporation are referred to as the Practice.

The Nurse Practitioner is licensed to practice in Georgia.

The Corporation desires to employ the Nurse Practitioner upon the terms and conditions hereinafter set forth, and the Nurse Practitioner desires to accept such employment.

Article I—Employment

1.1. Professional Services. The Corporation agrees to employ the Nurse Practitioner under this Agreement. The Nurse Practitioner agrees to render professional services for individuals who present themselves as patients of the Practice and to carry out the duties described in Schedule A, which is attached to and made as a part of this Agreement. In performing such services, the Nurse Practitioner shall comply with policies and procedures established by the Corporation, including participation in quality assurance and utilization review activities. The Nurse Practitioner shall render professional services at the Jamestown location.

1.2. Full-Time Employment. The Nurse Practitioner agrees to devote her full time and best efforts to the performance of the duties outlined in Schedule A attached to this Agreement.

1.3. Standards. The Nurse Practitioner shall exercise independent professional judgment with respect to the care and treatment of all patients. The Nurse Practitioner agrees that the patient care services will be provided promptly, efficiently, and in strict accordance with the ethical and professional standards for the provision of healthcare services adopted by the Practice. The Nurse Practitioner agrees that her patient care efficiency and productivity (for example, the number of outpatient visits per week) will be consistent with or better than past experience.

1.4. Authorization for Exchange of Information. The Nurse Practitioner authorizes the Corporation to obtain credentialing information from any necessary source. Credentialing information includes all information related to the Nurse Practitioner's education, training, qualifications, character, and experience, including patient care, quality assurance, utilization review, and risk management records.

1.5. Charges and Accounts Receivable. The Nurse Practitioner assigns to the Corporation the full right to bill for all professional, administrative, and clinical services performed by the Nurse Practitioner. The Nurse Practitioner agrees that all fees, when accrued or paid, are the sole property of the Corporation and that the Nurse Practitioner has no direct interest in any of these fees. All fee schedules shall be established by the Corporation.

1.6. Medical Records. All medical records of the Practice shall be the property of the Corporation, subject to applicable provisions of the medical records law of Georgia.

Article II—Compensation, Benefits, Disability, and Insurance

2.1. Nurse Practitioner Compensation. In consideration of the Nurse Practitioner rendering services under this Agreement, the Corporation will pay the Nurse Practitioner the compensation as set forth on Schedule B.

2.2. Vacation and Employee Benefits. In addition to the monetary compensation, the Corporation shall provide the Nurse Practitioner with the vacation and employment benefits listed on Schedule C.

2.3. Termination of Disability. If the Agreement is terminated because of the Nurse Practitioner's disability pursuant to Subsection 3.2.1, the Nurse Practitioner's compensation shall terminate after the twenty-six (26) week determination period, but the Nurse Practitioner shall have the right to claim benefits under the long-term disability insurance policy provided as an employee benefit.

2.4. Professional Liability Insurance. During the term of this Agreement and thereafter, the Corporation shall continuously maintain in effect professional liability malpractice insurance for the Nurse Practitioner in the amount of $1,000,000 per occurrence/$3,000,000 annual aggregate coverage.

2.5. General Liability. During the term of this Agreement, the Corporation shall include the Nurse Practitioner as a covered employee under the Corporation's general liability insurance policy.

Article III—Term and Termination

3.1. Term. The term of this Agreement shall be 1 year beginning _____, 2013, and, if not sooner terminated as provided below, ending _____ , 2014. Thereafter, this Agreement shall automatically renew on a year-to-year basis, unless sooner terminated as provided below.

3.2. Termination by Corporation—Without Cure Period. The Corporation may terminate this Agreement at the sole discretion of the Corporation by written notice to the Nurse Practitioner (or representative) upon the occurrence of any of the following:

   3.2.1. The Nurse Practitioner dies or becomes disabled. As used in this Agreement, disabled means the Nurse Practitioner's inability to perform the material and essential functions of clinical care for patients, despite reasonable accommodations by the Corporation, by reason of any medically determinable physical or mental impairment that has been determined to be terminal or that has lasted or can be expected to last for a period of not less than twenty-six (26) weeks, based on an examination by an independent physician selected by the Corporation.

   3.2.2. The revocation, suspension, or cancellation of the Nurse Practitioner's professional license.

   3.2.3. The imposition of any restriction or limitation on the Nurse Practitioner by any governmental authority having jurisdiction over the Nurse Practitioner to the extent that the Nurse Practitioner cannot render the required professional services.

   3.2.4. A final determination by any board, hospital, or other organization having jurisdiction over the Nurse Practitioner's right to practice that the Nurse Practitioner has engaged in unprofessional or unethical conduct.

   3.2.5. The Nurse Practitioner's clinical privileges at a hospital are involuntarily reduced, suspended, or revoked by final action of the hospital board under the bylaws, rules, or regulations of the hospital.

3.2.6. The Nurse Practitioner is convicted in a criminal or civil proceeding of fraud, misappropriation, embezzlement, or Medicare or Medicaid fraud and abuse.

3.2.7. The Nurse Practitioner is excluded from participation in the Medicare or Medicaid program by reason of fraud and/or abuse.

3.2.8. The Nurse Practitioner has misused assets of the Corporation by fraud.

3.3. Termination by Corporation—With Cure Period. The Corporation may terminate this Agreement based upon a failure of the Nurse Practitioner to comply with the terms and provisions of the Agreement after giving the Nurse Practitioner a notice of the alleged deficiency and allowing the Nurse Practitioner thirty (30) days to cure the alleged deficiency. The following are examples of deficiencies subject to the provisions of this Section:

3.3.1. The failure or refusal of the Nurse Practitioner to comply with the reasonable policies, work requirements, standards, and regulations of the Corporation that may be established from time to time.

3.3.2. The Nurse Practitioner breaches any obligation, covenant, or warranty under this Agreement, or the Nurse Practitioner fails to faithfully and diligently perform the services required by the provisions of this Agreement.

3.3.3. Notwithstanding the above, a 30-day notice shall not be required if the same deficiency has occurred more than twice in any 18-month period and written notice to cure was provided with respect to the previous occurrences, or if the deficiency is material and is incapable of being cured.

3.4. Termination by Nurse Practitioner. The Nurse Practitioner may terminate this Agreement:

3.4.1. Based upon a breach by the Corporation for failure to pay the compensation payable under the Agreement or failure to fulfill any other obligations under this Agreement, provided that the Corporation was given written notice of default and thirty (30) days to cure the specified breach.

3.4.2. The physicians of the Corporation are convicted in a criminal or civil proceeding of fraud, misappropriation, embezzlement, or Medicare or Medicaid fraud and abuse.

3.4.3. The physicians of the Corporation are excluded from participation in the Medicare or Medicaid program by reason of fraud and/or abuse.

3.4.4. The Nurse Practitioner moves out of the State of Georgia and gives thirty (30) days notice.

3.5. Effect of Termination. Upon termination of this Agreement as provided in this Article III, neither party shall have any further rights, duties, or obligations under this Agreement, except as otherwise provided herein. The termination or expiration shall not affect any liability or other obligation of either party that accrued prior to the termination or expiration.

Article IV—Management Support Systems and Personnel

4.1. The Corporation shall provide for or secure nonphysician personnel (including administrative, nursing, and other medical support personnel) and services that are reasonably needed by the Practice consistent with sound management standards for similar practices in the community. These services shall include administration, marketing and financial services, computerized management information systems, and computerized billing systems.

4.2. The Corporation shall provide the Nurse Practitioner with monthly statements of billings, collections, and accounts receivables attributable to the Nurse Practitioner. Should the Nurse Practitioner have questions about the data supplied, the Corporation shall provide access to the Corporation's accounting records and a clerk, who keeps these records, will answer the Nurse Practitioner's questions or supply further information as needed.

4.3. If the Nurse Practitioner's own records of patient visits and billings differ from the records of the Corporation, and the discrepancy cannot be resolved by the information seeking covered by Section 4.2, the Corporation agrees to designate one representative to negotiate a settlement acceptable to both parties within thirty (30) days. If no settlement can be reached internally, the Corporation agrees to submit any unresolved dispute to third-party arbitration, with the arbitrator selected from a list provided by the American Arbitration Association. The Corporation agrees to share equally with the Nurse Practitioner the expenses of arbitration.

4.4. The Corporation shall assign one physician to sign the Nurse Practitioner's written agreement, as required by Georgia law. The physician assigned shall be available or shall appoint a designate who will be available for consultation with the Nurse Practitioner when needed.

Article V—Notices

All notices shall be in writing and personally delivered or sent by certified or registered mail, postage prepaid, return receipt requested, addressed to the Corporation and the Nurse Practitioner at the addresses shown below. Any and all notices or other communication given pursuant to this Agreement shall be deemed duly given on the date personally delivered or on the date deposited in the U.S. Postal Service. The parties may change its or his or her address by specifying the change in a written notice to the other:

If to the Nurse Practitioner:
    Jane Doe, CRNP
    98 Merit Drive
    Jamestown, GA 20000-3000

If to the Corporation:
　　Jack Frost, MD
　　201 Medical Drive, Suite 100
　　Jamestown, GA 20000

Article VI—Miscellaneous

6.1. Entire Agreement. This Agreement embodies the entire agreement between the parties and supersedes all prior agreements, letters of intent, or understandings of any nature whatsoever between the parties with respect to the matters covered herein.

6.2. Amendment: Nonwaiver. Except as otherwise specifically provided, no amendment or modification of this Agreement shall be valid unless it is in writing and signed by the Nurse Practitioner and the designee of the Corporation as named in Article 5. No waiver of any of the provisions of this Agreement shall be valid unless it is in writing and signed by the party against whom it is sought to be enforced. Any waiver of breach of this Agreement shall not be considered to be a continuing waiver or consent to any subsequent breach on the part of either the Corporation or the Nurse Practitioner.

6.3. Counterparts. This Agreement may be executed in counterparts, and each counterpart shall be deemed an original.

6.4. Assignment. This Agreement may not be assigned by the Corporation to any entity without the prior written consent of the Nurse Practitioner. This Agreement is personal to the Nurse Practitioner and is not assignable by the Nurse Practitioner, in whole or in part, without the prior written consent of the Corporation. This Agreement is binding upon and inures to the benefit of the parties respective permitted successors and permitted assigns.

6.5. Governing Law. This Agreement shall be construed in accordance with and governed by the laws of the State of Georgia.

6.6. Governmental Requirements. This Agreement is subject to the requirements of all applicable laws and regulations and any government agency having jurisdiction. The parties agree to negotiate in good faith to amend this Agreement to comply with any governmental requirements affecting the Agreement or either party, including, without limitation, requirements affecting reimbursement for healthcare services. If the parties are unable to negotiate a mutually acceptable amendment to comply with any provision of law, regulation, or ruling, either party may initiate a voluntary termination of this Agreement on thirty (30) days notice.

6.7. Confidentiality. The parties agree not to disclose this Agreement or its contents to any person, firm, or entity, except the agents or representatives of the parties, and except as required by law.

6.8. Further Assurances. The Nurse Practitioner agrees to execute, acknowledge, seal, and deliver further assurances, instruments, and documents and to take such further actions as the Corporation may reasonably request in order to fulfill the intent of this Agreement.

IN WITNESS WHEREOF, the parties have caused this Agreement to be executed as of the day and year first above written, with the intent that this be a sealed instrument.

BY:

Jack Frost, MD
Jones Medical Clinic, PC
Date _____

Jane Doe, MS, CRNP
Date _____

WITNESS/ATTEST:
Date _____

Schedule A—Duties

1. The Nurse Practitioner shall provide clinical and professional medical services to patients within the scope of Nurse Practitioner's qualifications and consistent with accepted standards of medical practice and consistent with the reasonable productivity standards adopted by the Corporation and the Nurse Practitioner.

2. The Nurse Practitioner shall provide general patient care at the site specified by performance of accepted procedures and commonly used therapies and provision of appropriate support services. The Nurse Practitioner's duties shall include, but not be limited to, keeping and maintaining (or causing to be kept and maintained) appropriate records relating to all professional services rendered by Nurse Practitioner under this Agreement and preparing and attending to, in connection with such services, all reports, claims, and correspondence necessary and appropriate in the circumstances, all of which records, reports, claims, and correspondence shall belong to the Corporation. The Nurse Practitioner shall do all things reasonably desirable to maintain and improve her professional skills, including attendance at professional, postgraduate seminars and participation in professional societies. In addition, the Nurse Practitioner shall perform the following administrative, teaching, or professional services for the Corporation:
   a. Order medical supplies for the office.
   b. Review lab and radiology reports of office patients, and take appropriate follow-up action.
   c. Precept students from Georgia State University.

3. The Nurse Practitioner shall be responsible for the quality of medical care rendered by Nurse Practitioner to the patients of the Practice and for ensuring that such care meets or exceeds currently accepted standards of medical competence.

4. The Nurse Practitioner shall participate in the quality assurance and risk management program.

5. The Nurse Practitioner shall assist in the recruitment and hiring of professional personnel and support staff to work in the practice.
6. The Nurse Practitioner will relate to colleagues, staff, patients, and the public in a collegial manner and will abide by standards of conduct appropriate to the workplace.
7. The Nurse Practitioner shall assist in the marketing of the Practice and participate in the professional activities that promote the Practice.

Schedule B—Compensation

1. During the year of this Agreement (_____, 2013 to_____ , 2014), the Nurse Practitioner shall be paid a salary of $91,000, payable in biweekly installments. Salary is understood to include the Nurse Practitioner's share of collected billings, as determined in Paragraph 2 below, and the Nurse Practitioner's performance of administrative, teaching, and other professional duties as specified in Schedule A, Paragraph 2, previously listed.
2. Billings shall be apportioned as the Nurse Practitioner's share as follows:
   a. The Corporation and the Nurse Practitioner agree that efficiency at collections is outside of the control of the Nurse Practitioner, but within the control of the Corporation. Therefore, the Corporation and the Nurse Practitioner agree to apply a 95% collection rate (percentage of billings collected, as of 120 days after billing) for the purposes of determining the Nurse Practitioner's collected billings. The Corporation agrees to take responsibility for maintaining a 95% rate of billings collected. In the event that the Corporation does not collect 95% of its billings during the term of this Agreement, Corporation agrees to pay the Nurse Practitioner salary as if the Corporation had maintained a 95% collections rate.

   b. The Corporation and the Nurse Practitioner agree to a fee schedule for the Nurse Practitioner's services, which is attached.

3. The Nurse Practitioner agrees to bill a minimum of $270,000 per year.
   a. Billings shall include self-paying patients, third-party payers, and internal billings, which shall include surgical follow-up visits handled by the Nurse Practitioner for the Corporation.
   b. Surgical follow-up visits are assigned a value of $70.00.
4. The Corporation shall retain all but $91,000 of collected revenues from the first $270,000 of billings generated by the Nurse Practitioner.
5. The Nurse Practitioner shall receive bonus payments to be determined as follows:
   a. If the Nurse Practitioner's billings exceed $68,000 in any quarter, collected revenues exceeding $68,000 per quarter shall be shared jointly and equally by the Nurse Practitioner and the Corporation, and the Corporation shall pay the Nurse Practitioner's 50% share to the Nurse Practitioner as a bonus within 30 days of the last day of the quarter.
   b. If the Nurse Practitioner bills less than $68,000 in any quarter, the Nurse Practitioner shall receive no bonus for that quarter, and the difference between the

amount billed by the Nurse Practitioner in the deficient quarter, and $68,000 shall be deducted from any bonus the Nurse Practitioner shall receive in a future quarter. There shall be no deduction from the Nurse Practitioner's salary.

c. In the event that this Agreement is terminated prior to receipt of any bonus payment due the Nurse Practitioner, the Corporation agrees to pay the Nurse Practitioner the bonus earned within 15 days of termination. In the event that termination occurs mid-quarter, both parties agree that neither bonus nor deficiency will apply for the final quarter.

Schedule C—Benefits

1. The Nurse Practitioner shall be entitled to the following benefits:
   a. Health insurance: The Corporation shall pay directly to the health insurance company up to $5000 per year for premiums for health insurance.
   b. Malpractice insurance: The Corporation shall pay the malpractice insurance premiums for the Nurse Practitioner.
   c. Pension benefits: The Corporation will fund the Nurse Practitioner's pension benefits.
   d. Vacation: Four (4) weeks per year.
   e. Continuing medical education time: One (1) week.
   f. Continuing medical education expenses: Up to $1500.00 per year, paid for by the Corporation.
   g. Life insurance: In an amount equal to annual base salary.
   h. Salary continuation plan: Short-Term Disability—full pay continuation until Long-Term Disability coverage begins at ninety (90) days.
   i. Sick leave: Ten (10) days per year.
   j. Professional fees and medical staff dues: Professional journals in the amount of $350 per year, medical staff dues at hospitals where the Nurse Practitioner attends patients of the Practice, state license fee, state Controlled Dangerous Substances and DEA license fees, and Basic Cardiac Life Support/Advanced Cardiac Life Support recertification fees.

Legal Scope of Nurse Practitioner Practice

Having an adequate legal description of nurse practitioners' (NPs') scope of practice according to state law is important for the following reasons:

1. To allow NPs to perform at their level of education and training
2. To avoid any charges of practicing medicine without a license
3. To avoid imputation of liability for medical malpractice to someone other than the NP, usually a physician
4. To place accountability for both benefits and harm to patients squarely on the NP
5. To provide a basis for inclusion of NPs in the legal definition of primary care providers, which is necessary for admission to provider panels
6. To establish that the NP is a professional entity, not just a "nonphysician," a "physician extender," or whatever an agency, employer, or delegating physician decides an NP is
7. To get reimbursement for physician services, when provided by an NP

State law is the most powerful source of authority for professional practice. However, federal agencies and private businesses may have policies on NP scope of practice, and professional societies may have accepted certain tasks, functions, and decisions as part of NP scope of practice.

Professional Association Definition of Scope of Practice

Some associations define the scope of practice for NPs in general or for individual NPs. For example, the American Academy of Nurse Practitioners' statement on scope of practice says:

> Nurse practitioners are licensed independent practitioners who practice in ambulatory, acute, and long-term care settings as primary and/or specialty care providers. According to their practice specialty, they provide nursing and medical services to individuals, families, and groups. In addition to diagnosing and managing acute episodic and chronic illnesses, NPs emphasize health promotion and disease prevention. Services include but are not limited to ordering, conducting, and interpreting diagnostic and laboratory tests, prescription of pharmacologic agents and treatments and nonpharmacologic therapies. Teaching and counseling individuals, families, and groups are a major part of nurse practitioners'

practice. As licensed independent practitioners, nurse practitioners practice autonomously and in collaboration with healthcare professionals and other individuals to diagnose, treat, and manage the patient's health problems. They serve as healthcare resources, interdisciplinary consultants, and patient advocates.[1]

Statutory Versus Regulatory Scope of NP Practice

Some states define scope of practice in statutes enacted by the state legislature. In other states, the legislature gives the board of nursing the authority to define the scope of NP practice. Either way is enforceable, and regulations carry the same force of law as statutes.

Some states describe scope of practice specifically, and some define it generally. State statutes describing NP scope of practice fall into six categories:

1. Scope of practice is clearly defined by statute.
2. Scope of practice is clearly defined by regulation.
3. Scope of practice is vaguely defined by statute.
4. Scope of practice is not defined.
5. Scope of practice is defined by exception from a state law prohibiting the practice of medicine without a license.
6. Scope of practice is defined by the individual physician, who may delegate to an NP by law.

The first category is the most secure for the NP.

At a time when NPs are viewed by some physicians as competitors, the first response to competitive pressures is often for physicians to point to state law and ask for strict interpretation. For example, physicians' associations may counter NPs' efforts to be designated as primary care providers (PCPs) for managed-care organizations or a patient's "medical home" by claiming that state law does not explicitly authorize NPs to perform the necessary functions. Then, only NPs in states where the NP scope of practice is clearly defined as including medical diagnosis and treatment, prescription of medication, and oversight of comprehensive healthcare services for patients will have legal grounds for arguing that NPs should be admitted to provider panels as PCPs or designated a "medical home."

A vaguely worded nurse practice act that states, for example, that the scope of NP practice includes "acts of advanced nursing practice" will not provide sound legal basis for arguments that NPs should be admitted to managed-care provider panels or receive fees for providing physician services. It is difficult to argue to managed-care executives, state administrators, and legislators that "acts of nursing practice" are the acts necessary to perform physician services.

Physician Challenges to NPs' Scope of Practice

An example of a physician challenge to NPs' scope of practice is a 1984 Missouri court case, *Sermchief v. Gonzales* [660 S.W.2d 683 (Mo. 1984)]. That case, which the NPs won only after it went to the state's supreme court, could be repeated in other states today where state law is not specific enough about the authority of NPs to diagnose and treat.

In *Sermchief*, two obstetric-gynecologic NPs were working in a family planning clinic under written protocols with the clinic's physicians. The NPs were taking histories, performing physical examinations, treating minor illnesses, and prescribing contraceptives. There was no specific charge of malpractice, but rather the Missouri Board of Medicine charged that the NPs were practicing medicine without a license.

The lower court agreed and found that the NPs were practicing medicine without a license. However, the Missouri Supreme Court, after analyzing the nurse practice act, noted that the legislature had deleted a requirement that a physician directly supervise nursing functions and decided that by that deletion the legislature had intended to broaden the scope of nursing.

The NPs eventually prevailed in the case, but that will not necessarily help NPs in other states if there is no express statutory authority for NPs' medical functions. NPs need a clear statutory definition of the scope of practice that includes medical diagnoses and treatment and prescriptive authority.

Need for Clarity of Scope of Practice

Some state laws describe scope of practice succinctly and others go into great detail. Longer is not necessarily better, and vague language should be avoided. Consider Oklahoma's statute on nurse practitioner scope of practice.

> "Certified Nurse Practitioner" is an Advanced Practice Registered Nurse who performs in an expanded role in the delivery of health care:
>
> a.   consistent with advanced educational preparation as a Certified Nurse Practitioner in an area of specialty,
> b.   functions within the Certified Nurse Practitioner scope of practice for the selected area of specialization, and
> c.   is in accord with the standards for Certified Nurse Practitioners as identified by the certifying body and approved by the Board.
>
> A Certified Nurse Practitioner shall be eligible, in accordance with the scope of practice of the Certified Nurse Practitioner, to obtain recognition as authorized by the Board to prescribe, as defined by the rules promulgated by the Board pursuant to this section and subject to the medical direction of a supervising physician. This authorization shall not include dispensing drugs, but shall not preclude, subject to federal regulations, the receipt of, the signing for, or the dispensing of professional samples to patients.
>
> *Citation:* OKLA. STAT. ANN. tit. 59, § 567.3a(6).

Under Oklahoma's statutory definition of NP scope of practice, an NP can prescribe, but it is unclear what else an NP can do. To prove that the NP can make medical diagnoses, the NP would need to produce transcripts and course descriptions, as well as information from the certifying body on the scope of practice. Oklahoma's Administrative Code provides a detailed description of NP scope of practice, however. The Oklahoma Administrative Code states the following:

The Certified Nurse Practitioner's scope of practice includes the full scope of nursing practice and practice in an expanded role as follows:

1. The Certified Nurse Practitioner (CNP) provides comprehensive health care to clients across the life span.
2. The CNP is responsible and accountable for the continuous and comprehensive management of a broad range of health services, which include, but are not limited to:
   A. promotion and maintenance of health;
   B. prevention of illness and disability;
   C. diagnosis and prescription of medications, treatments, and devices for acute and chronic conditions and diseases;
   D. management of health care during acute and chronic phases of illness;
   E. guidance and counseling services;
   F. consultation and/or collaboration with other health care providers and community resources;
   G. referral to other health care providers and community resources.

Citation: Okla. Admin. Code § 485:10–15.6(b)

An example of a comprehensive description of scope of practice is Pennsylvania's law:

When acting in collaboration with a physician as set forth in a collaborative agreement and within the CRNP's specialty, a CRNP may:

1. Perform comprehensive assessments of patients and establish medical diagnoses.
2. Order, perform and supervise diagnostic tests for patients and, to the extent the interpretation of diagnostic tests is within the scope of the CRNP's specialty and consistent with the collaborative agreement, may interpret diagnostic tests.
3. Initiate referrals to and consultations with other licensed professional health care providers, and consult with other licensed professional health care providers at their request.
4. Develop and implement treatment plans, including issuing orders to implement treatment plans. However, only a CRNP with current prescriptive authority approval may develop and implement treatment plans for pharmaceutical treatments.
5. Complete admission and discharge summaries.
6. Order blood and blood components for patients.
7. Order dietary plans for patients.
8. Order home health and hospice care.
9. Order durable medical equipment.
10. Issue oral orders to the extent permitted by the health care facilities' by-laws, rules, regulations or administrative policies and guidelines.

11. Make physical therapy and dietitian referrals.
12. Make respiratory and occupational therapy referrals.
13. Perform disability assessments for the program providing temporary assistance to needy families (TANF).
14. Issue homebound schooling certifications.
15. Perform and sign the initial assessment of methadone treatment evaluations, provided that any order for methadone treatment shall be made only by a physician.

Citation: 49 PA CODE § 21.251.

See **Exhibit** **1** for a breakdown of elements of NP practice found in various state laws.
See **Appendix** **A** for the law of each of the states regarding NP scope of practice.

Exhibit **1**   Specific Functions Included in States' Definitions of NP Scope of Practice

Diagnose	OR	MT	IL	VT
AL	PA	ND	IN	WA
AZ	SC	ND	KS	WI
CO	SD	NE	KY	WY
CT	UT	NV	LA	
DC	VT	NH	MD	**Admit to Hospital**
FL	WA	NJ	MA	AL
GA		NY	ME	AZ
HI	**Treat**	NC	MN	HI
IA	AL	OK	MO	OR
ID	AZ	OR	MS	WA
IL	CO	PA	NC	
IN	CT	SC	NC	**Refer**
LA	DE	SD	ND	AL
ME	DC	UT	NE	AZ
MD	FL	VT	NH	CO
MA	GA	WA	NJ	DC
MN	ID		NM	DE
MS	IL	**Prescribe**	NV	HI
MT	IN	AL	NY	IN
NC	KS	AZ	OH	KY
ND	KY	CO	OK	LA
NE	LA	CT	OR	ME
NH	ME	DE	PA	MD
NH	MD	DC	RI	MN
NJ	MA	FL	SC	MT
NV	MS	GA	SD	NC
NY	MN	IA	TX	NE
OK	MO	ID	UT	NH

Refer	Order Tests	Assist in Surgery
NJ	AL	HI
NV	AZ	
OK	CO	**Perform Palliative Care**
OR	DC	IL
PA	DE	
SD	FL	**Order Durable Medical Equipment**
UT	GA	
WA	HI	MT
	IA	PA
Teach	IL	
AL	KY	**Order Restraints**
DE	MA	SD
HI	MD	
IA	ME	
IL	MT	
IN	NE	
KS	NJ	
LA	NC	
ME	PA	
MT	WA	
NV	WI	
NC		
ND	**Perform Procedures**	
NH	WA	
OK		
OR	**Remove Epidural Catheter**	
SD	DE	

NP Scope of Practice Compared with Registered Nurse Scope of Practice

NP scope of practice usually includes medical diagnosis and treatment, while registered nurse (RN) scope of practice usually includes "nursing diagnosis" and "nursing interventions" or "nursing treatments."

Compare Oregon's scope of practice for an RN to Oregon's scope of practice for an NP. Oregon's law on scope of practice for an RN states:

> The Board recognizes that the scope of practice for the registered nurse encompasses a variety of roles, including, but not limited to:
>
> a. Provision of client care;
> b. Supervision of others in the provision of care;

c. Development and implementation of health care policy;
d. Consultation in the practice of nursing;
e. Nursing administration;
f. Nursing education;
g. Case management;
h. Nursing research;
i. Teaching health care providers and prospective healthcare providers;
j. Specialization in advanced practice;
k. Nursing informatics.

Citation: Or. Admin. § R. 851-045-0060.

Oregon's board of nursing has elegantly defined the scope of NP practice as follows:

. . .

3. The nurse practitioner provides holistic health care to individuals, families, and groups across the life span in a variety of settings, including hospitals, long-term care facilities, and community-based settings.
4. Within his or her specialty, the nurse practitioner is responsible for managing health problems encountered by the client and is accountable for health outcomes. This process includes:
   a. Assessment;
   b. Diagnosis;
   c. Development of a plan;
   d. Intervention;
   e. Evaluation.
5. The nurse practitioner is independently responsible and accountable for the continuous and comprehensive management of a broad range of health care, which may include:
   a. Promotion and maintenance of health;
   b. Prevention of illness and disability;
   c. Assessment of clients, synthesis and analysis of data, and application of nursing principles and therapeutic modalities;
   d. Management of health care during acute and chronic phases of illness;
   e. Admission of his/her clients to hospitals and long-term care facilities and management of client care in these facilities;
   f. Counseling;
   g. Consultation and/or collaboration with other care providers and community resources;
   h. Referral to other healthcare providers and community resources;
   i. Management and coordination of care;
   j. Use of research skills;
   k. Diagnosis of health/illness status;

1. Prescribing, dispensing, and administration of therapeutic devices and measures, including legend drugs and controlled substances as provided in Division 56 of the Oregon Nurse Practice Act, consistent with the definition of the practitioner's specialty category and scope of practice.
6. The nurse practitioner's scope of practice includes teaching the theory and practice of advanced practice nursing.
7. The nurse practitioner is responsible for recognizing limits of knowledge and experience, and for resolving situations beyond his/her nurse practitioner expertise by consulting with or referring clients to other healthcare providers.
8. The nurse practitioner will only provide healthcare services within the nurse practitioner's scope of practice for which he/she is educationally prepared and for which competency has been established and maintained. Educational preparation includes academic course work, workshops or seminars, provided both theory and clinical experience are included.

Citation: OR. ADMIN. § R. 851-050-0005.

In California, the scope of practice of an NP is defined as that of an RN:

The nurse practitioner shall function within the scope of practice as specified in the Nursing Practice Act and as it applies to all registered nurses.

Citation: Cal. Code Reg. tit. 16 §1485.

An NP or RN gets the authority to perform medical acts through standardized procedures developed with physicians. Here is a statement from the California Board of Professional Nursing website about the scope of practice of a nurse practitioner:

The NP does not have an additional scope of practice beyond the usual RN scope and must rely on standardized procedures for authorization to perform overlapping medical functions (CCR Section 1485). Section 2725 of the Nursing Practice Act (NPA) provides authority for nursing functions that are also essential to providing primary health care which do not require standardized procedures. Examples include physical and mental assessment, disease prevention and restorative measures, performance of skin tests and immunization techniques, and withdrawal of blood, as well as authority to initiate emergency procedures.

Nurse practitioners frequently ask if they really need standardized procedures. The answer is that they do when performing overlapping medical functions. Standardized procedures are the legal authority to exceed the usual scope of RN practice. Without standardized procedures the NP is legally very vulnerable, regardless of having been certified as a RN, who has acquired additional skills as a certified nurse practitioner.[2]

In general, NPs may make medical diagnoses and initiate and perform medical treatments, while RNs may not. RNs may make nursing diagnoses, carry out physician or NP orders, and perform nursing treatments, as well as many other functions. Ideally, NPs have clear authority under state law to perform comprehensive evaluations, make medical diagnoses, order tests, initiate and perform medical therapies, including the prescribing of medication, and admit patients to hospitals.

NP and Physician Scope of Practice Compared

When NP scope of practice is defined to include medical diagnosis, medical treatment, prescriptive authority, and admission of patients to hospitals, as in Oregon law, there is little legal difference between NP and physician scope of practice. However, in most states, medical scope of practice is defined more broadly than the scope of practice for any other healthcare professional. Consider Mississippi's definition of the practice of medicine:

> The practice of medicine shall mean to suggest, recommend, prescribe, or direct for the use of any person, any drug, medicine, appliance, or other agency, whether material or not material, for the cure, relief, or palliation of any ailment or disease of the mind or body, or for the cure or relief of any wound or fracture or other bodily injury or deformity, or the practice of obstetrics or midwifery, after having received, or with the intent of receiving therefore, either directly or indirectly, any bonus, gift, profit, or compensation; provided, that nothing in this section shall apply to females engaged solely in the practice of midwifery.

> *Citation:* MISS. CODE ANN. § 73-25-33.

The liberal use of the word "any" differentiates the physician scope of practice from the NP scope of practice. There are no laws that authorize as wide a scope of practice for NPs as the Mississippi law authorizes for physician practice.

An Individual NP's Portfolio

Individual NPs may want to develop portfolios—compilations of documentation of the NP's education, training, and experience. The portfolio often is a binder containing pages, which may be removed and copied as needed.

There are at least three good reasons to keep a portfolio. First, in many states, NPs must submit to the Board of Nursing a written agreement stating the services the NP is authorized to perform. NPs may want to perform procedures, such as colposcopy or suturing. Boards require NPs to document that they are qualified to perform such procedures. Qualifications might include formal course work, informal course work, or formal or informal one-to-one preceptorship experience. NPs can find it difficult to document such training, especially if the NP learned how to perform a procedure years ago from a physician while on the job. If NPs document the teaching at the time it is done, through a letter or form signed and dated by the instructor, the NP can produce the document as needed many years later, assuming the NP keeps such documents in a safe place—in the portfolio.

Second, some states' laws defer to scope of practice statements adopted by professional organizations. For example, Texas law states the following:

> The advanced practice nurse provides a broad range of health services, the scope of which shall be based upon educational preparation, continued advanced practice experience, and the accepted scope of professional practice of the particular specialty area. Advanced practice nurses practice in a variety of settings and, according to their practice specialties and roles, they provide a broad range of healthcare services to a variety of patient populations.
>
> 1. The scope of practice of particular specialty areas shall be defined by national professional specialty organizations or advanced practice nursing organizations recognized by the Board. The advanced practice nurse may perform only those functions which are within that scope of practice and which are consistent with the Nursing Practice Act, Board rules, and other laws and regulations of the State of Texas.
>
> *Citation:* TX ADMIN. CODE § 221.12.

NPs living in states with laws similar to Texas should have the scope and standards of practice established by the national organization representing the NP's specialty in their portfolios.

For example, if an NP in Texas is certified by the American Academy of Nurse Practitioners (AANP), the NP should keep in his/her portfolio a 1-page document from the AANP website titled *Scope of Practice for Nurse Practitioners.* The document states, in part:

> Nurse Practitioners are licensed independent practitioners who practice in ambulatory, acute and long-term care as primary and/or specialty care providers. According to their practice specialty they provide nursing and medical services to individuals, families, and groups. In addition to diagnosing and managing acute episodic and chronic illnesses, nurse practitioners emphasize health promotion and disease prevention. Services include, but are not limited to ordering, conducting, supervising, and interpreting diagnostic and laboratory tests, and prescription of pharmacologic agents and nonpharmacologic therapies. Teaching and counseling individuals, families, and groups are a major part of nurse practitioner practice.[1]

Third, some nurses are using their portfolios in place of resumes when interviewing for jobs. A portfolio could include the following:

- Statement of career goals
- Description of special interests or abilities

- Description of special projects conducted by the individual
- Articles or reports written by the individual
- Articles written about the individual
- Brochures from previous practices
- Testimonials or letters of appreciation from patients
- Letters of reference from former employers or coworkers
- Awards, honors, or distinction earned by the individual
- Transcripts
- Diplomas
- Certificates of certification as advanced practice nurse
- Nursing and advanced practice nursing (APN) license
- Photo of the individual
- Certificates of continuing education or training
- Letters of recommendation
- Letters, forms, or photographs documenting one-on-one training
- Listing of former jobs or projects
- National Provider Identifier and any other provider numbers needed for reimbursement
- Drug Enforcement Agency (DEA) number and state controlled substances prescriber number
- Certificate of professional liability insurance
- Copy of state law addressing NP scope of practice, prescribing, qualifications, and physician collaboration requirements, if any
- Previous written agreements, if state law requires physician collaboration
- Outcomes data, if the NP or an employer has tracked the NP's outcomes
- Data on performance measures, if the NP has participated in Medicare's Quality Reporting System or other quality measurement programs
- Productivity data, if the NP or an employer has tracked visits, revenues, and collections
- Patient satisfaction data, if the NP or an employer has tracked patient satisfaction

Finally, it saves time if one keeps the documents related to one's professional practice in one place.

Mandated Physician Involvement with NP Practice

In some states, there is no legal requirement for physician involvement in NP practice. However, in the majority of states, there is some legal requirement for physician involvement. That involvement may be "supervision," "collaboration," or some other form. It may be limited to situations where the NP is prescribing medications, or it may be required for all advanced practice.

See **Exhibit 2** for a chart listing requirements of physician involvement by state. For text of state laws regarding physician involvement, see **Appendix B**.

Exhibit 2   Physician Involvement Required for NP Practice

Collaborate	Supervise	Protocols	None
AL	FL	AL	AK
AR	MI	AR	AZ
CT	ME*	CA	CO
DE	SC	FL	DC
GA	OK	GA	HI
IA+	TN	KS	ID
IL		MA	KY
IN	**Delegate**	NJ	ME**
KS	GA	NY	MT
LA	MI	SC	ND
MA	MN	TX	NH
MD	SC		NM
MN	WV	**Referral**	NV
MO		**Process**	OR
MS	**Direct**	AK	RI
NC	OK		UT***
ND	AR		VT**
NE			WA
NJ			WY
NY			
OH			
OH			
PA			
SD			
VA			
VT*			
WV			
WI			

+Iowa Administrative Code requires collaboration for medical functions; however, the Board of Nursing's position is that advanced registered nurse practitioners function independently.
*First 24 months of practice only.
**After 24 months.
***Consultation/referral plan required to prescribe Schedules II–III controlled substances.

Some states require that NPs practice using written protocols. Some states require a written agreement between the NP and the physician that states how the physician will participate in NP practice, what medications the NP may prescribe, what procedures an NP may perform, how often a physician will review NP documentation, and under what circumstances an NP must contact a physician. A protocol is a written instrument that guides the NP in collecting data from the patient and recommends specific action based upon the collected data. It consists of mutually agreed upon medical guidelines between the physician and the NP that define their individual and shared responsibilities. The protocol is considered a standard because it provides a guideline for a minimum level of safe practice in specific situations.[3]

Exhibit   3 is an example of a protocol.

Exhibit   3   Urinary Tract Infection Protocol: Initial Visit

I.   RATIONALE

This protocol will assist in the differentiation between pyelonephritis and urinary tract symptoms sufficiently to eradicate the symptoms per se rather than an attempt to eradicate any bacteriuria that may or may not be present. The design of the protocol for urinary tract infection (UTI) encompasses these principles.

II.   SYMPTOMS

A.   CYSTITIS

1.   FEMALE PATIENTS

Order a STAT clean catch urinalysis (UA) for female patients with any of the following symptoms;

a.   Dysuria

b.   Frequency

c.   Urgency

d.   Inability to empty bladder completely

2.   Male patients

Male patients with any of the above symptoms should be seen by a physician, not by an NP, unless they have a uretheral discharge (possible venereal disease (VD)—follow VD protocol).

B.   PYELONEPHRITIS

1.   In addition to the above symptoms, patients with pyelonephritis may have:

a.   Fever greater than 100.0° F, or

b.   Flank pains, or

c.   Chills, or

d.   Nausea, vomiting, or abdominal pain.

2.   Continue with protocol through the physical exam with these patients, but then consult supervising physician before deciding on treatment.

III.   HISTORY

A.   Consult supervising physician if patient has:

1.   A history of kidney problems, or

2.   Is currently pregnant. To ascertain this, always ask for last menstrual period (LMP) date and record for all female patients.

3.   Diabetes or insulin.

4.   Three or more UTIs in past 12 months.

B.   Continue with UTI protocol, but also refer patient to gynecology practitioner if history of:

---

1. Vaginal discharge, or
2. Perineal inflammation.

IV. PHYSICAL EXAM
    A. Perform the following examinations:
        1. Abdominal
        2. Costovertebral angle (CVA) tenderness
        3. Temperature

    B. Consult supervising physician if findings of:
        1. Fever greater than 100.0° F, or
        2. CVA tenderness.

V. LAB TESTS
INITIAL URINALYSIS

    A. Consult supervising physician if:
        1. Casts
        2. Red blood cells (RBCs) or protein are positive (with associated white blood cell (WBC) abnormality).

    B. If UA shows 10 or more WBCs/hpf and patient is symptomatic, give patient antibiotic prescription as described in the treatment section.

    C. If UA revealed 0–10 WBCs, review symptoms. If the symptoms are definite and very severe, treat with antibiotics; if symptoms are vague and poorly defined, then give patient symptomatic treatment as described in the treatment section and consider referral to gynecology for pelvic.

    D. Should the initial UA be "positive": (defined in guidelines below), then give patient a repeat UA slip for the abnormality found with instructions to have the UA one week following completion of treatment.

    Positive UA findings are defined as:

    Casts: any except occasional hyaline or rare granular
    RBCs > 3 (if not menstruating) and WBC < 5
    Protein > trace and WBC < 5

VI. TREATMENT
ANTIBACTERIAL TREATMENT
To be given if initial UA reveals 10 or more WBC/hpf, or in any case where symptoms are severe, even if UA revealed, WBC/hpf.

    A. Prescribe appropriate antibiotic drug (see below).

    B. Instruct patient to call in if symptoms do not subside within 72 hours. If patient does call back, information for treatment failure instructions.

SYMPTOMATIC TREATMENT
To be given only if initial UA reveals, 10 WBC/hpf, and patient has minimal or uncertain symptoms. Consider gynecology referral for pelvic.

    A. Prescribe either Propantheline 15 mg #20 sig: 1-2 QID prn or Belladonna with Pb tabs #15, sig: 1 tab QID prn.

B. Instruct patient to call in if symptoms persist beyond 72 hours or if symptoms worsen at any time.

VII. REPEAT URINALYSIS

A. Consult supervising physician if UA shows casts.

B. If repeat UA conforms abnormality (protein and/or RBC as listed below) refer to Proteinuria and/or Hematuria protocols.

Positive UA findings are defined as:

Casts: any, except occasional hyaline or rare granular
RBCs > 3 (if not menstruating) and WBC < 5
Protein > trace and WBC < 5

UTI PROTOCOL: ANTIBIOTIC TREATMENT

A. If organism found in patient's urine is not listed in the table below, consult supervising physician for treatment.

B. If this is the first antibiotic course (initial visit), assume E. coli and use the first listed drug to which patient is not allergic, as listed for E. coli in the drug table on the following page.

C. If this is a second antibiotic course (treatment failure), go to the first drug for the organism listed that is not the same as that previously used and to which the patient is not allergic. If the patient is allergic to all drugs listed, consult supervising physician for treatment.

D. Prescribe according to the prescription table which follows:
   1. If symptoms have been present within the past 48 hours, use 1 dose treatment.
   2. If symptoms have been present longer than 48 hours, use 5-day treatment.
   3. If symptoms persist after treatment with first drug, repeat UA and culture and consult supervising physician.

UTI PROTOCOL: TREATMENT FAILURE

If the patient calls in with persisted or recurrent symptoms after the first course of antibiotic treatment, obtain a clean catch urine specimen for UA and culture and sensitivity.

If the UA is negative, wait for the culture results before treating. If the UA is positive, treat with the next drug listed on the Antibiotic Prescription Table and review treatment choice when the culture and sensitivity results are available.

If culture is positive and patients symptoms are improving, stay with the same antibiotic. If not responding after 3 days, switch to a new antibiotic based on culture sensitivity.

Adapted from protocol developed by: _____, NP

_____, MD

(List names of nurse practitioners and physicians who developed the standardized procedure, including the protocol section.)

ANTIBIOTIC PRESCRIPTION TABLE

Organism	Drug	
E. Coli	Septra DS, AmoxicillinProteus mirabilis	Macrodantin, Keflex
Aerobacter	Septra DS, MacrodantinKlebsiella	Keflex, Ciprofloxacin
Enterococcus	Ampicillin	*Consult MD if allergic
Pseudomonas	Ciprofloxacin	(Usually not seen in out-patient setting)

Dosages	
SEPTRA DS	#3 PO at once or 1 bid × 5 days
AMOXICILLIN	500 mg 3 gms PO at once or 250 mg 1 tid × 5 days
MACRODANTIN	100 mg qid × 5 day
KEFLEX	250 mg qid × 5 day
CIPROFLOXACIN	250 mg qid × 5 day

Source: California Board of Registered Nursing. Available at http://www.rn.ca.gov. Retrieved May 30, 2013.

Notes

1. American Academy of Nurse Practitioners. (2013). Scope of practice for nurse practitioners. Retrieved from http://www.aanp.org/images/documents/publications/scopeofpractice.pdf
2. California Board of Registred Nursing. (2011.). General information: Nurse practitioner practice. Retrieved from http://www.rn.ca.gov/pdfs/regulations/npr-b-23.pdf
3. Phillips, R. S. (1985). Nurse practitioners: Their scope of practice and theories of liability. *Journal of Legal Medicine, 6,* 391–414.

Scope of Practice

In some states scope of practice is specified by statute; in other states it is specified by regulation. Both statutes and regulations carry the same legal weight. Statutes are laws made by the legislature; they are also changed by a vote of the legislature. Regulations are executive agency–made law; they can be changed by the agency or overridden by statute.

The following are excerpts from state law. For the complete language, see each state's Nurse Practice Act, usually available online through the state's Board of Nursing website.

Alabama

Practice as a certified registered nurse practitioner (CRNP) means the performance of nursing skills by a registered nurse who has demonstrated by certification that he or she has advanced knowledge and skills in the delivery of nursing services within a healthcare system that provides for consultation, collaborative management, or referral as indicated by the health status of the client.

Citation: ALA. CODE § 34-21-81(4a).

1. Functions and activities of certified registered nurse practitioners. The certified registered nurse practitioner is responsible for the continuous and comprehensive management of a broad range of health services for which the certified registered nurse practitioner is educationally prepared and for which competency is maintained, with physician collaboration as decribed in these rules. These services include but are not restricted to the following:
   a. Evaluate current health status and risk factors of individuals based on comprehensive health history and physical examination and assessment.
   b. Formulate a working diagnosis, develop and implement a treatment plan, and evaluate and modify therapeutic regimens to promote positive patient outcomes.
   c. Prescribe, administer and provide therapeutic measures, tests, procedures, and drugs.

    d. Counsel, teach and assist individuals and families to assume responsibility for self-care in prevention of illness, health maintenance, and health restoration.

    e. Consult with and refer to other healthcare providers as appropriate.

2. A standard protocol approved by the Board of Nursing and State Board of Medical Examiners shall address permissible functions and activities specific to the advanced practice of the certified registered nurse practitioner.

3. A certified registered nurse practitioner may, after the successful completion of an organized program of study and supervised clinical practice, carry out functions beyond the nurse practitioner educational preparation provided the functions are approved by the Board of Nursing as being within the legal scope of practice for a certified registered nurse practitioner. Such functions shall be submitted to the Joint Committee for consideration for inclusion on the standard protocol.

4. Request for additional functions to be added to the protocol may be submitted to the Joint Committee for consideration.

5. A certified registered nurse practitioner may write admission orders for inpatients as directed by the physician and subsequent orders in accordance with established protocols and institutional policies.

Citation: ALA. ADMIN. CODE r. 610-X-5-.10.

Alaska

The board recognizes advanced and specialized acts of nursing practice as those described in the scope of practice statements for nurse practitioners certified by national certification bodies recognized by the board.

Citation: ALASKA ADMIN. CODE, § 44.430.

Authority AS 08.68.100(a)

Arizona

Nurse practitioners

- Examine patients and establish medical diagnoses by client history, physical exam, and other criteria
- For a patient who requires the services of a health care facility: admit the patient to healthcare facilities, manage the care the patient receives in the facility, and discharge the patient from the facility
- Order and interpret laboratory, radiographic, and other diagnostic tests, and perform those tests that the RNP is qualified to perform
- Identify, develop, implement, and evaluate a plan of care for a patient to promote, maintain, and restore health

- Perform therapeutic procedures that the RNP is qualified to perform
- Prescribe treatments
- If authorized under R4-19-511, prescribe and dispense drugs and devices
- Perform additional acts that the RNP is qualified to perform

Citation: ARIZ. ADMIN. CODE § R4-19-508.

Arkansas

"Practice of advanced nurse practitioner nursing" means the performance for compensation of nursing skills by a registered nurse who, as demonstrated by national certification, has advanced knowledge and practice skills in the delivery of nursing services.

Citation: ARK. CODE ANN. § 17-87-102.(4)(B)(i).

"Practice of registered nurse practitioner nursing" means the delivery of health care services for compensation in collaboration with and under the direction of a licensed physician or under the direction of protocols developed with a licensed physician.

Citation: ARK. CODE ANN. § 17-87-102.(8)(A).

California

Nothing in this article shall be construed to limit the scope of practice of a registered nurse authorized pursuant to this chapter.

Citation: Cal. Bus. & Prof. Code § 2837.

Nothing in this article shall be construed to limit the scope of practice of the registered nurse authorized pursuant to the Business and Professions Code, Divison 2, Chapter 6. The nurse practitioner shall function within the scope of practice as specified in the Nurse Practice Act and as it applies to all registered nurses.

Citation: CAL. CODE REG. tit.16, § 1485.

Colorado

In order to enhance the cost efficiency and continuity of care, an advanced practice nurse may, within his or her scope of practice and within the advanced practice nurse-patient relationship, sign an affidavit, certification, or similar document that:

   I. Documents a patient's current health status;
  II. Authorizes continuing treatment, tests, services, or equipment; or
 III. Gives advance directives for end-of-life care.

b. Such affidavit, certification, or similar document may not:

    I. Be the prescription of medication unless the advanced practice nurse has been granted prescriptive authority pursuant to section 12-38-111.6; or

    II. Be in conflict with other requirements of law.

Citation: COLO. REV. STAT.§12-38-111.5(7)(A).

"Practice of professional nursing" means the performance of both independent nursing functions and delegated medical functions in accordance with accepted practice standards. Such functions include the initiation and performance of nursing care through health promotion, supportive or restorative care, disease prevention, diagnosis and treatment of human disease, ailment, pain, injury, deformity, and physical or mental condition using specialized knowledge, judgment, and skill involving the application of biological, physical, social, and behavioral science principles required for licensure as a professional nurse pursuant to section 12-38-111.

The "practice of professional nursing" shall include the performance of such services as:

I.   Evaluating health status through the collection and assessment of health data;

II.   Health teaching and health counseling;

III.   Providing therapy and treatment that is supportive and restorative to life and well-being either directly to the patient or indirectly through consultation with, delegation to, supervision of, or teaching of others;

IV.   Executing delegated medical functions;

V.   Referring to medical or community agencies those patients who need further evaluation or treatment;

VI.   Reviewing and monitoring therapy and treatment plans.

Citation: COLO. REV. STAT. ANN. § 12-38-103 (10)(a) and (b).

A nurse who meets the definition of advanced practice nurse . . . may be granted prescriptive authority as a function in addition to those defined in Section 12-38-103(10).

Citation: COLO. REV. STAT. ANN. § 12-38-111.5.

The scope of practice for an advanced practice nurse may be determined by the board in accordance with this article.

Citation: COLO. REV. STAT. ANN. § 12-38-111.6(8)(a).

Connecticut

Advanced nursing practice is defined as the performance of advanced level nursing practice activities, which by virtue of post-basic specialized education and experience are appropriate to and may be performed by an Advanced

Practice Registered Nurse. The advanced practice registered nurse performs acts of diagnosis and treatment of alteration in health status as described in subsection (a) of this section, and shall collaborate with a physician licensed to practice medicine in this state. In all settings, the advanced practice registered nurse may, in collaboration with a physician licensed to practice medicine in this state, prescribe, dispense, and administer medical therapeutics and corrective measures and may request, sign for, receive, and dispense drugs in the form of professional samples. . . .

Citation: CONN. GEN. STAT. ANN § 20-87a.

Delaware

"Independent practice by an advanced practice nurse" shall include those advance practice nurses who practice and prescribe without written guidelines or protocols but with a collaborative agreement with a licensed physician, dentist, podiatrist, or licensed Delaware health care delivery system and with the approval of the Joint Practice Committee.

Citation: DEL. CODE ANN. TIT. 24, § 1902(g).

Generic functions of the Advanced Practice Nurse with the Specialized Scope of Practice include, but are not limited to:

- Eliciting detailed health history(s)
- Defining nursing problem(s)
- Performing physical examination(s)
- Collecting and performing laboratory tests
- Interpreting laboratory data
- Initiating requests for essential laboratory procedures
- Initiating requests for essential x-rays
- Screening patients to identify abnormal problems
- Initiating referrals to appropriate resources and services as necessary
- Initiating or modifying treatment and medications within established guidelines
- Assessing and reporting changes in the health of individuals, families, and communities
- Providing health education through teaching and counseling
- Planning and/or instituting health care programs in the community with other health care professionals and the public
- Delegating tasks appropriately
- Prescribing medications and treatments independently pursuant to Rules and Regulations . . .
- Removing epidural catheters

Citation: DEL. NURSING REGS. tit. 24, ch 1900, § 8.7.

District of Columbia

The advanced practice registered nurse may perform actions of medical diagnosis, treatment, prescription, and other functions authorized by this subchapter.

Citation: D.C. Stat. § 3-1206.01(a).

An advanced practice registered nurse may:

1. Initiate, monitor, and alter drug therapies;
2. Initiate appropriate therapies or treatments;
3. Make referrals for appropriate therapies or treatments; and
4. Perform additional functions within his or her specialty determined in accordance with rules and regulations promulgated by the board.

Citation: D.C. Stat. § 3-1206.04.

"Practice of advanced practice registered nursing" means the performance of advanced-level nursing actions, with or without compensation, by a licensed registered nurse with advanced education, knowledge, skills, and scope of practice who has been certified to perform such actions by a national certifying body acceptable to the Board of Nursing. The practice of advanced practice registered nursing includes:

A. Advanced assessment;
B. Medical diagnosis;
C. Prescribing;
D. Selecting, administering, and dispensing therapeutic measures;
E. Treating alterations of the health status; and
F. Carrying out other functions identified in subchapter VI of this chapter and in accordance with procedures required by this chapter.

Citation: D.C. Stat. § 3-1201.02(2).

Florida

An advanced registered nurse practitioner shall perform those functions authorized in this section within the framework of an established protocol that is filed with the board upon biennial license renewal and within 30 days after entering into a supervisory relationship with a physician or changes to the protocol. The board shall review the protocol to ensure compliance with applicable regulatory standards for protocols. The board shall refer to the department licensees submitting protocols that are not compliant with the regulatory standards for protocols. A practitioner currently licensed under chapter 458, chapter 459, or chapter 466 shall maintain supervision for directing the specific course of medical treatment. Within the established framework, an advanced registered nurse practitioner may:

a. Monitor and alter drug therapies.
b. Initiate appropriate therapies for certain conditions.
c. Perform additional functions as may be determined by rule . . .
d. Order diagnostic tests and physical and occupational therapy.

Citation: FLA. STAT. Ch. 464.012(3).

All categories of Advanced Registered Nurse Practitioner may perform functions listed in Section 464.012(3), F.S. The scope of practice for all categories of ARNP's shall include those functions which the ARNP has been educated to perform including the monitoring and altering of drug therapies, and initiation of appropriate therapies, according to the established protocol and consistent with the practice setting.

Citation: FLA. ADMIN REGISTER & FLA. ADMIN CODE. Ch. 064B9-4.009.

Within the context of advanced or specialized nursing practice, the advanced registered nurse practitioner may perform acts of nursing diagnosis and nursing treatment of alterations of the health status. The advanced registered nurse practitioner may also perform acts of medical diagnosis and treatment, prescription, and operation which are identified and approved by a joint committee composed of three members appointed by the Board of Nursing, two of whom must be advanced registered nurse practitioners; three members appointed by the Board of Medicine, two of whom must have had work experience with advanced registered nurse practitioners; and the State Surgeon General or the State Surgeon General's designee.

Citation: FLA. STAT. Ch. 464.003(2).

Georgia

The nurse practitioner provides advanced practice nursing care and medical services specific to the nurse practitioner respective specialty to individuals, families, and groups, emphasizing health promotion and disease prevention as well as the diagnosis and management of acute and chronic diseases. The nurse practitioner collaborates as necessary with a variety of individuals to diagnose and manage clients' healthcare problems.

Citation: GA. COMP. R. & REGS. r. 410-12-.03(2)(a).

The advanced practice registered nurse is authorized to perform advanced nursing functions and certain medical acts which include, but are not limited to, ordering drugs, treatments, and diagnostic studies as provided in O.C.G.A. 43-24-26.1 and Chapter 410.13.

Citation: GA. COMP. R. & REGS. r. 410-12-.01(4b).

Hawaii

In addition to those functions specified for the registered nurse, and in accordance with appropriate nationally recognized standards of practice, the advanced practice registered nurse may perform the following generic acts which include, but are not limited to:

1. Provide direct nursing care by utilizing advanced practice scientific knowledge, skills, nursing and related theories to assess, plan, and implement appropriate health and nursing care to patients;
2. Provide indirect care. Plan, guide, evaluate, and direct the nursing care given by other personnel associated with the health care team;
3. Teach, counsel, or plan care for individuals or group, utilizing a synthesis of advanced skills, theories, and knowledge of biologic, pharmacologic, physical, sociocultural and psychological aspects of care to accomplish desired objectives;
4. Serve as a consultant and resource of advanced clinical knowledge and skills to those involved directly or indirectly in patient care;
5. Participate in joint and periodic evaluation of services rendered including, but not limited to, chart reviews, case reviews, patient evaluations, and outcome of case statistics;
6. Establish collaborative, consultative, and referral networks as appropriate with other health care professionals. Patients who require care beyond the scope of practice of an APRN shall be referred to an appropriate health care provider;
7. Manage the plan of care prescribed for the patient;
8. Initiate and maintain accurate records and authorize appropriate regulatory and other legal documents;
9. Recognize, develop, and implement professional and community educational programs related to health care;
10. Conduct research and analyze the health needs of individuals and populations and design programs which target at-risk groups and cultural and environmental factors which foster health and prevent illness;
11. Participate in policy analysis and development of new policy initiative in the area of practice specialty; and
12. Contribute to the development, maintenance, and change of health care delivery systems to improve quality of health care services and consumer access to services.

Citation: HAW. ADMIN. R. §16-89-81(b).

Nurse practitioner scope of practice, depending on area of specialty, may include, but is not limited to:

A. Evaluate the physical and psychosocial health status of patients through a comprehensive health history and physical examination, or mental status examination, using skills of observation, inspection, palpation, percussion, and auscultation, and using diagnostic instruments or procedures that are basic to the clinical evaluation of physical, developmental, and psychological signs and symptoms;

B. Order, interpret, or perform diagnostic, screening, and therapeutic examinations, tests and procedures.

C. Formulate a diagnosis;

D. Plan, implement, and evaluate care;

E. Order or utilize medical, therapeutic, or corrective measures, including, but not limited to, rehabilitation therapies, medical nutritional therapy, social services and psychological and other medical services;

F. Monitor the effectiveness of therapeutic interventions;

G. Assist in surgery; and

H. Admit and discharge clients for inpatient care at facilities licensed as hospitals, long term care facilities or hospice.

Citation: HAW. ADMIN. R. § 16-89-81(c)(1).

Practice as an advanced practice registered nurse means the scope of nursing in a category approved by the board, regardless of compensation or personal profit, and includes the registered nurse scope of practice. The scope of an advanced practice registered nurse includes but is not limited to advanced assessment and the diagnosis, prescription, selection, and administration of therapeutic measures including over the counter drugs, legend drugs, and controlled substances within the advanced practice registered nurse's role and specialty-appropriate education and certification.

Citation: HAW. REV. STAT. § 457-a.

Idaho

An advanced practice registered nurse is authorized to perform advanced nursing practice, which may include the prescribing, administering and dispensing of therapeutic pharmacologic agents, as defined by board rules. An advanced practice registered nurse shall perform only those acts as provided by the board and for which the individual is educationally prepared.

Citation: IDAHO CODE § 54-1402(1).

Advanced Practice Registered Nurse. Means a registered nurse licensed in this state who has gained additional specialized knowledge, skills and experience through a graduate or post-graduate program of study as defined herein and is authorized to perform advanced nursing practice, which may include acts of diagnosis and treatment, and the prescribing, administering and dispensing of therapeutic pharmacologic and non-pharmacologic agents, as defined herein.

Citation: IDAHO ADMIN. CODE §23.01.01: 271.02.

Illinois

a. Advanced practice nursing by certified nurse practitioners, certified nurse anesthetists, certified nurse midwives, or clinical nurse specialists is based on knowledge and skills acquired throughout an advanced practice nurse's nursing education, training, and experience.

b. Practice as an advanced practice nurse means a scope of nursing practice, with or without compensation, and includes the registered nurse scope of practice.

c. The scope of practice of an advanced practice nurse includes, but is not limited to, each of the following:

   1. Advanced nursing patient assessment and diagnosis.
   2. Ordering diagnostic and therapeutic tests and procedures, performing those tests and procedures when using health care equipment, and interpreting and using the results of diagnostic and therapeutic tests and procedures ordered by the advanced practice nurse or another health care professional.
   3. Ordering treatments, ordering or applying appropriate medical devices, and using nursing medical, therapeutic, and corrective measures to treat illness and improve health status.
   4. Providing palliative and end-of-life care.
   5. Providing advanced counseling, patient education, health education, and patient advocacy.
   6. Prescriptive authority as defined in Section 65-40 of this Act.
   7. Delegating selected nursing activities or tasks to a licensed practical nurse, a registered nurse, or other personnel.

Citation: 225 ILL. COMP. STAT. § 65/65-30.

Indiana

"Nurse practitioner" means an advanced practice nurse who provides advanced levels of nursing client care in a specialty role, who meets the requirements of the advanced practice nurse as outlined in Section 3 of this rule.

Citation: IND. ADMIN. CODE tit. 848, r. 4-1-4.

[Indiana law does not use the words "scope of practice," but describes "standards for each nurse practitioner" as follows:]

1. Assess clients by using advanced knowledge and skills to:
   A. identify abnormal conditions;
   B. diagnose health problems;
   C. develop and implement nursing treatment plans;

D. evaluate patient outcomes; and

E. collaborate with or refer to a practitioner, as defined in IC 25-23-1-19.4, in managing the plan of care.

2. Use advanced knowledge and skills in teaching and guiding clients and other health team members.

3. Use appropriate critical thinking skills to make independent decisions, commensurate with the autonomy, authority, and responsibility of a nurse practitioner.

4. Function within the legal boundaries of their advanced practice area and shall have and utilize knowledge of the statutes and rules governing their advanced practice area; including the following:

A. State and federal drug laws and regulations.

B. State and federal confidentiality laws and regulations.

C. State and federal medical records access laws.

5. Consult and collaborate with other members of the health team as appropriate to provide reasonable client care, both acute and ongoing.

6. Recognize the limits of individual knowledge and experience, and consult with or refer clients to other health care providers as appropriate.

7. Retain professional accountability for any delegated intervention, and delegate interventions only as authorized by IC 25-23-1 and this title.

8. Maintain current knowledge and skills in the nurse practitioner area.

9. Conduct an assessment of clients and families, which may include health history, family history, physical examination, and evaluation of health risk factors.

10. Assess normal and abnormal findings obtained from the history, physical examination, and laboratory results.

11. Evaluate clients and families regarding development, coping ability, and emotional and social well-being.

12. Plan, implement, and evaluate care.

13. Develop individualized teaching plans with each client based on health records.

14. Counsel individuals, families, and groups about health and illness and promote attention to wellness.

15. Participate in periodic or joint evaluations of services rendered, including, but not limited to, the following:

A. Chart reviews.

B. Client evaluations.

C. Outcome statistics.

16. Conduct and apply research findings appropriate to the area of practice.

17. Participate, when appropriate, in the joint review of the plan of care.

Citation: IND. ADMIN. CODE tit. 848, r. 4-2-1.

The board shall establish a program under which advanced practice nurses who meet the requirements established by the board are authorized to prescribe legend drugs, including controlled substances (as defined in IC 35-48-1).

b. The authority granted by the board under this section:
   1. expires on October 31 of the odd-numbered year following the year the authority was granted or renewed; and
   2. is subject to renewal indefinitely for successive periods of two (2) years.

c. The rules adopted under section 7 of this chapter concerning the authority of advanced practice nurses to prescribe legend drugs must do the following:
   1. Require an advanced practice nurse or a prospective advanced practice nurse who seeks the authority to submit an application to the board.
   2. Require, as a prerequisite to the initial granting of the authority, the successful completion by the applicant of a graduate level course in pharmacology providing at least two (2) semester hours of academic credit.
   3. Require, as a condition of the renewal of the authority, the completion by the advanced practice nurse of the continuing education requirements set out in section 19.7 of this chapter.

Citation: IND. CODE §25-23-1-19.5(a).

Iowa

In the advanced role, the nurse practices nursing assessment, intervention, and management within the boundaries of the nurse-client relationship. Advanced nursing practice occurs in a variety of settings within an interdisciplinary healthcare team, which provides for consultation, collaborative management, and referral. The ARNP may perform selected medically designated functions when a collaborative practice agreement exists.

Citation: IOWA ADMIN. CODE r. 655-6.1(152).

Kansas

Each "advanced practice registered nurse" (APRN), as defined by K.S.A. 65-1113 and amendments thereto, shall function in an expanded role to provide primary, secondary, and tertiary health care in the APRN's category of advanced practice. Each APRN shall be authorized to make independent decisions about advanced practice nursing needs of families, patients, and clients and medical decisions based on the authorization for collaborative practice with one or more physicians. This regulation shall not be deemed to require the immediate and physical presence of the physician when care is given by an APRN. Each APRN shall be directly accountable and responsible to the consumer.

Citation: KAN. ADMIN. REGS. § 60-11-101(a).

Each advanced registered nurse practitioner in the category of nurse practitioner shall function in an expanded role at a specialized level, through the application of advanced knowledge and skills and shall be authorized to perform the following:

a. Provide health promotion and maintenance, disease prevention, and independent nursing diagnosis, as defined in K.S.A. 65-1113(b) and amendments thereto, and treatment, as defined in K.S.A. 65-1113(c) and amendments thereto, of acute and chronic diseases;

b. develop and manage the medical plan of care for patients or clients, based on the authorization for collaborative practice;

c. provide health care services for which the nurse practitioner is educationally prepared and for which competency has been established and maintained. Educational preparation may include academic coursework, workshops, institutes, and seminars if theory or clinical experience, or both, are included;

d. provide health care for individuals by managing health problems encountered by patients and clients; and

e. provide innovation in evidence-based nursing practice based upon advanced clinical expertise, decision making, and leadership skills and serve as a consultant, researcher, and patient advocate for individuals, families, groups, and communities to achieve quality, cost-effective patient outcomes and solutions.

Citation: KAN. ADMIN. REGS. § 60-11-104.

An advanced practice registered nurse may prescribe drugs pursuant to a written protocol as authorized by a responsible physician.

Citation: KAN. STAT. ANN. § 65-1130(d).

Kentucky

"Advanced practice registered nursing" means the performance of additional acts by registered nurses who have gained added knowledge and skills through an approved organized postbasic program of study and clinical experience; and who are certified by the American Nurses' Association or other nationally established organizations or agencies recognized by the board to certify registered nurses for advanced practice registered nursing as a certified nurse practitioner, certified nurse anesthetist, certified nurse midwife, or clinical nurse specialist; and who are certified in at least one (1) population focus. The additional acts shall, subject to approval of the board, include but not be limited to, prescribing treatment, drugs, devices, and ordering diagnostic tests. Advanced practice registered nurses who engage in these additional acts shall be authorized to issue prescriptions for and dispense nonscheduled legend drugs as defined in KRS 217.905 and to issue prescriptions for but not to dispense Schedules II through V controlled substances as classified in KRS 218A.060, 218A.070, 218A.080,

218A.090, 218A.100, 218A.110, 218A.120, and 218A.130, under the conditions set forth in KRS 314.042 and regulations promulgated by the Kentucky Board of Nursing on or before August 15, 2006.

a. Prescriptions issued by advanced practice registered nurses for Schedule II controlled substances classified under KRS 218A.060 shall be limited to a seventy-two (72)-hour supply without any refill. Prescriptions issued under this subsection for psychostimulants may be written for a thirty (30)-day supply only by an advanced practice registered nurse certified in psychiatric-mental health nursing who is providing services in a health facility as defined in KRS Chapter 216B or in a regional mental health-mental retardation services program as defined in KRS Chapter 210.

b. Prescriptions issued by advanced practice registered nurses for Schedule III controlled substances classified under KRS 218A.080 shall be limited to a thirty (30)-day supply without any refill. Prescriptions issued by advanced practice registered nurses for Schedules IV and V controlled substances classified under KRS 218A.100 and 218A.120 shall be limited to the original prescription and refills not to exceed a six (6)-month supply. . . .

Citation: Ky. Rev. Stat. Ann. § 314.011(8).

The practice of the advanced practice registered nurse shall be in accordance with the standards and functions defined in the following scope and standards of practice statements for each specialty area.

- In the performance of advanced practice registered nursing, the advanced practice registered nurse shall seek consultation or referral in those situations outside the advanced practice registered nurse's scope of practice.
- Advanced practice registered nursing shall include prescribing medications and ordering treatments, devices, and diagnostic tests which are consistent with the scope and standard of practice of the advanced practice registered nurse.

Advanced practice registered nursing shall not preclude the practice by the advanced practice registered nurse of registered nursing practice as defined in KRS 314.011(5).

Citation: 201 Ky. Admin. Regs. § 20:057 Sections 2–5.

Louisiana

An advanced practice registered nurse shall practice as set forth in R.S. 37:913(3)(a) and the standards set forth in these administrative rules. The patient services provided by an APRN shall be in accord with the educational preparation of that APRN. . . .

Standards of practice are essential for safe practice by the APRN and shall be in accordance with the published professional standards for each recognized specialty and/or functional role. The core standards for all categories of advanced practice registered nurses include, but are not limited to:

1. an APRN shall meet the standards of practice for registered nurses as defined in LAC 46:XLVII.3901-3915;
2. an APRN shall assess patients at an advanced level, identify abnormal conditions, analyze and synthesize data to establish a diagnosis, develop and implement treatment plans, and evaluate patient outcomes;
3. the APRN shall use advanced knowledge and skills in providing patients and health team members with guidance and teaching;
4. an APRN shall use critical thinking and independent decision-making at an advanced level commensurate with the autonomy, authority, and responsibility of the specialty and functional role while working with patients and their families in meeting health care needs;
5. an APRN shall demonstrate knowledge of the statutes and rules governing advanced registered nursing practice and function within the legal boundaries of the appropriate advanced registered nursing practice role;
6. an APRN shall demonstrate knowledge of and apply current nursing research findings relevant to the advanced nursing specialty and functional role;
7. an APRN shall make decisions to solve patient care problems and select medical treatment regimens in collaboration with a licensed physician or dentist; and
8. an APRN shall retain professional accountability for his/her actions and/or interventions.

Citation: La. Admin. Code tit. 46, § XLVII-4513.

a. "Advanced practice registered nursing" means nursing by a certified registered nurse anesthetist, certified nurse midwife, clinical nurse specialist, or nurse practitioner which is based on knowledge and skills acquired in a basic nursing education program, licensure as a registered nurse, and a minimum of a master's degree with a concentration in the respective advanced practice nursing specialty which includes both didactic and clinical components, advanced knowledge in nursing theory, physical and psychosocial assessment, nursing interventions, and management of health care. Advanced practice registered nursing includes:

  i. Assessing patients, analyzing and synthesizing data, and knowledge of and applying nursing principles at an advanced level.
  ii. Providing guidance and teaching.
  iii. Working with patients and families in meeting health care needs.
  iv. Collaborating with other health care providers.
  v. Managing patients' physical and psychosocial health-illness status with regard to nursing care.
  vi. Utilizing research skills.

    vii. Analyzing multiple sources of data and performing certain acts of medical diagnosis in accordance with the collaborative practice agreement.

    viii. Making decisions in solving patient care problems and selecting treatment regimens in collaboration with a licensed physician, dentist, or other health care provider as indicated.

    ix. Consulting with or referring patients to licensed physicians, dentists, and other health care providers in accordance with a collaborative practice agreement.

b. Advanced practice registered nursing may include certain acts of medical diagnosis, in accordance with R.S. 37:913(8) and (9), or medical prescriptions of therapeutic or corrective nature, prescribing assessment studies, legend and certain controlled drugs, therapeutic regimens, medical devices and appliances, receiving and distributing a therapeutic regimen of prepackaged drugs prepared and labeled by a licensed pharmacist, and free samples supplied by a drug manufacturer, and distributing drugs for administration to and use by other individuals within the scope of practice as defined by the board and in accordance with this Paragraph.

Citation: La. Rev. Stat. § 37:913(3).

Maine

The certified nurse practitioner shall provide only those health care services for which the certified nurse practitioner is educationally and clinically prepared, and for which competency has been maintained. The Board reserves the right to make exceptions. Such health care services, for which the certified nurse practitioner is independently responsible and accountable, include:

1. obtaining a complete health data base that includes a health history, physical examination, and screening and diagnostic evaluation
2. interpreting health data by identifying wellness and risk factors and variations from norms
3. diagnosing and treating common diseases and human responses to actual and potential health problems
4. counseling individuals and families
5. consulting and/or collaborating with other healthcare providers and community resources
6. referring client to other health care providers and community resources.

Citation: Code Me. R. § 02 380 3.

"Advanced practice registered nursing" means the delivery of expanded professional health care by an advanced practice registered nurse that is:

94

B. Within the advanced practice registered nurse's scope of practice as specified by the board of rulemaking, taking into consideration any national standards that exists; and

C. In accordance with the standards of practice for advanced practice registered nurses as specified by the board by rulemaking, taking into consideration any national standards that may exist. Advanced practice registered nursing includes consultation with or referral to medical and other health care providers when required by client health care needs.

A certified nurse practitioner or a certified nurse midwife who qualified as an advanced practice registered nurse may prescribe and dispense drugs or devices, or both, in accordance with rules adopted by the board.

A certified nurse practitioner who qualified as an advanced practice registered nurse must practice, for at least 24 months, under the supervision of a licensed physician or a supervising nurse practitioner or must be employed by a clinic or hospital that has a medical director who is a licensed physician. The certified nurse practitioner shall submit written evidence to the board upon completion of the required clinical experience.

Citation: ME. REV. STAT. ANN. tit. 32, § 2102-2A.

Maryland

A. A nurse practitioner may perform independently the following functions:
   1. A comprehensive physical assessment of patients;
   2. In accordance with Family Law Article, §2-301, Annotated Code of Maryland, certify to the clerk of the court that a:
      a. 16 or 17 year old individual, who wants to get married without parental consent, has been examined and found to be pregnant or has given birth to a child; or
      b. 15 year old individual, who has parental consent to be married, has been examined and found to be pregnant or has given birth to a child;
   3. In accordance with Transportation Article, §13-704, Annotated Code of Maryland, certify to the Department of Transportation that an individual needs special consideration for certain health reasons;
   4. In accordance with Health General Article, §4-208, Annotated Code of Maryland, complete the date of birth and medical information required on a birth certificate;
   5. In accordance with Health General Article, §4-212, Annotated Code of Maryland, complete a death certificate if:
      a. The medical examiner does not take charge of the body; and
      b. The deceased was under the care of the nurse practitioner;

6. In accordance with Health General Article, §13-704, Annotated Code of Maryland, conduct education and training to certify individuals for the Insect Sting Emergency Treatment Program;
7. Establish medical diagnosis for common short-term and chronic stable health problems;
8. In accordance with Health General Article, §4-212, Annotated Code of Maryland, file a replacement death certificate;
9. In accordance with Health General Article, §5-601, Annotated Code of Maryland, issue a "do not resuscitate order" on a Maryland Emergency Medical Services form.
10. Order, perform, and interpret laboratory and diagnostic tests;
11. Order and perform diagnostic, therapeutic, and corrective measures;
12. Prescribe drugs;
13. Provide emergency care;
14. Refer patients to appropriate licensed physicians or other health care providers as needed; and
15. In accordance with Health General Article, §5-602, Annotated Code of Maryland, witness an advance directive.

B. A nurse practitioner may practice only in the area of specialization in which certified.

C. Nothing in this chapter limits or prohibits a registered nurse from performing those functions which constitute the practice of registered nursing as defined by law.

Citation: MD. REGS. CODE. 10 § 27.07.02.

Massachusetts

The practice of registered nurses shall include, but not be limited to:

1. the application of nursing theory to the development, implementation, evaluation, and modification of plans of nursing care for individuals, families and communities;
2. coordination and management of resources of care delivery;
3. management, direction and supervision of the practice of nursing, including the delegation of selected activities to unlicensed assistive personnel.

Advanced practice nurse regulations which govern the ordering of tests, therapeutics, and prescribing of medications shall be promulgated by the board of nursing and in conjunction with the board of medicine.

Citation: MASS. GEN LAWS CH 112 § 80B.

The area of practice of a nurse practitioner includes:

a. Assessing the health status of individuals and families by obtaining health and medical histories, performing physical examinations, diagnosing health and developmental problems, and caring for patients suffering from acute and chronic diseases by managing therapeutic regimens according to guidelines approved and developed in compliance with 244 CMR § 4.22.

Citation: Code Mass Regs Tit. 244 § 4.26(a).

Michigan

[There is no statutory or regulatory scope of practice for NPs. Physicians may delegate at their discretion.]:

Subject to subsections (2) to (6), a licensee who holds a license other than a health profession subfield license may delegate to a licensed or unlicensed individual who is otherwise qualified by education, training or experience the performance of selected acts, tasks or functions where the acts, tasks, or functions fall within the scope of practice of the licensee's profession and will be performed under the licensee's supervision. A licensee shall not delegate an act, task, or function under this section if the act, task, or function, under standards of acceptable and prevailing practice, requires the level of education, skill, and judgment required of the licensee under this article.

Citation: Mich. Comp. Laws § 333.16215(1).

Minnesota

"Nurse practitioner practice" means, within the context of collaborative management:

1. diagnosing, directly managing, and preventing acute and chronic illness and disease; and
2. promoting wellness, including providing non-pharmacologic treatment. The certified nurse practitioner is certified for advanced registered nurse practice in a specific field of nurse practitioner practice.

Citation: Minn. Stat. Ann. § 148.171(11).

The "practice of advanced practice registered nursing" means the performance of clinical nurse specialist practice, nurse-midwife practice, nurse practitioner, or registered nurse anesthetist practice as defined in subdivisions 5, 10, 11, and 21. The practice includes functioning as a direct care provider, case manager, consultant, educator, and researcher. The practice of advanced practice registered nursing also includes accepting referrals from, consulting with, cooperating with, or referring to all other types of health care providers, including but not limited to physicians, chiropractors, podiatrists, and dentists, provided that the advanced practice registered nurse and the other provider are practicing within their scopes of practice as defined in state law. The advanced practice registered nurse must practice within a health care system that provides for consultation, collaborative management, and referral as indicated by the health status of the patient.

Citation: Minn. Stat. Ann. § 148.171(13).

Mississippi

"Advanced nursing practice" means, in addition to the practice of professional nursing, the performance of advanced-level nursing approved by the board which, by virtue of graduate education and experience are appropriately performed by an advanced practice registered nurse. The advanced practice registered nurse may diagnose, treat, and manage medical conditions. This may include prescriptive authority as identified by the board.

Citation: Miss. Nursing Practice Law §73-15-5(4).

Missouri

RNs recognized by the MSBN as being eligible to practice as an APRN shall function clinically within the professional scope and standards of their advanced practice nursing clinical specialty area and consistent with their formal advanced nursing education and national certification, if applicable, or within their education, training, knowledge, judgment, skill, and competence as an RN.

Citation: Mo. Code Regs. Ann. tit. 20, § 2200-4.100(4)(A)(2).

The methods of treatment and the authority to administer, dispense, or prescribe drugs delegated in a collaborative practice arrangement between a collaborating physician and collaborating APRN shall be within the scope of practice of each professional and shall be consistent with each professional's skill, training, education, competence, licensure, and/or certification and shall not be further delegated to any person except that the individuals identified in sections 338.095 and 338.198, RSMo, may communicate prescription drug orders to a pharmacist.

Citation: Mo. Code Regs. Ann. tit. 20, § 2200-4.200.

(3)(A) When a collaborative practice arrangement is utilized to provide health care services for conditions other than acute self-limited or well-defined problems, the collaborating physician, or other physician designated in the collaborative practice arrangement, shall examine and evaluate the patient and approve or formulate the plan of treatment for new or significantly changed conditions as soon as is practical, but in no case more than two (2) weeks after the patient has been seen by the collaborating APRN or RN.

Citation: Mo. Code Regs. Ann. tit. 20, § 2200-4.200 (3)(H).

Montana

Nurse practitioner practice means the independent and/or collaborative management of primary and/or acute health care of individuals, families, and communities including:

a. assessing the health status of individuals and families using methods appropriate to the client population and area of practice such as health history taking, physical examination, and assessing developmental health problems;

b. instituting and facilitating continuity of health care to clients, including:
    i. ordering durable medical equipment, treatments and modalities, and diagnostic tests;
    ii. receiving and interpreting results of diagnostic procedures;
    iii. making medical and nursing diagnoses; and
    iv. working with clients to promote their understanding of and compliance with therapeutic regimens.

c. promoting wellness and disease prevention programs;

d. referring clients to a physician or other health care provider, when appropriate;

e. providing instruction and counseling to individuals, families, and groups in the areas of health promotion and maintenance, including involving such persons in planning for their health care; and

f. working in collaboration with other health care providers and agencies to provide and, where appropriate, coordinate services to individuals and families.

Citation: MONT. ADMIN. R. § 24.159.1470(1).

Nebraska

An advanced practice registered nurse practitioner may provide healthcare services within specialty areas.

1. A nurse practitioner may provide health care services within specialty areas. A nurse practitioner shall function by establishing collaborative, consultative, and referral networks as appropriate with other health care professionals. Patients who require care beyond the scope of practice of a nurse practitioner shall be referred to an appropriate health care provider.

2. Nurse practitioner practice means health promotion, health supervision, illness prevention and diagnosis, treatment, and management of common health problems and acute and chronic conditions, including:
   a. Assessing patients, ordering diagnostic tests and therapeutic treatments, synthesizing and analyzing data, and applying advanced nursing principles;
   b. Dispensing, incident to practice only, sample medication which are provided by the manufacturer and are provided at no charge to the patient; and

c. Prescribing therapeutic measures and medications, relating to health conditions within the scope of practice. Any limitation on the prescribing authority of the advanced practice registered nurse for controlled substances listed in Schedule II of Section 28-405 shall be recorded in the integrated practice agreement. . . .

Citation: Neb. Rev. Stat. § 38-2315.

Nevada

[**Effective through June 30, 2014.**]

1. The Board may issue a license to practice as an advanced practice registered nurse to a registered nurse who has completed an educational program designed to prepare a registered nurse to:
   a. Perform designated acts of medical diagnosis;
   b. Prescribe therapeutic or corrective measures; and
   c. Prescribe controlled substances, poisons, dangerous drugs and devices, and who meets the other requirements established by the Board for such licensure.
2. An advanced practice registered nurse may:
   a. Engage in selected medical diagnosis and treatment; and
   b. If authorized pursuant to NRS 639.2351, prescribe controlled substances, poisons, dangerous drugs and devices.
3. The Board shall adopt regulations:
   a. Specifying the training, education and experience necessary for licensure as an advanced practice registered nurse.
   b. Delineating the authorized scope of practice of an advanced practice registered nurse
   c. Establishing the procedure for application for licensure as an advanced practice registered nurse.

Citation: Nev. Rev. Stat. § 632.237, as amended May 2013 by AB 170.

An advanced practice registered nurse may perform the following acts in addition to the functions of a registered nurse if the advanced practice registered nurse is properly prepared and the acts are currently within the standard of practice for his or her role and population of focus:

1. Systematically assess the health status of person and families by:
   a. Taking, recording and interpreting medical histories and performing physical examinations; and
   b. Performing or initiating selected diagnostic procedures.

2. Based on information obtained in the assessment of a person's health, manage the care of selected persons and families with common, acute, recurrent or long-term health problems. Management may include:
   a. Initiation of a program of treatment;
   b. Evaluation of responses to health problems and programs of treatment;
   c. Informing a person or family of the status of the patient's health and alternatives for care;
   d. Evaluation of compliance with a program of treatment agreed upon by the person or family and the advanced practice registered nurse.;
   e. Modification of programs of treatment based on the response of the person or family to treatment;
   f. Referral to appropriate providers of health care; and
   g. Commencement of care required to stabilize a patient in an emergency.
3. Any other act if:
   a. The advanced practice registered nurse is certified to perform that act by an organization recognized by the Board;
   b. The performance of the act was taught in the program of education attended by the advanced practice registered nurse;
   c. The performance of the act was taught in a comprehensive program of instruction successfully completed by the advanced practice registered nurse, which included clinical experience;
   d. The act is within the scope of practice of an advanced practice registered nurse as determined by the Board; or
   e. The advanced practice registered nurse is trained to perform that act by a physician or another advanced practice registered nurse and the act:
      1. Has been described as being performed by an advanced practice registered nurse in two or more national nursing publications, national nursing practice guidelines or national standards for nursing practice, or any combination thereof, which are listed in the *Cumulative Index to Nursing and Allied Health Literature*, as adopted by referenced in NAC 632.1110; or
      2. Has been individually approved by the Board.

Citation: Nev. Admin. Code § 632.255.

New Hampshire

I. Advanced practice registered nursing by nurse practitioners shall consist of a combination of knowledge and skills acquired in basic nursing education. The APRN scope of practice, with or without compensation or personal profit, shall be limited to:

a. Performing acts of advanced assessment, diagnosing, prescribing, selecting, administering, and providing therapeutic measures and treatment regimes;

b. Obtaining consultation, planning, and implementing collaborative management, referral, or transferring the care of the client as appropriate; and

c. Providing such functions common to a nurse practitioner for which the APRN is educationally and experientially prepared and which are consistent with standards established by a national credentialing or certification body recognized by the National Council of State Boards of Nursing and approved by the board in the appropriate APRN role and specialty.

II. An APRN shall practice within standards consistent with standards established by a national credentialing or certification body recognized by the National Council of State Boards of Nursing and approved by the board in the appropriate APRN role and specialty. The board shall not approve a new advanced practice specialty category that has not been developed by a national credentialing or certifying body recognized by the National Council of State Board of Nursing without approval of the legislature under RSA 332-G:6. Each APRN shall be accountable to clients and the board:

a. For complying with this chapter and the quality of advanced nursing care rendered;

b. For recognizing limits of knowledge and experience and planning for the management of situations beyond the APRN's expertise; and

c. For consulting with or referring clients to other healthcare providers as appropriate.

III. An APRN shall have plenary authority to possess, compound, prescribe, administer, and dispense and distribute to clients controlled and non-controlled drugs within the scope of the APRN's practice as defined by this chapter. Such authority may be denied, suspended, or revoked by the board after notice and the opportunity for hearing, upon proof that the authority has been abused.

IV. Any expansion of the scope of practice shall be adopted by legislation in accordance with RSA 332-G:6.

Citation: N.H. Rev. Stat. Ann. § 326-B:11.

New Jersey

a. In addition to all other tasks which a registered professional nurse may, by law, perform, an advanced practice nurse may manage preventive care services, and diagnose and manage deviations from wellness and long-term illnesses, consistent with the needs of the patient and within the scope of practice of the advanced practice nurse, by:

1. initiating laboratory and other diagnostic tests;

2. prescribing or ordering medications and devices, as authorized by subsections b. and c. of this section;

3. prescribing and ordering treatments, including referrals to other licensed health care professionals, and performing specific procedures in accordance with the provisions of this subsection.

Citation: N.J. Stat. Ann. § 45:11-49.a.

New Mexico

Certified nurse practitioners who have fulfilled requirements for prescriptive authority may prescribe in accordance with the rules, regulations, guidelines, and formularies for individual certified nurse practitioners promulgated by the board.

Citation: N.M. Stat. Ann. § 61-3-23.2.C.

Certified nurse practitioners may:

1. Perform an expanded practice that is beyond the scope of practice of professional registered nursing;

2. Practice independently and make decisions regarding health care needs of the individual, family, or community and carry out health regimens, including the prescription and dispensing of dangerous drugs and controlled substances included in Schedule II through V of the Controlled Dangerous Substances Act; and

3. Serve as a primary acute, chronic long-term and end-of-life health care provider and as necessary collaborate with licensed medical doctors, osteopathic physicians, or podiatrists.

Citation: N.M. Stat. Ann. § 61-3-23.2.B.

New York

The practice of registered professional nursing by a nurse practitioner, certified under section six thousand nine hundred ten of this article, may include the diagnosis of illness and physical conditions and the performance of therapeutic and corrective measures within a specialty area of practice, in collaboration with a licensed physician qualified to collaborate in the specialty involved, provided such services are performed in accordance with a written practice agreement and written practice protocols.

Citation: N.Y. Educ. Law, Art. 139 § 6902.3(a).

Prescriptions for drugs, devices, and immunizing agents may be issued . . . in accordance with the practice agreement and practice protocols.

Citation: N.Y. Educ. Law Art. 139 § 6902.3(b).

North Carolina

A nurse practitioner shall be held accountable by both Boards for the continuous and comprehensive management of a broad range of personal health services for which the nurse practitioner is educationally prepared and for which competency has been maintained, with physician supervision as described in Rule .0810 of this Section. These services include but are not restricted to:

1. Promotion and maintenance of health;
2. Prevention of illness and disability;
3. Diagnosis, treating, and managing acute and chronic illnesses;
4. Guidance and counseling of both individuals and families;
5. Prescribing, administering, and dispensing therapeutic measures, tests, procedures and drugs;
6. Planning for situations beyond the nurse practitioner's expertise, and consulting with and referring to other health care providers as appropriate; and
7. Evaluating health outcomes.

Citation: N.C. ADMIN CODE tit. 21, r. 36.0802.

North Dakota

1. Practice as an advanced practice registered nurse may include:
   a. Perform a comprehensive assessment of clients and synthesize and analyze data within a nursing framework;
   b. Identify, develop, plan, and maintain evidence-based, client-centered nursing care;
   c. Prescribe a therapeutic regimen of health care, including diagnosing, prescribing, administering, and dispensing legend drugs and controlled substances;
   d. Evaluate prescribed health care regimen;
   e. Participate in nursing care management according to chapter 54-05-04 relating to standards for assignment and delegation and section 54-05-02-02.2 assigning of nursing interventions;
   f. Promote a safe and therapeutic environment;
   g. Provide health teaching and counseling to promote, attain, and maintain the optimum health level of clients;
   h. Communicate and collaborate with the interdisciplinary team in the management of health care and the implementation of the total health care regimen;
   i. Manage and evaluate the clients' physical and psychosocial health-illness status;
   j. Manage, supervise, and evaluate the practice of nursing;
   k. Utilize evolving client information management systems;

l. Integrate quality improvement principles in the delivery and evaluation of client care;

m. Teach the theory and practice of nursing;

n. Analyze, synthesize, and apply research outcomes in practice; and

o. Integrate the principles of research in practice.

2. Notwithstanding the above, all services rendered by the licensee shall be commensurate with the academic preparation, knowledge, skills, and abilities of the advanced practice licensed nurse's experience, continuing education, and demonstrated competencies. The nurse must recognize individual limits of knowledge, skills, and abilities and plan for situations beyond the licensee's expertise.

Citation: N.D. ADMIN. CODE § 54-05-03.1-03.2.

Ohio

A certified nurse-midwife, certified nurse practitioner, certified registered nurse anesthetist, or clinical nurse specialist shall do all of the following:

1. Function within the scope of practice of nursing for a registered nurse as set forth in division (b) of section 4723.01 of the Revised Code and the rules of the board.

2. Function within the nurse's applicable scope of practice as set forth in section 4723.43 of the Revised Code and the rules of the board.

3. Practice in accordance with section 4723.481 of the Revised Code and Chapter 4723-9 of the Administrative Code if the individual holds a certificate to prescribe.

Citation: OHIO REV. CODE ANN. § 4723-4-053(A).

Oklahoma

A Certified Nurse Practitioner shall be eligible, in accordance with the scope of practice of the Certified Nurse Practitioner, to obtain recognition as authorized by the Board to prescribe, as defined by the rules promulgated by the Board pursuant to this section and subject to the medical direction of a supervising physician. This authorization shall not include dispensing drugs, but shall not preclude, subject to federal regulations, the receipt of, the signing for, or the dispensing of professional samples to patients.

The Certified Nurse Practitioner accepts responsibility, accountability, and obligation to practice in accordance with usual and customary advanced practice nursing standards and functions as defined by the scope of practice/role definition statements for the advanced registered nurse practitioner.

Citation: OKLA. STAT. ANN. tit. 59, § 567.3a (6).

The Certified Nurse Practitioner's (CNP) scope of practice includes the full scope of nursing practice and practice in an expanded role as follows:

1. The Certified Nurse Practitioner (CNP) provides comprehensive health care to clients across the life span.
2. The CNP is responsible and accountable for the continuous and comprehensive management of a broad range of health services, which include, but are not limited to:
   A. promotion and maintenance of health;
   B. prevention of illness and disability;
   C. diagnosis and prescription of medications, treatments, and devices for acute and chronic conditions and diseases;
   D. management of health care during acute and chronic phases of illness;
   E. guidance and counseling services;
   F. consultation and/or collaboration with other healthcare providers and community resources;
   G. referral to other healthcare providers and community resources.
3. The CNP will provide services based upon education, experience, and national certification. It is the responsibility of the licensee to document competency of any act, based upon education, experience and certification.
4. The scope of practice as previously defined is incorporated into the following specialty categories and further delineates the population served:
   A. Adult CNP (acute and/or primary) provides health care to adolescents and adults.
   B. Family CNP provides health care to persons across the lifespan.
   C. Geriatric CNP provides health care to older adults.
   D. Neonatal CNP provides health care to neonates and infants.
   E. Pediatric CNP (acute and/or primary) provides health care to persons from newborn to young adulthood.
   F. Women's Health Care CNP provides health care to adolescent and adult females. Care may also be provided to males with reproductive health needs or problems.
   G. Acute Care CNP provides health care to adults who are acutely or critically ill.
   H. The Adult Psychiatric and Mental Health CNP provides acute and chronic psychiatric and mental health care to persons age 13 or older.
   I. The Family Psychiatric and Mental Health CNP provides acute and chronic psychiatric and mental health care to persons across the lifespan.
   J. The Acute Care Pediatric CNP provides health care to persons from newborn to young adulthood with complex acute, critical, and chronic health conditions.
5. Effective January 1, 2016, the applicant for initial APRN licensure or APRN licensure by endorsement as a CNP shall hold certification in at least one of the following population foci: family/individual across the lifespan,

adult-gerontology (acute and/or primary), neonatal, pediatrics (acute and/or primary), women's health/gender related, or psychiatric/mental health.

Citation: OKLA. ADMIN. CODE § 485:10-15-6(c).

Oregon

. . .

3. The nurse practitioner provides holistic health care to individuals, families, and groups across the life span in a variety of settings, including hospitals, long-term care facilities, and community-based settings.

4. Within his or her specialty, the nurse practitioner is responsible for managing health problems encountered by the client and is accountable for health outcomes. This process includes:
   a. Assessment;
   b. Diagnosis;
   c. Development of a plan;
   d. Intervention;
   e. Evaluation.

5. The nurse practitioner is independently responsible and accountable for the continuous and comprehensive management of a broad range of health care, which may include:
   a. Promotion and maintenance of health;
   b. Prevention of illness and disability;
   c. Assessment of clients, synthesis and analysis of data and application of nursing principles and therapeutic modalities;
   d. Management of health care during acute and chronic phases of illness;
   e. Admission of his/her clients to hospitals and/or health services including but not limited to home health, hospice, long term care, and drug and alcohol treatment;
   f. Counseling;
   g. Consultation and/or collaboration with other care providers and community resources;
   h. Referral to other health care providers and community resources;
   i. Management and coordination of care;
   j. Use of research skills;
   k. Diagnosis of health/illness status;
   l. Prescribing, dispensing, and administration of therapeutic devices and measures including legend drugs and controlled substances as provided in Division 56 of the Oregon Nurse Practice Act, consistent with the definition of the practitioner's specialty category and scope of practice.

6. The nurse practitioner scope of practice includes teaching the theory and practice of advanced practice nursing.

7. The nurse practitioner is responsible for recognizing limits of knowledge and experience, and for resolving situations beyond his/her nurse practitioner expertise by consulting with or referring clients to other health care providers.

8. The nurse practitioner will only provide health care services within the nurse practitioner's scope of practice for which he/she is educationally prepared and for which competency has been established and maintained. Educational preparation includes academic course work, workshops or seminars, provided both theory and clinical experience are included.

Citation: OR. ADMIN. R. § 851-050-0005.

Pennsylvania

A CRNP . . . while functioning in the expanded role as a professional nurse, performs acts of medical diagnosis or prescription of medical therapeutics or corrective measures in collaboration with a physician licensed to practice.

Citation: 49 PA. CODE § 21.251.

a. A CRNP may collaborate only with physicians who hold a current license to practice in this Commonwealth.

b. When acting in collaboration with a physician as set forth in a collaborative agreement and within the CRNP's specialty, a CRNP may:
   1. Perform comprehensive assessments of patients and establish medical diagnoses.
   2. Order, perform and supervise diagnostic tests for patients and, to the extent the interpretation of diagnostic tests is within the scope of the CRNP's specialty and consistent with the collaborative agreement, may interpret diagnostic tests.
   3. Initiate referrals to and consultations with other licensed professional health care providers, and consult with other licensed professional health care providers at their request.
   4. Develop and implement treatment plans, including issuing orders to implement treatment plans. However, only a CRNP with current prescriptive authority approval may develop and implement treatment plans for pharmaceutical treatments.
   5. Complete admission and discharge summaries.
   6. Order blood and blood components for patients.
   7. Order dietary plans for patients.
   8. Order home health and hospice care.
   9. Order durable medical equipment.

10. Issue oral orders to the extent permitted by the health care facilities' by-laws, rules, regulations or administrative policies and guidelines.
11. Make physical therapy and dietitian referrals.
12. Make respiratory and occupational therapy referrals.
13. Perform disability assessments for the program providing temporary assistance to needy families (TANF).
14. Issue homebound schooling certifications.
15. Perform and sign the initial assessment of methadone treatment evaluations, provided that any order for methadone treatment shall be made only by a physician.

Citation: 49 PA CODE §21.282a(a) and (b).

Rhode Island

"Certified registered nurse practitioner" (RNP) means an advanced practice nurse utilizing independent knowledge of physical assessment and management of health care and illnesses. The practice includes prescriptive privileges, and collaboration with other licensed healthcare professionals, including, but not limited to, physicians, pharmacists, podiatrists, dentists, and nurses. Such collaboration is not required to be pursuant to a written collaboration agreement, with a specific designation physician, or at the same physical location as a collaborating practitioner.

Citation: R.I. R. R5-34-NUR/ED 1.10.

South Carolina

In addition to those activities considered the practice of nursing, an APRN may perform delegated medical acts.

Citation: S.C. CODE ANN. § 40-33-20(5).

"Delegated medical acts" means additional acts delegated by a physician or dentist to the NP, CNM, or CNS and may include formulating a medical diagnosis and initiating, continuing, and modifying therapies, including prescribing drug therapy, under approved written protocols . . . Delegated medical acts must be agreed to jointly by both the Board of Nursing and the Board of Medical Examiners. Delegated medical acts must be performed under the general supervision of a physician or dentist who must be readily available for consultation.

Citation: S.C. CODE ANN. § 40-33-20(23).

South Dakota

A nurse practitioner may perform the following overlapping scope of advanced practice nursing and medical functions pursuant to § 36-9A-15, including:

1. The initial medical diagnosis and the institution of a plan of therapy or referral;
2. The prescription of medications and provision of drug samples or a limited supply of labeled medications, including controlled drugs or substances listed in Schedule II in Chapter 34-20B for one period of not more than thirty days for treatment of causative factors and symptoms. Medications or sample drugs provided to patients shall be accompanied with written administration instructions and appropriate documentation shall be entered in the patient's medical record;
3. The writing of a chemical or physical restraint order when the patient may do personal harm or harm others;
4. The completion and signing of official documents such as death certificates, birth certificates, and similar documents required by law;
5. The performance of a physical examination for participation in athletics and the certification that the patient is healthy and able to participate in athletics.

Citation: S.D. CODIFIED LAWS § 36-9A-12.

The nurse practitioner or nurse midwife advanced practice nursing functions include:

1. Providing advanced nursing assessment, nursing intervention, and nursing case management;
2. Providing advanced health promotion and maintenance education and counseling to clients, families, and other members of the health care team;
3. Utilizing research findings to evaluate and implement changes in nursing practice, programs, and policies; and
4. Recognizing limits of knowledge and experience, planning for situations beyond expertise, and consulting with or referring clients to other health care providers as appropriate.

These advanced practice nursing functions are under the jurisdiction of the Board of Nursing.

Citation: S.D. CODIFIED LAWS § 36-9A-13.1.

Tennessee

There is no description of the scope of practice for a nurse practitioner in Tennessee law, other than the authority to write and sign prescriptions and/or issue drugs.

Citation: [for prescriptive authority] TENN. CODE ANN. § 63-7-123(a) and (b)(2).

Texas

The advanced practice nurse provides a broad range of health services, the scope of which shall be based upon educational preparation, continued advanced practice experience and the accepted scope of professional practice of the particular specialty area. Advanced practice nurses practice in a variety of settings and, according to their practice specialty and role, they provide a broad range of health care services to a variety of patient populations.

1. The scope of practice of particular specialty areas shall be defined by national professional specialty organizations or advanced practice nursing organizations recognized by the Board. The advanced practice nurse may perform only those functions which are within that scope of practice and which are consistent with the Nursing Practice Act, Board rules, and other laws and regulations of the State of Texas.
2. The advanced practice nurse's scope of practice shall be in addition to the scope of practice permitted a registered nurse and does not prohibit the advanced practice nurse from practicing in those areas deemed to be within the scope of practice of a registered nurse.

Citation: 22 Texas Admin. Code § 221.12.

Utah

"Practice of advanced practice registered nursing" means the practice of nursing within the generally recognized scope and standards of advanced practice registered nursing as defined by rule and consistent with professionally recognized preparation and education standards of an advanced practice registered nurse by a person licensed under this chapter as an advanced practice registered nurse. Advanced practice registered nursing includes:

a. maintenance and promotion of health and prevention of disease;
b. diagnosis, treatment, correction, consultation, or referral for common health problems; and
c. prescription or administration of prescription drugs or devices, including:
    i. local anesthesia
    ii. schedule IV-V controlled substances; and
    iii. schedule II-III controlled substances in accordance with a consultation and referral plan.

Citation: Utah Code Ann. § 58-31b-102(13).

Vermont

"Advanced practice registered nurse" or "APRN" means a licensed registered nurse, authorized to practice in this state who, because of specialized education and experience is endorsed to perform acts of medical diagnosis and to prescribe medical, therapeutic, or corrective measures under administrative rules adopted by the board.

Citation: Vt. Stat. Ann. tit. 26, § 1572(4).

An APRN practices an expanded scope of nursing, which includes the registered nurse scope of practice. The scope of an APRN includes assessing at an advanced level, diagnosing, prescribing, giving medical and nursing orders, and evaluating care.

Citation: Vt. Board of Nursing Admin Rules 15.2(3).

Virginia

A nurse practitioner licensed in a category other than certified registered nurse anesthetist shall be authorized to render care in collaboration with a licensed patient care team physician as part of a patient care team.

Citation: 18 Va. Admin. Code § 90-30-120A.

Washington

An advanced registered nurse practitioner, under his license, may perform for compensation nursing care, as that term is usually understood, of the ill, injured, or infirm and in the course thereof, she or he may do the following things that shall not be done by a person not so licensed, except as provided in RCW 18.79.260 and 18.79.270:

1. Perform specialized and advanced levels of nursing as recognized jointly by the medical and nursing professions, as defined by the commission;
2. Prescribe legend drugs and Schedule V controlled substances, as defined in the Uniform Controlled Substances Act, chapter 69.50 RCW, and Schedule II through IV subject to RCW 18.79.240(1)(r) or (s) within the scope of practice defined by the commission;
3. Perform all acts provided in RCW 18.79.260;
4. Hold himself out to the public or designate himself as an advanced registered nurse practitioner or as a nurse practitioner.

Citation: Wash. Rev. Code § 18.79.250.

1. A licensed advanced registered nurse practitioner (ARNP) is a registered nurse prepared in a formal educational program to assume primary responsibility for continuous and comprehensive management of a broad range of patient care, concerns, and problems.
2. The ARNP is prepared and qualified to assume primary responsibility and accountability for the care of patients.

3. ARNP practice is grounded in nursing and incorporates the use of independent judgment as well as collaborative interaction with other health care professionals when indicated in the assessment and management of wellness and health conditions as appropriate to the ARNP's area of practice and certification.
4. The ARNP functions within his or her scope of practice according to the commission approved certification program and standards of care developed by professional organizations.
5. The ARNP shall obtain instruction, supervision, and consultation as necessary before implementing new or unfamiliar techniques or practices.
6. Performing within the scope of the ARNP's knowledge, experience, and practice, the licensed ARNP may perform the following:
   a. Examine patients and establish diagnoses by patient history, physical examination, and other methods of assessment;
   b. Admit, manage, and discharge patients to and from healthcare facilities;
   c. Order, collect, perform, and interpret diagnostic tests;
   d. Manage health care by identifying, developing, implementing, and evaluating a plan of care and treatment for patients;
   e. Prescribe therapies and medical equipment;
   f. Prescribe medications when granted authority under this chapter;
   g. Refer patients to other healthcare practitioners, services or facilities; and
   h. Perform procedures or provide care services that are within the scope of practice according to the commission approved certification program.

Citation: WASH. ADMIN. CODE § 246-840-300.

West Virginia

"Advanced Practice Registered Nurse" (APRN) means a registered nurse who has acquired clinical knowledge and skills preparing him or her to independently provide direct and indirect care to patients, who has completed a board approved graduate-level education program and who has passed a board approved national certification examination.

Citation: W.VA. CODE ST. R. tit. 19, § 19-7-2.1.Wisconsin.

The intent of the board of nursing in adopting rules in this chapter is to specify education, training, or experience that a registered nurse must satisfy to call himself or herself an advanced practice nurse; to establish appropriate education, training, and examination requirements that an advanced practice nurse must satisfy to qualify for a certificate to issue prescription orders; to define the scope of practice within which an advanced practice nurse prescriber may issue prescription orders; to specify the classes of drugs, individual drugs, or devices that may not be prescribed by an advanced practice nurse prescriber; to specify the conditions to be met for a registered nurse to administer a drug prescribed or directed by an advanced practice nurse prescriber; to establish procedures for maintaining a certificate to issue prescription orders, including requirements for continuing education; and to establish the minimum amount of malpractice insurance required of an advanced practice nurse prescriber.

Citation: Wis. Admin. Code § N8.01(2).

To promote case management, the advanced practice nurse prescriber may order laboratory testing, radiographs or electrocardiograms appropriate . . . to his or her education, training, or experience.

Citation: Wisc. Admin. Code § N8.10(6).

Wyoming

"Advanced practice registered nurse (APRN)" means a nurse who:

A. May prescribe, administer, dispense or provide nonprescriptive and prescriptive medications including prepackaged medications, except Schedule I drugs as defined in W.S. 35-7-1013 and 35-7-1014;

B. Has responsibility for the direct care and management of patients and clients in relation to their human needs, disease states and therapeutic and technological interventions;

C. Has a master's degree in nursing, or an advanced practice registered nurse specialty or has completed an accredited advanced practice registered nurse educational program prior to January 1, 1999; and

D. Has completed an advanced program of study in a specialty area in an accredited nursing program, has taken and passed a national certification examination in the same area, and has been granted recognition by the board to practice as an APRN.

Citation: Wyo. Stat. Ann. §33-21-120(a)(i).

a. The advanced practice registered nurse is subject at all times to the established Standards of Nursing Practice as stated in Chapter 3 of these rules and regulations, the standards and scope of practice established by national professional organizations, and/or accrediting agencies representing the various core, role and population focus areas of advanced practice registered nursing, and the Wyoming Nurse Practice Act.

b. The board recognizes advanced practice registered nurse core, role and population focus areas described in the scope of practice statements for advanced practice registered nurses issued by national professional organizations and/or accrediting agencies.

Citation: Wyo. Board of Nursing Rules Chapter 4 § Section 7.

Physician Collaboration

Alabama

COLLABORATION. A formal relationship between one or more certified registered nurse practitioners and certified nurse midwives and a physician or physicians under which these nurses may engage in advanced practice nursing as evidenced by written protocols approved in accordance with the requirements of this article or exempted in accordance with requirements of this article. The term collaboration does not require direct, on-site supervision of the activities of a certified registered nurse practitioner or a certified nurse midwife by the collaborating physician. The term does require such professional oversight and direction as may be required by the rules and regulations of the State Board of Medical Examiners and the Board of Nursing.

Citation: ALA. CODE § 34-21-81(5).

Requirements for collaborative practice by physicians and certified registered nurse practitioners:

1. The collaborating physician shall:
   a. Provide professional medical oversight and direction to the certified registered nurse practitioner.
   b. Be readily available for direct communication or by radio, telephone or telecommunications.
   c. Be readily available for consultation or referrals of patients from the certified registered nurse practitioner.
2. In the event the collaborating physician is not readily available, provisions shall be made for medical coverage by a physician who is pre-approved by the State Board of Medical Examiners and is familiar with these rules.
3. If the certified registered nurse practitioner is to perform duties at a site away from the collaborating physician, the written protocol shall clearly specify the circumstances and provide written verification of physician availability for consultation, referral, or direct medical intervention in emergencies and after hours, if indicated.

4. The collaborating physician shall be present with the certified registered nurse practitioner in an approved collaborative practice site for not less than ten percent (10%) of the certified registered nurse practitioner's scheduled hours in the collaborative practice as specified in the protocol application. In addition, the collaborating physician shall visit each approved collaborative practice site not less than quarterly. The collaborating physicians with the Alabama Department of Public Health and county health departments are exempt from this requirement.

5. The certified registered nurse practitioner's scheduled hours in licensed acute care hospitals, licensed skilled nursing facilities, licensed special-care assisted living facilities, and licensed assisted living facilities are not subject to the required minimum hours for physician presence.

6. If the certified registered nurse practitioner's scheduled weekly collaborative practice hours are:
   a. Thirty or more hours per week, the certified registered nurse practitioner shall be present in an approved practice site with the collaborating or covering physician for time equal to ten percent (10%) of the certified registered nurse practitioner's scheduled weekly hours. Cumulative hours may accrue on a monthly basis.
   b. Less than 30 hours per week, the certified registered nurse practitioner shall be present in an approved practice site with the collaborating or covering physician for time equal to ten percent (10%) of the certified registered nurse practitioner's scheduled weekly hours. Cumulative hours may accrue on a quarterly basis.

7. The collaborating physician shall provide notice in writing to the State Board of Medical Examiners of the commencement or termination of a collaborative practice agreement as required by Rule 540-X-8-.04(4).

8. The Joint Committee may, at its discretion, waive the requirements of written verification of physician availability upon documentation of exceptional circumstances. Employees of the Alabama Department of Public Health and county health departments are exempt from the requirements of written verification of physician availability.

9. A written standard protocol specific to the specialty practice area of the certified registered nurse practitioner and the specialty practice area of the collaborating physician, approved and signed by both the collaborating physician and the certified registered nurse practitioner, shall:
   a. Identify all sites where the certified registered nurse practitioner will practice within the collaboration protocol.
   b. Identify the physician's principal practice site.
   c. Be maintained at each practice site.
   d. Include a formulary of drugs, devices, medical treatments, tests and procedures that may be prescribed, ordered, and implemented by the certified registered nurse practitioner consistent with these rules and which are appropriate for the collaborative practice setting.

e. Include a pre-determined plan for emergency services.

f. Specify the process by which the certified registered nurse practitioner shall refer a patient to a physician other than the collaborating physician.

g. Specify a plan for quality assurance management with established patient outcome indicators for evaluation of the clinical practice of the certified registered nurse practitioner and include review of no less than ten percent (10%) of medical records plus all adverse outcomes. Documentation of quality assurance review shall be readily retrievable, identify records that were selected for review, include a summary of findings, conclusions, and, if indicated, recommendations for change. Quality assurance monitoring may be performed by designated personnel, with final results presented to the physician and certified registered nurse practitioner for review.

Citation: ALA. ADMIN. CODE r. 610-X-5-.08.

Alaska

If intending to deliver health care services to the public, must submit with the application for initial authorization a consultation and referral plan; the plan must

A. describe the applicant's clinical practice;

B. identify the expected client population focus area, which is within the scope of practice of the applicant;

C. list the applicant's method of routine consultations and referrals, the method of documenting routine consultations and referrals in the patient record, and the names and titles of health care providers that the applicant will use for routine consultations and referrals;

D. list the applicant's method for emergency referrals; and

E. *repealed 10/3/2011;*

F. describe the process for quality assurance the applicants will use to evaluate the applicant's practice, including

   i. the use of standards that apply to the area of practice;

   ii. present or past review of the practice;

   iii. use of preestablished criteria; and

   iv. a written evaluation of the quality assurance review with a plan for corrective action, if indicated, and follow-up;

Citation: ALASKA ADMIN. CODE tit. 12, § 44.400(5)(c).

Arizona

"Collaborate" means to establish a relationship for consultation or referral with one or more licensed physicians on an as-needed basis. Supervision of the activities of a registered nurse practitioner by the collaborating physician is not required.

Citation: ARIZ. ADMIN. CODE § R4-19-101.

Arkansas

A collaborative practice agreement shall include, but not be limited to, provisions addressing: (1) The availability of the collaborating physician for consultation or referral or both; (2) Methods of management of the collaborative practice, which shall include protocols for prescriptive authority; (3) Coverage of the health care needs of a patient in the emergency absence of the advanced practice nurse or physician; and (4) Quality assurance.

Citation: ARK. CODE ANN. § 17-87-310(C).

California

Neither this chapter nor any other provision of law shall be construed to prohibit a nurse practitioner from furnishing or ordering drugs or devices when all of the following apply:

a. The drugs or devices are furnished or ordered by a nurse practitioner in accordance with standardized procedures or protocols developed by the nurse practitioner and the supervising physician and surgeon when the drugs or devices furnished or ordered are consistent with the practitioner's educational preparation or for which clinical competency has been established and maintained.
b. The nurse practitioner is functioning pursuant to standardized procedure, as defined by Section 2725, or protocol. The standardized procedure or protocol shall be developed and approved by the supervising physician and surgeon, the nurse practitioner, and the facility administrator or the designee.
c. 1. The standardized procedure or protocol covering the furnishing of drugs or devices shall specify which nurse practitioners may furnish or order drugs or devices, which drugs or devices may be furnished or ordered, under what circumstances, the extent of physician and surgeon supervision, the method of periodic review of the nurse practitioner's competence, including peer review, and review of the provision of the standardized procedure.
   2. In addition to the requirements in paragraph (1), for Schedule II controlled substance protocols, the provision for furnishing Schedule II controlled substances shall address the diagnosis of the illness, injury, or condition for which the Schedule II controlled substance is to be furnished.
d. The furnishing or ordering of drugs or devices by a nurse practitioner occurs under physician and surgeon supervision. Physician and surgeon supervision shall not be construed to require the physical presence of the physician, but does include (1) collaboration on the development of the standardized procedure, (2) approval of the standardized procedure, and (3) availability by telephonic contact at the time of patient examination by the nurse practitioner.
e. For purposes of this section, no physician and surgeon shall supervise more than four nurse practitioners at one time.

f. 1. Drugs or devices furnished or ordered by a nurse practitioner may include Schedule II through Schedule V controlled substances under the California Uniform Controlled Substances Act . . . and shall be further limited to those drugs agreed upon by the nurse practitioner and physician and surgeon and specified in the standardized procedure.

   2. When Schedule II or III controlled substances . . . are furnished or ordered by a nurse practitioner, the controlled substances shall be furnished or ordered in accordance with a patient-specific protocol approved by the treating or supervising physician. A copy of the section of the nurse practitioner's standardized procedure relating to controlled substances shall be provided, upon request, to any licensed pharmacist who dispenses drugs or devices, when there is uncertainty about the nurse practitioner furnishing the order.

g. 1. The board has certified in accordance with Section 2836.3 that the nurse practitioner has satisfactorily completed (1) at least six month's physician and surgeon-supervised experience in the furnishing or ordering of drugs or devices, and (2) a course in pharmacology covering the drugs or devices to be furnished or ordered under this section.

   2. Nurse practitioners who are certified by the board and hold an active furnishing number, who are authorized through standardized procedures or protocols to furnish Schedule II controlled substances, and who are registered with the United States Drug Enforcement Administration, shall complete, as part of their continuing education requirements, a course including Schedule II controlled substances based on the standards developed by the board. The board shall establish the requirements for satisfactory completion of this subdivision.

h. Use of the term "furnishing" in this section, in health facilities defined in Section 1250 of the Health and Safety Code, shall include (1) the ordering of a drug or device in accordance with the standardized procedure and (2) transmitting an order of a supervising physician and surgeon.

i. "Drug order" or "order" for purposes of this section means an order for medication which is dispensed to or for an ultimate user, issued by a nurse practitioner as an individual practitioner, within the meaning of Section 1306.02 of Title 21 of the Code of Federal Regulations. Notwithstanding any other provision of law, (1) a drug order issued pursuant to this section shall be treated in the same manner as a prescription of the supervising physician; (2) all references to "prescription" in this code and the Health and Safety Code shall include drug orders issued by nurse practitioners; and (3) the signature of a nurse practitioner on a drug order issued in accordance with this section shall be deemed to be the signature of a prescriber for purposes of this code and the Health and Safety Code.

Citation: Ann. Cal. Bus. & Prof. Code § 2836.1.

Furnishing or ordering of drugs or devices by nurse practitioners is defined to mean the act of making a pharmaceutical agent or agents available to the patient in strict accordance with a standardized procedure. All nurse practitioners who are authorized pursuant to Section 2836.1 to furnish or issue drug orders for controlled substances shall register with the United States Drug Enforcement Administration.

Citation: Ann. Cal. Bus. & Prof. Code § 2836.2.

Colorado

An advanced practice nurse shall practice in accordance with the standards of the appropriate national professional nursing organization and have a safe mechanism for consultation or collaboration with a physician or, when appropriate, referral to a physician. Advanced practice nursing also includes, when appropriate, referral to other health care providers.

Citation: Colo. Rev. Stat. Ann. § 12-38-111.5(6).

Connecticut

…"[C]ollaboration" means a mutually agreed upon relationship between an advanced practice registered nurse and a physician who is educated, trained, or has relevant experience that is related to the work of such advanced practice registered nurse. The collaboration shall address a reasonable and appropriate level of consultation and referral, coverage for the patient in the absence of the advanced practice registered nurse, a method to review patient outcomes, and a method of disclosure of the relationship to the patient. Relative to the exercise of prescriptive authority, the collaboration between an advanced practice registered nurse and a physician shall be in writing and shall address the level of Schedule II and III controlled substances that the advanced practice registered nurse may prescribe and provide a method to review patient outcomes, including, but not limited to, the review of medical therapeutics, corrective measures, laboratory tests, and other diagnostic procedures that the advanced practice registered nurse may prescribe, dispense, and administer.

Citation: Conn. Gen. Stat. Ann. § 20-87(b).

Delaware

Advanced practice nurses shall operate in collaboration with a licensed physician, dentist, podiatrist, or licensed Delaware health care delivery system to cooperate, coordinate, and consult with each other as appropriate pursuant to a collaborative agreement defined in the rules and regulations promulgated by the Board of Nursing, in the provision of health care to their patients. Advanced practice nurses desiring to practice independently or to prescribe independently must do so pursuant to Title 24, § 1906(a)(20) of Title 24.

Citation: DEL. CODE ANN. tit. 24, § 1902(b)(1b).

The "Joint Practice Committee" with the approval of the Board of Medical Licensure and Discipline shall have the authority to grant, restrict, suspend or revoke practice or independent practice authority and the Joint Practice Committee with the approval of the Board of Medical Licensure and Discipline shall be responsible for promulgating rules and regulations to implement the provisions of this chapter regarding "advanced practice nurses" who have been granted authority for independent practice and/or independent prescriptive authority.

Citation: DEL. CODE ANN. tit. 24, § 1906(20).

Those individuals who wish to engage in independent practice without written guidelines or protocols and/or wish to have independent prescriptive authority shall apply for such privilege or privileges to the Joint Practice Committee and do so only in collaboration with a licensed physician, dentist, podiatrist, or licensed Delaware health care delivery system. This does not include those individuals who have protocols and/or waivers approved by the Board of Medical Licensure and Discipline.

Citation: DEL. CODE ANN. tit. 24, § 1902(b)(2).

District of Columbia

a. Generally, advanced practice registered nurses shall carry out acts of advanced registered nursing in collaboration with a licensed health care provider.
d. Notwithstanding the provisions of this section, hospitals, facilities, and agencies, in requiring specific levels of collaboration and licensed health care providers in agreeing to the levels of collaboration, shall apply reasonable, nondiscriminatory standards, free of anticompetitive intent or purpose, in accordance with Chapter 14 of Title 2, Chapter 45 of Title 28, and § 44-507.

Citation: D.C. STAT. § 3-1206.03.

Florida

An Advanced Registered Nurse Practitioner shall only perform medical acts of diagnosis, treatment, and operation pursuant to a protocol between the ARNP and a Florida-licensed medical doctor, osteopathic physician, or dentist. The degree and method of supervision, determined by the ARNP and the physician or dentist, shall be specifically identified in the written protocol and shall be appropriate for prudent health care providers under similar circumstances. General supervision by the physician or dentist is required, unless these rules set a different level of supervision for a particular act. The number of persons to be supervised shall be limited to insure that an acceptable standard of medical care is rendered in consideration of the following factors:

a. Risk to patient;
b. Educational preparation, specialty, and experience of the parties to the protocol;
c. Complexity and risk of the procedures;
d. Practice setting; and
e. Availability of the physician or dentist.

Citation: FLA. ADMIN. CODE Ch. 64B9-4.010(1).

Georgia

A nurse protocol agreement between a physician and an advanced practice registered nurse pursuant to this Code section shall:

1. Be between an advanced practice registered nurse who is in a comparable specialty area or field as that of the delegating physician;
2. Contain a provision for immediate consultation between the advanced practice registered nurse and the delegating physician; if the delegating physician is not available, the delegating physician for purposes of consultation may designate another physician who concurs with the terms of the nurse protocol agreement;
3. Identify the parameters under which delegated acts may be performed by the advanced practice registered nurse, including without limitation the number of refills which may be ordered, the kinds of diagnostic studies which may be ordered, the extent to which radiographic image tests may be ordered, and the circumstances under which a prescription drug order may be executed. In the event the delegating physician authorizes the advanced practice registered nurse to order an X-ray, ultrasound, or radiographic imaging test, the nurse protocol agreement shall contain provisions whereby such X-ray, ultrasound, or radiographic imaging test shall be read and interpreted by a physician who is trained in the reading and interpretation of such tests; a report of such X-ray, ultrasound, or radiographic imaging test may be reviewed by the advanced practice registered nurse; and a copy of such report shall be forwarded to the delegating physician, except that such provision for an ultrasound shall not be required for an advanced practice registered nurse acting within his or her scope of practice as authorized by Code Sections 43-26-3 and 43-26-5.
4. Require documentation either in writing or by electronic means or other medium by the advanced practice registered nurse or those acts performed by the advanced practice registered nurse which are specific to the medical act authorized by the delegating physician;

5. Include a schedule for periodic review by the delegating physician of patient records. Such patient records review may be achieved with a sampling of such records as determined by the delegating physician;

6. Provide for patient evaluation or follow-up examination by the delegating physician or other physician designated by the delegating physician pursuant to paragraph (2) of this subsection, with the frequency of such evaluation or follow-up examination based on the nature, extent, and scope of the delegated act or acts as determined by the delegating physician in accordance with paragraph (3) of this subsection and accepted standards of medical practice as determined by the board;

7. Be reviewed, revised, or updated annually by the delegating physician and the advanced practice registered nurse;

8. Be available for review upon written request to the advanced practice registered nurse by the Georgia Board of Nursing or to the physician by the board; and

9. Provide that a patient who received a prescription drug order for any controlled substance pursuant to a nurse protocol agreement shall be evaluated or examined by the delegating physician or other physician designated by the delegating physician pursuant to paragraph (2) of this subsection on at least a quarterly basis or at a more frequent interval as determined by the board.

d. A written prescription drug order issued pursuant to this Code section shall be signed by the advanced practice registered nurse and shall be on a form which shall include, without limitation, the names of the advanced practice registered nurse and delegating physician who are parties to the nurse protocol agreement, the patient's name and address, the drug or device ordered, directions with regard to the taking and dosage of the drug or use of the device, and the number of refills. A prescription drug order which is transmitted either electronically or via facsimile shall conform to the requirements set out in paragraphs (1) and (2) of Subsection (c) of Code Section 26-4-80, respectively.

Citation: GA CODE ANN. § 43-34-25(b).

Hawaii

"Collaborate" means a process in which an APRN works with other members of the health care team to deliver health care services.

Citation: HAW. ADMIN. R § 16-89-2.

Idaho

An advanced practice registered nurse collaborates with other health professionals in providing health care.

Citation: IDAHO CODE § 54-1402(1).

Illinois

a. A written collaborative agreement is required for all advanced practice nurses engaged in clinical practice, except for advanced practice nurses who are authorized to practice in a hospital or ambulatory surgical treatment center.

a-5. If an advanced practice nurse engages in clinical practice outside of a hospital or ambulatory surgical treatment center in which he or she is authorized to practice, the advanced practice nurse must have a written collaborative agreement.

b. A written collaborative agreement shall describe the working relationship of the advanced practice nurse with the collaborating physician or podiatrist and shall authorize the categories of care, treatment, or procedures to be performed by the advanced practice nurse. A collaborative agreement with a dentist must be in accordance with subsection (c-10) of this Section. Collaboration does not require an employment relationship between the collaborating physician and advanced practice nurse.

Collaboration means the relationship under which an advanced practice nurse works with a collaborating physician or podiatrist in an active clinical practice to deliver health care services in accordance with (i) the advanced practice nurse's training, education, and experience and (ii) collaboration and consultation as documented in a jointly developed written collaborative agreement.

The agreement shall promote the exercise of professional judgment by the advanced practice nurse commensurate with his or her education and experience. The services to be provided by the advanced practice nurse shall be services that the collaborating physician or podiatrist is authorized to and generally provides or may provide in his or her clinical medical or podiatric practice, except as set forth in subsections (b-5) or (c-5) of this Section.

The agreement need not describe the exact steps that an advanced practice nurse must take with respect to each specific condition, disease, or symptom but must specify which authorized procedures require the presence of the collaborating physician or podiatrist as the procedures are being performed. The collaborative relationship under an agreement shall not be construed to require the personal presence of a physician or podiatrist at the place where the services are rendered.

Methods of communication shall be available for consultation with the collaborating physician or podiatrist in person or by telecommunications in accordance with established written guidelines as set forth in the written agreement.

b-5. Absent an employment relationship, a written collaborative agreement may not (1) restrict the categories of patients of an advanced practice nurse within the scope of the advanced practice nurses training and experience, (2) limit third party payors or government health programs, such as the medical assistance program or Medicare with which the advanced practice nurse contracts, or (3) limit the geographic area or practice location of the advanced practice nurse in this State.

c. Collaboration and consultation under all collaboration agreements shall be adequate if a collaborating physician or podiatrist does each of the following:

1. Participates in the joint formulation and joint approval of orders or guidelines with the advanced practice nurse and he or she periodically reviews such orders and the services provided patients under such orders in accordance with accepted standards of medical practice or podiatric practice and advanced practice nursing practice.

2. Provides collaboration and consultation with the advanced practice nurse at least once a month. In the case of anesthesia services provided by a certified registered nurse anesthetist, an anesthesiologist, physician, dentist, or podiatrist must participate through discussion of and agreement with the anesthesia plan and remain physically present and available on the premises during the delivery of anesthesia services for diagnosis, consultation, and treatment of emergency medical conditions.

3. Is available through telecommunications for consultation on medical problems, complications, or emergencies or patient referral. In the case of anesthesia services provided by a certified registered nurse anesthetist, an anesthesiologist, physician, dentist, or podiatrist must participate through discussion of and agreement with the anesthesia plan and remain physically present and available on the premises during the delivery of anesthesia services for diagnosis, consultation, and treatment of emergency medical conditions.

The agreement must contain provisions detailing notice for termination or change of status involving a written collaborative agreement, except when such notice is given for just cause. [Portions omitted.]

> *Citation:* 225 ILL. COMP. STAT. § 60/54.5 as amended by Public Act 098-0192, enacted August 6, 2013.

Indiana

An advanced practice nurse shall operate in collaboration with a licensed practitioner as evidenced by a practice agreement, or by privileges granted by the governing board of a hospital ... with the advice of the medical staff of the hospital that sets forth the manner in which the advanced practice nurse and a licensed practitioner will cooperate, coordinate, and consult with each other in the provision of health care to their patients.

> *Citation:* IND. CODE ANN. § 25-23-1-19.4(b).

"Practitioner" means [for the purpose of the nurse practice act]:

- A licensed physician
- A veterinarian
- A dentist
- A podiatrist
- An optometrist
- An advanced practice nurse who meets the requirements of IC 25-23-1-19.5
- A physician assistant licensed under IC 25-27.5 who is delegated prescriptive authority under IC 25-27.5-5-6

Citation: IND. CODE ANN. § 16-42-19-5.

An advanced practice nurse may be authorized to prescribe legend drugs, including controlled substances, if the advanced practice nurse . . . (7) submits proof of collaboration with a licensed practitioner in the form of a written practice agreement that sets forth the manner in which the advanced practice nurse and licensed practitioner will cooperate, coordinate, and consult with each other in the provision of health care to patients. Practice agreements shall be in writing and shall also set forth provisions for the type of collaboration between the advanced practice nurse and the licensed practitioner and the reasonable and timely review by the licensed practitioner of the prescribing practices of the advanced practice nurse.

Citation: IND. ADMIN. CODE tit. 848, r. 5-1-1(7).

Iowa

The ARNP may perform selected medically designated functions when a collaborative practice agreement exists.

Citation: IOWA ADMIN. CODE r. 655-7.1(152).

Author's note: The Iowa Board of Nursing interprets Iowa law as not requiring physician involvement in nurse practitioner practice:

- "In Iowa, an ARNP may practice independently." *Source:* Iowa Board of Nursing website
- "An ARNP may have a collaborative agreement with a physician or physicians if their practice so warrants, but this agreement is not a requirement of the Iowa Board of Nursing."

Source: Iowa Board of Nursing Newsletter, Volume 28, Number 4

Author's note: The inconsistency between the regulatory language and the Board of Nursing statements seem to be related to whether an ARNP is performing medicine or nursing. Making medical diagnoses and treating with medical therapies (prescribing medications and ordering therapies) are medical functions, and therefore would require collaboration with a physician.

Kansas

An advanced practice registered nurse may prescribe drugs pursuant to a written protocol as authorized by a responsible physician. Each written protocol shall contain a precise and detailed medical plan of care for each classification of disease or injury for which the advanced practice registered nurse is authorized to prescribe and shall specify all drugs which may be prescribed by the advanced practice registered nurse. Any written prescription order shall include the name, address, and telephone number of the responsible physician. The advanced practice registered nurse may not dispense drugs, but may request, receive and sign for professional samples and may distribute professional samples to patients pursuant to written protocol as authorized by a responsible physician.

Citation: KAN. STAT. ANN. § 65-1130(d).

"Authorization for collaborative practice" shall mean that an ARNP is authorized to develop and manage the medical plan of care for patients or clients based upon an agreement developed jointly and signed by the ARNP and one or more physicians. Each ARNP and physician shall jointly review the authorization for collaborative practice annually. Each authorization for collaborative practice shall include a cover page containing the names and telephone numbers of the ARNP and the physician, their signatures, and the date of review by the ARNP and the physician. Each authorization for collaborative practice shall be maintained in either hard copy or electronic format at the ARNP's principal place of practice.

Citation: KAN. STAT. ANN. § 60-11-101(b).

Kentucky

Before an advanced practice registered nurse engages in the prescribing or dispensing of nonscheduled legend drugs as authorized under KRS 314.011(8), the advanced practice registered nurse shall enter into a written "Collaborative Agreement for Advanced Practice Registered Nurse's Prescriptive Authority for Nonscheduled Legend Drugs" (CAPA-NS) with a physician that defines the scope of the prescriptive authority for nonscheduled legend drugs.

Citation: [New legislation enacted February 2014 — no collaboration required for experienced NPs.] KY. REV. STAT. ANN. § 314.042(8).

Before an advanced registered nurse practitioner engages in the prescribing of Schedules II through V controlled substances as authorized by KRS 314.011(8), the advanced practice registered nurse practitioner shall enter into a written "Collaborative Agreement for the Advanced Practice Registered Nurse's Prescriptive Authority for Controlled Substances" (CAPA-CS) with a physician that defines the scope of the prescriptive authority for controlled substances [further requirements omitted].

Citation: KY. REV. STAT. ANN. § 314.042(9).

Louisiana

7. "Collaboration" means a cooperative working relationship with another licensed physician, dentist, or other health care providers to jointly contribute to providing patient care and may include, but not be limited to discussion of a patient's diagnosis and cooperation in the management and delivery of health care with each provider performing those activities that he is legally authorized to perform.

8. "Collaborative practice" means the joint management of the health care of a patient by an advanced practice registered nurse performing advanced practice registered nursing and one or more consulting physicians or dentists. Except as otherwise provided in R.S. 37:930, acts of medical diagnosis and prescription by an advanced practice registered nurse shall be in accordance with a collaborative practice agreement.

9. "Collaborative practice agreement" means a formal written statement addressing the parameters of the collaborative practice which are mutually agreed upon by the advanced practice registered nurse and one or more licensed physicians or dentists which shall include but not be limited to the following provisions:

   a. Availability of the collaborating physician or dentist for consultation or referral, or both.

   b. Methods of management of the collaborative practice which shall include clinical practice guidelines.

   c. Coverage of the health care needs of a patient during any absence of the advanced practice registered nurse, physician, or dentist.

   Citation: La. Rev. Stat. Ann. § 37:913.

vi. The applicant shall . . . provide evidence of . . . [a] collaborative practice agreement . . . which shall include, but not be limited to:

a. A plan of accountability among the parties that: (i) defines the limited prescriptive authority of the APRN and the responsibilities of the collaborating physician or physicians; (ii) delineates a plan for possible hospital admissions and privileges which includes a statement that the collaborating physician must have said privileges at the same institution before an APRN can receive this determination at said institution; (iii) delineates mechanisms and arrangements for diagnostic and laboratory requests for testing; and (iv) delineates a plan for documentation of medical records;

b. clinical practice guidelines . . . shall contain documentation of the types of categories or schedules of drugs available and generic substitution for prescription and be in accordance with current standards of care and evidence-based practice for the APRN specialty and functional role and be: (i) mutually agreed upon by the APRN and collaborating physician; (ii) specific to the practice setting; (iii) maintained on site; and (iv) reviewed and signed at least annually by the APRN and physician to reflect current practice.

c. documentation of the availability of the collaborating physician when the physician is not physically present in the practice setting. . . .

d. documentation shall be shown that patients are informed about how to access care when both the APRN and/or collaborating physicians are absent from the practice setting; and

e. an acknowledgment of the mutual obligation and responsibility of the APRN and collaborating physician to insure that all acts of limited prescriptive authority of the APRN are properly documented.

Citation: La. Admin. Code tit. 46, § XLVII.4513.

Maine

1. Requirements for initial approval to practice

   C. Submits evidence of a minimum of 1500 hours of practice in an expanded specialty nursing role within 5 years preceding application, or have completed a nurse practitioner program within 5 years preceding application. If more than 5 years have elapsed since completion of an advanced practice registered nurse program and the applicant does not meet the practice requirement of 1500 hours, the applicant shall complete 500 hours of clinical practice supervised by a physician or nurse practitioner in the same specialty area of practice.

2. For temporary approval [to practice] for graduates of nurse practitioner programs

   A. A nurse practitioner must practice for a minimum of 24 months under the supervision of a licensed physician, or a supervising nurse practitioner, or be employed by a clinic or hospital that has a medical director who is a licensed physician.

   B. The applicant shall identify a supervisory relationship with a licensed physician or nurse practitioner in the same practice category who will provide oversight for the nurse practitioner.

Citation: Code Me. R. § 02 380 008 (Section 2).

Maryland

A. Before commencing practice, a nurse practitioner shall complete a Board-approved written attestation that:

1. The nurse practitioner has an agreement for collaborating and consulting with a physician;

2. States the name and license number of the physician;

3. The nurse practitioner shall refer to and consult with physicians and other health care providers as needed; and
4. The nurse practitioner shall practice in accordance with the standards of practice of:
   a. The American Academy of Nurse Practitioners; or
   b. Any other national nurse practitioner certifying body recognized by the Board.
B. The Board shall:
   1. Maintain an approved written attestation; and
   2. Make the approved written attestation available to the Board of Physicians on the request of the Board of Physicians.
C. If a nurse practitioner terminates or changes an agreement to collaborate, a new written attestation stating the name of the physician shall be submitted immediately, by mail or facsimile, to the Board.

Citation: MD. CODE tit. 10 § 27.07.04.

Massachusetts

1. All nurses practicing in an expanded role . . . shall practice in accordance with the written guidelines developed in collaboration with and mutually acceptable to the nurse and to:
   a. a physician expert by virtue of training or experience in the nurse's area of practice; or
   b. the appropriate medical staff and nursing administration staff of the institution employing the nurse.
2. In all cases the written guidelines shall designate a physician who shall provide medical direction as is customarily accepted in the specialty area. Guidelines may authorize the nurse's performance of any professional activities included within her area of practice. The guidelines shall:
   a. specifically describe the nature and scope of the nursing practice;
   b. describe the circumstances in which physician consultation or referral is required;
   c. describe the use of established procedures for the treatment of common medical conditions which the nurse may encounter; and
   d. include provisions for managing emergencies.
3. In addition to the requirements of 244 CMR 4.22(2), the guidelines pertaining to prescriptive practice shall:
   a. include a defined mechanism to monitor prescribing practices, including documentation of review with a supervising physician at least every three months;
   b. include protocols for initiation of intravenous therapies and Schedule II drugs;

c. specify the frequency of review of initial prescription of controlled substances; the initial prescription of Schedule II drugs must be reviewed by the physician within 96 hours; and

d. conform to M.G.L. c.94C, 105 CMR 700.000 et seq., and M.G.L. c.112, § 80E or § 80G, as applicable.

Citation: CODE MASS. REGS. tit. 244, § 4.22.

Michigan

Subject to subsections (2) to (6), a licensee who holds a license other than a health profession subfield license may delegate to a licensed or unlicensed individual who is otherwise qualified by education, training or experience the performance of selected acts, tasks, or functions where the acts, tasks, or functions fall within the scope of practice of the licensee's profession and will be performed under the licensee's supervision. A licensee shall not delegate an act, task, or function under this section if the act, task, or function, under standards of acceptable and prevailing practice, requires the level of education, skill, and judgment required of the licensee under this article.

Citation: MICH. COMP. LAWS § 333.16215(1).

Minnesota

"Collaborative management" is a mutually agreed-upon plan between an advanced practice registered nurse and one or more physicians or surgeons licensed under chapter 147 that designates the scope of collaboration necessary to manage the care of patients. The advanced practice registered nurse and the one or more physicians must have experience in providing care to patients with the same or similar medical problems.

Citation: MINN. STAT. ANN. § 148.171(6).

Mississippi

An advanced practice registered nurse shall perform those functions authorized in this section within a collaborative/consultative relationship with a dentist or physician with an unrestricted license to practice dentistry or medicine in this state and within an established protocol or practice guidelines, as appropriate, that is filed with the board upon license application, license renewal, after entering into a new collaborative/consultative relationship or making changes to the protocol or practice guidelines or practice site. The board shall review and approve the protocol to ensure compliance with applicable regulatory standards. The advanced practice registered nurse may not practice as an APRN if there is no collaborative/consultative relationship with a physician or dentist and a board approved protocol or practice guidelines.

Citation: MISS. NURSING PRACTICE LAW §73-15-20(3).

Missouri

Collaborative practice arrangements—Refers to written agreements, jointly agreed upon protocols, or standing orders, all of which shall be in writing, for the delivery of healthcare services.

Citation: MO. CODE REGS. ANN. tit. 20, § 2200-4.200 (1)(C).

A. The collaborating physician in a collaborative practice shall not be so geographically distanced from the collaborating RN or APRN as to create an impediment to effective collaboration in the delivery of healthcare services or the adequate review of those services.
B. The use of a collaborative practice arrangement by an APRN who provides health care services that include the diagnosis and initiation of treatment for acutely or chronically ill or injured persons shall be limited to practice locations where the collaborating physician, or other physician designated in the collaborative practice arrangement, is no further than fifty (50) miles by road, using the most direct route available, from the collaborating APRN if the APRN is practicing in federally-designated health professional shortage areas (HPSAs). Otherwise, in non-HPSAs, the collaborating physician and collaborating APRN shall practice within thirty (30) miles by road of one another.
C. An APRN who desires to enter into a collaborative practice arrangement at a location where the collaborating physician is not continuously present shall practice together at the same location with the collaborating physician continuously for a period of at least one (1) month before the collaborating APRN practices at a location where the collaborating physician is not present. It is the responsibility of the collaborating physician to determine and document the completion of the same location practice described in the previous sentence.
D. A collaborating physician shall not enter into a collaborative practice arrangement with more than three (3) full-time equivalent APRNs. This limitation shall not apply to collaborative arrangements of hospital employees providing inpatient care service in hospitals as defined in Chapter 197, RSMo, or population-based public health services as defined in this rule.

Citation: MO. CODE REGS. ANN. tit. 20, § 2200-4.200(2).

The methods of treatment and the authority to administer, dispense, or prescribe drugs delegated in a collaborative practice arrangement between a collaborating physician and collaborating APRN shall be within the scope of practice of each professional and shall be consistent with each professional's skill, training, education, competence, licensure, and/or certification and shall not be further delegated to any person except that the individuals identified in sections 338.095 and 338.198, RSMo, may communicate prescription drug orders to a pharmacist.

Citation: Mo. Code Regs. Ann. tit. 20, § 2200-4.200(3)(A).

C. The collaborating physician shall consider the level of skill, education, training, and competence of the collaborating RN or APRN and ensure that the delegated responsibilities contained in the collaborative practice arrangement are consistent with that level of skill, education, training, and competence.
D. Guidelines for consultation and referral to the collaborating physician or designated health care facility for services or emergency care that is beyond the education, training, competence, or scope of practice of the collaborating RN or APRN shall be established in the collaborative practice arrangement.
E. The methods of treatment, including any authority to administer or dispense drugs, delegated in a collaborative practice arrangement between a collaborating physician and a collaborating RN shall be delivered only pursuant to a written agreement, jointly agreed-upon protocols, or standing orders that shall describe a specific sequence of orders, steps, or procedures to be followed in providing patient care in specified clinical situations.
F. The methods of treatment, including any authority to administer, dispense, or prescribe drugs, delegated in a collaborative practice arrangement between a collaborating physician and a collaborating APRN shall be delivered only pursuant to a written agreement, jointly agree-upon protocols, or standing orders that are specific to the clinical conditions treated by the collaborating physician and collaborating APRN.

Citation: Mo. Code Regs. Ann. tit. 20, § 2200-4.200(3).

Methods of treatment delegated and authority to administer, dispense, or prescribe drugs shall be subject to the following:

1. The physician retains the responsibility for ensuring the appropriate administering, dispensing, prescribing, and control of drugs utilized pursuant to a collaborative practice arrangement in accordance with all state and federal statues, rules, or regulations....

Citation: Mo. Code Regs. Ann. tit. 20, § 2200-4.200(3)(G).

A. In order to assure true collaborative practice and to foster effective communication and review of services, the collaborating physician, or other physician designated in the collaborative practice arrangement, shall be immediately available for consultation to the collaborating RN or APRN at all times, either personally or via telecommunications.

B. The collaborative practice arrangement between a collaborating physician and a collaborating RN or APRN shall be signed and dated by the collaborating physician and collaborating RN or APRN before it is implemented, signifying that both are aware of its content and agree to follow the terms of the collaborative practice arrangement. The collaborative practice arrangement and any subsequent notice of termination shall be in writing and shall be maintained by the collaborating professionals for a minimum of eight (8) years after termination of the collaborative practice arrangement. The collaborative practice arrangement shall be reviewed at least annually and revised as needed by the collaborating physician and collaborating RN or APRN. Documentation of the annual review shall be maintained as part of the collaborative practice arrangement.

C. Within thirty (30) days of any change and with each physician's license renewal, the collaborating physician shall advise the Missouri State Board of Registration for the Healing Arts whether he/she is engaged in any collaborative practice agreement, including collaborative practice agreements delegating the authority to prescribe controlled substances and also report to the board the name of each licensed RN or APRN with whom he/she has entered into such agreement. A change shall include, but not be limited to, resignation or termination of the RN or APRN; change in practice locations; and addition or new collaborating professionals.

D. An RN or an APRN practicing pursuant to a collaborative practice arrangement shall maintain adequate and complete patient records in compliance with section 334.097, RSMo.

E. The collaborating physician shall complete a review of a minimum of ten percent (10%) of the total health care services delivered by the collaborating APRN. If the APRN's practice includes the prescribing of controlled substances, the physician shall review a minimum of twenty percent (20%) of the cases in which the APRN wrote a prescription for a controlled substance. If the controlled substance chart review meets the minimum total ten percent (10%) as described above, then the minimum review requirements have been met. The collaborating APRN's documentation shall be submitted for review to the collaborating physician at least every fourteen (14) days. This documentation submission may be accomplished in person or by other electronic means and reviewed by the collaborating physician. The collaborating physician must produce evidence of the chart review upon request of the Missouri State Board of Registration for the Healing Arts. This subsection shall not apply during the time the collaborating physician and collaborating APRN are practicing together as required in subsection (2)(C) above.

F. If a collaborative practice arrangement is used in clinical situations where a collaborating APRN provides health care services that include the diagnosis and initiation or treatment for acutely or chronically ill or injured persons, then the collaborating physician shall be present for sufficient periods of time, at least once every two (2) weeks, except in extraordinary circumstances that shall be documented, to participate in such review and to provide necessary medical direction, medical services, consultations, and supervision of the health care staff. In such settings, the use of a collaborative practice arrangement shall be limited to only an APRN.

G. The collaborating physician and collaborating RN or APRN shall determine an appropriate process of review and management of abnormal test results which shall be documented in the collaborative practice arrangement.

Citation: Mo. Code Regs. Ann. tit. 20, § 2200-4.200(4).

Montana

Nurse practitioner (NP) practice means the independent and/or collaborative management of primary and/or acute health care of individuals, families, and communities including . . . working in collaboration with other health care providers and agencies to provide and, where appropriate, coordinate services to individuals and families.

Citation: Mont. Admin. R. § 24.159.1470(f).

Nebraska

Collaboration means a process and relationship in which a nurse practitioner, together with other health professionals, delivers health care within the scope of authority of the various clinical specialty practices.

Citation: Neb. Rev. Stat. § 38-2308.

1. Integrated practice agreement means a written agreement between a nurse practitioner and a collaborating physician in which the nurse practitioner and the collaborating physician provide for the delivery of health care through an integrated practice. The integrated practice agreement shall provide that the nurse practitioner and the collaborating physician will practice collaboratively within the framework of their respective scopes of practice. Each provider shall be responsible for his or her individual decisions in managing the health care of patients. Integrated practice includes consultation, collaboration, and referral.

2. The nurse practitioner and the collaborating physician shall have joint responsibility for patient care, based upon the scope of practice of each practitioner. The collaborating physician shall be responsible for supervision of the nurse practitioner to ensure the quality of health care provided to patients.

3. For the purposes of this section:
   a. Collaborating physician means a physician or osteopathic physician licensed in Nebraska and practicing in the same geographic area and practice specialty, related specialty, or field of practice as the nurse practitioner; and
   b. Supervision means the ready availability of the collaborating physician for consultation and direction of the activities of the nurse practitioner within the nurse practitioner's defined scope of practice.

Citation: NEB. REV. STAT. § 38-2310.

Nevada

Note: Section 632.2555 has been repealed as of December 10, 2013.

New Hampshire

There is no requirement for physician collaboration for NP practice in New Hampshire.

New Jersey

An advanced practice nurse may order medications and devices in the inpatient setting, subject to the following condition:

1. the collaborating physician and advanced practice nurse shall address in the joint protocols whether prior consultation with the collaborating physician is required to initiate an order for a controlled dangerous substance;
2. the order is written in accordance with standing orders or joint protocols developed in agreement between a collaborating physician and the advanced practice nurse, or pursuant to the specific direction of a physician;
3. the advanced practice nurse authorizes the order by signing his or her own name, printing the name and certification number, and printing the collaborating physician's name;
4. the physician is present or readily available through electronic communications;
5. the charts and records of the patients treated by the advanced practice nurse are reviewed by the collaborating physician and the advanced practice nurse within the period of time specified by rule adopted by the Commissioner of Health and Senior Services pursuant to section 13 of P.L.1991, c.377 (C.45:11-52);
6. the joint protocols developed by the collaborating physician and the advanced practice nurse are reviewed, updated and signed at least annually by both parties; and
7. the advanced practice nurse has completed six contact hours of continuing professional education in pharmacology related to controlled substances, including pharmacologic therapy and addiction prevention and management,

in accordance with regulations adopted by the New Jersey Board of Nursing. The six contact hours shall be in addition to the New Jersey Board of Nursing pharmacology education requirements for advanced practice nurses related to initial certification and recertification of an advanced practice nurse as set forth in N.J.A.C.13:37-7.2 and 12:37-7.5.

c. An advanced practice nurse may prescribe medications and devices in all other medically appropriate settings, subject to the following conditions:
1. the collaborating physician and advanced practice nurse shall address in the joint protocols whether prior consultation with the collaborating physician is required to initiate a prescription for a controlled dangerous substance;
2. the prescription is written in accordance with standing orders or joint protocols developed in agreement between a collaborating physician and the advanced practice nurse, or pursuant to the specific direction of a physician;
3. the advanced practice nurse writes the prescription on a New Jersey Prescription Blank pursuant to P.L.2003, c.280 (C.45:14-40 et seq.), signs his name to the prescription and prints his name and certification number;
4. the prescription is dated and includes the name of the patient and the name, address, and telephone number of the collaborating physician;
5. the physician is present or readily available through electronic communications;
6. the charts and records of the patients treated by the advanced practice nurse are periodically reviewed by the collaborating physician and the advanced practice nurse;
7. the joint protocols developed by the collaborating physician and the advanced practice nurse are reviewed, updated, and signed at least annually by both parties; and
8. the advanced practice nurse has completed six contact hours of continuing professional education in pharmacology related to controlled substances, including pharmacologic therapy and addiction prevention and management, in accordance with regulations adopted by the New Jersey Board of Nursing. The six contact hours shall be in addition to New Jersey Board of Nursing pharmacology education requirements for advanced practice nurses related to initial certification and recertification of an advanced practice nurse as set forth in N.J.A.C.13:37-7.2 and 13:37-7.5.

d. The joint protocols employed pursuant to Subsections b. and c. of this section shall conform with standards adopted by the Director of the Division of Consumer Affairs pursuant to Section 12 of P.L.1991, c. 377 (C.45:11–51) or Section 10 of P.L.1999, c. 85 (C.45:11–49.2), as applicable.

Citation: N.J. Stat. Ann. § 45:11-49.

New Mexico

The Certified Nurse Practitioner makes independent decisions regarding the health care needs of the client and also makes independent decisions on carrying out health care regimens.

Citation: N.M. Admin. Code § 16.12.2.13.N(1).

New York

[A practice agreement between NP and a physician is required.]

Each practice agreement shall provide for patient records review by the collaborating physician in a timely fashion but in no event less often than every three months. The names of the nurse practitioner and the collaborating physician shall be clearly posted in the practice setting of the nurse practitioner.

Citation: N.Y. Educ. Law, Art. 139 § 6902.3(c).

No physician shall enter into practice agreements with more than four nurse practitioners who are not located on the same physical premises as the collaborating physician.

Citation: N.Y. Educ. Law, Art. 139 § 6902.3(e).

The practice protocol shall reflect current accepted medical and nursing practice. The protocols shall be filed with the department within ninety days of the commencement of the practice and may be updated periodically. The commissioner shall make regulations establishing the procedure for the review of protocols and the disposition of any issues arising from such review.

Citation: N.Y. Educ. Law, Art. 139 § 6902.3(d).

North Carolina

The following are the quality assurance standards for a collaborative practice agreement:

1. Availability: The primary or back-up supervising physician(s) and the nurse practitioner shall be continuously available to each other for consultation by direct communication or telecommunication.
2. Collaborative Practice Agreement:
   a. shall be agreed upon and signed by both the primary supervising physician and the nurse practitioner, and maintained in each practice site;
   b. shall be reviewed at least yearly. This review shall be acknowledged by a dated signature sheet, signed by both the primary supervising physician and the nurse practitioner, appended to the collaborative practice

agreement and available for inspection by members or agents of either Board;

   c. shall include the drugs, devices, medical treatments, tests, and procedures that may be prescribed, ordered and performed by the nurse practitioner consistent with Rule .0809 of this Section; and

   d. shall include a pre-determined plan for emergency services.

3. The nurse practitioner shall demonstrate the ability to perform medical acts as outlined in the collaborative practice agreement upon request by members or agents of either Board.

4. Quality Improvement Process.

   a. The primary supervising physician and the nurse practitioner shall develop a process for the ongoing review of the care provided in each practice site including a written plan for evaluating the quality of care provided for one or more frequently encountered clinical problems.

   b. This plan shall include a description of the clinical problem(s), an evaluation of the current treatment interventions, and if needed, a plan for improving outcomes within an identified timeframe.

   c. The quality improvement process shall include scheduled meetings between the primary supervising physician and the nurse practitioner at least every six months. Documentation for each meeting shall:

      i. identify clinical problems discussed, including progress toward improving outcomes as stated in Sub-item (4)(b) of this Rule, and recommendations, if any, for changes in treatment plan(s);

      ii. be signed and dated by those who attended; and

      iii. be available for review by members or agents of either Board for the previous five calendar years and be retained by both the nurse practitioner and primary supervising physician.

5. Nurse Practitioner-Physician Consultation. The following requirements establish the minimum standards for consultation between the nurse practitioner and primary supervising physician(s):

   a. During the first six months of a collaborative practice agreement between a nurse practitioner and the primary supervising physician, there shall be monthly meetings for the first six months to discuss practice relevant clinical issues and quality improvement measures.

   b. Documentation of the meetings shall:

      i. identify clinical issues discussed and actions taken;

      ii. be signed and dated by those who attended; and

      iii. be available for review by members or agents of either Board for the previous five calendar years and be retained by both the nurse practitioner and primary supervising physician.

Citation: N.C. ADMIN. CODE tit. 21, r. 36.0810.

North Dakota

There is no requirement for physician collaboration for APRN practice in North Dakota.

Ohio

A ... certified nurse practitioner, in collaboration with one or more physicians or podiatrists, may provide preventive and primary care services, provide services for acute illness, and evaluate and promote patient wellness within the nurse's nursing specialty, consistent with the nurse's education and certification, and in accordance with rules adopted by the board. A certified nurse practitioner who holds a certificate to prescribe issued under Section 4723.48 of the Revised Code may, in collaboration with one or more physicians or podiatrists, prescribe drugs and therapeutic devices in accordance with Section 4723.481 of the Revised Code. When a certified nurse practitioner is collaborating with a podiatrist, the nurse's scope of practice is limited to the procedures that the podiatrist has the authority under Section 4731.51 of the Revised Code to perform.

Citation: OHIO REV. CODE ANN. § 4723.43(C).

Oklahoma

A Certified Nurse Practitioner shall be eligible, in accordance with the scope of practice of the Certified Nurse Practitioner, to obtain recognition as authorized by the Board to prescribe ... subject to the medical direction of a supervising physician.

Citation: OKLA. STAT. ANN. tit. 59, § 567.3a(6).

Oregon

There is no requirement of physician collaboration.

Pennsylvania

Collaboration—A process in which a CRNP works with one or more physicians to deliver health care services within the scope of the CRNP's expertise. The process includes all of the following:

i. Immediate availability of a licensed physician to a CRNP through direct communications or by radio, telephone or telecommunications.
ii. A predetermined plan for emergency services.
iii. A physician available to a CRNP on a regularly scheduled basis for referrals, review of the standards of medical practice incorporating consultation and chart review, drug and other medical protocols within the

practice setting, periodic updating in medical diagnosis and therapeutics and cosigning records when necessary to document accountability by both parties.

Citation: 49 Pa. Code § 21.251.

Rhode Island

"Certified registered nurse practitioner (RNP)" means an advanced practice nurse utilizing independent knowledge of physical assessment and management of health care and illnesses. The practice includes prescriptive privileges, and collaboration with other licensed healthcare professionals, including, but not limited to, physicians, pharmacists, podiatrists, dentists and nurses. Such collaboration is not required to be pursuant to a written collaboration agreement, with a specific designated physician, or at the same physical location as a collaborating physician.

Citation: R.I. R. § R5-34-NUR/ED 1.0(1.10).

South Carolina

... Nurse practitioners who perform delegated medical acts must have a supervising physician or dentist who is readily available for consultation and shall operate within the approved written protocols.

Citation: S.C. Code Ann. § 40-33-20(41).

"Approved written protocols" mean specific statements developed collaboratively by a physician or medical staff and a NP, CNM, or CNS that establishes physician delegation for medical aspects of care, including the prescription of medications.

Citation: S.C. Code Ann. § 40-33-20(10).

Delegated medical acts performed by a nurse practitioner, certified nurse-midwife, or clinical nurse specialist must be performed pursuant to an approved written protocol between the nurse and physician and must include ... (a) this general information:
   i. Name, address, and South Carolina license number of the nurse;
   ii. Name, address, and South Carolina license number of the physician;
   iii. Nature of practice and practice locations of the nurse and physician;
   iv. Date the protocol was developed and dates the protocol was reviewed and amended;
   v. Description of how consultation with the physician is provided and provision for backup consultation in the physician's absence.

   b. This information for delegated medical acts:

i. The medical conditions for which therapies may be initiated, continued, or modified;

ii. The treatments that may be initiated, continued, or modified;

iii. The drug therapies that may be prescribed;

iv. Situations that require direct evaluation by or referral to the physician.

2. The original protocol and any amendments to the protocol must be reviewed at least annually, dated and signed by the nurse and physician, and made available to the Board for review within 72 hours of request. Failure to produce protocols upon request of the board is considered misconduct and subjects the licensee to disciplinary action. A random audit of approved written protocols must be conducted by the board at least biennially.

3. Licensees who change practice settings or physicians, shall notify the board of the change within 15 business days and provide verification of approved written protocols. NPs, CNMs and CNSs who discontinue their practice shall notify the board within 15 days.

Citation: S.C. CODE ANN. § 43-33-34(D).

South Dakota

"Collaborative agreement" defined. The term, collaborative agreement, as used in this chapter, means a written agreement authored and signed by the nurse practitioner or nurse midwife and the physician with whom the nurse practitioner or nurse midwife is collaborating. A collaborative agreement defines or describes the agreed upon overlapping scope of advanced practice nursing and medical functions that may be performed, consistent with § 36-9A-12 or 36-9A-13, and contains such other information as required by the boards. A copy of each collaborative agreement shall be maintained on file with and be approved by the boards prior to performing any of the acts contained in the agreement.

Citation: S.D. CODIFIED LAWS § 36-9A-15.

Advanced practice nursing and medical functions—Collaborative agreement required. A nurse practitioner or nurse midwife may perform the overlapping scope of advanced practice nursing and medical functions only under the terms of a collaborative agreement with a physician licensed under Chapter 36-4. Any collaborative agreement shall be maintained on file with the boards. Collaboration may be by direct personal contact, or by a combination of direct personal contact and indirect contact via telecommunication, as may be required by the boards. If the collaborating physician named in a collaborative agreement becomes temporarily unavailable, the nurse practitioner or nurse midwife may perform the agreed upon overlapping scope of advanced practice nursing and medical functions in consultation with another licensed physician designated as a substitute.

Citation: S.D. CODIFIED LAWS § 36-9A-17.

Collaboration with a licensed physician or physicians. A nurse practitioner or nurse midwife may perform the overlapping scope of advanced practice nursing and medical functions defined in SDCL 36-9A-12 and 36-9A-13, in collaboration with a physician or physicians licensed under SDCL Chapter 36-4. Collaboration by direct personal contact with each collaborating physician must occur no less than twice each month unless it is established in the collaborative agreement that one of the twice monthly meetings may be held by telecommunication. Collaboration with each collaborating physician shall occur at least once per month by direct personal contact.

Citation: S.D. ADMIN. R. § 20:62:03:03.

Direct personal contact. For the purposes of this chapter, the term, direct personal contact, means that both the collaborating physician and the nurse practitioner or nurse midwife are physically present on site and available for the purposes of collaboration. When the collaborating physician is not in direct personal contact with the nurse practitioner or nurse midwife, the physician must be available by telecommunication. If the boards consider additional direct personal contact necessary for a nurse practitioner or nurse midwife, they shall set the terms of that additional collaboration and require inclusion of those terms in that nurse practitioner's or midwife's collaborative agreement as a condition for its approval.

Citation: S.D. ADMIN. R. § 20:62:03:04.

Collaboration—Separate practice location. In addition to the required two meetings per month, the collaborating physician must be physically present on-site every ninety days at each practice location. This requirement does not apply to locations where health care services are not routine to the setting, such as patient homes and school health screening events.

Citation: S.D. ADMIN. R. § 20:62:03:05.

Tennessee

b. 1. A nurse who has been issued a certificate of fitness as a nurse practitioner pursuant to § 63-7-207 and this section shall file a notice with the board, containing the name of the nurse practitioner, the name of the licensed physician having supervision, control, and responsibility for prescriptive services rendered by the nurse practitioner and a copy of the formulary describing the categories of legend drugs to be prescribed and/or issued by the nurse practitioner. The nurse practitioner shall be responsible for updating this information.

2. The nurse practitioner who holds a certificate of fitness shall be authorized to prescribe and/or issue controlled substances listed in Schedules II, III, IV, and V . . . upon joint adoption of physician supervisory rules concerning controlled substances. . . .

Citation: TENN. CODE ANN. § 63-7-123(b)(1)&(2).

Texas

The advanced practice nurse acts independently and/or in collaboration with the health team in the observation, assessment, diagnosis, intervention, evaluation, rehabilitation, care and counsel, and health teachings of persons who are ill, injured, or infirm or experiencing changes in normal health processes; and in the promotion and maintenance of health or prevention of illness.

Citation: 21 Tex. Admin. Code § 221.13(c).

When providing medical aspects of care, advanced practice nurses shall utilize mechanisms that provide authority for that care. These mechanisms may include, but are not limited to, protocols or other written authorization. This shall not be construed as requiring authority for nursing aspects of care.

1. Protocols or other written authorization shall promote the exercise of professional judgment by the advanced practice nurse commensurate with his/her education and experience. The degree of detail within protocols/policies/practice guidelines/clinical practice privileges may vary in relation to the complexity of the situations covered by such protocols, the advanced specialty area of practice, the advanced educational preparation of the individual, and the experience level of the individual advanced practice nurse.

2. Protocols or other written authorization:
   A. should be jointly developed by the advanced practice nurse and the appropriate physician(s);
   B. shall be signed by both the advanced practice nurse and the physician(s);
   C. shall be reviewed and re-signed at least annually;
   D. shall be maintained in the practice setting of the advanced practice nurse; and
   E. shall be made available as necessary to verify authority to provide medical aspects of care.

e. The advanced practice nurse shall retain professional accountability for advanced practice nursing care.

Citation: 21 Tex. Admin. Code § 221.13(d)&(e).

a. The APRN with full licensure and a valid prescription authorization number shall:
   1. order or prescribe only those drugs or devices that are:
      A. authorized by a prescriptive authority agreement or, if practicing in a facility-based practice, authorized by either a prescriptive authority agreement or protocols or other written authorization; and
      B. ordered or prescribed for patient populations within the accepted scope of professional practice for the APRN's license; and

2. comply with the requirements for chart reviews specified in the prescriptive authority agreement and periodic face to face meetings set forth in the prescriptive authority agreement; or

3. comply with the requirements set forth in protocols or other written authorization if ordering or prescribing drugs or devices under facility-based protocols or other written authorization.

b. Prescription Information. The format and essential elements of a prescription drug order shall comply with the requirements of the Texas State Board of Pharmacy. The following information must be provided on each prescription:

1. the patient's name and address;
2. the name, strength, and quantity of the drug to be dispensed;
3. directions to the patient regarding taking of the drug and the dosage;
4. the intended use of the drug, if appropriate;
5. the name, address, and telephone number of the physician with whom the APRN has a prescriptive authority agreement or facility-based protocols or other written authorization;
6. address and telephone number of the site at which the prescription drug order was issued;
7. the date of issuance;
8. the number of refills permitted;
9. the name, prescription authorization number, and original signature of the APRN who authorized the prescription drug order; and
10. the United States Drug Enforcement Administration numbers of the APRN and the delegating physician, if the prescription drug order is for a controlled substance.

c. Generic Substitution. The APRN shall authorize or prevent generic substitution on a prescription in compliance with the current rules of the Texas State Board of Pharmacy relating to generic substitution.

d. An APRN may order or prescribe medications for sexually transmitted diseases for partners of an established patient, if the APRN assesses the patient and determines that the patient may have been infected with a sexually transmitted disease. Nothing in this subsection shall be construed to require the APRN to issue prescriptions for partners of patients.

e. APRNs may order or prescribe only those medications that are FDA approved unless done through protocol registration in a United States Institutional Review Board or Expanded Access authorized clinical trial. "Off label" use, or prescription of FDA-approved medications for uses other than that indicated by the FDA, is permitted when such practices are:

1. within the current standard of care for treatment of the disease or condition; and
2. supported by evidence-based research.

f. The APRN with full licensure and a valid prescriptive authorization number shall cooperate with representatives of the Board and the Texas Medical Board during an inspection and audit relating to the operation and implementation of a prescriptive authority agreement.

Citation: 22 Tex. Admin. Code §224.4.

Utah

"Consultation and referral plan" means a written plan jointly developed by an advanced practice registered nurse and a consulting physician that permits the advanced practice registered nurse to prescribe schedule II-III controlled substances in consultation with the consulting physician.

Citation: Utah Code Ann. § 58-31b-102(5).

Vermont

Graduates with fewer than 24 months and 2,400 hours of license active advanced nursing practice shall have a formal agreement with a collaborating provider.

Citation: Vt. Board of Nursing Admin Rules 15.14.

a. A collaborating provider is:
   1. an APRN or
   2. a physician licensed to practice medicine under Title 26, Chapter 23, or
   3. an osteophathic physician licensed to practice under Title 26, Chapter 33.
b. The collaborating provider's license must be in good standing, and the collaborating provider shall practice in the same role and population focus or specialty as the new graduate APRN's area of certification.
c. An APRN collaborating provider shall have practiced in the same specialty for a minimum of four years. The Board, in its discretion, may waive the requirement that a collaborating provider be licensed in Vermont upon showing of necessity by the APRN. Any waiver granted under this section will only apply to providers currently licensed in the United States.

Citation: Vt. Board of Nursing Admin Rules 15.17.

Virginia

A nurse practitioner licensed in a category other than certified registered nurse anesthetist shall be authorized to render care in collaboration and consultation with a licensed patient care team physician as part of patient care team.

Citation: 18 Va. Admin. Code § 90-30-120.A.

A nurse practitioner with prescriptive authority may prescribe only within the scope of the written or electronic practice agreement with a patient care team physician.

Citation: 18 VA. ADMIN. CODE § 90-40-90.

"Practice agreement" means a written or electronic agreement jointly developed by the patient care team physician and the nurse practitioner for the practice of the nurse practitioner that also describes the prescriptive authority of the nurse practitioner, if applicable.

Citation: 18 VA. ADMIN. CODE § 90-40-10.

Washington

No physician collaboration is required by law for nurse practitioner practice in Washington.

West Virginia

The board may, in its discretion, authorize an advanced nurse practitioner to prescribe prescription drugs in a collaborative relationship with a physician licensed to practice in West Virginia and in accordance with applicable state and federal laws. An authorized advanced nurse practitioner may write or sign prescriptions or transmit prescriptions verbally or by other means of communication.

For purposes of this section an agreement to a collaborative relationship for prescriptive practice between a physician and an advanced practice registered nurse shall be set forth in writing. . . .

Collaborative agreements shall include, but not be limited to, the following:
1. Mutually agreed upon written guidelines or protocols for prescriptive authority as it applies to the advanced practice registered nurse's clinical practice;
2. Statements describing the individual and shared responsibilities of the advanced practice registered nurse and the physician pursuant to the collaborative agreement between them;
3. Periodic and joint evaluation of prescriptive practice; and
4. Periodic and joint review and updating of the written guidelines or protocols.

Citation: W.VA. CODE ANN. § 30-7-15(a).

Wisconsin

Advanced practice nurse prescribers shall facilitate collaboration with other health care professionals, at least one of whom shall be a physician, through the use of modern communication techniques.

Citation: WIS. ADMIN. CODE § N8.10(2).

Advanced practice nurse prescribers shall work in a collaborative relationship with a physician. The collaborative relationship is a process in which an advanced practice nurse prescriber is working with a physician, in each other's presence when necessary, to deliver health care services within the scope of the practitioner's professional expertise. The advanced practice nurse prescriber and the physician must document this relationship.

Citation: WIS. ADMIN. CODE § N8.10(7).

Wyoming

There is no requirement for physician collaboration or supervision.

Negligence and Malpractice

Nurse practitioners (NPs) carrying out their daily routines have one constant on their everyday "to do" list: "Do no harm." Nevertheless, when an NP, or any other healthcare provider, makes hundreds of decisions a day, it is inevitable that mistakes will be made.

For example, researchers studying medical errors at a major teaching hospital followed nurses and doctors for 9 months on three surgical units. They found that some medical error was made with almost half of the patients and that for at least 18% of the patients there was a serious consequence. Only 1% of these patients sued for malpractice, however.[1]

Though malpractice lawsuits against NPs are rare, the financial and emotional sequelae of being sued are so dire that it is worth dealing with this subject in depth. The meaning and incidence of lawsuits against NPs are difficult to state accurately, for a variety of reasons.

First, a filed lawsuit has no meaning other than to state that a person believes himself or herself to have been harmed. The belief may be unfounded. The blame may be placed on the wrong person. The complaint may not even meet the definition of malpractice. Thus, tracking the incidence of filed suits is of very limited value.

Second, some suits that are filed and that name NPs do so not because the plaintiff believes an NP caused harm but because an NP is a member of a team of caregivers who are being sued, and at the early stages of a lawsuit it is not clear who is responsible. On the other hand, some NPs who actually have been negligent may not be sued, for a variety of reasons.

Third, unless an insurance company reports a damage award—a successful lawsuit or a settlement for damages—against an NP to the National Practitioner Data Bank (NPDB), a lawsuit may come to light only through a search of county court or insurance company records. Insurance companies are required to report damage awards to the NPDB. If a suit is filed but the plaintiff is unsuccessful in proving the necessary elements for malpractice, there will be no report filed with the NPDB. Keeping a national tally of unsuccessful lawsuits filed against NPs is almost impossible.

That being said, one study comparing the incidence of successful lawsuits against advanced practice nurses (APNs), physicians, and physician assistants (PAs) found that in 2006, the chances of paying a malpractice award were 1 in 62 for physicians, 1 in 563 for PAs, and 1 in 1016 for APNs, based on the ratio of awards divided by the number of licensed providers.[2]

What Can Happen to an NP Who Is Sued?

An NP who is sued may feel like leaving the profession, may doubt his or her ability to make decisions, or may resort to over-referring and seeking unnecessary consultation. In addition, the NP may find that his or her insurance rates are increased, may miss days of work while testifying, may have to pay some legal expenses, and may have to mount a defense before the state licensing board.

Boards of nursing do not automatically investigate NPs who have lost malpractice lawsuits. However, if someone involved with the case reports the NP to the board of nursing, or the negligence approaches the level of gross negligence, the board of nursing likely will investigate. Gross negligence, for a professional, is the intentional failure to perform a professional duty in reckless disregard of the consequences.

Lifecycle of a Lawsuit

A lawsuit starts with the filing of pleadings with a state court, usually in the county where the incident occurred. Some states direct malpractice actions to an arbitration panel. The case is presented to the panel, and its members make a decision in favor of one party. Depending on state law, either party may appeal, in which case there will be a trial. At trial, a judge or jury decides in favor of one party. Either party may then appeal to a higher state court. Rarely, a party will seek an appeal to a federal court. Federal courts may accept or refuse appeals from the state courts. Although it is possible that a malpractice case could go all the way to the U.S. Supreme Court, it is highly unlikely. Usually, the highest state court of appeals is the highest level of consideration of a malpractice case, and often the parties will let the matter drop after the state trial court case. Because the holdings of state trial courts are not published, the public cannot easily access information on malpractice trials unless there is an appeal. The opinions of appeals courts are published, and that is the information attorneys and professionals can use to gain insight into malpractice cases.

What Is Malpractice?

Malpractice is the failure of a professional to exercise that degree of skill and learning commonly applied by the average prudent, reputable member of the profession. Negligence is the predominant legal theory of malpractice liability. Negligence includes failure to follow up, failure to refer when necessary, failure to disclose necessary information to a patient, and failure to give necessary care.

Elements of Malpractice

A plaintiff in a malpractice suit must prove the following elements:

1. The NP owed the plaintiff a duty.
2. The NP's conduct fell below the standard of care.
3. The NP's conduct caused the plaintiff's injury.
4. The plaintiff was injured.

Duty

A duty is established when there is a provider–patient relationship. A visit to the NP's office by a patient establishes an NP's duty to that patient. However, there need not be an office visit to establish duty. Duty can be established by a telephone conversation or casual discussion with a patient or with someone who is not officially a patient. If an NP gives professional advice or treatment in any setting, a duty may be established. If an injured party has reason to believe that there was a provider–patient relationship, there may in fact be such a relationship, even if the provider did not think of the interaction in that way.

What Is the Standard of Care for NPs?

NPs are duty bound to use such reasonable, ordinary care, skill, and diligence as NPs in good standing in the same general type of practice in similar cases.

An NP is held to the standard of care of a reasonably prudent NP, not necessarily to the standard of care expected of a physician. In many situations, however, the standards of care for physicians and NPs will be identical. For example, an NP providing primary care can be held to the same standard as a physician providing primary care.

If an NP is sued for malpractice, the standard of care will be argued in court. If an NP believes that she or he met the standard of care, the NP's attorney will enlist expert witnesses, usually other NPs, who will give testimony describing the steps that a reasonably prudent NP would take in a similar situation. The plaintiff's attorney also will enlist expert witnesses, who can be expected to testify that the standard of care called for other measures than those performed by the defendant NP. A judge or jury will accept either the plaintiff's or the defendant's explanation of the standard of care and will then decide whether the defendant NP met that standard.

Causation of Injury

For malpractice to have occurred, a breach of the standard of care must have caused an injury to the plaintiff. For example, a patient visits an NP and is diagnosed with otitis media. The NP prescribes penicillin, to which the patient is allergic. This allergy is marked on the patient's chart. The patient leaves the clinic with penicillin, but before she takes it, she is stung by a bee on the front steps of the clinic. She has an allergic reaction to the bee sting and falls and hits her head, causing a permanent scar on her face. The patient sues the clinic and the NP, claiming that the NP had a duty to the patient, the NP breached the standard of care (by prescribing penicillin for a penicillin-allergic patient), and the patient suffered an injury. All of these claims are true, but there is no malpractice because the breach of the standard of care (prescribing penicillin to an allergic patient) did not cause the injury (the wound to the head).

Injury

A provider may be terribly negligent, but if there is no injury, there is no malpractice. For example, if an NP prescribes penicillin to a patient who is allergic, and the patient takes the penicillin but has no reaction that injures them, then there is no malpractice, even though the standard of care has been breached and even though, if an injury occurred, there would have been a causal relationship between breach of the standard of care and injury.

Examples of Lawsuits Against NPs

Missed Diagnosis

Example 1

The patient, a middle-aged man, began experiencing chest pain at work. He called the clinic and got an appointment for 4 PM. He worked until 4 PM and went to the clinic. An NP evaluated the patient, took a history and examined him, and conferred with a physician. The NP diagnosed muscle spasm and initiated treatment with Valium.

The patient went home, went to sleep, and awakened at 1 AM with severe chest pain. He went to the emergency department, where he was examined by a physician. A chest X-ray was taken. The physician diagnosed muscle spasm. He ordered Demerol, intramuscularly, and prescribed oral codeine.

At noon the next day, the patient's chest pain returned and was more severe. He went to the emergency department. An electrocardiogram was done, which showed a myocardial infarction. Finally, a correct diagnosis was made. The patient recovered but did not return to full-time work for 18 months. The patient sued the NP and the medical group for lost wages and won. [*Fein v. Permanente Med. Group*, 38 Cal. 3d 137, 695 P.2d 665, 211 Cal. Rptr. 369 (1985).] This is an old case, but there have been several recent cases in which NPs (and physicians) missed myocardial infarctions because they did not perform electrocardiograms when the patient complained of chest pain.

What NPs Can Learn from This Case

Rule out the worse diagnosis early on, especially if it can be done easily and inexpensively, as with an electrocardiogram.

Example 2

An NP saw a young married female patient for symptoms of cramps, headache, dysmenorrhea, and lesions on the perineum during menses. The NP examined the patient and, on the basis of the physical exam, diagnosed genital herpes. The NP counseled the patient about causes, prevention, and treatment. A physician working with the NP prescribed an antiviral medication appropriate for treating genital herpes.

The symptoms continued, however. The patient saw another physician, who correctly diagnosed the lesions as severe candidiasis.

The patient sued the NP and the employing doctor, claiming pain and suffering and expenses of treatment. The patient's husband claimed loss of society, companionship, and conjugal relationship with his wife.

The court dismissed the case against the NP but found that the doctor associated with the NP had breached the standard of care. The plaintiff won against the doctor.

The physician appealed the case, asking whether the NP's mistake was correctly imputed to the physician. The appeals court said it was. [*Adams v. Kreuger*, 124 Idaho 74, 856 P.2d 864 (1993).]

What NPs Can Learn from This Case:

1. The diagnosis of a sexually transmitted infection carries with it an emotional component. A patient surely will discuss the matter with the partner, and relationships may break up as a result. Always confirm physical exam findings with laboratory testing, especially when diagnosing sexually transmitted infections.

2. Some courts do not consider NPs to be professionally responsible for their judgments. However, most judges and juries find NPs responsible for their own decisions. When an NP is sued, sometimes the physician collaborator also is sued. Usually, if the physician collaborator did not participate in the case, because, for example, the NP did not ask the physician for help, then the physician collaborator is dropped from the complaint. However, there is one recent case where an NP was sued and the physician collaborator was held liable, even though the physician did not participate in the care of the patient. The judge felt that the physician should have exercised more supervision over the NP.

Example 3

A patient saw a family NP for a complaint of discharge and constant scabbing of one of her nipples, of several months' duration. The NP ordered topical and oral antibiotics and a mammogram, which was negative. The patient returned 7 months later with continuing pain and discharge from the same nipple. The NP referred the patient to a dermatologist. The patient did not see the dermatologist.

Four months later, the patient saw her gynecologist, who again treated her breast symptoms with antibiotics and assured her that she did not have cancer.

The patient saw the NP several more times during the year following the first visit. Reasons for the patient's visits were varied. Eighteen months after the first visit, the patient came to the NP with unmistakable masses in her breast. The NP referred the patient to a surgical oncologist, who diagnosed Paget's disease. The cancer had metastasized, and the patient died shortly after the diagnosis. The patient's family sued the NP, the patient's family practitioner, and the gynecologist, and won damages against all three providers. The court said all three providers had breached the standard of care. [*Jenkins v. Payne*, 465 S.E.2d 795 (Va. 1996).]

What NPs Can Learn from This Case

An NP must follow up symptoms from past visits, even when a patient does not continue to complain about the symptoms. In this case, the NP should have continued to ask, on subsequent visits, whether the breast discharge had resolved and whether the patient had followed up with the dermatologist. Unless the patient stated that the breast discharge and scabbing had resolved (in which case the NP should have documented resolution of the symptom), the NP should have followed up with biopsy when the symptoms did not respond to the initial antibiotics.

Failure to Refer

Example 1

A young man went to an emergency room with acute pain caused by testicular trauma after being hit by a softball. He was urinating blood. He was evaluated by a family NP, who prescribed hydrocodone and naproxen. He was discharged 3 hours later with advice to keep ice on the injury and to schedule an elective ultrasound in 2 days. The patient had increasing pain and his right testicle continued to swell. He returned to the emergency department for re-evaluation. An emergency room physician immediately obtained a testicular ultrasound after an examination, which revealed significant bruising, swelling, and tenderness. The ultrasound revealed an adjacent hemorrhage or hydrocele. There also was questionable arterial flow to the right testicle. The physician recommended that the patient see a urologist urgently. The urologist admitted the patient for an immediate scrotal exploration and thereafter concluded that the right testicle was ruptured and not viable. The testicle was removed. The urologist's operative report included a comment that he may have been able to save the testicle if he had seen the patient on the day of the accident. The patient sued the NP, alleging negligence in the failure to order and review a testicular ultrasound before his discharge at the initial presentation. The plaintiff also claimed that the NP should have referred him to a urologist the same day. The defendant argued that the testicle may not have been salvageable even with earlier surgery. The parties settled for $100,000. [Laska, L. editor, *Malpractice Verdicts, Settlements and Experts*, October 2012.]

What NPs Can Learn from This Case

1. Know when to refer. Refer when the possibility of severe patient injury is high (testicular trauma, urinating blood, potential for loss of testicle) and the NP's expertise does not extend to the body area or system affected. (Urologic injuries are not something most primary care providers are expert at evaluating and managing.)
2. If deciding to evaluate an injury yourself, rather than refer, order the test most likely to rule out the worst possibility, and follow up.

Mishandling of Medicine

Example 1

A 49-year-old woman was attacked while at work at a psychiatric clinic. Her attacker was a patient, a schizophrenic woman who had become paranoid, psychotic, and convinced that someone was following her and possibly trying to kill her. The patient entered the clinic, filled out some paperwork, and then pulled a butcher knife out of her handbag and repeatedly stabbed the staff person. The employee suffered wounds to her hands, arms, face, eyes, torso, heart, lungs, liver, bowels, buttocks, and vagina, and she lost her eyesight as a result of the attack. The patient had a well-documented history of chronic schizophrenia and noncompliance with medications. She had a history of violent behavior. Her last psychotic attack had resulted in involuntary commitment. During her hospitalization she did not recognize the need to take medications. She was assessed as a moderately high risk of danger to others. She was released to the care of a community psychiatric clinic and saw an NP there. The NP had not reviewed the patient's history completely and lowered the dosage of antipsychotic medication because the woman said she did not like taking the medications. The injured worker sued the clinic. The parties settled for $5.5 million. A portion of the settlement was paid to an employee who witnessed the attack and suffered post-traumatic stress disorder due to seeing her coworker lying on the floor disemboweled with her eyes gouged out. [(Laska, L., editor, *Medical Malpractice Verdicts, Settlements and Experts*, January 2010.)]

What NPs Can Learn from This Case

Individuals with schizophrenia may not want to adhere to a prescribed regimen for a variety of reasons. While patient requests normally deserve consideration, when the patient is being treated for psychosis, there is justification and even necessity for refusing to comply with the patient's wishes. When a clinician encounters a recently discharged psychiatric patient who has been prescribed a medication regimen, it is a breach of the standard of care to decrease dosages without discussion with and approval by the patient's team, which should include the psychiatrist who supervised the patient's care in the hospital. There are a number of considerations clinicians should address related to decreasing antipsychotic medications, including the following:

- Likelihood of psychotic relapse
- SSRI discontinuation syndrome
- Antipsychotic discontinuation syndrome
- Anticholinergic withdrawal reaction
- Withdrawal dyskinesia
- Rebound dystonia
- Potential for adverse events related to abrupt discontinuation (e.g., dizziness, lightheadedness, nausea, tremors, insomnia, sedation, electric shock-like pains, and anxiety)

Another lesson: Spend the time to get old records on patients.

Failure to Provide Preventive Care

Example 1

A 35-year-old woman visited a primary care physician's office for various ailments in 2001 and 2002. She saw a primary care physician twice and an NP four times. The patient had a history of splenectomy in 1985. She had received Pneumovax following the procedure. She did not receive Haemophilus or Meningococcal vaccination. Subsequent to 2002, the patient developed a pneumococcal infection that required a 3-month hospitalization and a 2-month stay in a rehabilitation facility. During the hospitalization, she became septic, suffered organ failure and necrosis, and had partial amputation of toes. She can now walk only short distances and suffers from chronic infections and pain. The patient/plaintiff contended that the standard of care required the defendants to revaccinate the patient with a Pneumovax booster due to her asplenia. The plaintiff contended that if the defendants had complied with the accepted standard of care, then she would have avoided her subsequent pneumococcal infection. The clinicians argued that the patient's visits had all been for acute sick visits, not annual preventive and wellness physicals, which did not provide them with an opportunity to recommend or administer a pneumococcal vaccination. The defendants also claimed that the pneumococcal vaccination is not the standard of care, is not proven effective, and would not necessarily have prevented the plaintiff's infection. The parties reached a $3 million settlement. [(Laska, L., editor, *Medical Malpractice Verdicts, Settlements, and Experts*, January 2010.)]

What NPs Can Learn from This Case

Generally, patients get one Pneumovax per lifetime. However, patients without spleens need special consideration. The standard of care is to revaccinate asplenic patients. Furthermore, patients who come only for "sick visits" and never get a preventive care evaluation are risks to themselves and to their healthcare providers. The clinician who wants to decrease risk will either make time during sick visits for attention to preventive matters or will insist that all patients schedule a preventive visit every 1–3 years.

Failure to Perform Routine Screening

Example 1

A child visited a primary care center from birth to 9 months. At one visit (the case report does not specify the age of the child at this visit) the child's mother pointed out to an NP that one of the child's pupils was larger than the other. Two months later the parent told the NP that the child's eyes did not move in tandem. The parent claimed the NP said these symptoms were not important. Three months later the NP tested the child for "red reflex." The NP saw no light reflected back and referred the child to an ophthalmologist, who diagnosed retinoblastoma in both eyes. One eye was removed 3 months later and the other 3 years later. The mother claimed that the NP should have tested for red reflex earlier, which would have saved one eye. The mother admitted that one eye would have been lost in any event. The parties settled for $2 million. [Laska, L., editor, *Malpractice Verdicts, Settlements and Experts*, January 2013.]

What NPs Can Learn from This Case

Understand the standard of care for routine screening for your population. The standard of care calls for an NP or physician to perform a red reflex examination at every well child visit until a child can read. One source of the standard of care is the American Academy of Pediatrics (AAP). Here is a summary of the AAP recommendations: "All neonates, infants, and children should have an examination of the red reflex of the eyes performed by a pediatrician or other primary care clinician trained in this examination technique before discharge from the neonatal nursery and during all subsequent routine health supervision visits." [American Academy of Pediatrics, Section on Ophthalmology, American Association for Pediatric Ophthalmology and Strabismus, American Academy of Ophthalmology, and American Association of Certified Orthoptists, "Red Reflex Examination in Neonates, Infants and Children," *Pediatrics* 2008;122;1401 at http://pediatrics.aappublications.org/content/122/6/1401.full.pdf]

The National Practitioner Data Bank

The National Practitioner Data Bank (NPDB) is a repository for damage award data; that is, payments from professional liability insurance companies on behalf of their clients to injured parties for successful malpractice claims. NPDB also records adverse actions against providers by licensing boards, hospitals, and professional quality assurance committees.

The NPDB is the responsibility of the U.S. Department of Health and Human Services. It was established under a law that was intended to encourage hospitals, state licensing boards, and other healthcare entities to discipline those who engage in unprofessional behavior and to restrict the ability of incompetent physicians, dentists, and other healthcare practitioners to move from state to state without disclosure of their previous dangerous performance.

Under the law, any malpractice insurer who pays any amount to a plaintiff on behalf of an NP in a malpractice case must report that payment to the NPDB. If an NP pays an injured patient directly to settle a matter, that payment need not be reported. The insurer must also report damage awards to state licensing boards. A malpractice insurer must report to the NPDB any amount of dollars paid on behalf of a client to a plaintiff. If a healthcare provider pays an injured party directly, that need not be reported. In addition, state licensing boards are required to report adverse licensure actions, hospitals are required to report adverse clinical privilege actions, and professional societies are required to report adverse professional society membership actions.

Hospitals must check the NPDB data every 2 years before granting clinical privileges. Certain agencies may check the NPDB data. The general public does not have access to the NPDB data. Individual NPs may see their NPDB file and add a brief comment to give their version of an incident listed in the database.

Working with Practice Guidelines

An NP may be following practice guidelines as a matter of law, policy, or good practice. Some states require an NP to establish practice protocols or guidelines, with or without a physician's input.

NPs should consult state law to determine whether written guidelines are required. Written guidelines should meet these criteria:

1. Do not write guidelines so detailed that they cannot reasonably be followed in everyday practice.
2. Base guidelines on evidence and widely used resources, and reference those resources in the guidelines.
3. Practices may adopt an already published set of guidelines.
4. Follow the guidelines.
5. If the guidelines are inappropriate for a particular patient, document why an alternative tack is being taken.
6. If guidelines are not followed because a patient will not comply, document efforts to follow guidelines and patient noncompliance.

The federal Agency for Healthcare Research and Quality (AHRQ) establishes guidelines for practice and conducts research into what works and what does not work in healthcare prevention and treatment. AHRQ has established guidelines for the care of certain conditions. An NP who is caring for patients with conditions addressed by AHRQ should follow the AHRQ guidelines or document why the guidelines are inappropriate for a particular patient. AHRQ changes its guidelines fairly frequently to keep up with new evidence. Visit the AHRQ website (http://www.ahrq.gov) to check for new and retired guidelines.

How to Prevent Lawsuits

1. Be careful about establishing patient–provider relationships. If an NP gives medical advice to a person, for example in a social situation, that person is considered a patient and thus the NP should exercise all of the cautions and standards that they would exercise with a patient in an office or hospital setting.
2. Know the standard of care and practice within it.
3. If practice guidelines or protocols have been adopted by the office or agency, follow them.
4. When in doubt, take a conservative approach.
5. Rule out the worst diagnoses early on.
6. Know the limits of training and expertise.
7. Follow up.

What to Do If Sued

1. Call the NP's professional liability insurance company to report the lawsuit.
2. Do not talk about the suit with anyone but the NP's attorney. Specifically, do not talk with the plaintiff/patient or the plaintiff's attorney.
3. Consider retaining the NP's own attorney if the suit is against a group.
4. Never change a record after learning of a lawsuit (or for any other reason).
5. A deposition—a pretrial information-gathering session—can be as important as a trial in terms of the need for preparation. What an NP says in deposition can lock the NP into what he or she may say at trial.
6. Think carefully before agreeing to settle. Settlement awards will appear on an NP's NPDB record.

Communication

Researchers who compared the time physicians spent with patients with malpractice history found that primary care doctors with two or more malpractice claims against them spent 15 minutes on average with each patient, whereas doctors with no malpractice claims against them spent an average of 18.3 minutes with each patient. Quality-of-care ratings for the sued physicians were as good as ratings for physicians who had not been sued.[3]

Experienced NPs know that good provider–patient communication means better outcomes and higher patient satisfaction. Good communication also means fewer lawsuits. Satisfied patients generally do not sue.

Liability of Collaborating Physicians

In the past, some courts have found physicians liable for the negligent acts of NPs. In the majority of these cases, there was some element of physician involvement in the misdiagnosis. Nevertheless, physicians cannot expect to be fully free from the threat of lawsuit for the acts of the NPs they collaborate with or supervise until the legal requirements for collaboration are lifted.

Medical practices and agencies that set policies calling for supervision of NPs and other APNs can expect to be held liable when NPs are not, in fact, supervised.

Consider the following example: A Texas hospital had a contract with a group of anesthesiologists to provide anesthesia services. The anesthesia group employed certified registered nurse anesthetists (CRNAs). The contract between the hospital and the anesthesia group stated that all CRNAs would be supervised by the anesthesia group. The hospital's written policies and procedures required "direct and personal" supervision of CRNAs by physicians. Hospital policy also required that (1) patients be fully informed about the anesthesia providers who would be giving care, (2) an anesthesiologist prepare and evaluate patients about to have surgery, (3) CRNAs document and discuss the evaluation of their patients with a supervising anesthesiologist or surgeon, and (4) the supervising physician countersign all orders for medications.

One night, a CRNA working without an anesthesiologist onsite attempted to intubate a patient having respiratory distress during a Caesarean section. The CRNA called the anesthesiologist on call to come in right away. The anesthesiologist immediately headed for the hospital. The CRNA eventually was able to intubate, but the patient suffered irreversible brain injury.

The patient and her husband settled with the CRNA and physician. The plaintiff's suit against the hospital went to trial. The plaintiffs argued that the hospital was negligent for failing to adopt, implement, and enforce appropriate policies relating to providing an anesthesiologist, having an anesthesiologist evaluate the patient, supervising the CRNA, disclosing that a nurse was providing anesthesia, failing to exercise care in credentialing, and failing to ensure proper quality assurance and peer review in the anesthesia department.

The jury found that the hospital had not followed its own policies. The jury also found that the CRNA and physician were not negligent but found that the hospital was negligent, that the hospital's negligence was the cause of the patient's injuries, and that the hospital was liable for the injury to the patient.

The hospital appealed the case. The appeals court upheld the jury's decision. [*Denton Reg. Med. Ctr. v. LaCroix*, No. 2-95-003-CV (Tex. Ct. App. June 26, 1997).]

A physician is not automatically liable for the negligence of an NP with whom the physician has a written agreement to collaborate when called upon. Generally, some neglect by the physician has to be proven.

On the other hand, if a physician is required, by policy or law, to supervise, then a physician has the responsibilities of supervisors in general. In general, employers and supervisors must determine that their employees or supervisees are adequately trained and competent in the areas in which they practice. If employees or supervisees are not adequately trained or competent, then the employer or supervisor is obligated to provide further training and guidance or to replace the employee or supervisee. If policies are called for, by law or higher policy, supervisors are responsible for ensuring that policies are in place. If supervisors know that policies are not being followed by employees or supervisees, it is their responsibility to monitor supervised personnel until policies are followed, or to replace the personnel.

Guidelines for physicians who are required by law or policy to collaborate with or supervise NPs and who want to avoid malpractice based on the negligence of an employed NP include the following:

1. Ascertain that the NP is licensed, and verify the NP's education, training, and malpractice history.
2. Comanage patients with the NP until the physician can confirm that the NP is professionally competent.
3. Consult state law to determine what is required of a collaborating physician. Conform to state requirements.
4. Consult state law regarding scope of NP practice. Do not encourage the NP to go further than scope of practice allows unless the physician develops written protocols or is physically present.
5. Telephone diagnosis is risky for both the physician and the NP. If an after-hours call is a necessity of practice, establish a second level of call whereby NPs taking calls can get backup.
6. Consult state law to determine whether an NP is independent or dependent upon physician collaboration or supervision. If supervision is required by law, determine whether direct or indirect supervision is required. "Direct supervision" of an NP requires a physician to be immediately and physically available should the need arise. "Indirect supervision" or "general supervision" requires that the physician be on the premises or available by telephone in a timely and consistent manner.
7. If practice guidelines or protocols exist, follow them.
8. Consider supporting NP organizations in their efforts to eradicate legal requirements of supervision or collaboration. Support legal language that places responsibility for an NP's actions squarely on the NP. A physician who employs an NP who is independently responsible for their actions is less likely to be vicariously liable for an NP's malpractice, and a physician can spend less time in supervisory activities.

Malpractice Insurance

An NP cannot control everything. Everyone makes mistakes. Insurance provides a comfort factor that is well worth the money.

Four frequently asked questions about malpractice insurance are: (1) Do I need to have my employer cover me under the hospital/university/practice policy? (2) Will I be more likely to be sued if I have malpractice insurance? (3) Should I get "claims made" or "occurrence" insurance? and (4) Which company's policy is best?

Do I Need Insurance if My Employer Covers Me Under the Hospital, University, or Practice Policy?

NPs who treat patients outside of their work settings or who moonlight definitely need individual insurance policies. For example, many NPs are approached by neighbors, friends, and relatives for prescriptions. The wise NP will not only treat each of these encounters as thoroughly as if the friend was a patient at the office (or decline to become involved at all), but have malpractice insurance to cover the possibility of a mistake.

An NP who neither moonlights nor treats neighbors and friends may still want an individual policy, even if an employer covers an NP under an umbrella policy. Why? Because a lawsuit fractures collegial alliances. The human tendency is to deny one's own liability and blame others. In such an environment, each healthcare provider needs an advocate to protect his or her interests. Insurance will pay for that defense.

Am I More Likely to Be Sued if I Have Malpractice Insurance?

Possibly, but that is not a good reason to forego insurance. Patients do not usually know whether an NP has malpractice insurance. An injured patient who consults an attorney usually files suit before the patient or his or her attorney knows the insured status of the healthcare provider being sued. Information about the insurance usually comes out in the discovery process in preparation for trial.

However, an NP who tells patients about his or her malpractice coverage may provide an incentive for a litigious patient or may relieve a reluctant patient from any feeling of guilt over suing a respected healthcare provider.

Should I Get "Claims Made" or "Occurrence" Insurance?

Get "occurrence" insurance, which covers any incident that occurred while the NP was insured. Under a "claims made" policy, an NP is covered only when the insurance policy is active, no matter when the incident occurred. If an NP retires, leaves the profession, or no longer has need for active insurance, the NP must nevertheless keep a "claims made" insurance policy active (pay the premium) to receive coverage for incidents that happened in years past. A "claims made" policy is extended through purchasing of a "tail" policy.

Which Company's Policy Is Best?

NPs should choose a company that is located in the United States (in case the NP has to sue the insurance company), has been in business at least 10 years, and has a stable financial rating.

An NP will be able to judge the quality of his or her insurer only after a lawsuit is over. There are no surveys of sued NPs that provide guidance about which company provides the best service.

Notes

1. Andrews, L. B. (1997). An alternative strategy for studying adverse events in medical care. *Lancet, 349,* 309–313. A more recent study found that medical errors occurred in half of all hospital admissions for general pediatric surgery. See Proctor, M. L., et al. (2003). Incidence of medical errors and adverse outcomes on a pediatric general surgery service, *Journal of Pediatric Surgery, 38*(9), 1361–1365.
2. Hooker, R. S., Nicholson, J. G., & Le, T. (2009). Does the employment of physician assistants and nurse practitioners increase liability? *Journal of Medical Licensure Discipline, 95*(2),6–16.
3. Levinson, W., Roter, D., Mullooly, J., Dull, V., & Frankel, R. (1997). The relationship with malpractice claims among primary care physicians and surgeons. *JAMA, 227,* 553–559.

Resources

Buppert, C. (2010). Avoiding malpractice. Law Office of Carolyn Buppert, P.C. Available from the author's website at http://www.buppert.com/publications.html

Medical Malpractice Verdicts, Settlements, and Experts, newsletter, Lewis Laska, editor. Contact: 901 Church St., Nashville, TN 37203, 1-800-298-6288.

Risk Management

Risk management is what one does to avoid problems later. Compare risk management to preventive medicine; risk management prevents legal problems.

Nurse practitioners (NPs) are at risk for two categories of professional mishap: clinical mishap and business mishap. There can be great overlap between clinical and business problems; that is, a clinical problem can turn into a business problem and then into a legal problem. For example, when an NP makes a clinical error and a patient discovers the error, the patient is quite likely to tell friends, relatives, and coworkers. Then the problem evolves into a business problem for the NP because the friends, relatives, and coworkers of that patient are unlikely to visit the NP. If the patient is harmed by the NP's error and files a lawsuit based on malpractice, the NP also has a legal problem.

All NPs face certain risks associated with practice:

- Risk of making a clinical error
- Risk of being sued for malpractice when there was no clinical error
- Risk of public perception that the NP is a poor-quality provider
- Risk of breaching patient confidentiality and/or privacy
- Risk of failing to inform patients fully about treatment and to get informed consent to treat
- Risk of failing to disclose information that patients need to get follow-up
- Risk of poor quality ratings
- Risk of disciplinary action
- Risk of being accused of Medicare fraud for upcoding a patient visit
- Risk of business failure as a result of downcoding patient visits

Whether any of these risks becomes an actual problem is largely up to the NP.

Risk of Making a Clinical Error

Medical professionals who have been sued report that the experience soured their attitude toward their profession. NPs are rarely sued. Nevertheless, a lawsuit, even a lawsuit where the NP is not found to be liable, is a devastating personal experience. Therefore, every NP should incorporate into his or her practice an awareness of how to avoid malpractice.

NPs will maintain their positive attitudes toward their profession by practicing litigation avoidance techniques, just as they would advocate preventive medicine and healthcare maintenance to their patients. Avoidance measures include exercising caution about establishing patient–provider relationships and, when a patient–provider relationship has been established, practicing consistently in conjunction with the accepted standard of care for NPs.

What Is Malpractice?

Malpractice is a failure of professional skill that results in injury, loss, or damage. A claim of malpractice requires that a patient/plaintiff prove the following:

1. The existence of a client–professional relationship—a "duty of care."
2. Behavior below the appropriate standard of care for professionals dealing in like circumstances.
3. A causal link between the practitioner's failure to conform to treatment standards and harm to the patient.
4. Actual injury to the patient.

More detailed information on medical malpractice is provided elsewhere in the text.

Existence of a Professional Relationship

A patient–provider relationship is established when a patient arrives at an NP's office for a visit, when an NP undertakes the care of a hospitalized patient, or when an NP makes a home visit to a patient. However, patient–provider relationships also can arise in other less obvious ways, including the following:

- Over the telephone
- At a social gathering
- By supervising another's treatment
- By providing sample medication
- By giving advice or opinions to family or friends

When Is a Person a "Patient"?

Consider the following example: NP Jones receives a message to call Nurse Smith at home. Nurse Smith is a former colleague of NP Jones, and Jones remembers Smith as a very talented and competent nurse. Smith is calling about a personal health matter. Smith's son, James, age 6, has an earache. James has had several earaches in the past, all caused by infections, all cleared by amoxicillin. James is otherwise completely healthy, reports Smith.

Smith is working the evening shift, and James is in first grade all day. Smith does not have time to see James' pediatrician until the end of the month, 2 weeks away. Nor does Smith want to pay the $25 copay to see the pediatrician. NP Jones remembers that he met James once at a picnic, but he has never seen James in the office. Smith recalls that she has always respected NP Jones's judgment. Smith asks NP Jones, a family NP, to prescribe amoxicillin for James. Smith is asking a favor, as she and NP Jones both know that Smith's HMO insurance will not reimburse NP Jones for an office visit.

Is 6-year-old James NP Jones's patient? If NP Jones calls in a prescription for James, the answer is yes.

Managing Risk by Limiting Patient Relationships

If NP Jones gives any advice to Nurse Smith or prescribes any medication to James, NP Jones has taken on a professional relationship with James, and James is now NP Jones's patient. NP Jones will then be liable for any breach in the standard of care that leads to an injury to James. It does not matter that James is the patient of another provider. It does not matter that NP Jones will receive no compensation for treating James. It does not matter that the interaction occurs solely over the telephone.

NP Jones, to protect himself (manage his risk), should either: (1) politely refuse to give advice, other than that Smith should call James's pediatrician, or (2) require Smith to bring James to NP Jones's office to go through the usual new patient evaluation before Jones prescribes an antibiotic or otherwise treats James. NP Jones should then follow up with James as NP Jones would with any of his patients.

For 95 out of 100 times that NP Jones is presented with a situation like this, NP Jones could proceed to treat the child over the telephone with no ill effects to the child or to NP Jones's malpractice history. However, NP Jones will be liable in court for the 5% of cases where: (1) the mother makes an erroneous diagnosis, (2) the mother does not know that the organism in the child's ear is resistant to the antibiotic used in the past, or (3) there is some other problem that NP Jones would have discovered with a careful history and physical examination.

In short, NPs should say "no" to all requests they receive for care that skirt the normal, safe evaluation process. The lesson of this case may seem elementary to experienced NPs. However, it is included because the pressure is great to deliver care to people who "just want a little advice" but are not "patients." It is easy for an NP to forget that they bear professional responsibility for *any* healthcare advice given.

What Is the Standard of Care for NPs?

The standard of care in any clinical situation is discovered by answering the question: What reasonable and ordinary care, skill, and diligence would be given by practitioners in good standing, in the same geographic area, in the same general type of practice in similar cases?

NPs are held to the standard of care of the reasonable and diligent NP. Is this the same standard that pertains to physicians? It may be. If the NP is performing primary care services, for example, the standard of care for an NP and for a physician performing those services will be the same standard.

Consider the example of *Fein v. Kaiser Permanente* (discussed in detail elsewhere in the text). The Fein case is a good illustration of a missed diagnosis. In that case, Mr. Fein, a middle-aged attorney, called a Kaiser clinic at midday complaining of chest pains. He got a 4 PM appointment, at which time he was evaluated by an NP who incorrectly diagnosed musculoskeletal pain. Mr. Fein was having a myocardial infarction. Later in the evening,

Mr. Fein was evaluated by a physician, who also incorrectly diagnosed Mr. Fein's chest pain. It was not until Mr. Fein's third visit that an electrocardiogram was done.

The NP easily could have ruled out myocardial infarction through an electrocardiogram at the first visit. That would be risk management. A prudent NP faced with a middle-aged male patient with chest pain would rule out myocardial infarction before diagnosing musculoskeletal pain. In this case, the NP and physician shared the same standard of care.

How Does an NP Keep Up with the Standard of Care?

Sources of information about standards of care for any specific disease or healthcare maintenance effort include:

- Internet articles
- Newsletters and listserves
- Textbooks and reference books
- Professional journals
- Respected colleagues
- Continuing education presentations
- Government agency–generated guidelines, such as Agency for Healthcare Research and Quality guidelines

An NP who wishes to avoid breaching the standard of care will consult current books and journals on a day-to-day basis, will attend continuing education presentations regularly, will refer patients to specialists when necessary, and will seek consultation from attending or consulting physicians or from other NPs when necessary.

Risk of Being Sued for Malpractice When There Was No Clinical Error

Some patients sue healthcare providers when there was a poor outcome but no actual malpractice on the part of the provider. Whether a provider has, in fact, fulfilled the elements of malpractice is not determined until there is a trial on the matter or the matter is settled out of court.

NPs who have the opportunity to defuse a potential lawsuit through extra time spent with a dissatisfied patient should do so, even if they know that any threatened lawsuit is ultimately without merit. Therefore, risk management efforts aimed at avoiding lawsuits include keeping patients satisfied and appeasing dissatisfied patients. Patients are annoyed by long waits for appointments, long waits in the office waiting room, impersonal treatment, and constant busy signals when trying to call the office. Keeping in mind the estimate that 90% of dissatisfied patients will not complain, it is wise to pay attention to patient complaints and to attempt to resolve problems with patients.

Risk of Public Perception That the Individual NP Is a Poor-Quality Provider

The risk of being perceived as a poor-quality provider is perhaps more of a business risk than a legal risk. How could an NP get a reputation as a poor provider? Like any other professional, an NP can get a poor reputation by failing to follow up with clients; by being inattentive, late, forgetful, or sloppy in appearance, demeanor, language, or intellect; by being unreliable; or by being unable to make a decision.

Risk of Breaching Patient Confidentiality

Patients have a right to confidentiality. Breach of privacy is an intentional tort and can be the basis for a lawsuit by a patient. Breach of privacy also can be malpractice, the basis for a disciplinary action by a state's board of nursing, and a violation of state and federal law. And, under federal regulations, a patient who feels that his or her NP has violated his or her privacy rights can complain to the U.S. Office of Civil Rights. The Office may investigate, and, if an NP has not complied with the government's recommendations aimed at protecting patient privacy, the government may fine the NP.

NPs can breach a patient's confidentiality in the following ways:

- Talking about a patient within earshot of others
- Releasing medical information about a patient without prior written permission
- Leaving a telephone message on a patient's answering machine
- Discussing a patient's condition with family members
- Leaving patient records within view
- Discarding unshredded duplicate records
- Giving a patient's name and address to a vendor
- Accessing a patient's medical record unnecessarily, for curiosity purposes
- Leaving a laptop containing patient information on a subway train
- Faxing patient data to the wrong number, by mistake

It is unusual for patients to sue for breach of confidentiality and it may be difficult for patients to prove. However, patient word of mouth about perceived breaches of confidentiality can harm community perception of a medical practice or provider. Therefore, NPs should seek private places to discuss patients, arrange for discarded records to be shredded, keep records out of view of others, and decline to discuss patient conditions or send written documents on a patient unless the NP has the patient's written permission. An example of an authorization form to use when it is necessary to disclose information about patients to third parties for reasons other than patient treatment, payment, or healthcare operations is given in **Exhibit   1**.

Exhibit 1 Sample Authorization Form

This form allows a patient to authorize release of protected healthcare information for specified purposes other than treatment, payment, and operations, or to disclose protected healthcare information to a specified third party.

I authorize [Name of provider and/or class of person authorized to make the use or disclosure] to release my:

□ Name
□ Address
□ Telephone number
□ Email address
□ Social security number
□ Insurance policy information
□ Diagnosis or health status
□ Laboratory tests or results
□ X-rays
□ Immunization record
□ Physical exam results
or
□ Other information about my health status, described as follows:

_____

_____

To: [Name of authorized recipients or class of recipients to which information may be released]

via:

□ Fax to [Name and number]
□ Mail to [Name and address]
□ Telephone to [Name and telephone number]
□ Pick up in person

For the purposes of:

_____

_____

This authorization is effective on the date signed and continues until:

□ [Provide date]

I understand the following:

a. If I refuse to authorize release of my health information, [Name of practice and provider] may not refuse to treat me.
b. I may revoke this authorization at any time by notifying [Name and contact information of privacy officer].
c. The information disclosed pursuant to this authorization may be redisclosed by the recipient and therefore may be outside the protection of federal rules on privacy.
d. The healthcare provider named here:
   ☐ will
   ☐ will not
   receive remuneration for disclosing information about me.

_____
Signature

_____
Printed name

_____
Date

Risk of Violating a Patient's Right to Informed Consent

A patient has a right to consent to the care being given and a right to refuse care that is offered. An NP has a legal responsibility to give a patient enough information about the risks and benefits of the care being offered that the patient can make an informed decision about accepting the care.

Informed consent involves disclosure of material risks of care and requires that a patient be competent to understand the risks and make a judgment about accepting care. The doctrine of informed consent requires that there be no coercion in getting a patient to consent to care. The law of informed consent is physician oriented, but the doctrine can be expected to be upheld when an NP is the caregiver.

The doctrine of informed consent arose from a societal desire to discourage persons from unauthorized touching of others. The predisposition against nonconsensual touching expanded when applied to the practice of medicine. In medicine, the requirement is that a physician must inform a patient about what is to be done and obtain the patient's consent before treating. Even though the doctrine of informed consent is grounded in the law of battery, the objective of the courts in applying the doctrine of informed consent has been more involved than the simple avoidance of one person's unauthorized touching of another. The majority of courts have adopted a self-determination rationale for informed consent. That is, a person has a right to determine what shall be done with his or her body.[1]

Many cases where patients have complained that their right to informed consent was violated involved surgery. Of course, surgery is only one of many possible treatments, and physicians are only one of many possible healthcare providers. There are many decisions to be made when a person seeks medical attention, most of which are less dramatic than surgery. For example, prescription drugs have been known to have side effects not discovered until years after the drugs are in common use. Even when a treatment has been used for years with relatively few complications, patients subjected to treatment may want to know that they are taking a risk and that there may be side effects.

An NP who is trying to minimize personal risk and risk to a patient will give as much information as possible to a patient contemplating any therapy. How much information does a patient need? Enough to formulate a reasonable decision.

If an NP failed to get informed consent from a patient before treating the patient, the patient could sue the NP, basing a suit on battery or on negligence. A patient who sued an NP for battery would claim that the patient had not authorized the NP to touch the patient. A patient who sued on the basis of negligence would claim that the NP had not given the patient enough information to consent, in an informed way, to the treatment. In either case, a patient could win monetary damages from an NP.

Does an NP need to get consent for everything? It is well established that before a surgeon performs surgery, he or she must obtain the informed consent of the patient. It is less clear whether an NP must get informed consent before prescribing medication; whether minor but invasive procedures, such as blood transfusion, the starting of intravenous lines, and office incision and drainage, require informed consent; and whether noninvasive treatments carrying some risk, such as office psychotherapy, massage, or even an examination, require informed consent.

At least 25 states have legislation regarding informed consent.[2] An example of an informed-consent statute, one that is oriented toward the physician, is New York's. That law defines lack of informed consent as:

> Failure of the person providing the professional treatment or diagnosis to disclose to the patient such alternatives thereto and the reasonable, foreseeable risks and benefits involved as a reasonable medical, dental, or podiatric practitioner under similar circumstances would have disclosed, in a manner permitting the patient to make a knowledgeable evaluation.

> *Citation:* N.Y. Pub. Health Law § 2805-d.

The law limits the right of action to nonemergent therapies and diagnostic procedures that involve invasion or disruption of the integrity of the body. The statute conforms with New York's case law, which limits the cause of action to procedures that are invasive. The law lists defenses.

Another example of a statute addressing informed consent is Washington's (Wash. Rev. Stat. Ann. Code § 7.70.050). That law states the elements of informed consent as: (1) failure to inform regarding a material fact, (2) patient consented without being aware of the facts, (3) a reasonably prudent patient would not have consented if the information had been adequately conveyed, and (4) injury to the patient.

All states have case law requiring that physicians inform patients of the risks and benefits of surgery and obtain patient consent in writing before doing surgery.

Some courts have defined treatment broadly.[3] Among the nonsurgical treatments around which informed-consent issues have emerged are application of oxygen to a neonate [*Burton v. Brooklyn Doctor's Hosp.* 88 A.D.2d 217, 452 N.Y.S. 2d 875 (App. Div. 1982)],[4] radiation therapy [*Nelson v. Patrick*, 58 N.C. App. 546, 293 S.E.2d 829 (Ct. App. 1982), appeal after remand 73 N.C. App. 1, 326 S.E.2d 45 (1985)], and gastroscopy [*Cooper v. Roberts*, 220 Pa. Super. 260, 286 A.2d 647 (Super. Ct. 1971)]. The courts found that the plaintiffs had causes of action. The Supreme Court of Pennsylvania stated that a physician's duty to disclose a collateral risk involved in treatment is the same "whether or not the treatment can be technically termed operative" (*Cooper v. Roberts*, 220 Pa. Super. 260, 2, 286 A.2d).

Other courts, while not holding that the doctrine of informed consent applies to non-surgical treatments, have stated in an aside (dictum) that the term "treatment" can be broadly construed [*Pratt v. University of Minn. Affiliated Hosps. and Clinics*, 414 N.W.2d 399 (Minn. Ct. App. 1987)]. The state that defines treatment most broadly is Minnesota. According to the Minnesota Supreme Court, bed rest, when combined with special instructions, would constitute treatment [*Madsen v. Park Nicollet Med. Ctr.*, 431 N.W.2d 855 (Minn. 1988)]. At the opposite extreme is New York, where the need for informed consent is limited to invasive procedures [*Karlsons v. Guerinot*, 57 A.D.2d 73, 394 N.Y.S.2d 933 (App. Div. 1977)].

At least one court has declined to find the need for informed consent in a common, minor, invasive procedure. Informed consent was not applicable to the giving of a flu shot in a Louisiana medical clinic. The court stated that "medical or surgical procedure" did not extend to a flu shot and that to hold otherwise would lead to results in the day-to-day practice of medicine never intended by the legislature [*Novak v. Texada, Miller, Masterson and Davis Med. Clinic*, 514 So. 2d 524, writ denied, 515 So. 2d 807 (La. 1987)]. That one court found bed rest a treatment but another found an injection not a medical or surgical procedure demonstrates the inconsistency of viewpoint among jurisdictions.

The Minnesota Supreme Court, going a step further than most other jurisdictions, stated, "[We] believe there may be some nontreatment situations where the doctrine should be applicable" [*Pratt v. University of Minn. Affiliated Hosps. and Clinics*, 414 N.W.2d 399 (Minn. Ct. App. 1987)]. In *Pratt*, a case about genetic counseling, a plaintiff couple asserted that physicians had been negligent in not disclosing the risk of the couple's encountering a particular genetic abnormality in future children. The physicians, after interviewing the couple and obtaining the tests available, had rejected one possible diagnosis, autosomal recessive disorder, as highly unlikely. Therefore, they did not disclose to the parents the risks of that condition. A subsequent child of the couple was born with autosomal recessive disorder, the diagnosis thought unlikely by the physicians. The plaintiffs asked the Minnesota court to apply to genetic counseling a variation on the doctrine of informed consent [*Pratt v. University of Minn. Affiliated Hosps. and Clinics*, 414 N.W.2d 399 (Minn. Ct. App. 1987)]. Because diagnostic advice and counseling, not treatment, was the medical service involved, the term *negligent nondisclosure* was used. Negligent nondisclosure is discussed more fully in the next section.

The court held that the mere diagnosis of a condition, where all appropriate tests have been performed, does not give rise to a duty to disclose risks inherent in conditions not diagnosed [*Pratt v. University of Minn. Affiliated Hosps. and Clinics*, 414 N.W.2d 399 (Minn. Ct. App. 1987)]. While negligent nondisclosure did not apply in this case, the court stated that the doctrine could be applicable in some other nontreatment situations.

In summary, there is wide disparity among the states regarding how the doctrine of informed consent may be applied. At one end of the continuum, informed consent is needed only for invasive procedures. At the other end, it is needed for counseling.

In *Canterbury v. Spence* [464 F.2d 777 (D.C. Cir. 1972)] [See also *Sard v. Hardy* (281 Md. 432, 379 A.2d 1014)], the U.S. Court of Appeals for the District of Columbia Circuit gave some general advice to physicians that holds true today and can be applied to NPs. The court declined to adopt a standard of full disclosure, saying that it is prohibitive and unrealistic to expect physicians to discuss every risk of a proposed treatment and that such full information generally is unnecessary from a patient's viewpoint. However, the court listed physicians' responsibilities regarding disclosure:

1. Communicate information to the patient when the exigencies of reasonable care call for it.
2. Alert the patient to symptoms of bodily abnormality.
3. Inform the patient when the ailment does not respond to the physician's ministrations.
4. Instruct the patient about any limitations to be observed for his or her own welfare.
5. Inform the patient about precautionary therapy that he or she should seek in the future.
6. Advise the patient of the need for or desirability of any alternative treatments promising greater benefit than that being pursued.
7. Advise the patient regarding risks to his or her well-being that the contemplated therapy may involve.

Citation: *Canterbury v. Spence*, 464 F.2d 772 (D.C. Cir. 1972).

Many practices cover the risk of a claim of battery by having each patient sign a consent to an examination at the time of registration. Most practices have informed-consent policies that address invasive procedures, such as endometrial biopsy, cervical biopsy, and incision and drainage.

NPs who want to avoid the risk of violating the informed-consent doctrine should do the following:

- Give patients information on risks, benefits, and alternatives to any invasive procedure, and obtain written consent for any procedure.
- Find out what state law requires in the way of informed consent for specific tests, treatments, and procedures.

- Give patients information on the risks, benefits, and alternatives to any treatment, including prescription medications, and ask for their agreement to the treatment.
- Document that information about the risks, benefits, and alternatives to the treatment has been given to the patient and that the patient agrees to the treatment.

Does an NP Need to Get Consent in Writing?

Consent to surgery must be in writing. Consent for invasive procedures that could be considered surgery—endometrial biopsy, for example—should also be in writing. If state law requires consent for specific testing, it must be in writing. In general, however, consent to medical treatment need not be in writing.

Special Cases
Emergency Situations

In an emergency, care may be given to save a patient's life, even if consent cannot be obtained prior to treatment.

Incompetency

A patient who is unconscious or mentally retarded; who has been judged insane; who cannot read, write, or hear; or who is under the influence of sedative drugs or alcohol is not competent to give consent. With the exception of an emergency situation, NPs should avoid treating such patients unless a parent or a court-appointed guardian is available to give consent.

Minors

Minor children cannot consent to treatment. Parental consent is necessary.

Risk of Negligent Nondisclosure

The doctrine of negligent nondisclosure emerged when a physician found an abnormality but failed to sufficiently alert the patient. For example, in *Cornfeldt v. Tongen* [262 N.W.2d 684 (Minn. 1977)], a physician failed to inform a patient of abnormalities in blood testing prior to surgery.

The Minnesota Supreme Court defined the elements of negligent nondisclosure as: (1) nondisclosure of a risk inherent in the treatment, (2) harm materialized from that risk, and (3) proximate causation. The elements of lack of informed consent are the same. The terms *lack of informed consent* and *negligent nondisclosure* refer to the same concept, though they are applicable in different situations. Consent is applicable when a treatment is proposed. Nondisclosure is applicable when an omission of information leads to an injury.

Under the doctrine of negligent nondisclosure, a physician (or an NP), having examined a patient and having found an abnormality, has a duty to inform the patient of the abnormality so that the patient can choose whether to submit to further tests [*Gates v. Jensen*, 92 Wash. 2d 246, 595 P.2d (1979); *Canterbury v. Spence*, 464 F.2d 777 (D.C. Cir. 1972)]. All facts must be disclosed that the doctor (or, by inference, the NP) knows or should know for the patient to make a decision. Some examples include *Truman v. Thomas*, 165 Cal. Rptr. 308, 611 P.2d 902 (Cal. 1980), in which a patient sued a physician for failing to disclose the danger of refusing a Pap smear, and *Lauderdale v. United States*, 666 F. Supp. 1511 (D. Ala. 1987), in which a physician was found liable when he did not inform a patient of a heart problem, the seriousness of the problem, and the necessity for a return visit.

In *Gates*,[5] a physician discovered an increased pressure in a patient's eyes. This suggested glaucoma, a treatable eye disease. The physician failed to inform the patient of the abnormality and of diagnostic procedures that could be undertaken to determine the significance of the abnormality. This resulted in a delay in the diagnosis and treatment of the glaucoma. By the time glaucoma was diagnosed, the patient was functionally blind. The Supreme Court of Washington found that the physician had a duty of disclosure. The court held that the doctrine of informed consent required that the ophthalmologist inform the patient of an abnormality discovered during a routine examination and of diagnostic procedures that could be taken to determine the significance of that abnormality. The court reasoned that a physician has a fiduciary duty to inform a patient of abnormalities in his or her body.[6]

In *Truman*, the issue was whether a physician should have disclosed to his patient the risks of refusing a test. There, a physician had advised his patient to have a Pap smear, a test that detects the presence of cervical cancer, but did not inform her of the risks of refusing the test. She refused to have it. As a result, cancer of the cervix went undiscovered until it had become disseminated. The patient died at the age of 30. The Supreme Court of California held that the trial judge should have given an instruction to the jury that would have allowed the jury to consider whether the physician breached a duty by not disclosing to the patient the danger of failing to undergo a Pap smear.

From a healthcare provider's point of view, there are few guidelines. To give too much detail could be uneconomical. To give too little could be negligent. From a patient's point of view, a requirement that more information be given can be only beneficial.

Right of Patients to Refuse Treatment

Patients may refuse treatment. NPs caring for patients who refuse treatment that the NP believes is necessary should inform such patients of the risks of refusing treatment. After that, it is the patient's right to decide. NPs should document that they have explained the risks, benefits, and alternatives of treatment and the risks of refusing treatment and that the patient nevertheless refuses it.

Risk of Poor Quality Ratings

Increasingly, consumer-oriented groups and Medicare are compiling and reporting data on performance of healthcare providers using various measures. Consumer-oriented groups collect data from health plans, and health plans collect the data from medical practices. The National Committee on Quality Assurance's HEDIS (Health Plan Employer Data and Information Set) is currently the most commonly applied performance criterion among health plans. HEDIS data are gathered from patient surveys, patient charts, and billing forms. For more information or current HEDIS measures, visit the website (http://www.ncqa.org). Medicare collects quality data through its Physician Quality Reporting Initiative (PQRI). For more information on PQRI, visit the Center for Medicare and Medicaid Services (CMS) website (http://www.cms.hhs.gov).

An NP who wants to avoid the risk of poor quality ratings should:

- Understand what performance measures currently are being used
- Develop personal or practicewide systems for complying with performance guidelines and monitoring his or her performance
- Request and obtain feedback on performance

Risk of Disciplinary Action

A state board of nursing approves an NP's right to practice in a state. A board of nursing can suspend or revoke an NP's license.

A court cannot revoke an NP's license. A court can find against an NP in a malpractice lawsuit and direct an NP to pay an injured patient monetary damages, however. If, on the basis of what a judge hears in a case, the judge believes an NP to be grossly negligent, the judge may report the nurse to the board of nursing. *Gross negligence* is indifference to duty or the intentional failure to perform a manifest duty in reckless disregard of the consequences as affecting the life of another.

A board of nursing will respond not only to reports of gross nursing negligence, but also to reports of impairment, fraud, or criminal activity by nurses. Impairment could be reported by a patient, coworker, or supervisor, based on their observation of a nurse. Fraud might include falsifying the nurse's application to the board, falsifying medical records, or documenting that a patient has been seen when the patient has not. A nurse convicted of a felony can expect to be investigated by the board of nursing.

In general, the disciplinary process is as follows:

1. The NP receives a letter stating that he or she is being investigated by the board and requesting that the NP call the board to arrange a meeting.
2. The NP meets with an investigator. The investigator will produce records or other evidence of questionable care given by the NP and ask the NP to respond. The NP may explain why the NP conducted the care or documented the care as they did.
3. The investigator will gather information from other sources. The investigator may talk with auditors, colleagues, patients, or administrators.
4. The investigator will recommend to the board that the investigation be dropped or will recommend a hearing.
5. An administrative hearing, resembling a trial, will be held. The NP should be represented by an attorney. The board of nursing will be represented by a state attorney. Evidence may be presented. Witnesses may testify. Often, the board will give the nurse the option of a prehearing settlement conference. In that case, the nurse, his or her attorney, some board members, and some board staff meet in a less formal setting and discuss the matter. The board representatives may recommend a disposition of the matter without an evidentiary hearing.

6. A hearing officer (or board member present at the prehearing settlement conference) will make a recommendation to the board.
7. The board will decide to drop the matter or discipline the nurse.
8. Discipline may include probation, suspension of a license, or revocation of a license.
9. After the passage of a specified time period, the nurse whose license is revoked may reapply for licensure.

Only a small percentage of registered nurses have been subject to disciplinary action by boards of nursing. The percentage of NPs subject to disciplinary action is probably even smaller. However, NPs are subject to discipline, and it is not unusual for an NP to be called before the board of nursing for an investigatory meeting. For example, an NP might be reported to the board of nursing after an audit of a hospital or nursing home turned up irregularities.

An NP who receives a notice of investigation should be worried. Even if an investigator characterizes the meeting as nonadversarial and states that its purpose is strictly information gathering, an investigation is in fact adversarial and an NP has much to lose. NPs should know that state auditors of nursing homes are not NPs and may not be experienced in evaluating the work of NPs. Furthermore, board of nursing investigators usually are not NPs, though they are probably registered nurses (RNs). An RN investigator may ask such questions as, "This EKG [electrocardiogram] reading says 'abnormal EKG.' Why did you not call in a cardiologist, or send the patient to the emergency room?" The answer may well be: "That abnormality is a left axis deviation that was not clinically significant for that patient at that time. A cardiology consult or an emergency room visit was not clinically indicated." That response may end the inquiry about the abnormal EKG. The RN investigator may not know the nuances of EKG interpretation and may find that answer satisfactory. An NP who can explain all of his or her actions probably will find that the investigation ends with the meeting. However, an NP who is distraught by the nature of the investigation may not give clear explanations. An NP under the pressure and emotional upset of investigatory questioning may not be as assertive in defending his or her actions as is legally prudent.

An NP who receives a letter notifying him or her of an investigation by the board of nursing should retain an attorney immediately. The attorney should represent the NP at the initial meeting with the investigator for the board of nursing. Investigators may tell NPs that an attorney is not necessary. Investigators may also tell NPs that attorneys are not allowed at the meeting. Nevertheless, the NP should engage an attorney, and the attorney can communicate with the investigator about attending the meeting. Attorneys are comfortable with adversarial interactions, are experienced in advocating for clients, and are not likely to dissolve into tears when an investigator questions the NP's professional competency. Furthermore, an attorney will see that an NP's due process rights are protected through the investigation and hearing.

Risk of Medicare Fraud

In the past 15 years, the U.S. Justice Department has increased its investigative efforts into healthcare fraud and abuse. The level of fraudulent billing is such that an estimated 7% to 8% of total healthcare spending goes not for care given, but for care not given.[7]

NPs are responsible for ensuring that the billing for their services matches the level of care given and that their documentation matches the level of care billed. *Upcoding* is billing for a higher level of visit than actually was conducted. Upcoding is healthcare fraud.

Each Current Procedural Terminology (CPT) code has corresponding levels of required history taking, physical examination, and medical decision making, all of which must be supported in an NP's medical record documentation. For example, if an NP meets all of the criteria for a CPT 99214 visit and bills for a 99214 visit but documents only the criteria for a 99213 visit, the NP is at risk of being charged with Medicare fraud. Fraud is intentional deception. Billing a higher code than is supported by documentation may be unintentional. However, NPs are expected to know how to bill correctly. Ignorance is a poor defense. Furthermore, if a provider pleads ignorance but auditors find that more errors were made in overcoding than undercoding visits, a court will find that the upcoding was intentional. On the other hand, providers will not want to undercode. Undercoding will lead to low revenues for a practice.

Consequences of selecting an inappropriate code are Medicare or Medicaid audit failure, loss of Medicare or Medicaid provider status, a fine, and loss or restriction of the NP's license by the board of nursing. Obviously, the consequences also can include loss of one's job.

CMS and the American Medical Association have agreed upon a set of documentation guidelines. These guidelines went into effect in July 1998. Revisions have been proposed since then, but as of the publication of this text, clinicians should abide by the 1995 or 1997 guidelines, whichever the clinician finds to be most useful.

Business Risk Management

An NP who starts a business risks business failure. If the NP has partners or fellow directors or stockholders in a corporation, the NP also risks failure of those relationships.

Who Is the Boss?

Consider the following example: Nurse Practitioner Able and Nurse Practitioner Best have agreed to go into practice together. Able is an OB-GYN NP, and Best is a family NP. They are both very experienced. They have known each other for 5 years. They have never worked together, but each knows that the other is well respected in the community. They have carefully planned the business and have decided to be "equal partners."

A friend of Best's told Best that she should have a written agreement with Able. Best called Attorney Clodd, who told Best that he charged $350 an hour and that a partnership agreement usually ran about $900. Clodd also told Best that he would represent only Best and that Able should have her own attorney in the partnership-forming process. Able and Best wanted to forego the expenses of attorneys at this stage. They decided not to draw up a partnership agreement.

The practice opened. Able and Best had no problem choosing the location for the practice, the furniture, or the equipment. They agreed on a receptionist.

After 3 months, Best noticed that half of Able's patients were without insurance and that many did not pay for service at the time of service and owed the practice money. Best's patients had insurance for the most part. Furthermore, the lab was billing the practice for Pap smears and other expensive gynecologic tests, and the lab's bills were mounting. Best had been telling her patients that if there was no insurance to cover the visit and any necessary laboratory work, the patient, not the practice, was responsible for the office visit and lab charges.

Best told Able about the bills and the accounts receivable for Able's patients. Able, who saw her patient roster growing, did not want to offend patients by pressing about the bills. Best wanted to press the patients with outstanding bills for payment. Best's husband was tiring of Best being without a paycheck and was pressuring Best to be a better businessperson.

Who is the boss in this situation? Able and Best did not establish a method of resolving disagreements between them. Therefore, no one is the boss, and they could argue about this issue, or other issues, for years.

How to Avoid a Broken Partnership

When a practitioner starts a business alone, there is no confusion about who makes the administrative and business decisions. Whenever more than one person is involved, however, there will be more than one opinion on how the business should operate. Often, decisions must be made for which there is no "right" or "wrong" answer. Magazines on medical practice management and the civil courts are full of examples of partnerships gone sour. Often, the reasons for the breakup are differences of opinion on how practice collections are made and how practice money is spent. To avoid the risk of deadlocked disagreement, which can lead to hurt feelings, which in turn can lead to "wanting out," it is wise for the members of the group to agree upon a decision-making process from the outset.

Any private practice should have one of the following forms of business: sole proprietorship, partnership, or corporation. If the business is a corporation, the corporation's bylaws (or operating agreement, in the case of a limited liability corporation) describe the chain of command within the company. If the business is a partnership, the partners in the business should have an agreement between them specifying the decision-making process. Partners who fail to specify, early in the process of forming the practice, who is to make what decisions and how a deadlock will be resolved will be facing a short-lived association.

Drawing up an administrative chart should be one of the first tasks in the planning process. At minimum, all principal practitioners should agree to the administrative structure. It is prudent to consult an attorney.

Dealing with High-Risk Patients

Certain patient characteristics should alert an NP to be especially aware of risk management strategies. These characteristics are multisystem failure, low intelligence, polypharmacy, noncompliant behavior, positive review of systems, substance abuse, and litigiousness.

Multisystem Failure

Refer or work closely with a consultant when caring for patients with multisystem failure. The risk is failure to refer when the standard of care would call for referral.

Low Intelligence

Have a guardian present when counseling or teaching a patient with low intelligence. The risk is failure to get informed consent to treatment. A patient who does not have the intellectual capability to process information and make decisions about his or her own care cannot be assumed to have consented to treatment.

Polypharmacy

When patients are on many medications, list the medications, side effects, cautions, and dosing instructions for the patient, or coordinate with a pharmacist who will run computer printouts with the information. Review the dosing schedule with the patient at every visit. Ascertain that the patient can read—that the patient is literate and has adequate eyesight.

Noncompliant Patients

Document attempts and strategies for increasing compliance in the noncompliant patient. Document the patient's verbal responses to the NP's questions about why the patient has not taken the recommended medication, controlled the diet, or changed the dressings.

Positive Review of Systems

When a patient has a generally positive review of systems, consider expanding the patient's problem list even further to include somatization, need for social support, inability to cope with life's pressures, and dependency issues. Consider repeating the review of systems on another visit to see whether the complaints persist. If so, an NP should be prepared to dissect each complaint, taking the more risky complaints first. Whether the problem list is long or short, there is no difference in the standard of care expected of an NP.

Substance Abuse

Do not be lured into becoming a source for a patient who is abusing substances. Patients have sued their healthcare providers for contributing to their substance abuse by prescribing medication.

Litigiousness

Patients who bring up their ongoing lawsuits against another provider can be expected to repeat the performance by suing their current provider.

Notes

1. The right to self-determination was explained by J. Cardozo in 1914: "Every human being of adult years and sound mind has a right to determine what shall be done with his own body; and a [physician who administers treatment] without his patient's consent commits an assault for which he is liable in damages." *Schloendorff v. Society of N.Y. Hospital*, 211 N.Y. 25, 105 N.E. 92 (1914).

2. *Hospital Law Manual, Attorney's Vol. IIB*. (1983). Gaithersburg, MD: Aspen Publishers.

3. For example, in *Head v. Colloton* [331 N.W.2d 870, 875 (Iowa 1983)], the court said, "Treatment is broad enough to embrace all steps in applying medical arts to a person." In *Patrich v. Menorah Med. Ctr.* [636 S.W.2d 134 (1982)], the Missouri Court of Appeals defined treatment as "measures necessary for physical well-being of the patient." Black's Law Dictionary defines treatment as including "examination and diagnosis as well as application of remedies" (6th ed., 1990, p. 1502).

4. In this case, administration of oxygen in high doses caused blindness in the infant.

5. The court used the doctrine of informed consent, even though the issue was not one of consent but of knowledge of an abnormality requiring further evaluation.

6. A duty arises whenever a doctor becomes aware of an abnormality that may indicate risk or danger. The facts that must be disclosed are all those facts that the physician knows or should know that the patient needs to make a decision about treatment. Id. at 923.

7. Sparrow, M. K. (1996). *License to steal*. Boulder, CO: Westview Press.

Lawmaking and Health Policy

Health care is regulated for the public good, to ensure quality to a public that is powerless to assert quality control as individuals. That is the theory, at least. In the real world, health care is regulated for quality reasons, and because professional groups lobby for regulations that support their profession and businesses lobby for regulations that help their businesses. Regulation is imposed through statutes, regulations, and policies, and when a statute or regulation is challenged in court, through the judicial system.

The Legal Process

Statutes

A statute is a law enacted by a state legislature or Congress. Laws are found in state and federal codes. For example, Maryland statutes are found in the Maryland Code Annotated, and federal statutes are found in the U.S. Code Annotated (U.S.C.A.).

Citizens can influence the statutes that are enacted by electing representatives who they think will vote as they would and by lobbying those representatives for passage of bills about specific issues.

For example, in many states, nurse practitioners' (NPs') prescriptive authority is found in a statute. In those states, the legislatures have considered the issue of NP prescribing and have approved it.

Regulations

A regulation is law written by a state or federal agency in accordance with a statute. Agencies are a part of the executive branch of government. A regulation cannot directly contradict a statute but may expand upon a statute, supplying details not included in it. The divided responsibility—between the legislature to enact statutes and the executive branch agencies to write regulations—is part of the balance of power created by the U.S. Constitution.

Citizens have input into regulations in that regulations, prior to being adopted, usually are published for public review, with an opportunity for public comment. Agencies may or may not accept the comments. Further, citizens who are unhappy with a current regulation can enlist their legislators to enact laws that require agencies to change the regulations. For example, if state regulations addressing nursing homes do not address NP practice in nursing homes, a state NP organization can ask the director of the appropriate state agency for a change of regulation to include NPs as providers in nursing homes, ask legislators to request a regulation change, and, if necessary, ask legislators for a statute that requires the agency head to change regulations to allow NPs to practice in nursing homes.

Policies

Policies are rules made by companies or government agencies that do not have the force of law but that dictate day-to-day decisions. Citizens have input regarding policies only insofar as they can convince whomever has authority over a policy to change it. Citizens may also lobby legislators for a law that requires companies or government agencies to change a policy. For example, a health plan may have a policy of credentialing physicians only. Local NPs who want to be on a plan's provider panel will want to persuade the appropriate health plan decision maker, through facts, figures, and a presentation of projected benefits to the health plan, of the need to change policy and include NPs on the panel.

The Judicial System

A state court may hold that a state law is unconstitutional, and a federal court may hold that a federal law is unconstitutional. Courts may interpret laws and determine whether laws have been applied as the legislature, or Congress, meant them to be. A citizen who believes that a law has been misapplied and who has suffered damage as a result may bring suit in court in an effort to force correct application of a law. For example, in 1983, the medical board in Missouri brought legal action against two NPs practicing in a women's services clinic, arguing that the NPs were practicing medicine without medical licenses. The lower court agreed that the NPs were practicing medicine without a license, but the NPs took the case to the highest court in Missouri, and after reviewing historical documents, this court held that the intent of the legislature in expanding the nurse practice act had been to expand the scope of practice to include the activities performed by the NPs.

Health Policy

Policy is defined by the *Merriam-Webster Collegiate Dictionary* as "a definite course or method of action selected . . . to guide and determine present and future decisions."[1] Presidents and governors have policies on health care. Executive branch policies may influence the activities of federal and state agencies. However, unless policy becomes law, policy is like nursing theory: it may or may not have any effect on the way people do things.

An example of the influence of policy on the healthcare industry is President Clinton's 1994 effort at healthcare reform. The president had a definite course of action, a move toward a one-payer system; that is, government-run health care. The president's plan was not enacted, however. In fact, it was criticized so soundly that it was never even introduced as a bill in Congress. But the threat implied by the Clinton healthcare reform policies—that if the healthcare industry did not change itself, the government would impose changes— encouraged the private sector to reform. Health care today is quite different from health care in 1993. "Managed care" is now a household phrase. President Obama followed up on

President Clinton's efforts to reform health care, advocating for the Affordable Care Act (ACA), which passed Congress in 2010 and included some aspects of the Clinton plan. To date, however, it is unclear how the provisions of the ACA will ultimately change health-care policy and/or the industry and practice of health care.

Laws and Rules That Affect NPs

NPs are affected by laws, regulations, policies, and court decisions that address the following:

- The scope of NP practice
- Reimbursement for health services
- Qualifications for NP licensure and renewal
- Delegation of authority by physicians
- Quality of care
- Requirements for collaboration
- Confidentiality and patient privacy
- Electronic medical records and e-prescribing
- Medical homes

NPs have found laws, regulations, and policies to be barriers to the practice for which they were educated. How can NPs change these legal barriers?

Changing Laws

NPs who seek to change laws generally do so because they find that a statute, regulation, or policy keeps them from doing something necessary for practice. For example, NPs who were enrolled as Medicaid providers found that once Medicaid patients began enrolling in managed-care health plans, the NPs could no longer be the primary providers for their patients because the policies of the managed-care organizations (MCOs) precluded NPs from being admitted to primary care provider (PCP) panels.

In some states, the quest to change MCO policy has turned into an effort to enact new statutes. That is because MCOs, when asked to admit NPs to provider panels, said that the state law was unclear. Therefore, NPs have sought to clarify state laws such that they are specifically designated by statute as PCPs.

Understanding the Big Picture

Managed care is one aspect of the big picture that has and will affect NP practice.

What Is Going on in Managed Care?

Simply put, managed care is a system where the insurer is not only the payer, but also the provider of health care. Prior to managed care, insurance companies paid bills submitted by providers. The insurer had no control over the quality or quantity of care being given and had no responsibility to patients other than to pay bills. Under managed care, the insurer is responsible for the care given. The insurer keeps close tabs on the services provided. The insurer monitors how the healthcare services are utilized, as well as the costs of care, and sometimes denies, in advance or retrospectively, payment for services. Under fully developed managed care, insurers agree with purchasers to give care—whatever care is needed—for a fixed fee (monthly, yearly, or per procedure) and clinicians agree with insurers to give whatever care is needed for that fee. The clinician shares the financial risk that a patient will need more care than a payment covers with the insurer.

The bottom line is that insurers are not only concerned with cost; they now also monitor the quality of care given by providers and practices.

The healthcare industry has recently come under scrutiny regarding quality of care from the people who purchase the most services—employers who buy health care for employees—and from consumer-oriented groups. Employers are beginning to base decisions about which health plan services to offer employees based upon quality data gathered by such organizations as the National Committee for Quality Assurance (NCQA). Employers monitor the NCQA data, NCQA monitors health plans, health plans monitor practices, and, often, practices monitor individual providers.

State and national legislators, wanting to ensure that citizens' best interests are not overshadowed by the goals of employers and insurers to make money, are introducing bills to improve quality and to make sure that citizens get the care they want or need. For example, some state legislatures have passed bills requiring that health plans allow postpartum mothers to stay overnight in the hospital for 24 hours after delivery in response to the practice of health plans requiring mothers to go home shortly after delivery. Citizen groups felt that good care required that postpartum mothers have at least a 1-night hospital stay. Thus, legislatures have been delving into healthcare decisions formerly made only by clinicians, and lately made by insurers and clinicians.

Stages of Managed Care

An NP's place in the healthcare landscape depends on many factors. One factor is the stage of managed care in the region. In the early stages of managed care, most patients are covered by traditional insurers, and MCOs try to encourage employers who purchase health plans to enroll employees by offering premiums that cost less than those of traditional insurers. In the middle stages of development of managed care, more patients are enrolled, and MCOs try to control costs by decreasing the number of hospital visits, the length of stay in hospitals, and the number of emergency department visits, and by bargaining with medical practices for reduced rates on visits. In the advanced states of managed care, most patients are enrolled in managed care, and medical practices have agreed to share the risks. In other words, medical practices agree to take care of patients for a fixed amount of money per year. If care costs more than the set fee, providers lose money. If care costs less than the set fees, providers make a profit. In the later stages of development, much attention is paid to providing care that will prevent hospitalization and other high costs in the future, and to providing the nuts and bolts of care most cost effectively. It is at these later stages that NPs are most likely to fulfill the needs of MCOs.

Where Do NPs Appear in the Managed Care Landscape?

The position of NPs is well described by a favorite quote of the late Congressman Sonny Bono, "We have good soap to sell, but we have to go out and sell it." NPs are likely candidates for the position of PCPs, responsible for their own panels of patients. Consider the endorsement of NP practices given by Dr. Stephanie Seremetis, Director of the Women's Health Program at Mount Sinai Medical Center, "Probably in the future the best use will be nurse practitioners in independent practice, using a physician as a backup for complex conditions and for system analysis."[2] Or consider the endorsement by Joseph A. Califano, Jr., former U.S. Secretary of Health, Education, and Welfare:

> We should develop a three-tiered medical system: nonphysician practitioners, primary care physicians, and physician specialists. The first tier—the front line of delivery—should be the nonphysician practitioners: physician assistants, nurse practitioners, and certified nurse midwives. These professionals are capable, reliable and cost efficient.... They should be licensed to diagnose ailments, treat common diseases, prescribe drugs, admit patients to hospitals, and release them.... The second tier should be composed of primary care physicians: the family doctors, pediatricians, and general internists, including geriatric practitioners. These physicians should handle the more complex cases that do not require specialist care and be available to consult, guide, and, where appropriate, supervise the nonphysician practitioners.... The third tier should be specialists.[3]

Now that the United States, under the ACA, is in a situation where many previously uninsured people will soon become insured, many who follow health policy have begun to see NPs as a solution to an impending shortage of healthcare providers. Here is one comment to this effect, from a health policy brief in *Health Affairs*:

> With a predicted shortage of primary care as the population grows and as millions of people become newly insured starting in 2014, one proposed solution is to expand the role of nurse practitioners in many more areas of the country, and to allow them to provide a wider range of preventive and acute health care services.[4]

The views expressed by Dr. Seremetis, Mr. Califano, and *Health Affairs* concern the general welfare. What about the welfare of the NP? Consider the view of Joseph Tommasino, a physician assistant writing about both physician assistants and NPs:

> Our professional growth ... is essentially stunted by the simple fact that we have nowhere to go. We all grapple with, but seldom talk about, our lack of vertical mobility.... Want to change jobs? Submit your curriculum vitae and join the throng of PAs or NPs that apply for the job. True, your experience should ultimately speak for itself, but even if it does, will you get the salary you deserve? I doubt it, especially given the propensity of administrators to fill slots with the least expensive PAs or NPs.... One thing is certain, NPs and PAs must be proactive in designing their own career tracks.[5]

Salary aside, NPs who are practice owners have the opportunity to design a flow of care that makes sense from their point of view. It is not cast in stone that care must be given through an office visit. The office visit mode of healthcare delivery came about because of a physician-driven effort to tie reimbursement to physician services. Under capitated managed care and under the part of the ACA describing Accountable Care Organizations, a good model of care delivery is any model that keeps patients satisfied, meets quality standards, and is cost-effective. That could mean increased use of community health nurses, home visits, and school-based health care. Groups of creative NPs with open minds are capable of designing effective models that get out of the box established by fee-for-service medicine. Currently, however, in the majority of states, NPs are giving primary care under the auspices of a physician. The present situation is a function of past history, the present law, and public perceptions of physicians as givers of medical care.

Past History

Physicians "professionalized" their practice before nurses or other healthcare practitioners did and before the NP role even existed. Physicians convinced lawmakers to draw the legal lines such that only physicians could diagnose and treat and only physicians could order and perform tests and procedures, and prescribe medication. For many years, nurses went along with physician dominance.

NPs are now trying to climb a hill where physicians work at the top. The entrances are barricaded and are being shored up on all sides by physicians, who want to maintain their status as "king of the hill." Many state laws governing the practice of medicine and health care still contain protectionism for physicians, while other healthcare providers have had to fight for the right to provide the services they have been educated to provide. In some states, NPs are winning those fights.

Present Law

Third-party reimbursement goes to PCPs and specialists. Therefore, if NPs want to have their own practices, they need to be legally designated as PCPs or have cash-based practices.

In many states, physician collaboration is a matter of law, although it should be a matter of clinical and professional judgment. Nevertheless, the majority of states require physician collaboration for NP practice, especially if prescription writing is involved. Most states allow NPs to prescribe if they have a collaborative agreement with a physician.

Public Perceptions

While research indicates that patients are highly satisfied with the care given by NPs, and while some patients specifically request NPs as their providers, it is unclear whether there is a general awareness that NPs could be PCPs in their own right without physician oversight or collaboration.

Television shows have impressed the image of the kindly family physician on the minds of the public. The American Medical Association and the American Academy of Family Physicians have active public relations campaigns that seek to maintain the public perception of the physician as PCP.

MCO policies initially called for physician PCPs, even though NPs were delivering much of the care of patients enrolled in MCOs. Some MCOs, however, are changing their policies.

What Must Happen for NPs to Be PCPs?

For NPs to achieve PCP status, three things must happen. Laws have to permit NPs to be PCPs, the public must accept and be comfortable with the concept of the NP as PCP, and MCOs must agree to designate NPs as PCPs. States that do not define a PCP as an NP will need to be convinced to add this legal permission. Public relations efforts should be aimed at convincing the public that they are safe with NPs. Simultaneously, MCOs need to be convinced of the advantages of having NPs as PCPs.

Laws can prohibit NPs from practicing, say nothing about NPs, or permit NPs to practice and protect that NP practice. An example of a prohibitive law is: "A separate office for the nurse practitioner shall not be established." This language was enacted in 1995 by the Virginia legislature, but the legislature eliminated it in 2012. An example of a permissive law is: "APRNs may serve as primary care providers of record." (V.T. Nursing R. §15.2[f]).

An example of a protective law (protective of physicians) is:

> It shall be an improper practice for the governing body of a hospital to refuse to act upon an application for staff membership or professional privileges or to deny or withhold from a physician, podiatrist, optometrist, dentist or licensed midwife staff membership or professional privileges in a hospital, or to exclude or expel a physician, podiatrist, optometrist, dentist or licensed midwife from staff membership in a hospital or curtail, terminate or diminish in any way a physician's, podiatrist's, optometrist's, dentist's or licensed midwife's professional privileges in a hospital, without stating the reasons therefor, or if the reasons stated are unrelated to standards of patient care, patient welfare, the objectives of the institution or the character or competency of the applicant. It shall be an improper practice for a governing body of a hospital to refuse to act upon an application or to deny or to withhold staff membership or professional privileges to a podiatrist based solely upon a practitioner's category of licensure.

> *Citation:* N.Y. Pub. Health Law §§ 2801-b.1.

NPs need to work to erase the laws that are prohibitive. NPs need more laws that are permissive and protective. An example of a law protective of NPs would be:

> A managed-care organization may not refuse to act upon an application for staff membership or professional privileges, or deny privileges for a nurse practitioner, without stating the reasons therefor, or if the reasons stated are unrelated to standards of patient care, patient welfare, the objectives of the institution or the character or competency of the applicant.

This is a slight alteration of New York's law quoted here, which protects physicians, dentists, podiatrists, optometrists, and nurse midwives from being denied hospital privileges without fair reason.

The first step for state and national NP organizations is to have an attorney analyze the law to identify barriers. Sometimes, when arguing about a professional issue, competitors will cite laws of which NPs were not even aware as the basis for barring NP participation.

The top priority areas where laws need to be changed to reflect NP training and practice are as follows:

- Authorization of PCP status
- Reimbursement
- Hospital privileges
- Loosening of legal requirements for physician collaboration
- Authorization to admit patients to skilled nursing facilities
- Authorization to order home health services
- Authorization to serve as medical director for hospice
- Authorization for NP practices to be "medical homes"

Once prohibitions are erased from the law, and once permission is certain, NPs will want to work toward legal protection. Other professions, notably physicians, have remarkable professional legal protection. The legal protection of physicians has been so great that the public associated "healthcare provider" with "physician" until recently, when other providers began to be assertive about their roles.

The stage is set for more permission and protection of professions other than physicians. For example, Medicaid law requires an insurer to offer a variety of choices to enrollees. Some state laws require insurers to pay NPs for services.

The Process of Changing the Law

Law change involves certain steps, including these:

- Developing a set of goals and legislative strategies for achieving the goals
- Developing relationships with lawmakers
- Analyzing present state law for barriers to NP practice
- Monitoring law changes proposed by other groups
- Responding to proposed law that affects NPs adversely
- Following up to see how bills that have been introduced have progressed
- Arranging testimony when bills come up for a hearing
- Arranging for communication with legislative representatives
- Drafting and arranging support for legislation that supports the NP agenda
- Following through until the bill is written into regulations
- Debriefing to see how the process can be done better next time

Developing Goals and Strategies

Clinicians know what gets in their way. NPs who have considered starting practices or who have actually done so know what stopped them from getting paid, know how difficult it can be to get a good physician collaborator, and whether they need hospital privileges. NP organizations should poll their members to develop a list of goals for the organizations. Then, keeping in mind that law must be in place, public perception must be favorable, and payer policies must be permissive, organizations can develop strategies for overcoming barriers. Strategies might include hiring a lobbyist, drafting a bill, hiring a public relations firm, brainstorming about ideas for news articles on NPs, meeting with researchers about data collection on NP practices, meeting with groups to ask for support, or meeting with MCO executives to explain the benefits to their business of having NPs as providers.

Developing Relationships with Lawmakers

NPs who attend fundraisers, assist candidates at election time, and otherwise get to know the lawmakers in their districts find that cooperation is there when it comes time to sponsor and vote for a bill important to NPs.

Analyzing Law for Barriers to NP Practice

An attorney familiar with the NP role should analyze the law of each state for each state organization. First, the attorney will analyze the law that names NPs to determine whether any prohibitions exist or whether permission or protection is needed. The attorney will also look for laws that do not name NPs but that regulate health care in a way that affects NPs. For example, the attorney will analyze state insurance law even if it does not name NPs as reimbursable providers. The attorney can locate the clause that should name NPs as reimbursable providers. The attorney should also analyze state law that addresses healthcare quality. If a law says a physician must oversee all care of patients in MCOs, the attorney can locate the clause that neglects NPs and suggest language changes that will remedy the barrier for NPs.

Monitoring Changes to the Law Proposed by Other Groups

NPs are not the only group looking to change the law. NP organizations need to have someone monitoring proposed statutes and regulations to see how incoming law might affect NPs. Physicians have historically sought protective language and will continue to do so, as will physical therapists, physician assistants, chiropractors, and other professionals. It is frustrating enough that NPs must change laws that were enacted before NPs existed. It is doubly frustrating when NPs are caught off guard and a new law is made that excludes NPs.

Collaborating with Other Stakeholders

Sometimes a law is proposed that adversely affects NPs but is not a result of professional competition. Instead, the proposed law is aimed at solving some unrelated problem. For example, the agency that administers Medicare, the Center for Medicare and Medicaid Services (CMS), sets the rates of payment for visits by Medicare patients. Physicians, NPs, physical therapists, chiropractors, and many other groups all may be working toward the same end: increasing those rates. In such situations, NPs may find allies in other professional groups. Again, to participate, NPs must be aware of the proposed law changes.

Following Up on Bills in Progress

A bill may be changed many times between introduction and passage. The job of the lobbyist includes checking on bill status nearly every day to determine when the hearings are, what amendments have been proposed, when the votes will be held, who is in favor and who is opposed, and what bills have been introduced that may counteract any given bill. Sometimes an NP organization, to get the legislative support to pass its bill, will need to agree to support another group's bill. In that case, a lobbyist must know who backs which bills, who will give what support in return for support, and what the NP organization's parameters are in terms of what can be supported and what cannot.

Arranging Testimony

Legislative committees hear testimony on a bill before a vote is taken to pass the bill out of committee and to the full legislative body, house, or senate. At hearings, citizens are permitted to address the committee or legislative body about the effect a bill will have on a citizen or a group. Committee members may question those who testify. Often there are many people who want to testify on a particular bill. There may be several hearings in a day. Keeping in mind that legislators can only digest so much information, parties are advised to keep testimony short and to the point. Three minutes is often all an individual has to make their point.

Legislators will be more affected by testimony that a bill will affect many people or will affect some people greatly. For example, a legislator is likely to be more swayed by testimony that a particular bill will open health care to 17,000 uninsured citizens than by testimony that a bill will give reimbursement to five self-employed NPs. On the other hand, if an NP can show legislators how the number of self-employed NPs could, with release of barriers, soon grow to 2500 self-employed NPs who can participate in a state program for the uninsured by offering reduced rate services, legislators' interest is likely to be stimulated. Legislators, like the population in general, are moved by issues that affect mothers and children, the elderly, public safety, and public expenditures. Testimony that shows how a bill touches on these issues can be very effective.

Lobbyists often help NP organizations develop testimony and testifiers. If a bill affecting NPs also affects patients, it is often helpful to have patients testify on behalf of the bill.

Arranging for Communication with Legislative Representatives

Citizens can communicate their opinions to legislators through telephone calls, emails, and visits, as well as in hearings. Legislators make themselves available to citizens at such gatherings as "nurses' night at the legislature" and other receptions. All legislators have aides who can hear citizen concerns and pass those concerns along to the legislator. NPs who want to communicate with legislators about professional issues can arrange for a personal visit with their individual legislators in their districts, telephone the legislator or aide, ask patients to contact their legislators about an NP issue of interest to the patient, and/or hire a lobbyist to communicate with the legislators.

It is a fact of life that legislators need money to conduct reelection campaigns. Legislators do, in fact, take the time to listen to contributors. Legislators remember the individuals and groups who contribute to their campaigns. Many NP organizations have political action committee funds that they use to support legislative campaigns. This is an important use of association funds.

Drafting and Arranging Support for Legislation That Furthers the NP Agenda

The drafting of legislative language is an art. Lobbyists, legislators, and attorneys do it. Citizens and associations do not do it, or rather, they usually do not do it well. A bill has to take into account the existing law, the form that state law takes, possible unintended consequences of particular language, the state-defined meaning of particular words, the possible reaction to opponents and competitors to specific language, and the need for conciseness and clarity of expression.

NP associations usually begin a bill-drafting process by discussing the problem NPs are trying to solve with a lobbyist. The lobbyist then locates the section of law that needs to be changed and proceeds to draft language changes that will solve the problem. Lobbyists, when drafting bills for NPs, often will get opinions from selected legislators and other professional groups about possible language in an attempt to pretest reactions to specific language. Often, between the time a bill is conceptualized and the time it is introduced, the bill's language has been changed and rearranged many times. And after the bill is introduced, the language may be changed several times through amendments.

After there is a draft of language for a proposed bill, or during the drafting process, a lobbyist seeks sponsors. A bill's sponsor introduces it and shepherds it through the legislature. There can be companion bills in both houses of the legislature, in which case there should be a sponsoring senator and a sponsoring representative. The selection of a sponsor is crucial because their personality, committee position, affiliations, and popularity will affect how the bill progresses. For example, a well-positioned sponsor may decline because the legislator is trying to curry favor from an opposing group. It is not uncommon to "shop" for sponsors.

After a lobbyist gets a bill sponsor, the search is on for cosponsors. A bill with many cosponsors is likely to get passed. No legislator likes his or her name on a bill that fails. So, cosponsors can be expected not only to support the bills they cosponsor, but also to work for passage of those bills.

After obtaining sponsors and cosponsors, a lobbyist's next task is to line up testimony for committee hearings. Then, after a hearing, a lobbyist turns attention to locking in votes. Lobbyists ask legislators directly whether they intend to vote for or against a bill. If the vote is "no," a lobbyist can ask why. If something about the bill can be tweaked to change a "no" vote to a "yes," a lobbyist can draft an amendment and seek the approval of sponsors, cosponsors, and other favorable voters on the amended language.

Finally, a bill comes to a vote. A bill must pass each house of the legislature. A bill that passes both houses then goes to the governor for approval. The final hurdle is escaping a gubernatorial veto. Lobbying is done even at this final stage to convince the governor and his or her staff of the worth of the bill.

After a bill becomes a law, the bill is codified—that is, written into the state's code of laws. Many bills are further expanded upon in regulations written by the state agencies that carry out the laws. Regulations may include detail not specified in the law, but regulations cannot directly contradict a statute.

NPs who are working toward legal change will want to work closely with their lobbyist all the way through regulation writing. After it is over, they can debrief to see how things could be done better next time.

Hiring Lobbyists and Attorneys

Lobbyists and attorneys often serve many clients and may or may not know the issues that are most important to NPs. An NP association that is fortunate enough to have a lobbyist and an attorney who are well versed in NP issues and already familiar with the law regarding NPs has a head start.

When interviewing an attorney, or lobbyist, ask these questions:

- What is your experience with NP issues?
- Have you personally experienced the care of an NP?
- Who are your other clients? Might their issues conflict with NP issues?
- Do you have any opinions about NPs?
- What does an NP do?

One would think a lobbyist or attorney who has scheduled an interview with an NP organization would have done enough research to answer this last question. But surprisingly, that is not always the case. A prospective lobbyist or attorney who cannot answer this question should not be hired.

Do-It-Yourself Lobbying

Some NPs are very good at testifying. Usually the best testifiers are those who have had the most practice. When called to testify, ask who the committee members are and whether any are healthcare providers. Ask about a time limit. Ask who else will be testifying, and coordinate the testimony if possible. The best testimony has an introduction, a middle, and a conclusion, just like a speech. Polish is not a necessity, but preparation is essential.

Should NPs Join with the State Nurses' Association for Lobbying?

In some states, the NP association is a separate organization from the state nurses' association. In other states, NPs are an interest group within the state nurses' association. Ideally, from the point of view of an outsider, the state nurses' association would take care of legislative issues for all nurses. However, NPs sometimes find that their issues are a lower priority for the state nurses' association than they would like. NPs have sometimes formed their own organizations and hired their own lobbyists for this reason.

It is worth noting that in Oregon, where state law is quite favorable to NPs, lobbying has always been done by a strong state nurses' association, of which NPs are an interest group. Officers of NP associations should attempt to work with the state nurses' association on legislative issues. If, after attempting to work with the state nurses' association, NPs find they cannot get what they need, then NPs can hire their own lobbyist.

Dealing with Government Agencies

Many people who work for government agencies lack an understanding of health care and specifically the role of NPs. Though an NP might expect that a state or federal agency would research an issue when knowledge is lacking, many state agencies rely on citizens and their representatives to bring problems to light and to do the legal research to support the proponent's position. When NPs or their hired representatives become familiar with the personnel of state and federal agencies and seek person-to-person communication about an NP issue, questions and problems can often be taken care of efficiently at the agency level without resorting to legislative action. Further, NPs will be included in government policy making when they sit on the advisory panels and commissions making the policies. It is part of a lobbyist's job to know the influential policy-making commissions in a state and attempt to get NPs appointed to these commissions and boards.

The Competition

Change would be easy if there were no competition. There is competition, however, and it is useful to know where it comes from and what competitors' interests are.

Physician Competition

Physicians fought hard for their position in health care and now fight to maintain it. The fight is by no means limited to NPs. Physicians have fought against other providers, such as homeopathic physicians and optometrists, and now they fight against MCOs, which physicians perceive as threatening physician autonomy.

Through capturing the mechanisms of reimbursement, physicians were able to secure and maintain a dominant position among healthcare providers. They are not going to give up their position now.

Although NPs made significant strides in the 1970s because of a physician shortage in certain areas, and although NPs made some progress in the 1990s because of a funds shortage, there are still many legal and policy barriers to NPs, many of which were established by and are now maintained through physician influence.

Whereas the climate in the early 1970s was conducive to the proliferation of "physician extenders" due to the physician shortage, in recent years the NP has been increasingly viewed by some physicians as a competitor rather than simply an extender of physician services.

Competition is something NPs always will need to budget for in terms of time, energy, and money.

Competition from Physician Assistants

Physician assistants (PAs) have many of the same goals as NPs: professional recognition and respect, the ability to make a good living, and the ability to control one's work product. PAs will have to fight their own battles, as their profession was set up differently from its inception. By nature of their name and mission, PAs are not meant to be independent providers. While individual NPs may compete with individual PAs for specific jobs, it is not fruitful for NP professional organizations to engage PA organizations in competition in the public arena.

Competition from Other Nurses

Some NP associations find that when they go for inclusion in the law as PCPs, other nurses, particularly clinical nurse specialists (CNSs), want to be included as well. At that point, there is a possibility that the legislature will be hearing competitive arguments from NP and CNS groups about the relative merits of each group. As with PAs, NPs and CNSs have many of the same goals. It will not serve either group well to fight, and public fighting will definitely cause harm. Peaceful coexistence is the key. If NPs only put forth efforts to further their profession and do not engage in efforts to hold back other professions, not only will time and expenses be saved, but public relations will be better.

How Can Individual NPs Make a Difference?

Individuals can influence lawmakers and lawmaking in the following ways:

- Ask candidates in local elections about their position on NPs, and vote accordingly. Support good candidates with campaign contributions, noting on the check that you are an NP.
- When a bill concerns NPs or health issues of concern to NPs, call or write legislators, noting that you are an NP.
- When regulations are proposed that affect NPs, write and send comments on how the proposed regulations will affect NPs.
- Join an NP association.
- Write letters to the editor of the local newspaper about news events affecting NPs or affecting your patients.

Conclusion

The process for making law conform to NP goals for the profession is this:

1. Analyze the current law for prohibitions, lack of permission, and lack of protection where it matters. Have an attorney work with the NP organization to do the analysis.
2. Draft a bill that erases prohibition, gives permission, or affords protection for NP practice. Have an attorney, lobbyist, or legislator work with the organization to do this.
3. Gather support for the bill among lawmakers and the public. Enlist the participation of association members in each legislative district.
4. Introduce the bill, and follow its progress, testifying when necessary, educating lawmakers when necessary, and arranging give-and-take with other groups when necessary. At this stage, professional lobbyists should be running the show.
5. Follow the bill through to the regulation-writing stage, monitoring the language of proposed regulations and commenting on the proposed regulations through letters. Have an attorney do this.
6. Refine the approach, based on what was learned with previous law changes. Association officers, attorneys, and lobbyists should do this.

Notes

1. Merriam-Webster. (2005). Policy definition. In *Merriam-Webster collegiate dictionary* (11th ed., p. 960). Springfield, MA: Author.
2. Freudenheim, M. (1997, November 2). The future wears white: Nurses treading on doctors' turf. *The New York Times Week in Review*. Retrieved from http://www.nytimes.com/1997/11/02/weekinreview/the-future-wears-white-nurses-treading-on-doctors-turf.html
3. Califano J. A., Jr. (1994). *Radical surgery: What's next for America's health care?* (p. 218). New York, NY: New York Times Books.
4. Health policy brief, Health Affairs. (2013, May 15.). Nurse practitioners and primary care. Retrieved from http://www.healthaffairs.org/healthpolicybriefs/brief.php?brief_id=92
5. Tommasino, J. (1998). The dilemma of the one-rung ladder. *Clinician Reviews, 8,* 31.

Measuring Nurse Practitioner Performance

Standards of care and measures of performance are interrelated. Measures of performance are used to determine the extent to which standards of care are met. Measuring performance without standards is like playing a game without rules. Setting standards without measuring performance is like making laws when there are no police to enforce the laws.

Measuring Quality

In general, the quality of clinical care is assessed by asking and answering the following questions:

- Did the clinician do the right thing?
- Was the care effective?
- Was care given in an appropriate time frame?
- Was the outcome as good as could be expected, given each patient's condition and personal characteristics and the current state of medical science?

The standard of care for a particular episode of illness is assessed by asking and answering these questions:

- What was the correct treatment?
- What was the correct timing of treatment?
- What was the correct teaching or counseling?

Measures of the standard of care ask and answer these questions:

- Did the clinician follow the standard?
- Did the patient's problem resolve?
- Did the problem resolve within the expected time frame?
- If the problem did not resolve and the clinician did not expect that it would resolve, did the patient's quality of life improve or did bothersome symptoms decrease in severity?
- Were the resources used to solve the problem in line with what would be expected for that problem?
- Was the patient satisfied with the experience of care?
- Was the patient satisfied with the outcome?

Multiple Measures, Multiple Measurers

Nurse practitioner (NP) performance is evaluated on several levels: productivity, utilization, and patient satisfaction, as well as the quality of clinical decision making. An NP's performance is judged by employers, patients, health plan auditors, peers, and possibly even researchers.

If an NP's performance is employer defined, then the NP will need to ascertain the values of the employer. To one employer, good performance might be synonymous with high billings, which could, because of time constraints, preclude giving adequate attention to each patient. For another employer, good performance might mean high scores on surveys of patient satisfaction. An NP who satisfies patients might not be a high biller. To yet another employer, good performance might mean close communication with the physician consultant, while in another practice it might mean independent functioning without the need for communication with a physician.

If performance is defined by the health plan, then a good performer is one who uses expensive resources—hospitals and emergency rooms—relatively infrequently.

If an NP's performance is defined by present performance measures developed by consumer-oriented groups, such as the National Committee for Quality Asurance (NCQA), an NP who sees that all children are properly immunized, who gets patients to quit smoking, and who raises the functional status of elderly patients will be seen as a good performer.

If an NP's performance is defined by peers, a good performer is likely to be an expert diagnostician who shares knowledge willingly with other NPs and who is compatible with other clinicians and staff.

If performance is defined by researchers, a good performer is one who meets the particular testing criteria studied by the researcher.

Finally, if performance is defined by patients, a good performer is one who does not make the patient wait more than 20 minutes in the waiting room before being seen, who is patient and polite, and who does not miss a serious diagnosis.

There is no single, widely accepted set of measures of an NP's worth or performance. In this chapter, several measures of performance are summarized.

Productivity

Definitions

A definition of productivity may depend upon the setting and the method of payment to the practice.

In a practice that gets reimbursed according to a fee-for-service structure, a productive NP is one who sees many patients, at a 99213 level or above, and who bills often for additional services that generate revenue, such as suturing, incision and drainage, and endometrial biopsy.

In a practice that receives mostly capitated payments, an NP who efficiently handles a large panel of patients with little use of the practice's resources—staff, materials, time—is a good performer.

If an NP is employed by a nursing home, productivity may mean keeping elderly patients out of the hospital, while imparting to their families the feeling that their loved one is being closely monitored and well cared for.

Measurement

In a fee-for-service practice, a simple way of measuring performance is to set the number of visits conforming to the evaluation and management Current Procedural Terminology (CPT) codes. For example, good performance could be set at 20 visits at levels 99211 to 99215 per day. One would not want to set a specific code as a performance measure because it is the patient's need for evaluation and management services that determines the CPT code billed, and a provider cannot predict what level of visit will be needed.

In a capitated practice, good performance could be set at maintenance of an 1800-member panel of patients, with patient satisfaction, as measured by a particular tool, at 80% or above.

In a nursing home practice, good performance could be measured by decreasing, over a previous year, the number of hospital visits among the nursing home's residents.

For a detailed discussion of NP productivity, see "Productivity Incentive Plans for Nurse Practitioners: How and Why" by Carolyn Buppert (http://www.buppert.com).

Housekeeping Performance Measures

NPs may have more experience with "housekeeping" forms of performance measurement than with substantive forms such as the Physician Quality Report System or the Health Plan Employer Data and Information Set (HEDIS). For example, many NPs' charts are audited for such things as clear labeling of allergies, initialing and dating of laboratory results, patient name on every page, and a completed problem list. While these are important matters, in the future, NPs should expect that audits will become increasingly more oriented toward outcomes.

NCQA Measures of Clinical Performance

Nonclinicians have begun to get involved in measuring clinical performance. After putting out a call for performance measures, NCQA received 800 suggestions and developed HEDIS and a set of clinical performance measures aimed largely at primary care providers. Presumably HEDIS is some indication of what employers, consumers, and health plan executives think is important for healthcare providers to accomplish. The HEDIS measures are still being refined.

Among the evaluation measures set by HEDIS for primary care providers are these:

- At least 80 percent of female patients age 40 to 69 had at least one mammogram in the past 2 years.
- Eighty-two percent of women age 21 to 64 had at least one Pap smear during the past 3 years.
- Ninety-seven percent of pregnant women began prenatal care during the first trimester of pregnancy.

Some of these data are collected from the Center for Medicare & Medicaid Services 1500 (billing) forms. Other data are collected by auditors who review charts or from surveys.

HEDIS also looks at these indicators:

- Whether women had a postpartum visit 21 and 56 days after delivery
- Whether patients who were hospitalized for mental illness and were seen on an outpatient basis by a mental health provider within 30 days after discharge

HEDIS measures change from time to time. For the current measures and benchmarks, visit the website (http://www.ncqa.org/HEDISQualityMeasurement.aspx).[1]

Other Measures

HEDIS is not the only set of performance measures, and NCQA is not the only organization looking after consumer interests and rating health plans and providers. Among the other organizations publishing performance measures are the Centers for Medicare & Medicaid Services, The Joint Commission, certain managed-care plans, certain state health departments, and the Agency for Healthcare Research and Quality. The performance measures advocated by these organizations overlap to some extent.

Formal Research

Researchers who have studied NP performance and compared it with physicians' performance have looked at the following measures:

- Whether NPs took a thorough history and gave appropriate treatment to a patient with a particular set of symptoms and history.[2]
- Whether NPs performed or followed up on a set of primary care tasks, such as follow-up on a low hematocrit and obtaining appropriate cancer screening tests.[3]
- Whether patients reported, on a survey, that their experience of care was satisfactory.[4]
- Whether NPs' care was cost-effective when all of the costs of care were tallied.[5]
- Whether the level of care in nursing homes was improved by NP participation.[6]
- Whether NPs controlled the blood pressure of patients diagnosed with hypertension to below 140/90.[7]

The performance of NPs was found to be at least as good as physicians' on these measures.

Patient Ratings

Many difficulties and intervening factors become apparent when one attempts to get patients to rate NP performance. Patients have their own set of beliefs about health and illness, which may affect their interpretation of the quality of care given to them. Patients may focus on nonclinical aspects of care that affect their experience. Patients may feel compelled to give a provider a good rating, fearing a turn in the relationship if they are critical. And surveys may reach a patient at a date much later than the care was given, when a patient has forgotten the bad or the good aspects of the care.

Nevertheless, patient-rated measures of performance are to be taken seriously. Whether or not an NP believes a patient's rating to be valid, much information can be gleaned from patient survey results. For example, if a patient's experience of care was influenced negatively by a grouchy receptionist, then attitude adjustment on the part of the receptionist is a relatively easy alteration for a practice to make.

Health plans, practices, and facilities often conduct patient surveys, and NPs would be wise to get copies of these various surveys and their results and to conduct visits and make corrections in problem areas accordingly.

Consumers are able to review other patients' experience with clinicians through commercial websites and through health plan sites. NPs thus are also advised to search such sites for comments about themselves and to make adjustments if needed.

Peer Review

Some accrediting organizations require that medical offices conduct regular peer review. There are many peer review tools in the NP literature.

Utilization

Because hospitals, emergency rooms, and specialists are high cost centers for health plans, health plans want providers to keep admissions and referrals to the emergency room and specialists at a minimum. Whether an NP works for a physician or is in independent practice, the NP can expect that in the world of managed care, someone will be looking at the numbers of admissions and referrals.

How to Get an "A" on Performance Report Cards

An NP who wants to shine on performance evaluations will determine who in a work setting is interested in what measures and will adapt his or her practice accordingly. If there are no adopted performance measures, the NP may want to adopt the self-evaluation routine given in **Appendix   A.**

The number of hoops through which NPs must jump continues to rise. Many more tasks are coming under scrutiny than ever before.

NPs who are only given 15 minutes to take care of a patient's episodic problem know the frustration of quickly leafing through a patient record to check on details. Whether a patient has been a smoker, whether a patient has been advised to quit, or whether a patient is up to date on healthcare maintenance—mammograms, immunizations, and Pap smears—often takes longer than 15 minutes to ascertain, even when the patient is sitting in the adjacent chair. Electronic medical records may decrease the amount of time NPs spend on healthcare maintenance in that some systems alert the clinician about tests needed and questions to ask. On the other hand, NPs may spend more time in the future on healthcare maintenance because they are reminded what is needed and attend to these needs.

Documentation of health maintenance checks was a problem long before HEDIS, NCQA, and even the term primary care provider came into common usage. Every primary care provider is familiar with the feeling of uneasiness that comes from scanning a chart for an established patient that contains no record—all in one place—of routine screening efforts and results. Occasionally, some thoughtful physician assistant, NP, or physician will have summarized a patient's chart in a progress note. The trick then becomes finding that progress note.

Some practices keep flowcharts to document healthcare maintenance. Some electronic medical records track and/or remind clinicians to attend to healthcare maintenance tasks. Practices that track health maintenance are far ahead of those that do not keep such information in a central place. But even practices that keep flowcharts need to know how health plans and Medicare have decided to "grade."

Ensuring Compliance

A simple tool, kept in the front of a chart or in a special section called "Performance Measures" or some similar title, can prompt busy providers to ask the pertinent questions; arrange the pertinent screens, tests, medications, classes, or counseling; and note the date when the work was done. Some electronic medical records are programmed to prompt clinicians to address health maintenance. One format for a tool is given in **Appendix B**.

NPs who are employees can be motivated to keep checklists and flowcharts up to date by tying compliance to bonuses, conducting internal quality assurance audits and giving feedback to providers on their performance, and including this activity in job descriptions and evaluation tools.

Self-employed NPs will find their own rewards in keeping up with outside measures of performance. Finding a healthcare provider is no longer a matter of word of mouth. Patients usually go to providers who will be reimbursed by the patient's health plan. Retention on provider panels is likely to be contingent on satisfaction of performance measures. Those providers who meet the standards now being set by consumer-driven groups will end up with a thriving practice, which, after all, is the most traditional measure of performance.

The organizations doing the measuring, grading, and reporting have the mission of helping consumers. How logistically difficult it is for health plans and providers to comply with these measures is not the main concern of these organizations.

The hoops are not limited to clinical performance measures. HEDIS has included measures of access and availability of care, patients' satisfaction with their care experience, health plan stability, utilization of selected services, cost of care, and such services as new member orientation and translation services.

HEDIS details are not particularly accessible to consumers, health plans, or providers. Anyone can purchase HEDIS reports and explanations from the NCQA, but they are expensive.

Strategies for complying with the performance criteria set by the NCQA and Medicare include increasing clinicians' and administrators' knowledge of specific performance measures, delegating responsibility for continuous quality improvement, implementing systems for tracking compliance, attending to patient satisfaction, addressing the functional level of elderly patients, and rewarding clinicians and practice managers for compliance and high scores.

Notes

1. National Committee for Quality Assurance. (n.d.). The Health Plan Employer Data and Information Set (HEDIS). Retrieved from http://www.ncqa.org/HEDISQualityMeasurement.aspx
2. Avorn, J., Everitt, D. E., & Baker, M. W. (1991). The neglected medical history and therapeutic choices for abdominal pain: a nationwide study of 799 physicians and nurses. *Archives of Internal Medicine, 151,* 694–698.
3. Hall J. A., Palmer R. H., & Orav, E. J. (1990). Performance quality, gender and professional role. A study of physicians and nonphysicians in 16 ambulatory care practices. *Medical Care, 28,* 489–501.
4. Perry, K. (1995). Patient survey: Physician extenders. Why patients love physician extenders. *Medical Economics, 72,* 58, 63, 67.
5. Salkever D. S., Skinner E. A., Steinwachs D. M., & Katz, H. (1982). Episode-based efficiency comparisons for physicians and nurse practitioners. *Medical Care, 20,* 143–153.
6. Mahoney, D. F. (1994). The appropriateness of geriatric prescribing decisions made by nurse practitioners and physicians. *Image, 26,* 41–46.
7. Mundinger, M. O., Kane, R. L., Lenz, E. R., Totten, A. M., Wei-Yann, T., Cleary, P. D….Shelanski, M. L. (2000). Primary care outcomes in patients treated by nurse practitioners or physicians: A randomized trial. *Journal of the American Medical Association, 283,* 59–68.

NP Self-Evaluation

To fare well on clinical performance evaluations, an NP should set up a routine for self-evaluation. Tailor the questions to your own patients and practice. For example:

1. For each visit, have I asked the patient:
   - Are you smoking? (If so, advise patient to quit.)
   - Did you get an appointment promptly?
   - How long did you spend in the waiting room? Was the wait too long or was it acceptable?
   - Has this visit satisfied your expectations?

2. On each visit, have I consulted the chart for:
   - Up-to-date immunizations?
   - Up-to-date cancer screening: Pap, mammogram, colonoscopy?
   - Eye exam in the past year for diabetic patients?
   - Follow-up visit within 6 weeks of giving birth for postpartum patients?

3. If a patient has been hospitalized:
   - If for mental illness, was the patient seen by a mental health clinician within 30 days after discharge?

   To do utilization self-monitoring, for each quarter, keep a notebook with this information:

   - Patient admissions to hospitals
   - Referrals to the emergency department
   - Referrals to specialists
   - Number of patients seen per day

Name: _____

Patient number: _____

Date of Birth: _____

Female Cancer Screening	Date	Result	Date	Result	Date	Result
Pap (21–64)						
Mammo (50–69)						

Adult Immunizations	Date	Result	Date	Result	Date	Result
Tetanus (all patients, q 10 yrs)						
Flu (q yr. > 50 y.o.)						
Pneumococcal (only for individuals > 65 y.o).						

Childhood Immunizations	Date	Date	Date	Date	Date
Diphtheria-tetanus-pertussis					
Polio					
MMR					
HIB					
Hep B					
Chicken Pox					
Pneumococcal conjugate					

Prescribing

Nurse practitioners (NPs) in 50 states and the District of Columbia have the legal authority to prescribe. The independence of NPs' prescriptive authority varies widely, and, in several states, words other than "prescribe" are used.

In 17 states and the District of Columbia, NPs have explicit legal authority to "prescribe," with no requirement for physician involvement. In one state (Utah), NPs need physician involvement only when prescribing Schedules II–III. In 33 states, NPs have explicit legal authority to prescribe but must have a collaborative relationship with a specific physician. In one state (Michigan), NPs do not have specific legal authority to prescribe, but the law permits physicians to delegate medical functions (see **Exhibit 1**). In 48 states and the District of Columbia, NPs may prescribe controlled substances. (See **Exhibit 2** for the states that fall into this category.) **Appendix A** presents laws on prescriptive authority for each state.

Controlled Substances

Controlled dangerous substances are narcotics, depressants, stimulants, and hallucinogenic drugs covered under the Controlled Substances Act, a federal law. In 49 states and the District of Columbia, NPs may prescribe controlled substances.

Classification of Controlled Substances

There are five "schedules" of controlled substances:

- *Schedule I*: Schedule I substances have no accepted medical use in the United States and have high abuse potential. Examples are heroin, LSD, MDMA ("ecstasy"), marijuana, and peyote.
- *Schedule II*: Schedule II drugs have a high abuse potential with severe psychic or physical dependence liability and in general are substances that have therapeutic utility. Schedule II narcotics include morphine, codeine, fentanyl, hydromorphone (Dilaudid), meperidine (Demerol), methadone, pantopon, and opium. Stimulants such as amphetamines are included in Schedule II, as well as depressants such as pentobarbital.
- *Schedule III*: Schedule III drugs are stimulants and depressants with an abuse potential that is less than those drugs in Schedules I and II. Schedule III narcotics include mixtures of limited specified quantities of codeine with noncontrolled active ingredients (such as

Tylenol with codeine), and mixtures of amobarbital, pentobarbital, or secobarbital with other noncontrolled medicinal ingredients.

- *Schedule IV*: Schedule IV drugs have less abuse potential than Schedule III and include depressants such as alprazolam, phenobarbital, and chloral hydrate.
- *Schedule V*: Schedule V substances have less abuse potential than Schedule IV and include preparations containing limited quantities of certain narcotic and stimulant drugs generally given for antitussive, antidiarrheal, and analgesic purposes. Examples are buprenorphine and propylhexedrin.

A complete listing of the drugs controlled under the Controlled Substances Act may be found in Title 21, Code of Federal Regulations, Part 1300 to end, Sections 1308.11 through 1308.15. Prescribing references usually provide the class of each drug listed.

Exhibit 1 Forms of Prescriptive Authority

Explicit Legal Authority to Prescribe/ No Physician Involvement Required	Arkansas
Alaska	California
Arizona	Connecticut
Colorado	Delaware
District of Columbia	Florida
Hawaii (Schedules III–V)	Georgia
Idaho	Illinois
Iowa	Indiana
Kentucky	Kansas
Maine	Louisiana
Montana	Maryland
New Hampshire	Massachusetts
New Mexico	Minnesota
North Dakota	Mississippi
Oregon	Missouri
Rhode Island	Nebraska
South Dakota	Nevada
Utah—except for Schedules II–III	New Jersey
Vermont	New York
Washington	North Carolina
Wyoming	Ohio
Physician May Delegate Authority to Prescribe	Oklahoma
Georgia	Pennsylvania
Michigan	South Carolina
Texas	Tennessee
	Texas
Explicit Legal Authority to Prescribe/ Physician Collaboration Required	Virginia
	West Virginia
Alabama	Wisconsin

| Exhibit 2 | State Regulations of NPs' Prescriptive Activity |

NP May Prescribe Controlled Substances (except Schedule I, which are not used medically)	
Alabama (Schedules III–V)	Missouri (not Schedule I–II)
Alaska	Montana
Arizona	Nebraska
Arkansas (not Schedule I–II)	Nevada
California	New Hampshire
Colorado	New Jersey
Connecticut	New Mexico
Delaware	New York
District of Columbia	North Carolina
Georgia (not Schedule I–II)	North Dakota
Hawaii	Ohio
Idaho	Oklahoma (not Schedule I–II)
Illinois	Oregon
Indiana	Pennsylvania
Iowa	Rhode Island
Kansas	South Carolina (not Schedule I–II)
Kentucky	South Dakota
Louisiana (not Schedule I–II, except for attention deficit disorder medications)	Tennessee
	Texas (not Schedule I–II)
	Utah
Maine	Vermont
Maryland	Virginia
Massachusetts	Washington
Michigan	West Virginia (not Schedule I–II)
Minnesota	Wisconsin
Mississippi	Wyoming

Drug Enforcement Administration Registration

The federal government—the Drug Enforcement Administration (DEA)—oversees NPs' prescribing of controlled substances. To prescribe controlled substances, an NP must register with the DEA and obtain a DEA number. The NP must use the DEA number on prescriptions for scheduled drugs.

DEA registration is one method of tracking healthcare providers' prescribing practices related to controlled substances. The DEA number is also a method of minimizing unauthorized prescribing; a person who is not authorized to prescribe but who wants to write a prescription for a controlled substance, has a prescription pad, and signs the name of an authorized prescriber will be unable to get the prescription filled if it does not include a DEA number.

Federal registration is based on the applicant's compliance with state and local laws. If a state requires a separate controlled substances license, an NP must obtain that license and submit a copy with the application for a DEA number. If state law does not authorize NPs to prescribe controlled substances, the DEA will not issue DEA numbers.

DEA registration costs $731 for a 3-year term. States may charge for registration as well. To apply for DEA registration, visit the DEA's website (http://www.deadiversion.usdoj.gov /drugreg). Once a DEA number is issued, a renewal application is automatically issued 45 days prior to expiration. Registrants must report, in writing, any change in business location to the DEA. DEA registration is issued in the NP's name at the business address.

Guidelines for Prescribing Legally

NPs should follow these general guidelines when prescribing:

1. Prescribe the right medicine at the right time for the right indication for the right patient.
2. If there is a practice protocol or guidelines in the facility, follow it.
3. If there is no facility-wide protocol, adhere to the standard of care in prescribing. The standard of care for prescribing may be assumed to be the *Physician's Desk Reference* or Epocrates (http://www.epocrates.com).
4. Before prescribing, ask a patient:
   - Are you pregnant?
   - Are you breastfeeding?
   - Are you allergic to any medications?
   - Have you taken [this medicine] before? Did it work? Did it give you any ill effects?
   - Do you have any liver or kidney problems?
   - What other medications are you on?
   - What other medical problems do you have?
5. Address any cross-sensitivities. For example, if a patient is allergic to penicillin, an NP probably should not prescribe Keflex, which has cross-sensitivities with penicillin.
6. Address any contraindications. For example, a patient with chronic hepatitis should not be prescribed a medication that has potential for liver damage unless it is a life or death situation and there is no other choice.
7. Address any drug interactions. For example, theophylline is antagonized by phenytoin and potentiated by macrolide antibiotics.
8. Inform the patient of potential side effects, and ask whether the patient wants to accept the risk of experiencing those side effects.
9. Instruct the patient to call or return if he or she notices any adverse change in his or her condition.

Other considerations when prescribing include the following:

- Can the patient afford the medication? If not, the NP should not count on the patient getting the prescription filled.
- Is the drug to be prescribed in the formulary for the agency or health maintenance organization?
- Is there potential for abuse of the medication? For example, a depressed patient may over-dose on a prescribed medication, and a patient with a history of substance abuse may be seeking to continue the habit through a request for pain medication.

- Can the patient read? For example, the author had a personal experience where a patient was not responding to a variety of blood pressure medications. After much trial and error as well as discussion, it was revealed that the patient was not literate. The patient kept his wide assortment of medications on top of the refrigerator. He depended on his wife to dole out the proper medication to him, at the proper time and in the proper dose. When she was not available, which was often, he did not get his medication.

Resources

Buppert, C. (2010). *Prescribing: Avoiding legal pitfalls for NPs.* Law Office of Carolyn Buppert, P.C. Available for purchase at http://www.buppert.com/publications.html

State-by-State Law
Prescriptive Authority

Alabama

[The] joint committee shall recommend model practice protocols to be used by certified registered nurse practitioners and certified nurse midwives and a formulary of legend drugs that may be prescribed by these advanced practice nurses, subject to approval by both the State Board of Medical Examiners and the Board of Nursing. The joint committee shall also recommend rules and regulations to establish the ratio of physicians to certified registered nurse practitioners and certified nurse midwives; provided, however, that the rules and regulations shall not limit the ratio to less than two nurse practitioners or midwives to one physician or one certified registered nurse practitioner and one certified nurse midwife to one physician and shall provide for exceptions. The joint committee shall also recommend rules and regulations that establish the manner in which a collaborating physician may designate a covering physician when temporarily unavailable as the collaborating physician.

Citation: Ala. § 34-21-87.

a. Certified registered nurse practitioners and certified nurse midwives, engaged in collaborative practice with physicians practicing under protocols approved in the manner prescribed by this article may prescribe legend drugs to their patients, subject to both of the following conditions:
   1. The drug type, dosage, quantity prescribed, and number of refills shall be authorized in an approved protocol signed by the collaborating physician; and
   2. The drug shall be on the formulary recommended by the joint committee and adopted by the State Board of Medical Examiners and the Board of Nursing.
b. A certified registered nurse practitioner or a certified nurse midwife may not initiate a call-in prescription in the name of a collaborating physician for any drug, whether legend or controlled substance, which the nurse practitioner

or certified nurse midwife is not authorized to prescribe under the protocol signed by the collaborating physician and certified registered nurse practitioner or certified nurse midwife and approved under this section unless the drug is specifically ordered for the patient by the physician, either in writing or by a verbal order which has been reduced to writing, and which has been signed by the physician within a time specified in the rules and regulations approved by the State Board of Medical Examiners and the Board of Nursing.

c. Registered nurses and licensed practical nurses are authorized to administer any legend drug that has been lawfully ordered or prescribed by an authorized practitioner including certified registered nurse practitioners, certified nurse midwives, and/or assistants to physicians.

Citation: Ala. Code § 34-21-86.

1. Certified registered nurse practitioners engaged in collaborative practice with physicians may be granted prescriptive authority upon submission of evidence of completion of an academic course in pharmacology or evidence of integration of pharmacology theory and clinical application in the certified registered nurse practitioner curriculum.

2. Certified registered nurse practitioners practicing under protocols approved in the manner prescribed by Code of Alabama, 1975, Section 34-21-80 et seq. may prescribe legend drugs to their patients, subject to the following conditions:

   a. The drug type, dosage, quantity prescribed, and number of refills shall be authorized in an approved protocol signed by the collaborating physician and the certified registered nurse practitioner. This requirement may be met if written prescriptions adhere to the standard recommended doses of legend drugs as identified in the *Physician's Desk Reference* or Product Information Insert, not to exceed the recommended treatment regimen periods.

   b. The drug shall be included in the formulary recommended by the Joint Committee and adopted by the Board of Nursing and the State Board of Medical Examiners.

3. A certified registered nurse practitioner shall not initiate a call-in prescription in the name of a collaborating physician for any drug, whether legend or controlled substance, which the certified registered nurse practitioner is not authorized to prescribe under the protocol signed by the collaborating physician and certified registered nurse practitioner and approved under this section unless the drug is specifically ordered for the patient by the physician, either in writing or by a verbal order which has been transcribed in writing, and which has been signed by the physician within seven working days or as otherwise specified by the Board of Nursing and the State Board of Medical Examiners.

4. A written prescription for any drug that the certified registered nurse practitioner is authorized to prescribe may be called in to a pharmacy, provided the prescription is entered into the patient's record and signed by the certified registered nurse practitioner.
5. The certified registered nurse practitioner in collaborative practice with prescriptive privileges shall not engage in prescribing for:
   a. Self.
   b. Immediate family members.
   c. Individuals who are not patients of the practice.
6. The certified registered nurse practitioner who is in collaborative practice and has prescriptive privileges may receive and sign for samples of legend drugs that are authorized in the approved formulary for the collaborative practice, provided the certified registered nurse practitioner complies with all applicable state and federal laws and regulations.
7. When prescribing legend drugs a certified registered nurse practitioner shall use a prescription format that includes all of the following:
   a. The name, medical practice site address and telephone number of the collaborating physician or covering physician.
   b. The certified registered nurse practitioner's name printed below or to the side of the physician's name.
   c. The medical practice site address and telephone number of the certified registered nurse practitioner if different from that of the collaborating physician.
   d. The certified registered nurse practitioner's registered nurse license number and identifying prescriptive authority number assigned by the Board of Nursing.
   e. The words "Product Selection Permitted" printed on one side of the prescription form directly beneath a signature line.
   f. The words "Dispense as written" printed on one side of the prescription form directly beneath a signature line.
   g. The date the prescription is issued to the patient.

Citation: Ala. Admin. Code r. 610-X-5-.11.

Upon receipt of a Qualified Alabama Controlled Substances Registration Certificate (QACSC) and a valid registration number issued by the United States Drug Enforcement Administration, a certified registered nurse practitioner (CRNP) or certified nurse midwife (CNM) may prescribe, administer, authorize for administration, or dispense only those controlled substances listed in Schedules III, IV, and V of Article 2, Chapter 2, of this title in accordance with rules adopted by the Board of Medical Examiners and any protocols, formularies, and medical regimens established by the board for regulation of a QACSC.

Citation: Ala. Code §20-2-253(a).

Alaska

a. The Board will, in its discretion, authorize an advanced nurse practitioner or "ANP" to prescribe and dispense legend drugs in accordance with applicable state and federal laws.
b. *Repealed 3/28/2008.*
c. An advanced nurse practitioner who applies for authorization to prescribe and dispense drugs
   1. must be currently designated as an ANP in Alaska at the time of application;
   2. shall provide evidence of completion of 15 contact hours of education in advanced pharmacology and clinical management of drug therapy within the two-year period immediately before the date of application; and
   3. shall submit a completed application, as required in 12 AAC 44.400(a)(6) accompanied by the application fee established by 12 AAC 02.280.

Citation: Alaska Admin. Code tit. 12, § 44.440.

There is no requirement for physician collaboration.

a. In addition to the legend drug prescriptive and dispensing authority under 12 AAC 44.440, the board will, in its discretion, authorize an advanced nurse practitioner or "ANP" to prescribe and dispense schedule 2-5 controlled substances in accordance with applicable state and federal laws if an applicant
   1. submits a completed application on a form provided by the department; the completed application must include the applicant's
      A. name, address, and phone number;
      B. authorization number as an ANP;
      C. date of birth;
      D. *repealed 12/27/2012*; and
      E. notarized signature certifying that the information in the application is correct to the best of the applicant's knowledge;
   2. *repealed 12/27/2012*; and
   3. pays the application fee established by 12 AAC 02.280.

Citation: Alaska Admin. Code tit. 12, § 44.445.

Arizona

A. The Board shall authorize an RNP to prescribe and dispense (P&D) drugs and devices within the RNP's specialty area and category of practice only if the RNP does all of the following:
   1. Obtains authorization by the Board to practice as a registered nurse practitioner;
   2. Applies for prescribing and dispensing privileges on the application for registered nurse practitioner certification;

3. Submits a completed application on a form provided by the Board that contains all of the following information:
    a. Name, address, and home phone number;
    b. Arizona registered nurse license number, or copy of compact license;
    c. Nurse practitioner specialty;
    d. Nurse practitioner certification number issued by the Board;
    e. Business address and telephone number; and
    f. A sworn statement verifying the truthfulness of the information provided;
4. Submits evidence of completion of a minimum of 45 contact hours of education within the three years immediately preceding the application, covering one or both of the following topics:
    a. _____ Pharmacology
    b. _____ Clinical management of drug therapy, and
5. Submits the required fee.
B. An applicant who is denied P & D authority may request a hearing by filing a written request with the Board within 30 days of service of the Board's order denying the application for P & D authority. Board hearings shall comply with A.R.S. Title 41, Chapter 6, Article 10, and 4 A.A.C. 19, Article 6.

Citation: Ariz. Admin. Code R4-19-511.

A. An RNP granted P & D authority by the Board may:
    1. Prescribe drugs and devices;
    2. Provide for refill of prescription-only drugs and devices for one year from the date of the prescription.
B. An RNP with P & D authority who wishes to prescribe a controlled substance shall obtain a DEA registration number before prescribing a controlled substance. The RNP shall file the DEA registration number with the Board.
C. An RNP with a DEA registration number may prescribe:
    1. A Class II controlled substance as defined in the federal Uniform Controlled Substances Act, 21 U.S.C. § 801 et seq., or Arizona's Uniform Controlled Substances Act, A.R.S. Title 36, Chapter 27, but shall not prescribe refills of the prescription;
    2. A Class III or IV controlled substance, as defined in the federal Uniform Controlled Substances Act or Arizona's Uniform Controlled Substances Act, and may prescribe a maximum of five refills in six months; and
    3. A Class V controlled substance, as defined in the federal Uniform Controlled Substances Act or Arizona's Uniform Controlled Substances Act, and may prescribe refills for a maximum of one year.
D. An RNP whose DEA registration is revoked or expires shall not prescribe controlled substances. An RNP whose DEA registration is revoked or limited shall report the action to the Board.

E. In all outpatient settings or at the time of hospital discharge, an RNP with P & D authority shall personally provide a patient or the patient's representative with the name of the drug, directions for use, and any special instructions, precautions, or storage requirements necessary for safe and effective use of the drug if any of the following occurs:
   1. A new drug is prescribed or there is a change in the dose, form, or direction for use in a previously prescribed drug;
   2. In the RNP's professional judgment, these instructions are warranted; or
   3. The patient or patient's representative requests instruction.
F. An RNP with P & D authority shall ensure that all prescription orders contain the following:
   1. The RNP's name, address, telephone number, and specialty area;
   2. The prescription date;
   3. The name and address of the patient;
   4. The full name of the drug, strength, dosage form, and directions for use;
   5. The letters "DAW," or "dispense as written," "do not substitute," "medically necessary" or any similar statement on the face of the prescription form if intending to prevent substitution of the drug;
   6. The RNP's DEA registration number, if applicable; and
   7. The RNP's signature.

Citation: Ariz. Admin. Code R4-19-512.

Arkansas

An advanced practice nurse with a certificate of prescriptive authority may receive and prescribe drugs, medications, or therapeutic devices appropriate to an advanced practice nurse's area of practice in accordance with rules established by the Board.

Citation: Ark. Code Ann. § 17-87-310(b)(1).

An advanced practice nurse may prescribe Schedule III-V drugs.

Citation: Ark. Code Ann. § 17-87-310(b)(2).

The Arkansas State Board of Nursing may grant a certificate of prescriptive authority to an advanced practice nurse who:

- Submits proof of successful completion of a board-approved advanced pharmacology course that shall include preceptorial experience in the prescription of drugs, medicine, and therapeutic devices; and
- Has a collaborative practice with a physician, who is licensed under the Arkansas Medical Practices Act, §§ 17-95-201–7-95-207, 17-95-301–17-95-305, and 17-95-401–17-95-411, and who has a practice comparable in scope, specialty or expertise to that of the advanced practice nurse on file with the board.

Citation: Ark. Code Ann. § 17-87-310(a).

California

Neither this chapter nor any other provision of law shall be construed to prohibit a nurse practitioner from furnishing or ordering drugs or devices when all of the following apply:

a. The drugs or devices are furnished or ordered by a nurse practitioner in accordance with standardized procedures or protocols developed by the nurse practitioner and the supervising physician and surgeon when the drugs or devices furnished or ordered are consistent with the nurse practitioner's educational preparation or for which clinical competency has been established and maintained.

b. The nurse practitioner is functioning pursuant to standardized procedure, as defined by Section 2725, or protocol. The standardized procedure or protocol shall be developed and approved by the supervising physician and surgeon, the nurse practitioner, and the facility administrator or the designee.

c. 1. The standardized procedure or protocol covering the furnishing of drugs or devices shall specify which nurse practitioner may furnish or order drugs or devices, which drugs or devices may be furnished or ordered, under what circumstances, the extent of physician and surgeon supervision, the method of periodic review of the nurse practitioner's competence, including peer review, and review of the provisions of the standardized procedure.

   2. In addition to the requirements in paragraph (1), for Schedule II controlled substance protocols, the provision for furnishing Schedule II controlled substances shall address the diagnosis of the illness, injury, or condition for which the Schedule II controlled substance is to be furnished.

d. The furnishing or ordering of drugs or devices by a nurse practitioner occurs under physician and surgeon supervision. Physician and surgeon supervision shall not be construed to require the physical presence of the physician, but does include: (1) collaboration on the development of the standardized procedure, (2) approval of the standardized procedure, and (3) availability by telephonic contact at the time of patient examination by the nurse practitioner.

e. For purposes of this section, no physician and surgeon shall supervise more than four nurse practitioners at one time.

f. 1. Drugs or devices furnished or ordered by a nurse practitioner may include Schedule II through Schedule V controlled substances under the California Uniform Controlled Substances Act . . . and shall be further limited to those drugs agreed upon by the nurse practitioner and physician and surgeon and specified in the standardized procedure.

   2. When Schedule II or III controlled substances . . . are furnished or ordered by a nurse practitioner, the controlled substances shall be

furnished or ordered in accordance with a patient-specific protocol approved by the treating or supervising physician. A copy of the section of the nurse practitioner's standardized procedure relating to controlled substances shall be provided, upon request, to any licensed pharmacist who dispenses drugs or devices, when there is uncertainty about the nurse practitioner furnishing the order.

g. 1. The board has certified that in accordance with Section 2836.3 the nurse practitioner has satisfactorily completed (1) at least 6 month's physician and surgeon-supervised experience in the furnishing or ordering of drugs or devices and (2) a course in pharmacology covering the drugs or devices to be furnished or ordered under this section.

   2. Nurse practitioners, who are certified by the board and hold an active furnishing number, who are authorized through standardized procedures or protocols to furnish Schedule II controlled substances, and who are registered with the United States Drug Enforcement Administration, shall complete, as part of their continuing education requirements, a course including Schedule II controlled substances based on the standards developed by the board. The board shall establish the requirements for satisfactory completion of this subsection.

h. Use of the term "furnishing" in this section, in health facilities defined in Section 1250 of the Health and Safety Code, shall include (1) the ordering of a drug or device in accordance with the standardized procedure and (2) transmitting an order of a supervising physician and surgeon.

i. "Drug order" or "order," for purposes of this section, means an order for medication which is dispensed to or for an ultimate user, issued by a nurse practitioner as an individual practitioner, within the meaning of Section 1306.02 of Title 21 of the Code of Federal Regulations. Notwithstanding any other provision of law, (1) a drug order issued pursuant to this section shall be treated in the same manner as a prescription of the supervising physician; (2) all references to "prescription" in this code and the Health and Safety Code shall include drug orders issued by nurse practitioners; and (3) the signature of a nurse practitioner on the drug order issued in accordance with this section shall be deemed to be the signature of a prescriber for purposes of this code and the Health and Safety Code.

Citation: Cal. Bus. & Prof. Code § 2836.1.

Furnishing or ordering of drugs or devices by nurse practitioners is defined to mean the act of making a pharmaceutical agent or agents available to the patient in strict accordance with a standardized procedure. All nurse practitioners who are authorized pursuant to Section 2836.1 to furnish or issue drug orders for controlled substances shall register with the United States Drug Enforcement Administration.

Citation: Cal. Bus. & Prof. Code § 2836.2.

Colorado

An advanced practice nurse who is listed on the advanced practice registry, has a license in good standing without disciplinary sanctions issued pursuant to Section 12-38-111, and has fulfilled requirements established by the board pursuant to this section may be authorized by the board to prescribe controlled substances or prescription drugs as defined in article 22 of this title.

Citation: Colo. Rev. Stat. Ann. § 12-38-111.6(1).

For detailed requirements, see the Colorado Board of Nursing Rules, Ch. XV.

Connecticut

In all settings, the advanced practice registered nurse may, in collaboration with a physician licensed to practice medicine in this state, prescribe, dispense, and administer medical therapeutics and corrective measures and may request, sign for, receive, and dispense drugs in the form of professional samples. . . .

Citation: Conn. Gen. Stat. Ann. § 20-87a(b).

Relative to the exercise of prescriptive authority, the collaboration between an advanced practice registered nurse and a physician shall be in writing and shall address the level of schedule II and III controlled substances that the advanced practice registered nurse may prescribe and provide a method to review patient outcomes, including, but not limited to, the review of medical therapeutics, corrective measures, laboratory tests and other diagnostic procedures that the advanced practice registered nurse may prescribe, dispense and administer.

Citation: Conn. Gen. Stat. Ann. §20-87a(b).

Delaware

Those individuals who wish to engage in independent practice without written guidelines or protocols and/or wish to have independent prescriptive authority shall apply for such privilege or privileges to the Joint Practice Committee and do so only in collaboration with a licensed physician, dentist, podiatrist, or licensed healthcare delivery system. This does not include those individuals who have protocols and/or waiver approved by the Board of Medical Licensure and Discipline.

Citation: Del. Code Ann. tit. 24, § 1902(b)(2).

The "Joint Practice Committee" with the approval of the Board of Medical Licensure and Discipline, shall have the authority to grant, restrict, suspend, or revoke practice or independent practice authorization, and the Joint Practice Committee with the approval of the Board of Medical Licensure and Discipline shall be responsible for promulgating rules and regulations to implement the provisions of this chapter regarding "advanced practice nurses" who have been granted authority for independent practice and/or independent prescriptive authority.

Citation: Del. Code Ann. tit. 24, § 1906(20).

APNs may prescribe, administer, and dispense legend medications including Schedule II-V controlled substances, (as defined in the Controlled Substance Act and labeled in compliance with 24 Del.C. §2536(C), parenteral medications, medical therapeutics, devices and diagnostics.

Citation: DEL. ADMIN. CODE, TIT. 24, §8.18.1.

District of Columbia

An advanced practice registered nurse may initiate, monitor, and alter drug therapies.

Citation: D.C. Stat. § 3-1206.4(1).

The advanced practice registered nurse may perform actions of medical diagnosis, treatment, prescription, and other functions authorized by this subchapter.

Citation: D.C. Stat. § 3-1206.1.

A nurse-practitioner shall have authority to prescribe those drugs on Schedules II through V established pursuant to the District of Columbia Uniform Controlled Substances Act of 1981, D.C. Code §§ 33-501 et seq., that are authorized by the protocol under which the nurse-practitioner is practicing.

Citation: D. C. Municipal Regs. §5910.1.

Florida

The scope of practice for all categories of advanced registered nurse practitioner's (ARNP) shall include those functions which the ARNP has been educated to perform including the monitoring and altering of drug therapies, and initiation of appropriate therapies, according to the established protocol and consistent with the practice setting.

Citation: Fla. Admin. Code Ch. 64B9-4.009.

Georgia

    b. 1. A physician may delegate to:
           A. A physician's assistant in accordance with a job description; or
           B. A nurse recognized by the Georgia Board of Nursing as a certified nurse midwife, certified registered nurse anesthetist, certified nurse practitioner, or clinical nurse specialist, psychiatric/mental health in

accordance with a nurse protocol the authority to order controlled substances selected from a formulary of such drugs established by the Composite State Board of Medical Examiners and the authority to order dangerous drugs, medical treatments, and diagnostic studies.

Citation: Ga. Code Ann. 43-34-26.1 (b)(1)(A) and (B).

In addition to and without limiting the authority granted pursuant to Code Section 43-34-23, a physician may delegate to an advanced practice registered nurse in accordance with a nurse protocol agreement the authority to order drugs, medical devices, medical treatments, diagnostic studies, or in life-threatening situations, radiographic imaging tests.

Citation: Ga. Code Ann. § 43-34-25(b).

"Nurse protocol agreement" means a written document mutually agreed upon and signed by an advanced practice registered nurse and a physician, by which document the physician delegates to that advanced practice registered nurse the authority to perform certain medical acts pursuant to this Code section, and which acts may include, without being limited to, the ordering of drugs, medical devices, medical treatments, diagnostic studies, or in life-threatening situations radiographic imaging tests. Such agreements shall conform to the provisions set forth in Subsection (c) of this Code section.

Citation: Ga. Code Ann. § 43-34-26.3(a)(10).

"Order" means to prescribe pursuant to a nurse protocol agreement which drug, medical device, medical treatment, diagnostic study, or in life-threatening situations, radiographic imaging test is appropriate for a patient and to communicate the same in writing, orally, via facsimile, or electronically.

Citation: Ga. Code Ann. § 43-34-26.3(a)(11).

Hawaii

The board shall grant prescriptive authority to qualified advanced practice registered nurses and shall designate the requirements for advanced nursing practice related to prescriptive authority. The board shall determine the exclusionary formulary for qualified advanced practice registered nurses who are granted prescriptive authority.

Citation: Haw. Statutes § 457-8.6(a).

Advanced practice registered nurses shall be considered qualified if they have met the requirements of section 457-8.5(a), and have met the advanced pharmacology requirements for initial prescriptive authority pursuant to rules adopted by the board. Only qualified advanced practice registered nurses authorized to diagnose, prescribe, and institute therapy or referrals of patients to health care agencies, health care providers, and community resources and, only as appropriate, to the practice specialty in which the advanced practice nurse is qualified, may:

1. Prescribe and administer over the counter drugs, legend drugs, and controlled substances pursuant to this chapter and to chapter 329 and request, receive, and dispense manufacturers' prepackaged samples of over the counter and non-controlled legend drugs to patients under their care; provided that an advanced practice registered nurse shall not request, receive, or sign for professional controlled substance samples;
2. Prescribe, order, and dispense medical devices and equipment; and
3. Plan and initiate a therapeutic regimen that includes nutritional, diagnostic, and supportive services including home health care, hospice, and physical and occupational therapy.

Citation: Haw. Statutes § 457-8.6(d).

a. The requirements for prescriptive authority are as follows:
  1. A completed application for prescriptive authority for controlled or non-controlled substances provided by the board and submitted with all appropriate documents (unless currently filed with the board) and required fees;
  2. Proof of a current, unencumbered license as a registered nurse in this State and in all other states in which the nurse has a current and active license;
  3. Proof of a current, unencumbered recognition or license as an advanced practice registered nurse in this State and in all other states in which the nurse has a current and active recognition or license as an advanced practice registered nurse or similar designation;
  4. Proof of a current, unencumbered certification for specialized and advanced nursing practice from a national certifying body recognized by the board;
  5. Proof of successful completion of an accredited graduate-level nursing program with a significant educational and practical concentration on the direct care of patients, recognized by the board, leading to a master's degree as a certified registered nurse anesthetist, a nurse midwife, a clinical nurse specialist, or a nurse practitioner;
  6. Proof of successful completion of at least thirty contact hours, as part of a master's degree program from an accredited, board-recognized college or university, of advanced pharmacology education, including advanced pharmacotherapeutics that is integrated into the curriculum, within the three-year time period immediately preceding the date of application. If completed more than the three-year time period, then one of the following shall be completed within the three-year time period immediately preceding the date of application for initial prescriptive authority:

A. At least thirty contact hours of advanced pharmacology, including advanced pharmacotherapeutics, from an accredited, board-recognized college or university; or

B. At least thirty contact hours of continuing education ("CE") approved by board-recognized national certifying bodies in advanced pharmacology, including advanced pharmacotherapeutics related to the applicant's scope of nursing practice specialty; and

7. Payment of a non-refundable application fee.

b. APRNs authorized to prescribe non-controlled substances and who subsequently wish to prescribed controlled substances shall submit the appropriate application for prescriptive authority for controlled substances and meet the requirements of this chapter.

c. Upon satisfying all requirements in chapter 457, HRS, and this chapter, and payment of required fees, the board shall grant prescriptive authority to the APRN.

d. Nothing in this section shall preclude a registered nurse, a licensed practical nurse, or an APRN from carrying out the prescribed medical orders of a license dentist, physician, osteopath, or podiatrist license in accordance with chapters 448, 453, or 463E, HRS, or the orders of a recognized APRN granted prescriptive authority in accordance with this chapter.

Citation: Haw. Admin. R. § 16-89-119.

a. The board of nursing shall consider the recommendations of the joint formulary advisory committee to determine the drugs or categories of drugs listed in the exclusionary formulary for APRNs granted prescriptive authority. The current formulary, attached to this chapter as "Exhibit A", lists the drugs or categories of drugs that shall be prescribed by the APRN.

b. The Exclusionary Formulary, and any revised formularies, shall be made available to licensed pharmacies at the request of the pharmacy at no cost.

c. The APRN shall comply with all applicable state and federal laws and rules relating to prescribing and administering of drugs. The APRN with prescriptive authority shall only prescribe, order, and dispense medical devices and equipment appropriate to the APRN's specialty.

d. Prescriptions by an APRN with prescriptive authority shall be written in accordance with 16-95-82.

Citation: Haw. Admin. R. § 16-89-122.

Prescriptive authority renewal for recognized advanced practice registered nurses.

a. Prescriptive authority for each APRN shall expire on June 30 of every odd-numbered year and shall be renewed biennially. APRNs seeking renewal of prescriptive authority shall also satisfy the renewal requirements for APRN recognition pursuant to section 16-89-87 and submit the following:

1. Evidence of current certification in the nursing practice specialty by a board-recognized national certifying body; and

2. Documentation of successful completion, during the prior biennium, of thirty contact hours of appropriate continuing education as determined by the board in the practice specialty area, eight contact hours of which shall be in pharmacology, including pharmacotherapeutics, related to the APRN's clinical practice specialty area, approved by board-recognized national certifying bodies, the American Nurses Association, the American Medical Association, or accredited colleges or universities. Documentation of successful completion of continuing education required for recertification by a recognized national certifying body, earned within the current renewal biennium, may be accepted in lieu of the thirty hours of continuing education required for renewal.

b. Failure, neglect, or refusal to renew the prescriptive authority by a recognized APRN on or before June 30 of each odd-numbered year shall result in automatic forfeiture of prescriptive authority. Failure of the APRN to renew prescriptive authority shall cause the APRN prescriptive authority to forfeit on the day after the expiration date. The APRN shall not prescribe until prescriptive authority has been restored. Renewal application deadlines shall be as established by the board. Prescriptive authority may be restored within six months from the date of forfeiture, provided the restoration application is in compliance with subsection (a) and is submitted with an additional payment of a restoration fee. Failure to restore within the time frame provided shall constitute an automatic termination of the prescriptive authority. Thereafter, to be eligible for prescriptive authority, the applicant shall meet the requirements of section 16-89-119.

c. Any APRN subject to this chapter who fails to renew his or her prescriptive authority and continues to practice as a recognized APRN with prescriptive authority shall be considered an illegal practitioner and shall be subject to penalties provided for by law.

Citation: Haw. Admin. R. § 16-89-123.

Idaho

Advanced practice registered nurses... are authorized to perform advanced nursing practice, which may include the prescribing, administering and dispensing of therapeutic pharmacologic agents, as defined by board rules.

Citation: Idaho Code § 54-1402(1).

Prescriptive and Dispensing Authorization. Means the legal permission to prescribe, deliver, distribute and dispense pharmacologic and non-pharmacologic agents to a client in compliance with Board rules and applicable federal and state laws. Pharmacologic agents include legend and Schedule II through V controlled substances.

Citation: IDAHO ADMIN. CODE §23.01.01.271.15.

An application for the authority to prescribe and dispense pharmacologic and non-pharmacologic agents may be made as part of initial licensure application or by separate application at a later date. Advanced practice registered nurses who complete their APRN graduate or post-graduate educational program after December 31, 2015, will automatically be granted prescriptive and dispensing authority with the issuance of their Idaho licensure.

a. An advanced practice professional nurse who applies for authorization to prescribe pharmacologic and non-pharmacologic agents within the scope of practice for the advanced practice role, shall:
   i. Be currently licensed as an advanced practice professional nurse in Idaho;
   ii. Provide evidence of completion of thirty (30) contact hours of post-basic education in pharmacotherapeutics. . . .
   iii. Submit a completed, notarized application form provided by the Board; and
   iv. Remit fees prescribed in Section 901 of these rules.

Citation: Idaho Admin. Code § 23.01.01.315.01(a).

Illinois

(Section scheduled to be repealed on January 1, 2018.)

a. A collaborating physician or podiatrist may, but is not required to, delegate prescriptive authority to an advanced practice nurse as part of a written collaborative agreement. This authority may, but is not required to, include prescription of, selection of, orders for, administration of, storage of, acceptance of samples of, and dispensing over the counter medications, legend drugs, medical gases, and controlled substances categorized as any Schedule III through V controlled substances, as defined in Article II of the Illinois Controlled Substances Act, and other preparations, including, but not limited to, botanical and herbal remedies. The collaborating physician or podiatrist must have a valid current Illinois controlled substance license and federal registration to delegate authority to prescribe delegated controlled substances.

b. To prescribe controlled substances under this Section, an advanced practice nurse must obtain a mid-level practitioner controlled substance license. Medication orders shall be reviewed periodically by the collaborating physician or podiatrist.

c. The collaborating physician or podiatrist shall file with the Department notice of delegation of prescriptive authority and termination of such delegation, in accordance with rules of the Department. Upon receipt of this notice delegating authority to prescribe any Schedule III through V controlled substances, the licensed advanced practice nurse shall be eligible to register for a mid-level practitioner controlled substance license under Section 303.05 of the Illinois Controlled Substances Act.

d. In addition to the requirements of Subsections (a), (b), and (c) of this Section, a collaborating physician may, but is not required to, delegate authority to an advanced practice nurse to prescribe any Schedule II controlled substances, if all of the following conditions apply:

1. Specific Schedule II controlled substances by oral dosage or topical or transdermal application may be delegated, provided that the delegated Schedule II controlled substances are routinely prescribed by the collaborating physician or podiatrist. This delegation must identify the specific Schedule II controlled substances by either brand name or generic name. Schedule II controlled substances to be delivered by injection or other route of administration may not be delegated.

2. Any delegation must be controlled substances that the collaborating physician or podiatrist prescribes.

3. Any prescription must be limited to no more than a 30-day supply, with any continuation authorized only after prior approval of the collaborating physician or podiatrist.

4. The advanced practice nurse must discuss the condition of any patients for whom a controlled substance is prescribed monthly with the delegating physician.

5. The advanced practice nurse meets the education requirements of Section 303.05 of the Illinois Controlled Substances Act.

e. Nothing in this Act shall be construed to limit the delegation of tasks or duties by a physician to a licensed practical nurse, a registered professional nurse, or other persons. Nothing in this Act shall be construed to limit the method of delegation that may be authorized by any means, including, but not limited to, oral, written, electronic, standing orders, protocols, guidelines, or verbal orders.

Citation: Ill. Comp. Stat. § 65/65-40.

a. A collaborating physician or podiatrist who delegates prescriptive authority to an advanced practice nurse shall include that delegation in the written collaborative agreement. This authority may include prescription of, selection of, orders for, administration of, storage of, acceptance of samples of, and dispensing over the counter medications, legend drugs, medical gases, and controlled substances categorized as Schedule III, III-N, IV, or V controlled substances, as defined in Article II of the Illinois Controlled Substances Act, and other preparations, including, but not limited to, botanical and herbal remedies. The collaborating physician or podiatrist must have a valid current Illinois controlled substance license and federal registration to delegate authority to prescribed delegated controlled substances.

b. Pursuant to Section 65-40(d) of the Act, a collaborating physician may, but is not required to, delegate authority to an advanced practice nurse to prescribe Schedule II or II-N controlled substances under the following conditions:

1. No more than 5 Schedule II or II-N controlled substances by oral dosage may be delegated. For the purposes of this Section generic substitution pursuant to Section 25 of the Pharmacy Practice Act shall be allowed under this Section when not prohibited by a prescriber's indication on the prescription that the pharmacist "may not substitute."
2. The collaborating physician can only delegate controlled substances that the collaborating physician prescribes.
3. Any prescription must be limited to no more than a 30-day oral dosage, with any continuation authorized only after prior approval of the collaborating physician.
4. The advanced practice nurse must discuss the condition of any patients for whom a controlled substance is prescribed monthly with the delegating physician.

c. An APN who has been given controlled substances prescriptive authority shall be required to obtain an Illinois mid-level practitioner controlled substance license in accordance with 77 Ill. Adm. Code 3100. The physician or podiatrist shall file a notice of delegation of prescriptive authority with the Division. The delegation of authority form shall be submitted to the Division prior to the issuance of a controlled substance license.

d. The APN may only prescribe and dispense within the scope of practice of the collaborating physician or podiatrist. Licensed dentists may not delegate prescriptive authority.

e. All prescriptions written and signed by an advanced practice nurse shall indicate the name of the collaborating physician or podiatrist. The collaborating physician's or podiatrist's signature is not required. The APN shall sign his/her own name.

f. An APN may receive and dispense samples per the collaborative agreement.

g. Medication orders shall be reviewed periodically by the collaborating physician or podiatrist.

Citation: Ill. Admin. Code. tit. 68, § 1300.430.

Indiana

An advanced practice nurse may be authorized to prescribe legend drugs, including controlled substances, if the advanced practice nurse does the following:

1. Submits an application with the required fee;
2. Submits proof of an active, unrestricted registered nurse license;

3. Submits proof of having met the requirements of all applicable laws for practice as advanced practice nurse in the state of Indiana;
4. Submits proof of a baccalaureate or higher degree in nursing;
5. If the applicant holds a baccalaureate degree only, submits proof of certification as a nurse practitioner or certified nurse midwife by a national organization recognized by the board and which requires a national certifying examination.
6. Submits proof of having successfully completed a graduate level pharmacology course, consisting of at least two (2) semester hours of academic credit from a college or university accredited by the commission on Recognition of Postsecondary Accreditation:
   A. within five (5) years of the date of application; or
   B. if the pharmacology course was completed more than five (5) years immediately preceding the date of the application, the applicant must submit proof of the following:
      i. completing at least thirty (30) actual contact hours of continuing education during the two (2) years immediately preceding the date of application, including a minimum of at least eight (8) actual contact hours of pharmacology, all of which must be approved by a nationally approved sponsor of continuing education for nurses.
      ii. Prescriptive experience in another jurisdiction within the five (5) years immediately preceding the date of application.
7. Submits proof of collaboration with a licensed practitioner in the form of a written practice agreement that sets forth the manner in which the advanced practice nurse and licensed practitioner will cooperate, coordinate, and consult with each other in the provision of health care to patients. . . .
8. Written practice agreements for advanced practice nurses applying for prescriptive authority shall not be valid until prescriptive authority is granted by the board.

Citation: Ind. Admin. Code tit. 848, r. 5-1-1.

Iowa

"Prescriptive authority" is the authority granted to an ARNP registered in Iowa in a recognized nursing specialty to prescribe, deliver, distribute, or dispense prescription drugs, devices, and medical gases when the nurse is engaged in the practice of that nursing specialty. Registration as a practitioner with the Federal Drug Enforcement Administration and the Iowa board of pharmacy examiners extends this authority to controlled substances. ARNPs shall access the Iowa board of pharmacy examiners Web site for Iowa pharmacy law and administrative rules and the Iowa Board of Pharmacy Examiners Newsletter.

Citation: Iowa Admin. Code r. 655-7.1(152).

Kansas

An advanced practice registered nurse may prescribe drugs pursuant to a written protocol as authorized by a responsible physician. Each written protocol shall contain a precise and detailed medical plan of care for each classification of disease or injury for which the advanced practice registered nurse is authorized to prescribe and shall specify all drugs which may be prescribed by the advanced practice registered nurse. Any written prescription order shall include the name, address, and telephone number of the responsible physician. The advanced practice registered nurse may not dispense drugs, but may request, receive, and sign for professional samples and may distribute professional samples to patients pursuant to a written protocol as authorized by a responsible physician. In order to prescribe controlled substances, the advanced practice registered nurse shall

1. register with the federal drug enforcement administration; and
2. notify the board of the name and address of the responsible physician or physicians. In no case shall the scope of authority of the advanced practice registered nurse exceed the normal and customary practice of the responsible physician. An advanced practice registered nurse certified in the category of registered nurse anesthetist while functioning as a registered nurse anesthetist under K.S.A. 1988 Supp. 65-1151 to 65-1164, including, and amendments thereto, shall be subject to the provisions of K.S.A. 65-1151 and 65-1164, inclusive and amendments thereto, with respect to drugs and anesthetic agents and shall not be subject to the provisions of this subsection. For the purposes of this subsection, "responsible physician" means a person licensed to practice medicine and surgery in Kansas who has accepted responsibility for the protocol and the actions of the advanced registered nurse practitioner when prescribing drugs.

Citation: Kan. Stat Ann. § 65-1130(d).

a. Each written protocol pursuant to which an advanced registered nurse practitioner may transmit prescription orders shall:
    1. Specify for each classification of disease or injury the corresponding class of drugs for which the advanced registered nurse practitioner is permitted to prescribe;
    2. Be maintained in either a looseleaf notebook or a book of published protocols. The notebook or book of published protocols shall include a cover page containing the following data:
        A. The names, telephone numbers, and signatures of the advanced registered nurse practitioner and a responsible physician who has authorized the protocol; and
        B. The date on which the protocol was adopted or last reviewed, and
    3. Be kept at the advanced registered nurse practitioner's principal place of practice.

Each written protocol that an advanced practice registered nurse is to follow when prescribing, administering, or supplying a prescription-only drug shall meet the following requirements:

1. Specify for each classification of disease or injury the corresponding class of drugs that the advanced practice registered nurse is permitted to prescribe;
2. Be maintained in either a loose-leaf notebook or a book of published protocols. The notebook or book of published protocols shall include a cover page containing the following data:
   A. The names, telephone numbers, and signatures of the advanced practice registered nurse and a responsible physician who has authorized the protocol; and
   B. The date on which the protocol was adopted or last reviewed; and
3. Be kept at the advanced practice registered nurse's principal place of practice.

b. Each advanced practice registered nurse shall ensure that each protocol is reviewed by the advanced practice registered nurse and physician at least annually.

c. Each prescription order in written form shall meet the following requirements:
   1. Include the name, address, and telephone number of the practice location of the advanced practice registered nurse;
   2. include the name, address, and telephone number of the responsible physician;
   3. be signed by the advanced practice registered nurse with the letters A.P.R.N.;
   4. be from a class of drugs prescribed pursuant to protocol; and
   5. contain any D.E.A. registration number issued to the advanced practice registered nurse when a controlled substance, as defined in K.S.A. 65-4101(e) and amendments thereto, is prescribed.

d. Nothing in this regulation shall be construed to prohibit any registered nurse or licensed practical nurse or advanced practice registered nurse from conveying a prescription order orally or administering a drug if acting under the lawful direction of a person licensed to practice either medicine and surgery or dentistry, or certified as an advanced registered nurse practitioner.

Citation: Kan. Admin. Regs. § 60-11-104a.

Kentucky

Advanced practice registered nurse shall include prescribing medications and ordering treatments, devices, and diagnostic tests, which are consistent with the scope and standard of practice of the advanced practice registered nurse.

Citation: 201 Ky. Admin. Regs. § 20:057 (Section 4).

KRS 314.011(8)(c) authorizes the Controlled Substances Formulary Development Committee to make recommendations to the Board of Nursing concerning any limitations for the prescription of specific controlled substances by advanced practice registered nurses. This administrative regulation establishes limitations for the prescription of specific controlled substances by advanced practice registered nurses.

Section 1. Specific Controlled Substances. The following controlled substances have been identified as having the greatest potential for abuse or diversion:
1. Diazepam (Valium), a Schedule IV medication;
2. Clonazepam (Klonopin), a Schedule IV medication;
3. Lorazepam (Ativan), a Schedule IV medication;
4. Alprazolam (Xanax), a Schedule IV medication; and
5. Carisoprodol (Soma), a Schedule IV medication.

Section 2. Limitations. Prescriptions for the medications listed in Section 1 of this administrative regulation shall be limited to a thirty (30) day supply without any refill.

Citation: 201 KY. ADMIN. REGS. §20:059.

Louisiana

An APRN may be granted prescriptive authority to prescribe assessment studies, including pharmaceutical diagnostic testing (e.g., dobutamine stress testing), legend and certain controlled drugs, therapeutic regimens, medical devices and appliances, receiving and distributing a therapeutic regimen of prepackaged drugs prepared and labeled by a licensed pharmacist, and free samples supplied by a drug manufacturer, and distributing drugs for administration to and use by other individuals within the scope of practice as defined by the board in R.S. 37.913(3)(b).

Requirements for prescriptive privileges:

- Hold a current; unencumbered, unrestricted, and valid RN licensure
- Hold a current, unencumbered, unrestricted, and valid APRN licensure
- Evidence of 500 hours of clinical practice as a licensed APRN within 1 year prior to applying for prescriptive and distributing authority
- 45 hours of education in pharmacotherapeutics
- 45 contact hours of pathophysiology/physiology in formal educational program
- Collaborative practice agreement with one or more licensed collaborating physicians
- Each year . . . six hours of continuing education in pharmacotherapeutics

Citation: La. Admin. Code tit. 46, § XLVII.4513.

Maine

A. Certified nurse practitioners and certified nurse–midwives are authorized to prescribe the following:
   1. over the counter drugs
   2. appliances and devices
   3. drugs related to the specialty area of certification
   4. drugs prescribed off label according to common and established standards of practice.
B. Regardless of the schedules indicated on the certificate issued by the Drug Enforcement Administration, the certified nurse practitioner and certified nurse–midwives shall prescribe only those controlled drugs from Schedules II, III, IIIN, IV, and V. A Drug Enforcement Agency (D.E.A.) number is required to prescribe these Drugs.

Citation: Code Me. R. § 02 380 008 (Section 7).

Maryland

A nurse practitioner may perform independently the following functions:

...Prescribe drugs...

Citation: Md. Regs. Code. 10 § 27.07.02A(12).

"Nurse practitioners certified by the Maryland Board of Nursing as Advanced Practice are automatically given prescriptive authority for non-controlled substances. The Advanced Practice Certification also allows them to apply for permission to prescribe Schedules II through V Controlled Dangerous Substances (CDS)."

Citation: Maryland Board of Nursing, *Instructions for Completing and Submitting the Nurse Practitioner (NP) Attestation Form & Supporting Documents.* Retrieved from http://www.mbon.org /adv_prac/attestation_instructions.pdf

Massachusetts

A nurse practitioner ... may issue written prescriptions and order tests and therapeutics pursuant to guidelines mutually developed and agreed upon by the nurse and the supervising physician in accordance with regulations promulgated jointly by the board and the board of registration in medicine after consultation with the board of registration in pharmacy. A prescription made by a nurse practitioner or psychiatric nurse mental health clinical specialist shall include the name of the physician with whom such nurse has developed and signed mutually agreed upon guidelines approved by said board and said board of registration in medicine pursuant to Section 80B.

Citation: Mass. Ann. Laws, Ch. 112, § 80E.

A nurse engaged in prescriptive practice means a nurse with: (a) authorization to practice in an expanded role; (b) a minimum of 24 contact hours in pharmacotherapeutics which are beyond those acquired in a generic nursing program ..., (c) valid registration to issue written or oral prescriptions or medication orders for controlled substances from the Massachusetts Department of Public Health ... and, where required, by the US Drug Enforcement Administration.

Citation: Mass. Regs. Code tit. 244, § 4.05.

The guidelines for prescriptive practice shall:

- Include a defined mechanism to monitor prescribing practices, including documentation of review with a supervising physician at least every three months;
- Include protocols for initiation of intravenous therapies and Schedule II drugs;
- Specify the frequency of review of initial prescription of controlled substances; the initial prescription of Schedule II drugs must be reviewed within 96 hours;
- Conform to M.G.L. c.94C, the regulations of the Department of Public Health at 105 CMR 700.000 et seq., and M.G.L. c.112 §§ 80E or 80H, as applicable.

Citation: Mass. Regs. Code tit. 244, § 4.22(3).

A supervising physician shall review and provide ongoing direction for the APN's prescriptive practice in accordance with written guidelines mutually developed and agreed upon with the APN pursuant to M.G.L. c. 112, §§ 80B, 80C, 80E, 80G, 80H, and the regulations of the Board of Registration in Nursing (244 CMR) and 243 CMR 2.10. This supervision shall be provided as is necessary, taking into account the education, training and experience of the APN, the nature of the APN's practice, and the physician's availability to provide clinical backup to ensure that the APN is providing patient care in accordance with accepted standards of practice.

(b) A supervising physician shall sign prescriptive practice guidelines only with those APNs for whom he or she is able to provide supervision consistent with 243 CMR 2.10(2) and (3), taking into account factors including, but not limited to geographical proximity, practice setting, volume and complexity of the patient population, and the experience, training and availability of the supervising physician and the APN(s).

(c) A supervising physician shall not enter into guidelines, pursuant to M.G.L. c. 112, §§ 80B, 80C, 80E, 80G, or 80H and 243 CMR 2.10, unless the APN has professional malpractice liability insurance as required by the BORN regulations.

5. a. A physician who supervises an APN engaged in prescriptive practice shall do so in accordance with written guidelines mutually developed and agreed upon with the APN.

    b. In all cases, the written guidelines shall:

      1. identify the supervising physician and APN;

      2. include a defined mechanism for the delegation of supervision to another physician including, but not limited to, the duration and scope of the delegation;

      3. describe the nature and scope of the APN's prescribing practice;

      4. identify the types of medication(s) to be prescribed, specify any limitations on medications to be prescribed; and describe the circumstances in which physician consultation or referral is required;

      5. describe the use of established procedures for the treatment of common medical conditions which the nurse may encounter;

      6. include provisions for managing emergencies;

      7. include a defined mechanism and time frame to monitor prescribing practices;

      8. include protocols for the initiation of intravenous therapies and Schedule II drugs;

      9. specify that the initial prescription of Schedule II drugs must be reviewed within 96 hours;

     10. specify that the guidelines must be kept on file in the workplace and be reviewed and re-executed every two years; and

     11. conform to M.G.L. c. 94C, the regulations of the Department of Public Health at 105 CMR 700.000.

Citation: Mass. Regs. Code tit. 243 §2.10 (4) and (5)

Michigan

A licensee who holds a license other than a health profession subfield license may delegate to a licensed or unlicensed individual who is otherwise qualified by education, training, or experience the performance of selected acts, tasks, or functions where the acts, tasks, or functions fall within the scope of practice of the licensee's profession and will be performed under the licensee's supervision. A licensee shall not delegate an act, task, or function under this section if the act, task, or function, under standards of acceptable and prevailing practice, requires the level of education, skill, and judgment required of the licensee under this article.

Citation: Mich. Comp. Laws § 333.16215(1).

A supervising physician may delegate in writing to a registered professional nurse the ordering, receipt, and dispensing of complimentary starter dose drugs other than controlled substances as defined by article 7 or federal law. When the delegated ordering, receipt, or dispensing of complimentary starter dose drugs occurs, both the registered professional nurse's name and the supervising physician's name shall be used, recorded, or otherwise indicated in connection with each order, receipt, or dispensing.

Citation: Mich. Comp. Laws § 333.17212(1).

1. A physician may delegate the prescription of controlled substances listed in schedules 3 to 5 to a registered nurse who holds specialty certification under section 17210 of the code, with the exception of a nurse anesthetist, if the delegating physician establishes a written authorization that contains all of the following information:
   a. The name, license number, and signature of the delegating physician.
   b. The name, license number, and signature of the nurse practitioner or nurse midwife.
   c. The limitations or exceptions to the delegation.
   d. The effective date of the delegation.
2. A delegating physician shall review and update a written authorization on an annual basis from the original date or the date of amendment, if amended. A delegating physician shall note the review date on the written authorization.
3. A delegating physician shall maintain a written authorization in each separate location of the physician's office where the delegation occurs.
4. A delegating physician shall ensure that an amendment to the written authorization is in compliance with subrule (1) (a) to (d) of this rule.
5. A delegating physician may delegate the prescription of schedule 2 controlled substances only if all of the following conditions are met:
   a. The delegating physician and nurse practitioner or nurse midwife are practicing within a health facility as defined in section 20106(d), (g), or (i) of the code; specifically, freestanding surgical outpatient facilities, hospitals, and hospices.
   b. The patient is located within the facility described in subdivision (a) of this subrule.
   c. The delegation is in compliance with this rule.
6. A delegating physician may not delegate the prescription of schedule 2 controlled substances issued for the discharge of a patient for a quantity for more than a 7-day period.
7. A delegating physician shall not delegate the prescription of a drug or device individually, in combination, or in succession for a woman known to be pregnant with the intention of causing either a miscarriage or fetal death.

Citation: Michigan Board of Medicine Rules R338.2305.

Minnesota

A certified nurse practitioner who has a written agreement with a physician based on standards established by the Minnesota Nurses Association and the Minnesota Medical Association that defines the delegated responsibilities related to the prescription of drugs and therapeutic devices, may prescribe and administer drugs and therapeutic devices within the scope of the written agreement and within practice as a nurse practitioner. The written agreement required under this subdivision shall be based on standards established by the Minnesota Nurses Association and the Minnesota Medical Association as of January 1, 1996, unless both associations agree to revisions.

Citation: Minn. Stat. Ann. § 148.235(2).

An advanced practice registered nurse who is authorized under this section to prescribe drugs is authorized to dispense drugs subject to the same requirements established for the prescribing of drugs. This authority to dispense extends only to those drugs dispensed in the written agreement entered into under this section. The authority to dispense includes, but is not limited to, the authority to receive and dispense sample drugs.

Citation: Minn. Stat. Ann. § 148.235(4b).

A licensed doctor of medicine, a doctor of osteopathy, duly licensed to practice medicine, a doctor of dental surgery, a doctor of dental medicine, a licensed doctor of podiatry, or a licensed doctor of optometry limited to Schedules IV and V, and in the course of professional practice only, may prescribe, administer, and dispense a controlled substance included in Schedules II through V of section 152.02, may cause the same to be administered by a nurse, an intern or an assistant under the direction and supervision of the doctor, and may cause a person who is an appropriately certified and licensed health care professional to prescribe and administer the same within the expressed legal scope of the person's practice as defined in Minnesota Statutes.

Citation: Minn. Stat. §152.12.

Mississippi

Certified nurse midwives and certified nurse practitioners may apply for controlled substance prescriptive authority after completing a board approved educational program. Certified nurse midwives and certified nurse practitioners who have completed the program and received prescription authority from the board may prescribe Schedules II-V. The words "administer," "controlled substances," and "ultimate user," shall have the same meaning as set forth in Section 41-29-105, unless the context otherwise requires. The board shall promulgate rules governing prescribing of controlled substances, including distribution, record keeping, drug maintenance, labeling and distribution requirements and prescription guidelines for controlled substances and all medications. Prescribing any controlled substance in violation of the rules promulgated by the board shall constitute a violation of Section 73-15-29(1) (f), (k) and (l) and shall be grounds for disciplinary action. The prescribing, administering or distributing of any legend drug or other medication in violation of the rules promulgated by the board shall constitute a violation of Section 73-15-29(1) (f), (k) and (l) and shall be grounds for disciplinary action.

Citation: Miss. Nursing Practice Law §73-15-20(8).

Missouri

The methods of treatment and the authority to administer, dispense, or prescribe drugs delegated in a collaborative practice arrangement between a collaborating physician and collaborating APRN shall be within the scope of practice of each professional and shall be consistent with each professional's skill, training, education, competence, licensure, and/or certification and shall not be further delegated to any person except that the individuals identified in sections 338.095 and 338.198, RSMo, may communicate prescription drug orders to a pharmacist.

Citation: Mo. Code Regs. Ann. tit. 20, § 2200-4.200(3)(A).

The collaborating physician shall consider the level of skill, education, training, and competence of the collaborating RN or APRN and ensure that the delegated responsibilities contained in the collaborative practice arrangement are consistent with that level of skill, education, training, and competence.

Citation: Mo. Code Regs. Ann. tit. 20, § 2200-4.200(3)(C).

The methods of treatment, including any authority to administer and dispense drugs, delegated in a collaborative practice arrangement between a collaborating physician and a collaborating RN shall be delivered only pursuant to a written agreement, jointly agreed-upon protocols, or standing orders that shall describe a specific sequence of orders, steps, or procedures to be followed in providing patient care in specified clinical situations.

Citation: Mo. Code Regs. Ann. tit. 20, § 2200-4.200(3)(E).

Methods of treatment delegated and authority to administer, dispense, or prescribe drugs shall be subject to the following:

1. The physician retains the responsibility for ensuring the appropriate administering, dispensing, prescribing, and control of drugs utilized pursuant to a

collaborative practice arrangement in accordance with all state and federal statutes, rules, or regulations;

2. All labeling requirements outlined in Section 338.059, RSMo shall be followed;
3. Consumer product safety laws and Class B container standards shall be followed when packaging drugs for distribution;
4. All drugs shall be stored according to the *United States Pharmacopeia* (USP) recommended conditions;
5. Outdated drugs shall be separated from the active inventory;
6. Retrievable dispensing logs shall be maintained for all prescription drugs dispensed and shall include all information required by state and federal statutes, rules, or regulations;
7. All prescriptions shall conform to all applicable state and federal statutes, rules, or regulations and shall include the name, address, and telephone number of the collaborating physician and collaborating APRN.

Citation: Mo. Code Regs. Ann. tit. 20, § 2200-4.200((3)G).

In addition to administering and dispensing controlled substances, an APRN, as defined in section 335.016, RSMo, may be delegated the authority to prescribe controlled substances listed in Schedules III, IV, and V of section 195.017, RSMo, in a written collaborative practice arrangement, except that, the collaborative practice arrangement shall not delegate the authority to administer any controlled substances listed in Schedules III, IV, and V of section 195.017, RSMo, for the purpose of inducing sedation or general anesthesia for therapeutic, diagnostic, or surgical procedures. Schedule III narcotic controlled substance prescriptions shall be limited to a one hundred twenty (120)-hour supply without refill.

Citation: Mo. Code Regs. Ann. tit. 20, § 2200-4.200(3)(G)9.

An APRN may not prescribe controlled substances for his or her own self or family. Family is defined as spouse, parents, grandparents, great-grandparents, children, grandchildren, great-grandchildren, brothers and sisters, aunts and uncles, nephews and nieces, mother-in-law, father-in-law, brothers-in-law, sisters-in-law, daughters-in-law, and sons-in-law. Adopted and step members are also included in family.

Citation: Mo. Code Regs. Ann. tit. 20, § 2200-4.200(3)(G)10.

An APRN or RN in a collaborative practice arrangement may only dispense starter doses of medication to cover a period of time for seventy-two (72) hours or less with the exception of Title X family planning providers or publicly funded clinics in community health settings that dispense medications free of charge.

Citation: Mo. Code Regs. Ann. tit. 20, § 2200-4.200(G)11.

Montana

Initial Application for Prescriptive Authority

1. The APRN shall submit a completed application for prescriptive authority and a nonrefundable fee as specified in ARM 24.159.401. The application for all APRNs except practicing CRNAs must include:
   a. evidence of successful completion of a graduate level course that provides a minimum of the equivalent of three academic semester credit hours (equaling a minimum of 45 contact hours) from an accredited program in pharmacology, pharmacotherapeutics, and the clinical management of drug therapy related to the applicant's area of specialty. The academic credits must be obtained within a three-year period immediately prior to the date the application is received at the board office and must meet the following requirements:
      i. no more than six of the 45 contact hours may concern the study of herbal or complementary therapies;
      ii. a minimum of 18 of the 45 contact hours must have been obtained within one year immediately prior to the date of application; and
      iii. a minimum of one-third of all contact hours must be face-to-face or interactive instruction.
   b. evidence of the course content and clinical preceptorship;
   c. a copy of the current certification from the APRN's national certifying body;
   d. a description of the proposed practice sites and typical caseload; and
   e. an updated quality assurance plan, if needed, as required by ARM 24.159.1466.

   Citation: Mont. Admin. R § 24.159.1463.

Prescribing Practices

1. Prescriptions must comply with all applicable state and federal laws.
2. All written prescriptions must include the following information:
   a. name, title, address, and phone number of the APRN who is prescribing;
   b. name of client;
   c. date of prescription;
   d. the full name of the drug, dosage, route, amount to be dispensed, and directions for its use;
   e. Drug Enforcement Administration (DEA) number of the prescriber on all scheduled drugs; and
   f. all requirements of state and federal regulations regarding prescriptions.
3. Records of all prescriptions must be documented in client records.

4. An APRN with prescriptive authority shall comply with federal DEA requirements for controlled substances and shall file DEA registrations and numbers with the board.
5. An APRN with prescriptive authority may not prescribe controlled substances for self or members of the APRN's immediate family.
6. In an emergency situation, Schedule II drugs may be phoned in to the pharmacist pursuant to 21 CFR 1306.11(d).
7. An APRN with prescriptive authority may not delegate the prescribing or dispensing of drugs to any other person.

Citation: Mont. Admin. R. § 24-159.1464.

Quality Assurance of APRN Practice

1. Within one month of initiating an APRN practice involving direct patient care the APRN shall submit a quality assurance plan to the board.
2. A quality assurance plan includes the following elements:
   a. location of the APRN's practice site(s);
   b. identification of the APRN's peer-reviewer or peer review organization. Peer review must occur on a quarterly basis and include review of 15 charts or 5 percent of all charts handled by the APRN, whichever is fewer. The peer-reviewer must work in the same practice specialty as the APRN and must hold an unencumbered license. If the APRN has prescriptive authority, the peer-reviewer must also have prescriptive authority;
   c. standards of practice set by the APRN's national professional organization, which the peer-reviewer will use to evaluate the APRN's practice;
   d. criteria for client referrals, patient outcomes, and chart documentation set by the APRN's national professional organization that the peer-reviewer will use to evaluate the APRN's practice; and
   e. description of the method the peer-reviewer will use to address areas in need of attention or improvement, if indicated, and to ensure follow-up evaluation.
3. By December 31 of each license renewal year, the APRN shall submit a quality assurance report to the board on the form provided by the department. The biennial quality assurance report shall:
   a. provide verification that each quarterly peer review has occurred;
   b. provide verification that area(s) identified by the peer reviewer as needing attention and improvement have been appropriately addressed according to the APRN's stated plan; and
   c. inform the board of any change in the location of the APRN's practice site(s), the identity of the peer-reviewer, or the quality assurance criteria

established by the national professional organization in the APRN's specialty area of practice.

Citation: Mont. Admin. R. § 24.159.1466.

Nebraska

2. Nurse practitioner means health promotion, health supervision, illness prevention and diagnosis, treatment, and management of common health problems and acute and chronic conditions, including:
   a. Assessing patients, ordering diagnostic tests and therapeutic treatments, synthesizing and analyzing data, and applying advanced nursing principles;
   b. Dispensing, incident to practice only, sample medications which are provided by the manufacturer and are provided at no charge to the patient; and;
   c. Prescribing therapeutic measures and medications relating to health conditions within the scope of practice. Any limitation on the prescribing authority of the nurse practitioner for controlled substances listed in Schedule II of Section 28-405 shall be recorded in the integrated practice agreement established pursuant to Section 38-2310.

Citation: Neb. Rev. Stat. Ann. § 38-2315.

Nevada

An advanced practice registered nurse may only prescribe controlled substances, poisons, dangerous drugs or devices which are currently within the standard of practice in his or her identified medical specialty.

Citation: Nev. Admin. Code § 632.259.

The State Board of Nursing will issue a certificate to dispense controlled substances, poisons, dangerous drugs and devices to an advanced practice registered nurse if the practitioner:
a. Successfully completes an examination administered by the State Board of Nursing on Nevada law relating to pharmacy; and
b. Submits to the State Board of Nursing his or her affidavit verifying that he or she has made application with the State Board of Pharmacy for a certificate of registration.

Citation: Nev. Admin. Code § 632.2595.

*A protocol must:

1. Reflect the ongoing collaborative relationship between the advanced practice registered nurse and the physician;
2. Reflect the current practice of the advanced practice registered nurse;

3. Reflect established national or customary standards for his or her medical specialty;
4. Be maintained at the place of his or her practice; and
5. Be available for review by the Board.

Citation: NEV. ADMIN. CODE § 632.2555.

This regulation (632.2555) was proposed for repeal as of November 2013 but had not yet been formally adopted as of February 2014.

New Hampshire

An APRN shall have plenary authority to possess, compound, prescribe, administer, dispense and distribute controlled and non-controlled drugs within the scope of the APRN's practice as defined by this chapter. Such authority may be denied, suspended, or revoked by the board after notice and the opportunity for hearing, upon proof that the authority has been abused.

Citation: N.H. Rev. Stat. Ann. § 326-B:11.III.

New Jersey

a. In addition to all other tasks which a registered professional nurse may, by law, perform, an advanced practice nurse may manage preventive care services, and diagnose and manage deviations from wellness and long-term illnesses, consistent with the needs of the patient and within the scope of practice of the advanced practice nurse, by:
   1. initiating laboratory and other diagnostic tests;
   2. prescribing or ordering medications and devices, as authorized by subsections b. and c. of this section; and
   3. prescribing or ordering treatments, including referrals to other licensed healthcare professionals, and performing specific procedures in accordance with the provisions of this subsection.
b. An advanced practice nurse may order medications and devices in the inpatient setting, subject to the following conditions:
   1. the collaborating physician and advanced practice nurse shall address in the joint protocols whether prior consultation with the collaborating physician is required to initiate an order for a controlled dangerous substance;
   2. the order is written in accordance with standing orders or joint protocols developed in agreement between a collaborating physician and the advanced practice nurse, or pursuant to the specific direction of a physician;
   3. the advanced practice nurse authorizes the order by signing his or her own name, printing the name and certification number, and printing the collaborating physician's name;

4. the physician is present or readily available through electronic communications;

5. the charts and records of the patients treated by the advanced practice nurse are reviewed by the collaborating physician and the advanced practice nurse within the period of time specified by rule adopted by the Commissioner of Health and Senior Services pursuant to Section 13 of P.L.1991, c.377 (C.45:11–52);

6. the joint protocols developed by the collaborating physician and the advanced practice nurse are reviewed, updated, and signed at least annually by both parties; and

7. the advanced practice nurse has completed six contact hours of continuing professional education in pharmacology related to controlled substances, including pharmacologic therapy and addiction prevention and management, in accordance with regulations adopted by the New Jersey Board of Nursing. The six contact hours shall be in addition to New Jersey Board of Nursing pharmacology education requirements for advanced practice nurses related to initial certification and recertification of an advanced practice nurse as set forth in N.J.A.C. 13:37-7.2 and 13:37-7.5.

c. An advanced practice nurse may prescribe medications and devices in all other medically appropriate settings, subject to the following conditions:

1. the collaborating physician and advanced practice nurse shall address in the joint protocols whether prior consultation with the collaborating physician is required to initiate a prescription for a controlled dangerous substance;

2. the prescription is written in accordance with standing orders or joint protocols developed in agreement between a collaborating physician and the advanced practice nurse, or pursuant to the specific direction of a physician;

3. the advanced practice nurse writes the prescription on a New Jersey Prescription Blank pursuant to P.L.2003, c.280 (C.45:14-40 et seq.), signs his name to the prescription and prints his name and certification number;

4. the prescription is dated and includes the name of the patient and the name, address, and telephone number of the collaborating physician;

5. the physician is present or readily available through electronic communications;

6. the charts and records of the patients treated by the advanced practice nurse are periodically reviewed by the collaborating physician and the advanced practice nurse;

7. the joint protocols developed by the collaborating physician and the advanced practice nurse are reviewed, updated, and signed at least annually by both parties; and

8. the advanced practice nurse has completed six contact hours of continuing professional education in pharmacology related to controlled substances, including pharmacologic therapy and addiction prevention and

management, in accordance with regulations to New Jersey Board of Nursing. The six contact hours shall be in addition to New Jersey Board of Nursing pharmacology education requirements for advanced practice nurses related to initial certification and recertification of an advanced practice nurse as set forth N.J.A.C. 13:37-7.2 and 13:37-7.5.

d. The joint protocols employed pursuant to Subsections b. and c. of this section shall conform with standards adopted by the Director of the Division of Consumer Affairs pursuant to Section 12 of P.L.1991, c.377 (C.45:11–51) or Section 10 or P.L.1999, c.85 (C.45-49.2), as applicable.

Citation: N.J. Stat. Ann. § 45:11-49.

An advanced practice nurse shall include the following information on each prescription blank issued:

1. The prescribing advanced practice nurse's full name, designation, that is, APN, address, telephone number, and certification number.
2. The full name, date of birth and address of the patient;
3. The date of issuance;
4. The name, strength, route and quality of the medication prescribed;
5. The number of refills permitted or time limit for refills, or both;
6. A handwritten, original signature;
7. An explicit indication, by initials placed next to "do not substitute," if a specified brand name drug is to be dispensed;
8. The full name, title, address, telephone number, and license number of the collaborating physician
9. Words, in addition to numbers, to indicate the drug quantity authorized if the prescription is for a controlled dangerous substance, for example: "ten (10) Percodan" or "five (5) Ritalin 5mg"; and
10. If the prescription is for a controlled dangerous substance, the advanced practice nurse's DEA number and instructions as to the frequency of use.

Citation: N.J. Admin. Code tit.13, § 37-7.9.

New Mexico

Certified nurse practitioners may . . . practice independently and make decisions regarding health care needs of the individual, family, or community and carry out health regimens, including the prescription and distribution of dangerous drugs and controlled substances included in Schedules II through V of the Controlled Substances Act. . . .

Citation: N.M. Stat. Ann. § 61-3-23.2.B(2).

Certified nurse practitioners who have fulfilled requirements for prescriptive authority may prescribe in accordance with the rules, regulations, guidelines, and formularies for individual certified nurse practitioners promulgated by the board.

Citation: N.M. Stat. Ann. § 61-3-23.2.C.

New York

Prescriptions for drugs, devices, and immunizing agents may be issued by a nurse practitioner . . . in accordance with the practice agreement and practice protocols. The nurse practitioner shall obtain a certificate from the department upon successfully completing a program including an appropriate pharmacology component, or its equivalent, as established by the commissioner's regulations, prior to prescribing under this subdivision. The certificate issued under Section 6910 shall state whether the nurse practitioner has successfully completed such a program or equivalent and is authorized to prescribe under this subdivision.

Citation: N.Y. Educ. Law § 6902.3(b).

An NP must obtain a DEA number in order to prescribe or dispense controlled substances.

Citation: New York State Nursing Board Office, Practice
Information: Prescription Privileges, February 2013.

North Carolina

b. Prescribing and dispensing stipulations are as follows:
   1. Drugs and devices that may be prescribed by the nurse practitioner in each practice site shall be included in the collaborative practice agreement as outlined in Rule .0810(b) of this Section.
   2. Controlled Dangerous Substances (Schedules II, IIN, III, IV, and V) defined by the State and Federal Controlled Substances Acts may be procured, prescribed or ordered as established in the collaborative practice agreement, providing all of the following restrictions are met:
      A. The nurse practitioner has an assigned DEA number which is entered on each prescription for a controlled substance;
      B. Dosage units for Schedules II, IIN, III, and IIIN are limited to a 30 day supply; and
      C. The supervising physician(s) must possess the same schedule(s) of controlled substances as the nurse practitioner's DEA registration. [Additional conditions omitted.]

Citation: N.C. Admin. Code tit. 21, r. 36.0809.

North Dakota

Requirements for prescriptive authority.
   Applicants for prescriptive authority shall:

1. Be currently licensed as an advanced practice registered nurse in North Dakota.
2. Submit a complete, notarized prescriptive authority application and pay the fee of fifty dollars.

3. Submit a completed transcript with degree posted from an accredited graduate level advanced practice registered nurse program and which includes evidence of completion of advanced pharmacotherapy, physical assessment, and pathophysiology.
4. Provide evidence of completion of thirty contact hours of education or equivalent in pharmacotherapy related to the applicant's scope of advanced practice that:
   a. Have been obtained within a three-year period of time immediately prior to the date of application for prescriptive authority; or
   b. May otherwise be approved by the board.

Citation: N.D. Admin. Code § 54-05-03.1-9.

The advanced practice registered nurse plans and initiates a therapeutic regimen that includes ordering and prescribing medical devices and equipment, nutrition, diagnostic and supportive services including home health care, hospice, and physical and occupational therapy.

1. A permanent advanced practice registered nurse license with the addition of prescriptive authority shall be issued following review and approval of the completed application by the board.
2. Between meetings of the board, board staff may review the prescriptive authority application and grant a temporary permit to prescribe if all the requirements are met.
3. The advanced practice registered nurse with prescriptive authority may prescribe drugs as defined by chapter 43-15-01 pursuant to applicable state and federal laws. Notice of the prescriptive authority granted will be forwarded to the board of pharmacy.
4. A prescriptive authority advanced practice registered nurse license does not include drug enforcement administration authority for prescribing controlled substances. Each licensee must apply for and receive a drug enforcement administration number before writing prescriptions for scheduled drugs.
5. The licensee may prescribe, administer, sign for, dispense over-the-counter, legend, and controlled substances, and procure pharmaceuticals, including samples following state and federal regulations.
6. The signature on documents related to prescriptive practices must clearly indicate that the licensee is an advanced practice registered nurse.
7. The advanced practice registered nurse with prescriptive authority may not prescribe, sell, administer, distribute, or give to oneself or to one's spouse or child any drug legally classified as a controlled substance or recognized as an addictive or dangerous drug.
8. Notwithstanding any other provision, a practitioner who diagnoses a sexually transmitted disease, such as chlamydia, gonorrhea, or any other sexually transmitted infection, in an individual patient may prescribe or dispense,

and a pharmacist may dispense, prescription antibiotic drugs to that patient's sexual partner or partners, without there having been an examination of that patient's sexual partner or partners.

Citation: N.D. Admin. Code § 54-05-03.1-10.

Ohio

Under a certificate to prescribe issued under Section 4723.48 of the Revised Code, a . . . certified nurse practitioner is subject to all of the following:

A. The nurse shall not prescribe any drug or therapeutic device that is not included in the types of drugs and devices listed on the formulary established in rules adopted under Section 4723.50 of the Revised Code;

B. The nurse's prescriptive authority shall not exceed the prescriptive authority of the collaborating physician or podiatrist;

C. The nurse may prescribe a Schedule II controlled substance only if all of the following are the case:
   a. The Patient has a terminal condition, as defined in section 2133.01 of the Revised Code
   b. The collaborating physician of the nurse initially prescribed the substance for the patient
   c. The prescription is for an amount that does not exceed the amount necessary for the patient's use in a single, twenty-four period. [Sections omitted.]

E. A . . . certified nurse practitioner may personally furnish to a patient a sample of any drug or therapeutic device included in the types of drugs and devices listed in the formulary. . . .[conditions apply].

Citation: Ohio Rev. Code Ann. § 4723.481.

Oklahoma

A Certified Nurse Practitioner shall be eligible, in accordance with the scope of practice of the Certified Nurse Practitioner, to obtain recognition as authorized by the Board to prescribe, as defined by rules promulgated by the Board pursuant to this section and subject to the medical direction of a supervising physician. This authorization shall not include dispensing drugs, but shall not preclude, subject to federal regulations, the receipt of, the signing for, or the dispensing of professional samples to patients.

Citation: Okla. Stat. Ann. tit. 59, § 567.3a.(6)(c).

The advanced practice nurse with prescriptive authority who prescribes Schedule III-V drugs will comply with state and Federal Drug Enforcement Administration (DEA) requirements prior to prescribing controlled substances.

1. The advanced practice nurse with prescriptive authority will submit in writing the assigned DEA number to the Board of Nursing within fourteen (14) days of receipt.
2. No more than a 30-day supply for Schedule III-V drugs shall be prescribed by the advanced practice nurse with prescriptive authority.

Citation: Okla. Admin. Code §485:10-16-5(c).

Oregon

The Oregon State Board of Nursing may grant to a certified nurse practitioner or certified clinical nurse specialist the privilege of writing prescriptions including prescriptions for controlled substances listed in schedules II, III, IIIN, IV, and V.

Citation: Or. Rev. Stat. § 678.390(1).

The nurse practitioner is independently responsible and accountable for the continuous and comprehensive management of a broad range of health care, which may include:

… Prescribing, dispensing, and administration of therapeutic devices and measures, including legend drugs and controlled substances as provided in Division 56 of the Oregon Nurse Practice Act, consistent with the definition of the practitioner's specialty category and scope of practice.

Citation: Or. Admin. R. § 851-050-0005(5)(l).

1. A written prescription shall include the date, printed name, legal signature, specialty category/title, business address, and telephone number of the prescribing nurse practitioner or clinical nurse specialist in addition to the required patient and drug information.
2. An electronically transmitted prescription as defined in OAR 855-006-0015 of the Pharmacy Act shall include the name and immediate contact information of the prescriber and be electronically encrypted or in some manner protected by up-to-date technology from unauthorized access, alteration, or use. Controlled substances have additional restrictions as defined by the DEA, which shall be followed.
3. A tamper resistant prescription shall meet criteria as defined in OAR 855-006-0015 of the Pharmacy Act.
4. Prescriptions may be written for over the counter drugs, durable medical equipment (DME), and devices.
5. Prescriptions shall be signed by the prescriber with the abbreviated specialty title of the nurse practitioner as per OAR 851-050-0005(9) or the title CNS as per 851-054-0015.
6. The nurse practitioner or clinical nurse specialist shall comply with all applicable laws and rules in prescribing, administering, and distributing drugs, including compliance with the labeling requirements of ORS Chapter 689.

7. A nurse practitioner or clinical nurse specialist shall only prescribe controlled substances in conjunction with their own valid and current DEA registration number appropriate to the classification level of the controlled substance.
8. Clinical nurse specialists and nurse practitioners with prescriptive authority are authorized to prescribe legend and controlled substances in Schedule II-V. Additionally, they may prescribe:
   a. Over-the-counter drugs;
   b. Appliances and devices;
   c. Orphan drugs;
   d. Limited access drugs;
   e. Antibiotics to partner(s) of patients diagnosed with a sexually transmitted infection without first examining the partner of the patient, consistent with Department of Human Services guidelines regarding Expedited Partner Therapy;
   f. Off label.

Citation: Or. Admin. R. § 851-056-0010.

1. Evaluation of appropriate prescribing by the Board is constructed based on the following premises:
   a. Nurse practitioners may provide care for specialized client populations within each nurse practitioner category/scope of practice;
   b. Clinical nurse specialists may provide care for individuals and populations within their specialty scope of practice;
   c. Prescribing is limited by the individual's scope of practice and knowledge base within that scope of practice;
   d. Clinical nurse specialists and nurse practitioners may prescribe the drugs appropriate for patients within their scope of practice as defined by OAR 851-050-0005; or 851-054-0020 and 0021;
   e. Clinical nurse specialists and nurse practitioners shall be held independently accountable for their prescribing decisions;
   f. All drugs prescribed shall have Food and Drug Administration (FDA) approval unless mentioned as an exception in OAR 851-056-0010.

Citation: Or. Admin. R. § 851-056-0012.

Pennsylvania

Collaborative Agreement—the written and signed agreement between a CRNP and a collaborating physician in which they agree to the details of their collaboration including the elements in the definition of collaboration.

Citation: 49 Pa Code § 21.251.

b. A CRNP with current prescriptive authority approval from the Board may prescribe, dispense, and administer drugs and therapeutic or corrective measures consistent with the prescriptive authority collaborative agreement and relevant to the CRNP's specialty from the following categories:

1. Antihistamines.
2. Anti-infective agents.
3. Antineoplastic agents, unclassified therapeutic agents, devices, and pharmaceutical aids.
4. Autonomic drugs.
5. Blood formation, coagulation and anticoagulation drugs, and thrombolytic and antithrombolytic agents.
6. Cardiovascular drugs.
7. Central nervous system agents.
8. Contraceptives including foams and devices.
9. Diagnostic agents.
10. Disinfectants for agents used on objects other than skin.
11. Electrolytic, caloric, and water balance.
12. Enzymes.
13. Antitussive, expectorants, and mucolytic agents.
14. Gastrointestinal drugs.
15. Local anesthetics.
16. Eye, ear, nose, and throat preparations.
17. Serums, toxoids, and vaccines.
18. Skin and mucous membrane agents.
19. Smooth muscle relaxants.
20. Vitamins.
21. Hormones and synthetic substitutes.

c. A CRNP may not prescribe or dispense a drug from the following categories:

1. Gold compounds.
2. Heavy metal antagonists.
3. Radioactive agents.
4. Oxytocics.
5. Schedule I controlled substances as defined by Section 4 of the Controlled Substance, Drug, Device, and Cosmetic Act (35 P.S. § 780-104).

d. Restrictions on CRNP prescribing and dispensing practices are as follows:

1. A CRNP may write a prescription for a Schedule II controlled substance for up to a 30-day supply as identified in the collaborative agreement.
2. A CRNP may prescribe a Schedule III or IV controlled substance for up to a 90-day supply as identified in the collaborative agreement.

e. A CRNP may not delegate prescriptive authority.

Citation: 49 Pa Code § 21.284.

Rhode Island

a. Prescriptive privileges for the certified registered nurse practitioner:
   1. Shall be granted under the governance and supervision of the department, board of nurse registration and nurse education; and
   2. Shall include prescription of legend medications and prescription of controlled substances from Schedules II, III, IV, and V that are established in regulation; and
   3. Must not include controlled substances from Schedule I.
b. To qualify for prescriptive privileges an applicant must submit on forms provided by the board of nurse registration and nursing education, verified by oath, that the applicant has evidence of completion of thirty (30) hours of education in pharmacology within the three (3) year period immediately prior to date of application. To maintain prescriptive privileges the certified registered nurse practitioner (R.N.P.) must submit upon request of the board of nurse registration and nursing education evidence of thirty (30) hours continuing education in pharmacology every six (6) years.

Citation: R.I. Gen. Laws § 5-34-39.

South Carolina

A. An advanced practice registered nurse applicant shall furnish evidence satisfactory to the board that the applicant:
   1. has met all qualifications for licensure as a registered nurse; and
   2. holds current specialty certification by a board-approved credentialing organization. New graduates shall provide evidence of certification within one year of program completion; however, psychiatric clinical nurse specialists shall provide evidence of certification within two years of program completion; and
   3. has earned a master's degree from an accredited college or university, except for those applicants who:
      a. provide documentation as requested by the board that the applicant was graduated from an advanced, organized formal education program appropriate to the practice and acceptable to the board before December 31, 1994; or
      b. graduated before December 31, 2003, from an advanced, organized formal education program for nurse anesthetists accredited by the national accrediting organization of that specialty. CRNAs who graduate after December 31, 2003, must graduate with a master's degree from a formal CRNA education program for nurse anesthetists accredited by the national accreditation organization of the CRNA specialty. An advanced practice registered nurse must achieve

and maintain national certification, as recognized by the board, in an advanced practice registered nursing specialty;

4. has paid the board all applicable fees; and
5. has declared specialty area of nursing practice and the specialty title to be used must be the title which is granted by the board-approved credentialing organization or the title of the specialty area of nursing practice in which the nurse has received advanced educational preparation.

B. An APRN is subject, at all times, to the scope and standards of practice established by the board-approved credentialing organization representing the specialty area of practice and shall function within the scope of practice of this chapter and must not be in violation of Chapter 47.

C. 1. A licensed nurse practitioner, certified nurse–midwife, or clinical nurse specialist must provide evidence of approved written protocols, as provided in this section. A licensed NP, CNM, or CNS performing delegated medical acts must do so under the general supervision of a licensed physician or dentist who must be readily available for consultation.

2. When application is made for more than three NP's, CNM's, or CNS's to practice with one physician or when an NP, CNM, or CNS is performing delegated medical acts in a practice site greater than forty-five miles from the supervising physician, the Board of Nursing and Board of Medical Examiners shall each review the application to determine if adequate supervision exists.

D. 1. Delegated medical acts performed by a nurse practitioner, certified nurse–midwife, or clinical nurse specialist must be performed pursuant to an approved written protocol between the nurse and the physician and must include, but is not limited to:

a. this general information:
   i. name, address, and South Carolina license number of the nurse;
   ii. name, address, and South Carolina license number of the physician;
   iii. nature of practice and practice locations of the nurse and physician;
   iv. date the protocol was developed and dates the protocol was reviewed and amended;
   v. description of how consultation with the physician is provided and provision for backup consultation in the physician's absence;

b. this information for delegated medical acts:
   i. the medical conditions for which therapies may be initiated, continued, or modified;
   ii. the treatments that may be initiated, continued, or modified;
   iii. the drug therapies that may be prescribed;
   iv. situations that require direct evaluation by or referral to the physician.

2. The original protocol and any amendments to the protocol must be reviewed at least annually, dated and signed by the nurse and physician, and made available to the board for review within seventy-two hours of request. Failure to produce protocols upon request of the board is considered misconduct and subjects the licensee to disciplinary action. A random audit of approved written protocols must be conducted by the board at least biennially.

3. Licensees who change practice settings or physicians shall notify the board of the change within fifteen business days and provide verification of approved written protocols. NP's, CNM's, and CNS's who discontinue their practice shall notify the board within fifteen business days.

E. 1. An NP, CNM, or CNS who applies for prescriptive authority:
   a. must be licensed by the board as a nurse practitioner, certified nurse–midwife, or clinical nurse specialist;
   b. shall submit a completed application on a form provided by the board;
   c. shall submit the required fee;
   d. shall provide evidence of completion of forty-five contact hours of education in pharmacotherapeutics acceptable to the board, within two years before application or shall provide evidence of prescriptive authority in another state meeting twenty hours in pharmacotherapeutics acceptable to the board, within two years before application;
   e. shall provide at least fifteen hours of education in controlled substances acceptable to the board as part of the twenty hours required for prescriptive authority if the NP, CNM, or CNS has equivalent controlled substance prescribing authority in another state;
   f. shall provide at least fifteen hours of education in controlled substances acceptable to the board as part of the forty-five contact hours required for prescriptive authority if the NP, CNM, or CNS initially is applying to prescribe in Schedules III through V controlled substances.

2. The board shall issue an identification number to the NP, CNM, or CNS authorized to prescribe medications. Authorization for prescriptive authority is valid for two years unless terminated by the Board for cause. Initial authorization expires concurrent with the expiration of the Advanced Practice Registered Nurse license.

3. Authorization for prescriptive authority must be renewed after the applicant meets requirements for renewal and provides documentation of twenty hours acceptable to the board of continuing education contact hours every two years in pharmacotherapeutics. For an NP, CNM, or CNS with controlled substance prescriptive authority, two of the twenty hours must be related to prescribing controlled substances.

F. 1. Authorized prescriptions by a nurse practitioner, certified nurse–midwife, or clinical nurse specialist with prescriptive authority:

a. must comply with all applicable state and federal laws;

b. is limited to drugs and devices utilized to treat common well-defined medical problems within the specialty field of the nurse practitioner or clinical nurse specialist, as authorized by the physician and listed in the approved written protocols. The Board of Nursing, Board of Medical Examiners, and Board of Pharmacy jointly shall establish a listing of classifications of drugs that may be authorized by physicians and listed in approved written protocols;

c. do not include prescriptions for Schedule II controlled substances; however, Schedules III through V controlled substances may be prescribed if listed in the approved written protocol and as authorized by Section 44-53-300;

d. must be signed by the NP, CNM, or CNS with the prescriber's identification number assigned by the board and all prescribing numbers required by law. The prescription form must include the name, address, and phone number of the NP, CNM, or CNS and physician and must comply with the provisions of Section 39-24-40. A prescription must designate a specific number of refills and may not include a nonspecific refill indication;

e. must be documented in the patient record of the practice and must be available for review and audit purposes.

2. An NP, CNM, or CNS who holds prescriptive authority may request, receive, and sign for professional samples, except for controlled substances in Schedule II, and may distribute professional samples to patients as listed in the approved written protocol, subject to federal and state regulations.

G. Prescriptive authorization may be terminated by the board if an NP, CNM, or CNS with prescriptive authority has:

1. not maintained certification in the specialty field;

2. failed to meet the education requirements for pharmacotherapeutics;

3. prescribed outside the scope of the approved written protocols;

4. violated a provision of Section 40-33-110; or

5. violated any state or federal law or regulations applicable to prescriptions.

. . . 4. A person who changes primary practice settings or physician or dentist shall notify the Board of this change within fifteen business days and provide verification of approved written guidelines.

Citation: S.C. Code Ann. § 40-33-44.

South Dakota

A nurse practitioner may perform the following overlapping scope of advanced practice nursing and medical functions pursuant to § 36-9A-15, including:

. . . The prescription of medications and provision of drug samples or a limited supply of labeled medications, including controlled drugs or substances listed on Schedule II in Chapter 34-20B for one period of not more than thirty days, for treatment of causative factors and symptoms. Medications or sample drugs provided to patients shall be accompanied with written administration instructions and appropriate documentation shall be entered in the patient's medical record.

Citation: S.D. Codified Laws § 36-9A-12(2).

Tennessee

The nurse practitioner who holds a certificate of fitness shall be authorized to prescribe and/or issue controlled substances listed in Schedules II, III, IV, and V of title 39, chapter 17, part 4, upon joint adoption of physician supervisory rules concerning controlled substances pursuant to Subsection (d).

Citation: Tenn. Code Ann. § 63-7-123(2).

Any prescription written and signed or drug issued by a nurse practitioner under the supervision and control of a supervising physician shall be deemed to be that of the nurse practitioner. Every prescription issued by a nurse practitioner pursuant to this section shall be entered in the medical records of the patient and shall be written on a preprinted prescription pad bearing the name, address, and telephone number of the supervising physician and of the nurse practitioner, and the nurse practitioner shall sign each prescription so written. Where the preprinted prescription pad contains the names of more than one (1) physician, the nurse practitioner shall indicate on the prescription which of those physicians is the nurse practitioner's primary supervising physician by placing a checkmark beside or a circle around the name of that physician.

Citation: Tenn. Code Ann. § 63-7-123(3)(A).

The Nurse Practice Act T.C.A. § 63-7-101 et seq. requires a certification process for a nurse practitioner to prescribe and/or issue noncontrolled legend drugs.

Citation: Tenn. Comp. R. & Regs. Ch. 1000-4-.01(3).

Texas

A physician may delegate to an advanced practice registered nurse or a physician assistant, acting under adequate physician supervision, the act of prescribing or ordering a drug or device as authorized through a prescriptive authority agreement between the physician and the advanced practice registered nurse or physician assistant, as applicable.

b. A physician and an advanced practice registered nurse or physician assistant are eligible to enter into or be parties to a prescriptive authority agreement only if:
   1. if applicable, the Texas Board of Nursing has approved the advanced practice registered nurse's authority to prescribe or order a drug or device as authorized under this subchapter;
   2. the advanced practice registered nurse or physician assistant:
      A. holds an active license to practice in this state as an advanced practice registered nurse or physician assistant, as applicable, and is in good standing in this state; and
      B. is not currently prohibited by the Texas Board of Nursing or the Texas Physician Assistant Board, as applicable, from executing a prescriptive authority agreement; and
   3. before executing the prescriptive authority agreement, the physician and the advanced practice registered nurse or physician assistant disclose to the other prospective party to the agreement any prior disciplinary action by the board, the Texas Board of Nursing, or the Texas Physician Assistant Board, as applicable.
c. Except as provided by Subsection (d), the combined number of advanced practice registered nurses and physician assistants with whom a physician may enter into a prescriptive authority agreement may not exceed seven advanced practice registered nurses and physician assistants or the full-time equivalent of seven advanced practice registered nurses and physician assistants.
d. Subsection (c) does not apply to a prescriptive authority agreement if the prescriptive authority is being exercised in:
   1. a practice serving a medically underserved population; or
   2. a facility-based practice in a hospital under Section 157.054.
e. A prescriptive authority agreement must, at a minimum:
   1. be in writing and signed and dated by the parties to the agreement;
   2. state the name, address, and all professional license numbers of the parties to the agreement;
   3. state the nature of the practice, practice locations, or practice settings;
   4. identify the types or categories of drugs or devices that may be prescribed or the types or categories of drugs or devices that may not be prescribed;
   5. provide a general plan for addressing consultation and referral;
   6. provide a plan for addressing patient emergencies;
   7. state the general process for communication and the sharing of information between the physician and the advanced practice registered nurse or physician assistant to whom the physician has delegated prescriptive authority related to the care and treatment of patients;
   8. if alternate physician supervision is to be utilized, designate one or more alternate physicians who may:

A. provide appropriate supervision on a temporary basis in accordance with the requirements established by the prescriptive authority agreement and the requirements of this subchapter; and

B. participate in the prescriptive authority quality assurance and improvement plan meetings required under this section; and

9. describe a prescriptive authority quality assurance and improvement plan and specify methods for documenting the implementation of the plan that includes the following:

A. chart review, with the number of charts to be reviewed determined by the physician and advanced practice registered nurse or physician assistant; and

B. periodic face-to-face meetings between the advanced practice registered nurse or physician assistant and the physician at a location determined by the physician and the advanced practice registered nurse or physician assistant.

f. The periodic face-to-face meetings described by Subsection (e)(9)(B) must:

1. include:

A. the sharing of information relating to patient treatment and care, needed changes in patient care plans, and issues relating to referrals; and

B. discussion of patient care improvement; and

2. be documented and occur:

A. except as provided by Paragraph (B):

i. at least monthly until the third anniversary of the date the agreement is executed; and

ii. at least quarterly after the third anniversary of the date the agreement is executed, with monthly meetings held between the quarterly meetings by means of a remote electronic communications system, including videoconferencing technology or the Internet; or

B. if during the seven years preceding the date the agreement is executed the advanced practice registered nurse or physician assistant for at least five years was in a practice that included the exercise of prescriptive authority with required physician supervision:

i. at least monthly until the first anniversary of the date the agreement is executed; and

ii. at least quarterly after the first anniversary of the date the agreement is executed, with monthly meetings held between the quarterly meetings by means of a remote electronic communications system, including videoconferencing technology or the Internet.

g. The prescriptive authority agreement may include other provisions agreed to by the physician and advanced practice registered nurse or physician assistant.

h. If the parties to the prescriptive authority agreement practice in a physician group practice, the physician may appoint one or more alternate supervising physicians designated under Subsection (e)(8), if any, to conduct and document the quality assurance meetings in accordance with the requirements of this subchapter.

i. The prescriptive authority agreement need not describe the exact steps that an advanced practice registered nurse or physician assistant must take with respect to each specific condition, disease, or symptom.

j. A physician, advanced practice registered nurse, or physician assistant who is a party to a prescriptive authority agreement must retain a copy of the agreement until the second anniversary of the date the agreement is terminated.

k. A party to a prescriptive authority agreement may not by contract waive, void, or nullify any provision of this section or Section 157.0513.

l. In the event that a party to a prescriptive authority agreement is notified that the individual has become the subject of an investigation by the board, the Texas Board of Nursing, or the Texas Physician Assistant Board, the individual shall immediately notify the other party to the prescriptive authority agreement.

m. The prescriptive authority agreement and any amendments must be reviewed at least annually, dated, and signed by the parties to the agreement. The prescriptive authority agreement and any amendments must be made available to the board, the Texas Board of Nursing, or the Texas Physician Assistant Board not later than the third business day after the date of receipt of request, if any.

n. The prescriptive authority agreement should promote the exercise of professional judgment by the advanced practice registered nurse or physician assistant commensurate with the advanced practice registered nurse's or physician assistant's education and experience and the relationship between the advanced practice registered nurse or physician assistant and the physician.

o. This section shall be liberally construed to allow the use of prescriptive authority agreements to safely and effectively utilize the skills and services of advanced practice registered nurses and physician assistants.

p. The board may not adopt rules pertaining to the elements of a prescriptive authority agreement that would impose requirements in addition to the requirements under this section. The board may adopt other rules relating to physician delegation under this chapter.

q. The board, the Texas Board of Nursing, and the Texas Physician Assistant Board shall jointly develop responses to frequently asked questions relating to prescriptive authority agreements not later than January 1, 2014. This subsection expires January 1, 2015.

> *Citation:* SB 406 (excerpt), enacted June 2013, with rules under development.

Utah

"Practice of advanced practice registered nursing" means . . . Prescription or administration of prescription drugs or devices, including:

   i. Local anesthesia;
  ii. Schedule IV-V controlled substances; and
 iii. Schedule II-III controlled substances in accordance with a consultation and referral plan.

Citation: Utah Code Ann. § 58-31b-102(13).

Vermont

"Advanced practice registered nurse" or "APRN" means a licensed registered nurse authorized to practice in this state who, because of specialized education and experience, is endorsed to perform acts of medical diagnosis and to prescribe medical, therapeutic, or corrective measures under administrative rules adopted by the board.

Citation: Vt. Stat Ann. tit. 26, § 1572(4).

Virginia

In accordance with the provisions of this section and pursuant to the requirements of Chapter 33 (§ 54.1-3300 et seq.) of this title, a licensed nurse practitioner, other than a certified registered nurse anesthetist, shall have the authority to prescribe controlled substances and devices as set forth in Chapter 34 (§ 54.1-3400 et seq.) of this title as follows: (i) Schedule V and VI controlled substances on and after July 1, 2000; (ii) Schedules IV through VI on and after January 1, 2002; and (iii) Schedules II through VI controlled substances on and after July 1, 2006. Nurse practitioners shall have such prescriptive authority upon the provision to the Board of Medicine and the Board of Nursing of such evidence as they may jointly require that the nurse practitioner has entered into and is, at the time of writing a prescription, a party to a written agreement with a licensed physician, which provides for the direction and supervision by such physician of the prescriptive practices of the nurse practitioner. Such written agreements shall include the controlled substances the nurse practitioner is or is not authorized to prescribe and may restrict such prescriptive authority as deemed appropriate by the physician providing direction and supervision. . . .

Citation: Va. Code Ann. § 54.1-2957.01.A.

The following restriction shall apply to any nurse practitioner authorized to prescribe drugs and devices pursuant to this section:

1. The nurse practitioner shall disclose to his patients the name, address and telephone number of the supervising physician, and that he is a licensed nurse practitioner.
2. Physicians, other than physicians employed by, or under contract with, local health departments, federally funded comprehensive primary care clinics, or nonprofit health care clinics or programs to provide supervisory services, shall not supervise and direct at any one time more than four nurse practitioners. In the case of nurse practitioners, other than nurse midwives, the supervising physician shall regularly practice in any location in which the nurse practitioner exercises prescriptive authority pursuant to this section. A separate office for the nurse practitioner shall not be established. . . .
3. Physicians employed by, or under contract with, local health departments, federally funded comprehensive primary care clinics, or nonprofit health care clinics or programs to provide supervisory services, shall not supervise and direct at any one time more than four nurse practitioners who provide services on behalf of such entities. Such physicians either shall regularly practice in such settings or shall make periodic site visits to such settings as required by regulations promulgated pursuant to this section. . . .

Citation: Va. Code Ann. § 54.1-2957.01.E.

A. A nurse practitioner with prescriptive authority may prescribe only within the scope of the written or electronic practice agreement with a patient care team physician.
B. At any time there are changes in the patient care team physician, authorization to prescribe, or scope of practice, the nurse practitioner shall revise the practice agreement and maintain the revised agreement.
C. The practice agreement shall contain the following:
   1. A description of the prescriptive authority of the nurse practitioner within the scope allowed by law and the practice of the nurse practitioner.
   2. An authorization for categories of drugs and devices within the requirements of § 54.1-2957.01 of the Code of Virginia.
   3. The signature of the patient care team physician who is practicing with the nurse practitioner or a clear statement of the name of the patient care team physician who has entered into the practice agreement.

Citation: 17 Va. Admin. Code § 90-40-90.

Washington

An advanced registered nurse practitioner under his or her license may perform for compensation nursing care, as that term is usually understood, of the ill, injured, or infirm and in the course thereof, she or he may do the following things that shall not be done by a person not so licensed, except as provided in RCS 18.79.260 and 18.79.270:

1. Perform specialized and advanced levels of nursing as recognized jointly by the medical and nursing professions, as defined by the commission;
2. Prescribe legend drugs and Schedule V controlled substances, as defined in the Uniform Controlled Substances Act, Chapter 69.50 RCW, and Schedule II through IV subject to RCW 18.79.240(1)(r) or (s) within the scope of practice defined by the commission;
3. Perform all acts provided in RCS 18.79.260;
4. Hold herself or himself out to the public or designate herself or himself as an advanced registered nurse practitioner or as a nurse practitioner.

Citation: Wash. Rev. Code § 18.79.250.

An ARNP may not . . . prescribe controlled substances in Schedule I.

Citation: Wash. Admin. Code § 246-840-420(3).

1. An advanced registered nurse practitioner licensed under chapter 18.79. RCW when authorized by the nursing commission may prescribe drugs, medical equipment and therapies pursuant to applicable state and federal laws.
2. The ARNP when exercising prescriptive authority is accountable for competency in:
   a. Patient selection;
   b. Problem identification through appropriate assessment;
   c. Medication or device selection;
   d. Patient education for use of therapeutics:
   e. Knowledge of interactions of therapeutics, if any;
   f. Evaluation of outcome; and
   g. Recognition and management of complications and untoward reactions.

Citation: Wash. Admin. Code § 246-840-400.

West Virginia

a. The board may, in its discretion, authorize an advanced practice registered nurse to prescribe prescription drugs in a collaborative relationship with a physician licensed to practice in West Virginia and in accordance with applicable state and federal laws. An authorized advanced practice registered nurse may write or sign prescriptions or transmit prescriptions verbally or by other means of communication.
b. For purposes of this section an agreement to a collaborative relationship for prescriptive practice between a physician and an advanced practice registered nurse shall be set forth in writing. . . .Collaborative agreements shall include, but not be limited to, the following:
   1. Mutually agreed upon written guidelines or protocols for prescriptive authority as it applies to the advanced practice registered nurse's clinical practice;

2. Statements describing the individual and shared responsibilities of the advanced practice registered nurse and the physician pursuant to the collaborative agreement between them;

3. Periodic and joint evaluation of prescriptive practice; and

4. Periodic and joint review and updating of the written guidelines or protocols.

(c) The board shall promulgate legislative rules . . . governing the eligibility and extent to which an advanced practice registered nurse may prescribe drugs. Such rules shall provide, at minimum, a state formulary classifying those categories of drugs, which shall not be prescribed by advanced practice registered nurse, including, but not limited to, Schedules I and II of the Uniform Controlled Substances Act, antineoplastics, radiopharmaceuticals, and general anesthetics. Drugs listed under Schedule III shall be limited to a 72-hour supply without refill. . . .

Citation: W.V. Code Ann. § 30-7-15a.

3.1. The board shall grant prescriptive authority to an advanced practice registered nurse applicant who meets all eligibility requirements specified in W. Va. Code §30-7-15b and the following:

3.1.a. Prior to application to the board for approval for limited prescriptive authority, the applicant shall:

3.1.a.1. Successfully complete an accredited course of instruction in pharmacology during undergraduate study;

3.1.a.2. Successfully complete an advanced pharmacotherapy graduate level course approved by the board of not less than 45 pharmacology contact hours;

3.1.a.3. Provide documentation of the use of pharmacotherapy in clinical practice in the education program;

3.1.a.4. Provide evidence of 15 pharmacology contact hours in advanced pharmacotherapy completed within 2 years prior to application for prescriptive authority;

3.1.a.5. Submit official transcripts or certificates documenting completion of pharmacology and pharmacotherapy course work.

3.1.a.6. The board may request course outlines and/or descriptions of courses if necessary to evaluate the pharmacology course content and objectives.

3.1.b. The advanced practice registered nurse shall submit a notarized application for prescriptive authority on forms provided by the Board with the following:

3.1.b.1. A fee set forth in the board's Fees rule, 19CSR12.

3.1.b.2. Written verification of an agreement to a collaborative relationship with a licensed physician holding an unencumbered

West Virginia license for prescriptive practice on forms provided by the board. The applicant shall certify on this form that the collaborative agreement includes the following:

3.1.b.2.A. Mutually agreed upon written guidelines or protocols for prescriptive authority as it applies to the advanced practice registered nurse's clinical practice;

3.1.b.2.B. Statements describing the individual and shared responsibilities of the advanced practice registered nurse and the physician pursuant to the collaborative agreement between them;

3.1.b.2.C. A provision for the periodic and joint evaluation of the prescriptive practice; and,

3.1.b.2.D. A provision for the periodic and joint review and updating of the written guidelines or protocols.

3.1.b.2.E. Additional documentation at the request of the board.

3.2. If the board obtains information that an applicant for prescriptive authority was previously addicted to or dependent upon alcohol or the use of controlled substances, the board may grant prescriptive authority with any limitations it considers proper. The limitations may include, but are not limited to, restricting the types of schedule drugs a nurse may prescribe.

3.3. The board shall forward a copy of the verification specified in Subdivision 3.1.b.2. of this rule to the Board of Medicine or to the Board of Osteopathy, whichever is indicated.

3.4. Upon satisfactory evidence that the advanced practice registered nurse applicant has met all above requirements for prescriptive authority, the Board shall assign an identification number to that nurse.

3.5. The board shall notify the Board of Medicine, the Board of Osteopathy, and the Board of Pharmacy of those advanced practice registered nurses who have been granted prescriptive authority, and shall also provide the prescriber's identification number and effective date of prescriptive authority.

3.6. The advanced practice registered nurse shall file with the board any restrictions on prescriptive authority that are not imposed by W. Va. Code §60A-3-301 et seq., or this rule, but which are within the written collaborative agreement and the name of the collaborating physician for each advanced practice registered nurse on the approved list.

3.7. The advanced practice registered nurse with prescriptive authority who wishes to prescribe Schedules III through V drugs shall comply with federal Drug Enforcement Agency requirements prior to prescribing controlled substances.

3.8. The advanced practice registered nurse shall immediately file any and all of his or her Drug Enforcement Agency registrations and numbers with the board.

3.9. The board shall maintain a current record of all advanced practice registered nurses with Drug Enforcement Agency registrations and numbers.

3.10. Any information filed with the board under the provisions of this rule shall be available, upon request, to any pharmacist, regulatory agency or board or shall be made available pursuant to other state or federal law.

3.11. The APRN shall maintain with the board a current mailing and, if available, a current e-mail address.

...

5.1. The advanced practice registered nurse shall not prescribe from the following categories of drugs:

5.1.a. Schedules I and II of the Uniform Controlled Substances Act;

5.1.b. Antineoplastics;

5.1.c. Radio-pharmaceuticals; or

5.1.d. General anesthetics.

5.1.e. MAO Inhibitors, except when in a collaborative agreement with a psychiatrist.

5.2. Drugs listed under Schedule III and benzodiazepines are limited to a 72 hour supply without refill.

5.3. The advanced practice registered nurse may prescribe drugs from Schedules IV through V in a quantity necessary for up to a 90 day supply, with only 1 refill, and shall provide that the prescription expires in 6 months, with the following exceptions:

5.3.a. Prescriptions for phenothiazines shall be limited to up to a 30 day supply and shall be non- refillable;

5.3.b. Prescriptions for non-controlled substances of antipsychotics, and sedatives prescribed by the advanced practice registered nurse shall not exceed the quantity necessary for a 90 day supply, shall provide for no more than 1 prescription refill and shall expire in 6 months.

5.4. Pursuant to a collaborative agreement as set forth in the law governing prescriptive authority the advanced practice registered nurse may prescribe an annual supply of any drug, with the exception of controlled substances, which is prescribed for the treatment of a chronic condition, other than chronic pain management.

5.5. The maximum dosage of any drug, including antidepressants, prescribed by the advanced practice registered nurse shall be consistent with the advanced practice registered nurse's area of practice.

5.6. Each prescription and subsequent refills given by the advanced practice registered nurse shall be entered on the patient's chart.

5.7. Advanced practice registered nurses shall not prescribe other prescription drugs or refill for a period exceeding 6 months; provided, that this limitation shall not include contraceptives or those treating a chronic condition as defined in WV Code §30-7-15a and section 19-8-5.4 of this rule.

5.8. An advanced practice registered nurse may administer local anesthetics.

5.9. The advanced practice registered nurse who has been approved for limited prescriptive authority by the board may sign for, accept, and provide to patients samples of drugs received from a drug company representative.

5.10. The prescription authorized by an advanced practice registered nurse shall comply with all applicable state and federal laws and regulations; must be signed by the prescriber with the legal designation or the designated certification title of the prescriber and must include the prescriber's identification number assigned by the board or the prescriber's national provider identifier assigned by the National Provider System pursuant to 45 CFR §162.408.

   5.10.a. All prescriptions shall include the following information:

      5.10.a.1. The name, title, address and phone number of the prescribing advanced practice registered nurse;

      5.10.a.2. The name and date of birth of the patient;

      5.10.a.3. The date of the prescription;

      5.10.a.4. The full name of the drug, the dosage, the route of administration and directions, for its use;

      5.10.a.5. The number of refills;

      5.10.a.6. The Drug Enforcement Agency number of the prescriber, when required by federal laws; and

      5.10.a.7. The prescriptive authority identification number issued by the board.

   5.10.b. An advanced practice registered nurse shall at the time of the initial prescription record in the patient record the plan for continued evaluation of the effectiveness of the controlled substances prescribed.

   5.10.c. An advanced practice registered nurse shall prescribe refills of controlled substances according to current laws and standards.

   5.10.d. Drugs considered to be proved human teratogens shall not be prescribed during a known pregnancy by the advanced practice registered nurse. This prohibition includes all Category D and X drugs from the Federal Drug Administration Categories of teratogen risks (21 CFR 201.57). Category C drugs should be given only if the patient benefit justifies the potential risks to the fetus and only after consultation with the collaborating physician.

5.11. The board may approve a formulary classifying pharmacologic categories of all drugs which may be prescribed by an advanced practice registered nurse with prescriptive authority.

Citation: W. Va. Code St. R. tit 19 §19-8-3 and 19-8-5.

Wisconsin

The board shall grant a certificate to issue prescription orders to an advanced practice nurse who meets the education, training, and examination requirements established by the board for a certificate to issue prescription orders. . . .

Citation: Wis. Stat. § 441.16(2).

1. Advanced practice nurse prescribers shall communicate with patients through the use of modern communication techniques.
2. Advanced practice nurse prescribers shall facilitate collaboration with other healthcare professionals, at least 1 of whom shall be a physician, through the use of modern communication techniques.
3. Advanced practice nurse prescribers shall facilitate referral of patient health care records to other health care professionals and shall notify patients of their right to have their health care records referred to other health care professionals.
4. Advanced practice nurse prescribers shall provide a summary of a patient's health care records, including diagnosis, surgeries, allergies, and current medications to other health care providers as a means of facilitation case management and improved collaboration.

Citation: Wis. Admin. Code § N8.10(1), (2), (3), and (4).

The advanced practice nurse prescriber:

1. May issue only those prescription orders appropriate to the advanced practice nurse prescriber's areas of competence, as established by his or her education, training or experience.
2. May not issue a prescription order for any schedule I controlled substance.
3. May not prescribe, dispense or administer any amphetamine, sympatho-mimetic amine drug or compound designated as a schedule II controlled substance pursuant to the provisions of s. 961.16(5), Stats., to or for any person except for any of the following:
   a. Use as an adjunct to opioid analgesic compounds for the treatment of cancer-related pain.
   b. Treatment of narcolepsy.
   c. Treatment of hyperkinesis.
   d. Treatment of drug-induced brain dysfunction.
   e. Treatment of epilepsy.
   f. Treatment of depression shown to be refractory to other therapeutic modalities.

4. May not prescribe, order, dispense or administer any anabolic steroid for the purpose of enhancing athletic performance or for other nonmedical purpose.
5. Shall, in prescribing or ordering a drug for administration by a registered nurse or licensed practical nurse under s. 441.16 (3)(cm), Stats., present evidence to the nurse and to the administration of the facility where the prescription or order is to be carried out that the advanced practice nurse prescriber is properly certified to issue prescription orders.

Citation: Wis. Admin Code §N 8.06.

1. Prescription orders issued by an advanced practice nurse prescriber shall:
   a. Specify the date of issue.
   b. Specify the name and address of the patient.
   c. Specify the name, address and business telephone number of the advanced practice nurse prescriber.
   d. Specify the name and quantity of the drug product or device prescribed, including directions for use.
   e. Bear the signature of the advanced practice nurse prescriber.
2. Prescription orders issued by advanced practice nurse prescribers for a controlled substance shall be written in ink or indelible pencil or shall be typewritten, and shall contain the practitioner's controlled substances number.

Citation: Wis. Admin Code §N 8.07.

1. Advanced practice nurse prescribers who prescribe independently shall maintain in effect malpractice insurance evidenced by one of the following:
   a. Personal liability coverage in the amounts specified in s. 655.23(4), Stats.
   b. Coverage under a group liability policy providing individual coverage for the nurse in the amounts set forth in s. 655.23 (4), Stats. An advanced practice nurse prescriber covered under one or more such group policies shall certify on forms provided by the board that the nurse will independently prescribe only within the limits of the policy's coverage, or shall obtain personal liability coverage for independent prescribing outside the scope of the group liability policy or policies.
2. Notwithstanding sub. (1), an advanced practice nurse prescriber who practices as an employee of this state or a governmental subdivision, as defined under s. 180.0103, Stats., is not required to maintain in effect malpractice insurance coverage, but the nurse shall certify on forms provided by the board that the nurse will prescribe within employment policies.
3. An advanced practice nurse prescriber who prescribes under the supervision and delegation of a physician or CRNA shall certify on forms provided by the board that the nurse complies with s. N 6.03 (2) and (3), regarding delegated acts.
4. An advanced practice nurse prescriber who prescribes in more than one setting or capacity shall comply with the provisions of subs. (1), (2) and (3) applicable to each setting or capacity. An advanced practice nurse prescriber

who is not an employee of this state or a governmental subdivision, and who prescribes independently in some situations and prescribes under the supervision and delegation of a physician or CRNA in other situations, shall meet the requirements of sub. (1) with respect to independent prescribing and the requirements of sub. (3) with respect to delegated prescribing.

5. Every advanced practice nurse who is certified to issue prescription orders shall annually submit to the board satisfactory evidence that he or she has in effect malpractice insurance required by sub. (1).

Citation: WIS. ADMIN CODE §N 8.08.

1. Except as provided in sub. (2), advanced practice nurse prescribers shall restrict their dispensing of prescription drugs to complimentary samples dispensed in original containers or packaging supplied by a pharmaceutical manufacturer or distributor.

2. An advanced practice nurse prescriber may dispense drugs to a patient if the treatment facility at which the patient is treated is located at least 30 miles from the nearest pharmacy.

Citation: WIS. ADMIN CODE §N 8.09 (1).

1. Advanced practice nurse prescribers shall communicate with patients through the use of modern communication techniques.

2. Advanced practice nurse prescribers shall facilitate collaboration with other health care professionals, at least 1 of whom shall be a physician, through the use of modern communication techniques.

Citation: WIS. ADMIN CODE §N 8.10(1).

Wyoming

"Advanced practice registered nurse (APRN)" means a nurse who:

A. May prescribe, administer, dispense, or provide nonprescriptive and prescriptive medications including prepackaged medications, except Schedule I drugs as defined in W.S. 35-7-1013 and 35-7-1014.

Citation: Wyo. Stat. Ann. § 33-21-120(a)(i).

a. The board may authorize an advanced practice registered nurse to prescribe medications and devices, within the recognized scope of advanced practice registered nurse and population focus, and in accordance with all applicable state and federal laws including, but not limited to the Wyoming Pharmacy Act [WS 33-24-101 through 33-24-204], the Wyoming Controlled Substances Act of 1971 [WS 35-7-1001 through 35-7-1101], the Federal Controlled Substances Act [21 U.S.C. § 801 et seq.], their applicable Rules and Regulations.

Citation: Wyo. Board of Nursing Rules, Ch. 4, § Section 8(a).

Strategies for Nurse Practitioners

The difference between making do and advancing is like the difference between eating all of what is put on one's plate and deciding what to have for dinner. Unfortunately, many of today's nurse practitioners (NPs) are simply making do.

NPs faced with restrictive or outdated laws often report at professional meetings that they are proud of how they are able to function despite the law. For example, NPs who want to own their own businesses can construct a private practice that conforms to the law by hiring a physician consultant. NPs practicing in states where the law requires physician oversight to prescribe can do so as long as a physician takes the necessary steps to conform to the state's requirements. NPs who cannot be designated as primary care providers (PCPs) and handle panels of managed-care patients may actually perform the patient care if a physician is designated as the PCP. In these cases, NPs say their reward is that patients know that they are providing their care and appreciate NPs' efforts.

Although many NPs are making the best of existing law, in many states, the law is still unsatisfactory. The states where NPs are free to practice their profession without mandatory participation by physicians are still in the minority.

Opportunities in a Changing Field

In states where barriers to NP practice have been lifted and where reimbursement is attainable from third-party payers, there are opportunities for healthcare delivery systems that increase attention to preventive medicine, increase access to citizens, and provide alternatives to expensive physician-oriented systems.

Under a see-a-nurse-first system, patients initially are seen by a registered nurse or NP. The nurses take care of as many of a patient's healthcare problems as is prudent, and then seek consultation and referral for those problems that exceed the scope of their practice. **Figure** 1 depicts a see-a-nurse-first system.

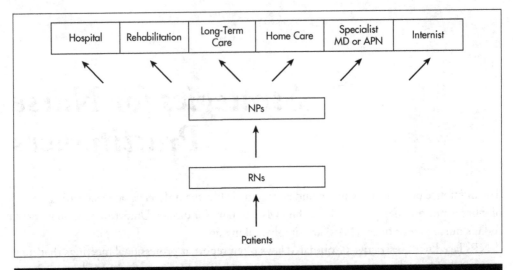

Opponents of the See-a-Nurse-First System

Physicians often oppose the see-a-nurse-first system of healthcare delivery. The American Academy of Family Physicians (AAFP) issued the following policy regarding NP practice: "The nurse practitioner should not function as an independent health practitioner. The AAFP position is that the nurse practitioner should only function in a collaborative practice arrangement under the direction and responsible supervision of a practicing, licensed physician."[1]

Some patients may be suspicious of a see-a-nurse-first system as well. For that reason, patients should be offered a choice of nurse and/or physician providers. Once the law offers a level playing field, both physicians and NPs will have incentives to improve their services to patients and will advance their respective professions.

Challenges for NPs Attempting to Advance the Profession

First, there is the matter of the energy required. NPs are accustomed to relying on volunteer organizations. Now is the time to hire professionals, however. Public relations experts, not volunteers, develop public relations campaigns for physician organizations. Physicians do not expect to see 30 patients at the office, stop by the hospital on the way home, and then get together at 8 PM to develop public relations campaigns. Physician organizations hire public relations firms or retain in-house staff whose sole job is to attend to the public image of physicians. NPs can hire professionals, too, and they should. Much publicity can be gained with a small budget and creative public relations professionals.

Second, there is the challenge of publicizing the good in NPs and comparing NP services to physician services without denigrating physicians. The solution to that challenge is to continue to publicize the studies that have shown that NPs are as competent providers of primary care as physicians.

Third, there is the phenomenon that every action generates a reaction. When physicians see NPs step up efforts to advance the profession, they may feel it necessary to react with more aggressive efforts. NPs who are intimidated by this should focus on their goal of advancing the profession to stay on course.

The major focus of physician arguments—that only physicians should have the authority to direct primary care—is the educational differential between NPs and physicians. However, physicians set their own educational level, and there has been no major study of physician education and training since 1910, when Abraham Flexner published a report commissioned by the Carnegie Foundation that called for medical training to be university-affiliated programs rather than 8-month programs where students came without a high school diploma.[2] There are no studies showing that the appropriate education for providing primary care is 4 years of medical school and 3 years of residency, which is the education for all physicians, whether they are brain surgeons, researchers into neurotransmitters, or providers of primary care. On the contrary, there are many studies showing that NPs are quite appropriate providers of primary care.

Strategies to Implement Collectively

NPs are familiar with the advantages of working collectively toward change. First, individuals can pool money and thus gain more purchasing power than an individual NP. Second, groups are taken more seriously by lawmakers and political parties than are individuals.

Marshalling support of even homogeneous groups is no small accomplishment. In the case of NPs, a stumbling block to collective action is the heterogeneity of NPs, as not every NP has the same professional interests, the same viewpoint, or the same goals. For example, NPs who are professors have professional goals that include getting government funding for their educational programs. NPs who are clinicians do not have educational funding as a top-priority goal. Instead, they have the goal of being able to practice with few barriers.

Nevertheless, organizations are necessary for the advancement of the NP profession. NPs inspire, encourage, and rejuvenate other NPs, which is necessary when the goals are long term.

Ten Organizational Strategies

The following ten strategies are suggested for NPs who want to advance the profession and/or their own opportunities.

Set a Goal

For example, one NP set herself a goal of becoming a PCP credentialed by health plans. She built up a base of loyal patients, became an excellent clinician, and worked with the state's organization of NPs to change the law so that an NP could be designated by a health maintenance organization (HMO) as a PCP. She succeeded.

Of course, NPs work not only in primary care, but also in specialty practices and tertiary care. In every setting, NPs need to choose an achievable and reasonable goal, one that affects not only themselves, but also other NPs.

Analyze the Law for Barriers

There is much ignorance and confusion about the law as it affects NPs. Some NPs say, "The law says we need to be supervised, but we really practice independently." By participating in a practice situation where the limits of the law are stretched, NPs are taking a risk. In some states, the law puts responsibility squarely on the NP for ensuring that supervisory requirements are met. Clinics, hospitals, and medical groups have little to lose if they provide little or no supervision and let NPs go as far as their desire for intellectual adventure and their professional judgment allows. NPs are bringing in at least $150 per hour and getting paid about $40 per hour. If an NP makes few mistakes and no one enforces the law, everything runs smoothly. However, the better an NP does with independent decision making, the more momentum builds for more independence, and pretty soon the NP is out on a limb, with no physician available to answer telephone calls to help, much less supervise. As soon as an NP makes a mistake, the burden is back on the NP for not seeking supervision. If the NP is a practice owner making $150 per hour and willing to take a risk, that is one thing, but if the NP is an employee earning $40 per hour, the risk outweighs the benefits.

Some NPs have argued that current law and custom permit them to practice in a satisfying manner and ask, "Why open a can of worms by attempting to change the law?" This argument not only offends a sense of legal "neatness," where law and current practice jibe, but also condones a timidity that is incongruent with the level of assertion needed to perform as an NP. Why would NPs participate in life-and-death decisions for patients and yet retreat from challenging statutory omissions that relegate NPs to the invisible category of "others" or "nonphysicians"?

Every NP needs a copy of every law that affects their practice. That includes law that does not mention NPs but that affects NPs because of the omissions. For example, every NP needs a copy of the NP scope of practice in the state where they are licensed and practicing.

National NP organizations need fact sheets that cover federal law regarding:

- Delegation of duties in nursing home care
- Direction of the care of hospitalized patients
- Anti-kickback laws
- Definition of medical care and medical care provider
- Application for Drug Enforcement Administration numbers
- Reimbursement by Medicare and Medicaid
- Coding and billing of Medicare and Medicaid visits
- Documentation guidelines
- Definition of collaboration

Because the officers and board members of NP organizations change from year to year, NP organizations should maintain a current file of the relevant law for each new officer to review at the start of the term. Much anxiety will be avoided if NPs have copies of the exact language of the law.

Lobby for Eradication of the Barriers

Once the barriers are known, organizations can enlist lobbyists to help eradicate them. NPs may make progress in one area, such as convincing managed-care organizations (MCOs) to admit NPs to panels, only to find that there is some phrase in state law that a state administrator interprets as barring NPs from becoming PCPs.

NPs should not expect to win passage of new legislation the first time it is introduced. Each time an issue is lobbied, more information comes out about NPs, and the idea of NPs becomes more familiar and palatable to lawmakers.

NPs may argue that if certain issues are brought up, they may lose ground in the law rather than gain it. NPs ask, "What if we introduce a law, but it is amended and passed at the last minute, and our authority to prescribe is lost?" While that is a possibility, it is not probable. Compare a situation an NP faces every day in clinical practice: A patient arrives complaining of low back pain. In 99% of cases, the back pain is due to musculoskeletal strain and will respond to rest and nonsteroidal anti-inflammatory drugs. In one case out of 100, the back pain will be something else, and in a very minuscule percentage of cases, the low back pain will be cancer. Does the NP rush all patients who complain of low back pain to magnetic resonance imaging at the first visit? No. Likewise, the chance that NPs, by introducing legislation to advance the profession, will actually fall backward is minuscule, for the following reasons. First, NPs are valuable to medical groups, hospitals, HMOs, and health departments. Second, a good lobbyist, as well as a sponsor of a bill, will follow it very closely. It is unlikely that a bill that was introduced on behalf of NPs will be amended without the knowledge of the NPs' lobbyist. Because the lobbyist is hired by an NP organization, it is unlikely that a lobbyist will be caught unaware or will fail to rally the NP organization client when necessary. Third, there is virtually no opposition to NPs as healthcare providers other than from organized physician groups, and then only when NPs are striving to release the legal apron strings that tie NPs to physicians. NPs should not be deterred by the prospect of introducing a bill five times before it is passed. If it takes 5 years to get a bill passed, so be it.

Sell MCOs and Purchasers of Health Services on NPs as PCPs

NPs can offer MCOs and employers, who purchase healthcare services for their employees, quality services at a reasonable cost. However, NPs cannot depend on health plan purchasers to know what NPs can do unless they educate them.

MCOs and business executives are used to listening to business presentations from those who want to sell services. NPs are not used to giving business presentations, but they can learn. Alternatively, NP organizations can retain the services of professionals who make business presentations to do the work on their behalf.

The basic message of a business presentation on why MCOs and businesses should contract with NPs as PCPs is that NPs give high-quality care at a reasonable price. The message should be supported by data demonstrating the quality of NP care and numbers demonstrating the rationale of the pricing schedule. Finally, MCOs and businesses need to know how they can contract with NPs, that is, where the NPs are located and whom to contact.

Promote NPs to the Public

For the most part, individuals who have experienced the care of an NP have been satisfied. However, there is still too great a number of people who have never experienced the care of NPs. Promotional efforts need to be aimed at the "unconvinced" segment of the population.

Further, some individuals who have experienced the care of NPs and been satisfied may not know that NPs are responsible for the care they provide. People may believe that NPs simply relay what a physician has decided and that NPs are simply physician helpers. NPs need to establish themselves as experts. That can be done, for example, through newspaper articles where NPs give advice on healthcare topics, through talk radio, through television public service announcements, through paid advertising, through presentations at community events, through journal articles, and through one-on-one interactions between NPs and patients.

Work the Data

All studies done on the care given by NPs are supportive of NPs. This includes many studies done by physicians and operations researchers, as well as studies done by nurses. NPs need to cite and recite the data in language that a layperson can understand. NPs also need to compile their own data on the effectiveness of their care. For example, electronic medical records systems now allow clinicians who treat diabetes to produce data that compare the effectiveness of individual clinicians at controlling patients' HgA1c. While physicians are hashing and rehashing the educational differences between NPs and physicians, NPs need to be repeating the data that support the assertion that NPs give good care. Therefore, the educational differential, while significant, must not be relevant. As mentioned earlier, to date, physicians have no data to prove that their additional years of education make them better PCPs than NPs.

Hire Professionals to Do the Association's Work

It is time to hire professionals and time for NP associations to act like businesses. It is time for board members to be relieved of the hands-on "doing" of association business so they can do what board members are supposed to do: decide how the association money is spent and evaluate the performance of the hired help.

Why? Because NPs are operating in an industry where changes are coming fast. NPs stand to gain ground, but progress will not come easily. Other professional groups are spending large sums to have experts monitor changes and ensure that their members' interests are represented when policy is made, law is enacted, and contracts are signed.

NPs have great potential because they combine nursing and medical knowledge. In volatile times, there are great opportunities. However, no laws will be enacted that designate NPs as PCPs unless bills are drafted expertly, hard lobbying is done successfully, and public relations efforts are increased and well targeted. No state regulations will be changed in NPs' favor without carefully drafted, persistent requests to state agencies. No health plans will open themselves to additional providers unless they can be shown how doing so will benefit them.

How are NP organizations going to fund all this expert help? By developing revenue streams other than membership dues. Each NP organization that does not have an annual continuing education conference for which the registration fee is at least $150 per day should work on creating one. Putting on a conference may require hiring a part-time conference coordinator. The budget for a conference should support a conference coordinator, the speakers' time, and the expenses of room rental and coffee, and the conference should make a profit. Each organization should charge for the use of its name and the use of its directory. When files of laws are sent out on request, the organization should charge for that service.

NP organizations need public relations specialists, lobbyists, and attorneys, either on retainer or on a per-project basis. Each organization also needs a paid executive director who answers to the board of directors.

Volunteer officers, board members, and committee chairs of NP organizations are running themselves ragged and burning out. These volunteers are making the day-to-day decisions about their organizations; often they also are talking with newspaper reporters, trying to recruit new members, trying to make sense of laws, folding flyers, licking stamps, and answering nonstop questions from individual NPs.

At a time when NPs are defending themselves, in the press and to the legislatures, and fighting for their spot in the managed-care landscape, they need to hire expert assistance, not rely on do-it-yourself operations. It is time to hire professionals and to get appropriate service.

Do Not Be Timid

Nurses, as a group, have lacked confidence and assertiveness in the past. NPs are trying to overcome barriers that were erected long before their title and position existed, barriers that resulted from this history of timidity in nursing. For example, in 1955, the American Nurses Association's (ANA's) model definition of nursing stated that nursing "shall not be deemed to include any acts of diagnosis or prescription of therapeutic or corrective measures."[3] In 1955, however, nurses were already performing acts that clearly were within the definition of diagnosis and prescription of corrective measures. Nevertheless, by 1967, 22 states had incorporated the ANA model language into state law.[4] To cover hospitals and agencies where nurses were engaging in "acts of diagnosis or prescription of therapeutic measures," joint statements of hospital, medical, and nursing associations were written that allowed nurses to perform certain acts, such as venipuncture or initiating intravenous fluids.[5] The joint statements were at odds with the law, yet no one challenged the law or the policy statements.

Today, NPs find that they can practice independently, meaning that they make decisions about patient care without consulting physicians. However, if state and federal regulations call for collaboration and define collaboration as supervision, NPs who push the envelope without also pushing for changes in legal language that supports their independent practice will be going nowhere.

It is time for NPs to affirm that NPs are experts in primary care. They should make statements such as "I am an expert in managing diabetes," rather than "NPs do primary care in collaboration with physicians."

Erase Collaboration from the Legal Vocabulary

NPs, like other healthcare providers, cannot function without collaboration with other experts. Nevertheless, nurses are virtually the only profession that has "collaboration" as a legal mandate.

NPs have considered the word collaboration an improvement on the word supervision. However, a close reading of federal law reveals that the law defines collaboration as supervision.

When arguing for erasure of barriers to NP practice, NPs have had difficulty convincing legislators of the difference between collaboration and supervision, and with good reason. Although there is a difference in the definitions of the two words—the dictionary defines collaboration as "work jointly with others" (and alternatively as "cooperate with or willingly assist an enemy force occupying one's country")[6] and supervision as "superintend, oversee"[7]—a legal mandate to collaborate suggests that the group given the mandate is not the final authority on a matter. Although NPs are not so arrogant as to consider themselves final authorities on all matters of health care, certainly NPs can and should consider themselves final authorities on primary care and other areas of medicine where they have specialized and have extensive education and experience. Consultation is appropriate, but a legal requirement for collaboration is not.

Insist Upon Legal Clarity of NP Authority to Practice

Compare Laws A and B on NP scope of practice:

Law A:
The board recognizes advanced and specialized acts of nursing practice as those described in the scope of practice statements for nurse practitioners certified by national certifying bodies recognized by the board.

Citation: Alaska Admin. Code tit. 12, § 44.430.

Law B:
The nurse practitioner provides holistic health care to individuals, families, and groups across the life span in a variety of settings, including hospitals, long-term care facilities, and community-based settings. Within his or her specialty, the nurse practitioner is responsible for managing health problems encountered by the client and is accountable for health outcomes. This process includes:

    a. Assessment
    b. Diagnosis
    c. Development of a plan
    d. Intervention
    e. Evaluation

The nurse practitioner is independently responsible and accountable for the continuous and comprehensive management of a broad range of health care, which may include:

a. Promotion and maintenance of health

b. Prevention of illness and disability

c. Assessment of clients, synthesis and analysis of data, and application of nursing principles and therapeutic modalities

d. Management of health care during acute and chronic phases of illness

e. Admission of his/her clients to hospitals and long-term care facilities and management of client care in these facilities

f. Counseling

g. Consultation and/or collaboration with other care providers and community resources

h. Referral to other healthcare providers and community resources

i. Management and coordination of care

j. Use of research skills

k. Diagnosis of health/illness status

l. Prescription and/or administration of therapeutic devices and measures including legend drugs and controlled substances . . . consistent with the definition of the practitioner's specialty category and scope of practice...

The nurse practitioner is responsible for recognizing limits of knowledge and experience, and for resolving situations beyond his/her nurse practitioner expertise by consulting with or referring clients to other healthcare providers. The nurse practitioner will only provide healthcare services within the nurse practitioner's scope of practice for which he/she is educationally prepared and for which competency has been established and maintained. Educational preparation includes academic course work, workshops or seminars, provided both theory and clinical experience are included.

Citation: Or. Admin. R. § 851-050-0005.

There is no question what an NP in Law B can do. Many questions are left unanswered by Law A, however. For example: What is "advanced and specialized acts of nursing practice?" Do such acts include medical services, or is an advanced practice nurse the same as a registered nurse? While Law B is specific and permissive of NP practice, Law A is unclear.

NPs need to insist upon clarity. Without clarity, other groups may decide what the law addressing NPs means.

Notes

1. American Academy of Family Physicians. (2009). Policy statement on nurse practitioners. Retrieved from http://www .aafp.org/about/policies/all/nurse-practitioners.html

2. Starr, P. (1992). *The social transformation of American medicine* (Chapter 3). New York, NY: Basic Books.

3. American Nurses' Association. (1955). ANA board approves a definition of nursing practice. *American Journal of Nursing, 55,* 1474.

4. Phillips, R. S. (1985). Nurse practitioners: Their scope of practice and theories of liability. *Journal of Legal Medicine, 6,* 391–414.
5. Bullough, B. (1975). The first two phases in nursing licensure. In: *The law and the expanding nursing role,* Vol. 7. New York, NY: Appleton-Century-Crofts.
6. Merriam-Webster. (2005). Collaboration definition. In: *Merriam-Webster collegiate dictionary* (11th ed.). Springfield, MA: Author.
7. Merriam-Webster. (2005). Supervision definition. In: *Merriam-Webster collegiate dictionary* (11th ed.). Springfield, MA: Author.

Common EENT Disorders in Primary Care

Karen S. Moore

Chapter Outline

Case 1 - Otitis

A. History and Physical Exam

B. Recommended Labs/Diagnostics

C. Pathophysiology

D. Treatment Plan

E. Guidelines to Direct Care:

Clinical Practice Guideline: Acute Otitis Externa, American Academy of Otolaryngology—Head and Neck Surgery Foundation. Original issued in 2006, revised in 2013.

Case 2 - Rhinitis

A. History and Physical Exam

B. Recommended Labs/Diagnostics

C. Pathophysiology

D. Treatment Plan

E. Guidelines to Direct Care:

The diagnosis and management of rhinitis: An updated practice parameter by the Joint Task Force on Practice Parameters, representing the American Academy of Allergy, Asthma & Immunology; and the Joint Council of Allergy, Asthma and Immunology.

American Academy of Allergy, Asthma and Immunology (AAAAI) Allergy and Asthma Medication Guide (2014).

Case 3 - Conjunctivitis

A. History and Physical Exam

B. Additional Assessments/Diagnostics Needed

C. Pathophysiology

D. Treatment Plan?

E. Guidelines to Direct Care:

American Academy of Ophthalmology (2009). Policy Statement: Guidelines for appropriate referral of persons with possible eye disease or injury.

Case 4 - Sinusitis

A. Physical Exam

B. Additional Assessments/Diagnostics Needed

C. Pathophysiology

D. Treatment Plan

E. Guidelines to Direct Care:

Infectious Disease Society of America (IDSA) Clinical Practice Guideline for Acute Bacterial Rhinosinusitis in Children and Adults (2012)

Case 5 - Pharyngitis

A. History and Physical Exam

B. Additional Assessments/Diagnostics Needed

C. Pathophysiology

D. Treatment Plan

E. Guidelines to Direct Care:

Clinical Practice guideline for the diagnosis and management of group A streptococcal pharyngitis: 2012 update by the Infectious Disease Society of America.

Learning Objectives

Using a case-based approach, the learner will be able to:

1. Identify key history and physical examination parameters for common ear, eye, nose, and throat (EENT) disorders seen in primary care, including otitis, allergic rhinitis, conjunctivitis, sinusitis, and pharyngitis.

2. Summarize recommended laboratory and diagnostic studies indicated for the evaluation of common EENT disorders seen in primary care.

3. State the pathophysiology of common EENT disorders.

4. Document a clear, concise SOAP note for patients with common EENT disorders.

5. Identify relevant education and counseling strategies for patients with common EENT disorders.

6. Develop a treatment plan for common EENT disorders utilizing current evidence-based guidelines.

Case 1

Jeremy is a 22-year-old male triathlete who presents with complaints of irritation and fullness in his right ear. He has been training 6 to 8 hours a day for an upcoming event. His training regimen includes running, swimming, cycling, weight lifting, and a strict nutritional regimen. He is very concerned that the fullness and irritation could require him to limit or curtail his training. He denies recent upper respiratory infection, denies illness in training partners and roommates, and denies nausea, vomiting, and dizziness. Immunizations up to date.

Physical Exam

Vital Signs: blood pressure (BP) 118/76, heart rate (HR) 64, respiratory rate (RR) 12, temperature (T) 98.5, height (Ht) 6'2", weight (Wt) 170 lbs

General (GEN): No acute distress

Head, eyes, ears, nose, and throat (HEENT): Normocephalic, pupils equal, round, react to light, accommodation

(PERRLA), sclera and conjunctiva clear without redness or injection. Ear canal reddened, edematous. Tympanic membrane (TM) clear, pearly, bony landmarks visible. No discharge; pain noted with traction on tragus.

Cardiovascular (CV): S_1 and S_2, regular rate and rhythm (RRR), no murmurs, no gallops, no rubs

Lungs: Clear to auscultation

Abdomen: Soft, nontender, nondistended, bowel sounds present $\times$ 4 quadrants, no organomegaly

Neuro: Rhine/Weber normal, Romberg negative

What additional assessments/diagnostics do you need?
What is your differential diagnoses list?
What is your working diagnosis?

Additional Assessments/Diagnostics Needed

ROS

Ask about common signs and symptoms of otitis and other conditions that may cause ear pain and irritation:[1-2]

- ► Cough
- ► Runny nose
- ► Throat irritation
- ► Hearing loss
- ► Ringing in the ears (tinnitus)
- ► Discharge from ears, nose, or throat
- ► Pressure or fullness in ears
- ► Swelling or fullness along the jawline, under the ears, or along the neck
- ► Pain, pressure, or difficulty with swallowing
- ► Chills or fever
- ► Pain along bony prominences of the head and neck

Physical Exam

The examination for this patient should include:[1-2]

- ► Careful inspection of the ear canal and TM to determine whether TM is intact and canal is obstructed
- ► Assessment of comorbid conditions that may require a modification in treatment (i.e., nonintact TM, immunocompromise, prior radiotherapy, tympanostomy tube)
- ► Evaluation of prior immunizations for adequate coverage of mumps

Common signs and symptoms of otitis externa may include:[1-2]

- Ear pain (otalgia)
- Irritation or itching in the external auditory canal
- Hearing loss
- Fullness or pressure in the ear
- Swelling, redness, and narrowing of the external auditory canal
- Tinnitus
- Possible discharge from ear that ranges from clear to purulent
- History of recent water activities such as swimming
- History of trauma to ear canal from use of cotton swabs and vigorous cleaning
- Fever may or may not be present

Routine Labs/Diagnostics

Otitis externa (OE) is typically diagnosed by history and physical examination, including otoscopy.[1-3] If a fungal causative agent is suspected, the patient is immunocompromised, the patient has a history of prior radiotherapy, or the examination suggests necrotizing OE, the following diagnostics may be considered:

- Gram stain and culture of discharge from the ear to determine causative agent
- Blood glucose level and urine dipstick to assess for diabetes
- Complete blood count (CBC) to assess white blood cells (WBCs) with CD4 count if necessary to assess for immunocompromise

Imaging studies are also not required or commonly done but may be necessary in the case of necrotizing OE, if mastoiditis or extensive cellulitis is suspected.

- Because of its ability to better detect bony erosion, high-resolution computed tomography (CT) scanning is preferred if assessing for mastoiditis[4]
- Magnetic resonance imaging (MRI) may be considered if soft tissue extension is a primary concern[5]

Differential Diagnoses List

Acute otitis externa

Chronica otitis externa

Otitis media

Ear canal obstruction

Mumps

Dental abscess

Working Diagnosis

Uncomplicated acute otitis externa

Pathophysiology

Acute otitis externa (AOE) is caused primarily by bacterial pathogens in the ear canal such as *Pseudomonas aeruginosa* and *Staphylococcus aureus*.[1-3] Many infections are polymicrobial. Fungal infection is very uncommon in primary AOE but may be seen in immunocompromised patients, patients previously unsuccessfully treated for AOE, and those with chronic otitis. AOE is characterized by acute inflammation and edema of the ear canal and surrounding tissues.

What Is Your Treatment Plan?

Pharmacologic

- Analgesic treatment based on the severity of pain
- Topical agents including antibiotics and anti-inflammatory agents
  - Acetic acid 2% solution
  - Acetic acid 2%, hydrocortisone 1% solution
  - Ciprofloxacin 0.2%, hydrocortisone 1% solution[6]
  - Ciprofloxacin 0.3%, dexamethasone 0.1%
  - Neomycin, polymyxin B, hydrocortisone
  - Ofloxacin 0.3%
- Oral/systemic antibiotics, antifungals, and anti-inflammatory agents should be reserved for complicated otitis that includes extension to surrounding soft tissue or bony involvement.[1-3]

Nonpharmacologic

- Ear hygiene: Avoid use of cotton swabs; keep ear canal dry
- Avoid swimming and submerging ear canal in water.
- If canal is obstructed, consider aural toileting, wicking, or both to encourage mobilization of drainage.
- Surgical debridement is reserved for necrotizing otitis or severe inflammation that prevents instillation of ear drops.
  - A wick may be placed to help with drop instillation.[1-3]

Education/Counseling

- Proper ear drop instillation requires appropriate positioning and patience. Patients should be instructed to:
  - Lie down with affected ear up
  - Instill enough drops to fill ear canal
  - Stay lying down with affected ear up for 3–5 minutes
  - Massage the tragus or gently move the ear back and forth to ensure proper placement of drops

- If a wick was placed, instruct the patient that the wick will fall out on its own as the inflammation recedes.
  - Do not pull or tug at the wick.
- Symptoms should begin to resolve in 48–72 hours. If symptoms worsen or do not improve in that time frame, additional care should be sought.
- Avoid swimming or submerging ear in water for 2–3 days following completion of treatment. Treatment regimens last from 7 to 10 days.[1-3]

SOAP Note

S: Jeremy is a 22-year-old male triathlete who reports a 3-day history of irritation and fullness in his right ear. He has been training 6–8 hours a day for an upcoming event with two hours per day swimming. He denies recent upper respiratory infection, denies illness in training partners and roommates, and denies nausea, vomiting, and dizziness. Immunizations up to date.

O: *Vital Signs:* BP 118/76, HR 64, RR 12, T 98.5, Ht 6'2", Wt 170 lbs

GEN: No acute distress

HEENT: Normocephalic, PERRLA, sclera and conjunctiva without redness. Ear canal reddened, edematous. TM clear, pearly, bony landmarks visible. No discharge, pain noted with traction on tragus.

CV: S_1 and S_2, RRR, no murmurs, no gallops, no rubs

Lungs: Clear to auscultation

Abdomen: Soft, nontender, nondistended, bowel sounds present × 4 quadrants, no organomegaly

Neuro: Rhine/Weber normal, Romberg negative

A: Acute otitis externa

P: Prescriptions provided for otic drops: ciprofloxacin 0.2%, hydrocortisone 1.0%, 3 gtts in affected ear three times daily × 7 days.[6] Use over-the-counter acetaminophen as directed. If no improvement in 48–72 hours, return for further evaluation. Avoid swimming, water sports, ear plugs, ear buds, cotton swabs, or mechanical irritation of ear canal during treatment and for 3 days following completion of otic antibiotic. Instruction provided on proper instillation of drops.

Health Promotion Issues

- Good ear hygiene[1-3]
- Discussion of sexually transmitted infection (STI) prevention, safety, depression, alcohol/drug use, skin cancer prevention/screening[7,8]
- Annual influenza vaccine[9]

Guidelines to Direct Care

Centers for Disease Control and Prevention. Recommended adult immunization schedule, by vaccine and age group. 2014. http://www.cdc.gov/vaccines/schedules/hcp/imz/adult.html. Accessed September 2, 2015.

Rosenfeld RM, Schwartz SR, Cannon CR, et al. Clinical practice guideline: acute otitis externa. *Otolaryngol Head Neck Surg.* 2014;150(1 suppl):S1–S24. Originally issued in 2006, revised in 2013. http://www.guideline.gov/content.aspx?id=47795&search=otitis. Accessed September 2, 2015.

US Preventive Services Task Force Recommendations for primary care practice: published recommendations. http://www.uspreventiveservicestaskforce.org/BrowseRec/Index/browse-recommendations. Accessed September 2, 2015.

Case 2

Oscar is a 42-year-old African American male who reports he has "had a cold for three weeks." States he has nasal congestion, a runny nose, nasal irritation, and sneezing. Denies frequent colds, but states he seems to "get sick every fall." Denies chest pain, reports "irritating cough" primarily at night, which he believes is due to "drainage." Past medical history (PMH) is significant for eczema, asthma symptoms in childhood, and allergy to strawberries. Denies facial pain or pressure, fever, night sweats, nausea, or vomiting. Denies recent illness in family members. Patient is married. He denies tobacco use in self or spouse. Reports childhood immunizations completed with a tetanus vaccination received 3 years ago. He refuses an annual influenza vaccination.

Physical Exam

Vital Signs: BP 130/84, HR 88, RR 16, T 98.8, Ht 6'0", Wt 192 lbs

GEN: No acute distress

HEENT: Normocephalic, PERRLA, sclera and conjunctiva clear without redness or injection. TMs intact bilaterally with bony landmarks visible, no discharge, no pain on palpation. Nares erythematous and edematous bilaterally. Inferior and middle turbinates gray and boggy with clear drainage noted. Posterior pharynx slightly erythematous without exudate. No lymphadenopathy. No pain on palpation of sinuses.

CV: S_1 and S_2, RRR, no murmurs, no gallops, no rubs

Lungs: Clear to auscultation

Abdomen: Soft, nontender, nondistended, bowel sounds present × 4 quadrants, no organomegaly

What additional assessments/diagnostics do you need?

What is the differential diagnoses list?

What is your working diagnosis?

Additional Assessments/Diagnostics Needed

ROS

The examination of this patient should include:

▶ Detailed history of the onset of symptoms, pattern of illness, chronicity and possible seasonality of symptoms, association with allergens/triggers, environmental and occupational history, as well as any medications used to alleviate symptoms.

Physical Exam

▶ Careful examination of the EENT system will help rule out any anatomic malformations and provide clues based on color of drainage, condition and color of nasal turbinates and pharynx.

▶ A complete respiratory examination is also necessary with a focus on any signs or symptoms of respiratory compromise.

Routine Labs/Diagnostics

▶ Determination of the offending allergen via immunoglobulin E (IgE) skin testing is recommended to provide a basis of treatment. For some patients, avoidance of the offending allergen is possible; others may require medication and allergen immunotherapy.[11]

▶ Fiber-optic nasal endoscopy or rhinomanometry may be indicated in cases in which obstruction of the nasal passages is suspected.

▶ Nasal smears for eosinophilia and nasal biopsies are reserved for cases in which the diagnosis of allergic rhinitis is uncertain.

▶ If a polyp found during nasal endoscopy requires further evaluation, a biopsy is performed.[10]

Differential Diagnoses List

Allergic rhinitis

Vasomotor rhinitis

Mechanical obstruction of nares

Chronic inflammatory rhinitis

Viral influenza

Acute sinusitis

Chronic sinusitis

Working Diagnosis

Allergic rhinitis

Pathophysiology

Rhinitis can be defined as one or more nasal symptoms of congestion, rhinorrhea, sneezing, and itching.[10] Rhinitis may be classified as allergic, nonallergic, or mixed. Although typically viewed as an inflammatory condition, some nonallergic types of rhinitis such as vasomotor and atrophic rhinitis are not primarily inflammatory. Allergic rhinitis is estimated to impact 10% to 30% of US adults annually. Risk factors for development of allergic rhinitis include a family history of allergies, presence of allergies in the patient documented by skin prick allergy testing, higher socioeconomic class, and a serum IgE > 100 U/mL noted before the age of 6 years. Although commonly viewed as a troublesome symptom rather than a disease in need of treatment, rhinitis is associated with significant morbidity, including lost time from school or work and decreased quality of life from fatigue and sleep disturbance. Allergic rhinitis is also implicated as a comorbidity for asthma exacerbation, sinusitis, and sleep apnea.

What Is Your Treatment Plan?

Pharmacologic

Intranasal pharmacologic agents are generally preferred over oral medications as the primary treatment modality for allergic rhinitis. In addition to efficacy of each category of medication and specific agents, side effects must be considered when making prescribing decisions.

▶ *Antihistamines:* Intranasal antihistamines are considered first-line treatment for allergic rhinitis. Second-generation antihistamines are preferred over first generation because of decreased sedative side effects. Intranasal antihistamines can be systemically absorbed, so sedation and interference with skin allergy testing must be considered in both intranasal and oral preparations.

▶ *Corticosteroids:* Intranasal corticosteroids are the most effective drug class in the management of allergic rhinitis. Corticosteroids provide consistent relief of inflammation when used on a routine basis. As-needed dosing of corticosteroids is not quite as effective as routine dosing regimens. Concerns over systemic side effects of corticosteroids are not generally seen when the intranasal medications are given in recommended doses. Oral corticosteroids are generally not recommended for management of allergic rhinitis.

▶ *Decongestants:* Decongestants such as pseudoephedrine and phenylephrine are alpha-adrenergic agonists that can be effective in reducing nasal congestion but also commonly result in troubling side effects such as insomnia, palpitation, and irritability. Decongestants should be used cautiously in patients with cardiac disease, hypertension, bladder neck obstruction, glaucoma, and hyperthyroidism.

▶ *Anticholinergics:* Anticholinergics may reduce rhinorrhea, but they are not effective in reduction of any other symptoms of allergic rhinitis.

▶ *Other:* Cromolyn, leukotriene antagonists (LT), and intranasal saline preparations are effective adjuvant treatments in the management of allergic rhinitis with minimal side effects noted.

Allergen immunotherapy may be recommended for patients with a documented IgE antibody to specific allergens if the burden of medication use is thought to be onerous or if the amount and types of medications can be significantly reduced, resulting in lowering of side effects.

Nonpharmacologic

Allergen avoidance is the primary prevention method for allergic rhinitis. Patients should be encouraged to keep a symptom diary and associated potential environmental and food triggers. Imaging studies are not routinely performed for allergic rhinitis unless comorbidities of sinus infection or mechanical obstruction are suspected.

Education/Counseling

- Allergen avoidance
- Treatment methodologies
    - Discuss choice of medications and side effect profile
    - Discuss the need for daily management
    - Consider special circumstances of each patient when prescribing
        - *Pregnancy:* Follow pregnancy risk categories
        - *Advanced age:* Important to differentiate type of rhinitis prior to management
        - *Specific disease states:* Cardiac disease, hypertension, bladder neck obstruction, glaucoma, and hyperthyroidism
        - *Athletes:* Competitive athletes must be given medications that comply with antidoping testing standards of international sports organizations
- Instruct in proper instillation of intranasal medications

SOAP Note

S: Oscar is a 42-year-old African American male with a 3-week history of nasal congestion, runny nose, nasal irritation, sneezing, nocturnal cough, and post-nasal drip. Reports spring exacerbation of symptoms annually. PMH is significant for eczema, asthma symptoms in childhood, and allergy to strawberries. Denies facial pain or pressure, and denies fever, night sweats, nausea, or vomiting. Denies recent illness in family members. Denies tobacco use in self or spouse. Tetanus vaccination 3 years ago, but refuses annual influenza vaccination.

O: *Vital Signs:* BP 130/84, HR 88, RR 16, T 98.8, Ht 6'0", Wt 192 lbs

GEN: No acute distress

HEENT: Normocephalic, PERRLA, sclera and conjunctiva clear without redness or injection. TMs intact bilaterally with bony landmarks visible, no discharge, no pain on palpation. Nares erythematous and edematous bilaterally. Inferior and middle turbinates gray and boggy with clear drainage noted. Posterior pharynx slightly erythematous without exudate. No lymphadenopathy. No pain on palpation of sinuses.

CV: S_1 and S_2, RRR, no murmurs, no gallops, no rubs

Lungs: Clear to auscultation

Abdomen: Soft, nontender, nondistended, bowel sounds present $\times$ 4 quadrants, no organomegaly

A: Allergic rhinitis

P: Referral provided for skin prick allergy testing. Following allergy testing, patient is instructed to begin taking fluticasone propionate intranasal 50 mcg/spray, two sprays in each nostril one time each day.[11]

Health Promotion Issues

- Discussion of STI prevention, depression, alcohol/drug use, skin cancer prevention/screening[7,8]
- Dyslipidemia screening[7,8]
- Annual influenza vaccine[9]

Guidelines to Direct Care

American Academy of Allergy Asthma and Immunology. AAAAI allergy and asthma medication guide. 2014. http://www.aaaai.org/conditions-and-treatments/drug-guide/nasal-medication.aspx. Accessed September 2, 2015.

Centers for Disease Control and Prevention. Recommended adult immunization schedule, by vaccine and age group. 2014. http://www.cdc.gov/vaccines/schedules/hcp/imz/adult.html. Accessed September 2, 2015.

US Preventive Services Task Force. Recommendations for primary care practice: published recommendations. http://www.uspreventiveservicestaskforce.org/BrowseRec/Index/browse-recommendations. Accessed September 2, 2015.

Wallace DV, Dykewicz MS, Bernstein DI. The diagnosis and management of rhinitis: an updated practice parameter. *J Allergy Clin Immunol*, 2008;122(2). http://www.aaaai.org/Aaaai/media/MediaLibrary/PDF%20Documents/Practice%20and%20Parameters/rhinitis2008-diagnosis-management.pdf. Accessed September 2, 2015.

Case 3

Emily is a 17-year-old white female who reports she awakened today with a red eye and feeling like her eyelashes were "stuck together." States initially upon awakening she felt like something was in her eye and her vision was blurry, but after she was able to fully open her eye and wash the eyelashes and eyelid, her vision was normal. Reports a history of recent "cough and stuffy nose" that she believes is improving. Denies sore throat, ear pain, or eye trauma. She is a nonsmoker and is not sexually active. Admits to occasional champagne at New Year's or weddings. Last menstrual period (LMP) was 20 days ago. She lives at home with her parents and two younger siblings. She is very active in sports in her high school, playing soccer and softball, and hopes to get a scholarship to attend college out of state next year. When asked about sick contacts, reports a teammate was treated for "pink-eye a few days ago." Childhood immunizations including human papillomavirus (HPV) vaccination series completed; tetanus booster received last year. Does not receive annual influenza vaccination.

Physical Exam

Vital Signs: BP 106/74, HR 72, RR 12, T 98.6, Ht 5'4", Wt 135 lbs

GEN: No acute distress

HEENT: Normocephalic, ear canal without redness, discharge, or edema noted. TM clear, pearly, bony landmarks visible. No pain on palpation of pinna or with traction. PERRLA with positive red reflex bilaterally. Oculus sinister (OS) visual acuity 20/20, sclera and conjunctiva clear and without redness, injection, or discharge noted. Fundoscopic exam with discs well marginated. No AV nicking. No photosensitivity noted. Oculus dexter (OD) 20/20, bulbar and palpebral conjunctiva reddened and injected with yellow-green discharge noted on lashline.

CV: S_1 and S_2, RRR, no murmurs, no gallops, no rubs

Lungs: Clear to auscultation

Abdomen: Soft, nontender, nondistended, bowel sounds present × 4 quadrants, no organomegaly

What additional assessments/diagnostics do you need?

What is the differential diagnoses list?

What is your working diagnosis?

Additional Assessments/Diagnostics Needed

ROS

When assessing a patient with red eye, it is important to differentiate between emergent, urgent, and routine eye issues.[12,13] Visual impairment necessitates immediate referral.

Eye Issues That Do Not Commonly Impair Vision

▶ Viral conjunctivitis

▶ Bacterial conjunctivitis

▶ Nongonococcal or nonchlamydial conjunctivitis

▶ Allergic conjunctivitis

▶ Blepharitis

▶ Episcleritis

▶ Peripheral corneal pterygium

▶ Subconjunctival hemorrhage

Eye Issues That Can Impair Vision

▶ Corneal injection (gonococcal infection/chlamydia/herpes simplex virus/herpes zoster virus)

▶ Corneal ulcer

▶ Anterior uveitis

▶ Scleritis

▶ Superficial keratitis

▶ Pterygium or corneal abrasion that encroaches on central cornea

Physical Exam

The examination for a complaint of a red eye should include the following:[12,13]

▶ A thorough health history to explore:

  ▶ Any causes of injury if they exist

  ▶ When the irritation and redness first began

  ▶ Visual changes

  ▶ Level of pain

  ▶ Light sensitivity

  ▶ Possible exposure to allergens and environmental causative agents

  ▶ Narrowing the causative agents in possible infectious exposures

▶ A review of the patient's medical record allows for comparison of current visual acuity with baseline visual acuity if the patient is well known to your practice.

▶ An undilated ophthalmoscopic examination should be performed, with the addition of fluorescein staining if available. Introduction of fluorescein and illumination with the blue or green light of the ophthalmoscope cause abrasions and dendritic lesions to be visualized more clearly by the examiner.

Routine Labs/Diagnostics

Laboratory testing is not routinely performed in acute, uncomplicated conjunctivitis.[12,13] If infection is resistant or recurring, a culture may be performed.

If the patient reports a sudden onset of severe eye redness with copious purulent discharge from the eye, hyperacute bacterial conjunctivitis associated with *Neisseria gonorrhoeae* infection should be suspected. Cultures of the eye and urgent referral should be initiated related to the propensity of *N. gonorrhoeae* to cause corneal perforation.

Differential Diagnoses List

Viral conjunctivitis

Bacterial conjunctivitis

Nongonococcal or nonchlamydial conjunctivitis

Allergic conjunctivitis

Blepharitis

Episcleritis

Peripheral corneal pterygium

Subconjunctival hemorrhage

unlike viral conjunctivitis, bacterial conjunctivitis is typically unilateral, but can sometimes spread to both eyes. The biggest d/c bacterial is purulent c̄ exam it is very noticeable c̄ and continuous and persists t/o day.

Working Diagnosis

Bacterial conjunctivitis

Pathophysiology

Bacterial conjunctivitis is caused by introduction of bacteria into the bulbar or palpebral conjunctiva.[12] Defense mechanisms within the eye trigger inflammation and the resultant redness as well as an increase in the viscosity and amount of lacrimal secretions. The offending organism impacts the amount of discharge, degree of redness and injection, and rapidity of progression of the infection.

What Is Your Treatment Plan?

Pharmacologic

Pharmacologic therapy and antibiotic choice are based on bacteria suspected to be causing the infection and clinician preference.[12–14] A significant difference in outcomes based on antibiotic selection in uncomplicated acute bacterial conjunctivitis has not been shown. With acute uncomplicated bacterial conjunctivitis in adults who do not wear contact lenses, pharmacologic treatment could include one of the following:

- Azithromycin 1% ophthalmic drops
- Trimethoprim/polymyxin B ophthalmic drops
- Sulfacetamide 10% ophthalmic drops or ointment
- Tobramycin 0.3% ophthalmic ointment
- Erythromycin 0.5% ophthalmic ointment

If the patient wears contact lenses, antibiotic coverage for *Pseudomonas aeruginosa* must be considered in the antibiotic selection process. A broad-spectrum antibiotic ophthalmic solution such as levofloxacin 1.5% ophthalmic drops should be selected.

Topical glucocorticoids have no role in the management of acute conjunctivitis by primary care clinicians. They can cause sight-threatening complications (corneal scarring, melting, and perforation) when used inappropriately in herpes simplex or bacterial keratitis.

Nonpharmacologic

- Wet compresses, cool or warm per patient preference
- Attention to patient education and counseling

Education/Counseling

- Advise contact lens wearers to discontinue lens wear. Contaminated lenses should be discarded, as should all contact lens solution and cases.
- All eye makeup should be discarded.

- New makeup may be purchased but should not be worn, until 24 hours after completion of treatment, when the eye is no longer pink and no discharge is observed.
- Clean the eye prior to medication administration.
- Instruct on proper medication administration.
- If an adult is prescribed ointment, remind the person not to drive or perform activities requiring good visual acuity for at least 20 minutes following administration as a result of blurring of vision.
- Instruct on good hand washing for all family members.
- Keep linens and washcloths separate from other household members' linens.
- Use linens one time only.
- Wash the affected eye area and side of the face last to avoid contamination of the noninfected eye if possible.
- Bacterial conjunctivitis is highly contagious and spread by direct contact with secretions or contact with contaminated objects.
- No work or school until 24 hours after complete resolution of eye redness and no discharge is observed.
- Call in 2 days if no improvement is seen or if symptoms worsen or vision decreases.
- Patients who do not respond should be referred to an ophthalmologist.

SOAP Note

S: Emily is a 17-year-old white female with a history of recent upper respiratory infection who awakened today with a red eye, matting of eyelashes, foreign body sensation, and blurry vision. Emily states her vision clears after washing eye region and eyelashes. Denies sore throat, ear pain, or eye trauma. She is a nonsmoker, is not sexually active, and does not use tobacco. Denies regular, frequent ETOH use. Reports a teammate was treated for "pinkeye a few days ago." Childhood immunizations including HPV vaccination series completed, tetanus booster received last year.

O: *Vital Signs:* BP 106/74, HR 72, RR 12, T 98.6, Ht 5'4", Wt 135 lbs

GEN: No acute distress

HEENT: Normocephalic, ear canal without redness, discharge, or edema noted. TM clear, pearly, bony landmarks visible. No pain on palpation of pinna or with traction. PERRLA with positive red reflex bilaterally. OS visual acuity 20/20, sclera and conjunctiva clear and without redness, injection, or discharge noted. Fundoscopic exam with discs well marginated. No AV nicking. No photosensitivity noted. OD 20/20, bulbar and palpebral conjunctiva reddened and injected with yellow-green discharge noted on lashline.

CV: S_1 and S_2, RRR, no murmurs, no gallops, no rubs

Lungs: Clear to auscultation

Abdomen: Soft, nontender, nondistended, bowel sounds present × 4 quadrants, no organomegaly

A: Acute bacterial conjunctivitis

P: Patient instructed on application of sulfacetamide 10% ophthalmic drops (1–2 gtts every 2–3 hours × 7 days). Hygiene, hand washing, and back to school education discussed with patient. Follow-up for conjunctivitis if the infection is not improving within 48 hours as evidenced by decreased irritation, decreased redness, and decreased discharge, or if not fully resolved within 7 days, or if condition worsens.

Health Promotion Issues

▶ Discussion of STI prevention, depression, alcohol/drug use, skin cancer prevention/screening, safety[8]

▶ Meningitis vaccine, annual influenza vaccine[9]

Guidelines to Direct Care

American Academy of Ophthalmology. Policy statement: referral of persons with possible eye diseases or injury. 2014. http://www.aao.org/clinical-statement/guidelines-appropriate-referral-of-persons-with-po. Accessed September 2, 2015.

Centers for Disease Control and Prevention. Recommended adult immunization schedule, by vaccine and age group. 2014. http://www.cdc.gov/vaccines/schedules/hcp/imz/adult.html. Accessed September 2, 2015.

US Preventive Services Task Force. Recommendations for primary care practice: published recommendations. http://www.uspreventiveservicestaskforce.org/BrowseRec/Index/browse-recommendations. Accessed September 2, 2015.

Case 4

Susan is a 54-year-old white female who reports she has had a "stuffy head" for "about two weeks" that will not go away. Reports nasal congestion, facial pain, facial pressure, and dental pain that worsens when bending forward. Reports she has intermittent nasal fullness and facial pain that have been treated successfully with antibiotics in the past. She is unsure of which antibiotic she was given previously, but states she "needs them about once or twice a year." She usually uses over-the-counter nasal spray when she starts to feel congestion "for about a week until it stops working." Admits to coughing intermittently throughout the day. States she usually has straw-colored sputum but has noticed it is a brownish green "for about a week." Denies allergies, denies recent well-woman exam, denies recent immunizations. States she has not been to see a healthcare provider other than at urgent care centers for antibiotics "in about ten years." Reports childhood immunizations were completed. PMH of varicella, rubella, rubeola, and mumps diseases in childhood. LMP 5 years ago. Reports alcohol use of about eight drinks per week. Twenty-pack-year history of tobacco use. Denies illicit drug use. Lives with husband of 15 years, no children. Denies illness in close contacts.

Physical Exam

Vital Signs: BP 110/76, HR 80, RR 12, T 99.1, Ht 5'6", Wt 160 lbs

GEN: No acute distress

HEENT: Normocephalic, PERRLA, sclera and conjunctiva clear without redness or injection. Ear canal slightly reddened, no discharge. TM clear, pearly, bony landmarks visible. Posterior pharynx slightly erythematous without exudate. No lymphadenopathy. Maxillary and frontal sinuses tender to palpation. Toothache increases with percussion. Dull transillumination of right maxillary sinus, left opaque. Frontal sinuses show dull transillumination. Nares erythematous and edematous bilaterally. Inferior and middle turbinates patent bilaterally. Mucopurulent mucus visible bilaterally. Neck: Supple. Thyroid without nodules or prominence noted.

CV: Point of maximal impact (PMI) located at 5th intercostal space (ICS) midclavicular line (MCL), S_1 and S_2, RRR, no murmurs, no gallops, no rubs. Pedal pulses 2+, no peripheral edema noted, no jugular vein distention (JVD) noted.

Lungs: Coarse crackles that clear with coughing noted throughout. No wheeze, no stridor, no tactile fremitus.

Abdomen: Soft, nontender, nondistended, bowel sounds present × 4 quadrants, no organomegaly

Skin turgor normal, mucous membranes moist.

What additional assessments/diagnostics do you need?

What is the differential diagnoses list?

What is your working diagnosis?

Additional Assessments/Diagnostics Needed

ROS

Ask about common signs and symptoms of sinus infection as well as other conditions that may cause the symptoms she describes, including:

▶ Cough

▶ Nasal drainage

▶ Throat irritation

▶ Ear pressure or pain

- ► Difficulty swallowing
- ► Chills or fever
- ► Altered taste, bad taste in the mouth
- ► Nausea
- ► Vomiting

Physical Exam

The examination for this patient should include:[15–16]

- ► Detailed history of the onset of symptoms, pattern of illness, chronicity, and possible seasonality of symptoms, association with allergens/triggers, environmental and occupational history, as well as any medications used to alleviate symptoms.
- ► Careful examination of the EENT system will help rule out any anatomic malformations and provide clues based on color of drainage, condition and color of nasal turbinates and pharynx.
- ► A complete respiratory examination is also necessary with focus on any signs or symptoms of respiratory compromise.

Clinical presentation leading to a diagnosis of sinusitis would include:[15]

- ► Onset with persistent symptoms of sinusitis that last for >10 days without clinical improvement
- ► Onset with severe symptoms of fever >39°C (102°F) and purulent nasal discharge or facial pain lasting 3–4 consecutive days at the beginning of illness
- ► Onset with worsening of symptoms characterized by initial illness with improvement and then 5–6 days later worsening of fever, headache, and increased nasal discharge referred to as double sickening

Once the clinical diagnosis is made, antibiotic therapy is recommended.[15–16]

Routine Labs/Diagnostics

Labs

In acute bacterial rhinosinusitis (ABRS), routine labs are generally not performed.[15–16] If indicated, the following labs may be helpful:

- ► A CBC with differential may help differentiate cause. Allergic causes of ongoing symptoms would appear as increased eosinophils, and primarily bacterial causes will show an increase in neutrophils.
- ► Skin prick allergy testing identifies the allergen that may precipitate sinus infections, allowing for allergen control to decrease frequency of exacerbations.
- ► Culture of direct sinus aspiration should be reserved for patients who experience antibiotic treatment failure.

Imaging Studies

Imaging studies in this case may include the following:

- ► Plain sinus radiographs provide a gross exam of the paranasal sinuses in an easily available and cost-effective manner. Air fluid levels can be seen in acute sinusitis, and mucosal thickening can be seen in chronic sinusitis. Although this is commonly done in practice, current guidelines do not recommend plain radiographs as the best imaging choice.[15–16]
- ► CT is the most useful imaging study in sinusitis. Imaging should be reserved for patients with suppurative complications of sinusitis. CT is much more specific than plain films and provides more detailed information about the type and level of sinus involvement, especially if surgical intervention is being considered. CT also shows surrounding tissues such as the orbits and brain.[15–16]
- ► MRI is more specific than CT scan in differentiating soft tissue densities and also more expensive. This imaging is reserved for differentiating benign and malignant lesions and is not generally recommended in cases of sinusitis alone.[15–16]
- ► Fiber-optic nasal endoscopy or rhinomanometry provides direct visualization of the sinus cavity, allowing the practitioner to visualize causes of mechanical obstruction. Polyps, foreign bodies, and anatomic anomalies can be directly visualized. Additionally, endoscopy allows for a specific culture of the middle meatus, which can be helpful in guiding treatment.[10,15,16]

Differential Diagnoses List

Upper respiratory infection

Allergic rhinitis

Vasomotor rhinitis

Mechanical obstruction of nares

Chronic inflammatory rhinitis

Viral influenza

Acute bacterial rhinosinusitis

Chronic sinusitis

Periodontal disease

Working Diagnosis

Acute bacterial rhinosinusitis

Pathophysiology

Sinusitis is a disease characterized by inflammation, edema, and infection.[15] Sinusitis and its treatment methodologies are subdivided into acute, subacute, chronic, and recurrent as follows:

- ► Acute—sudden onset runny, stuffy nose, facial pain that does not go away after 10–14 days. Acute sinusitis typically lasts 4 weeks or less.
- ► Subacute—an inflammation lasts 4–8 weeks.

- Chronic—a condition characterized by sinus inflammation symptoms lasting 8 weeks or longer.
- Recurrent—several attacks within a year.

Main goals in the treatment of sinusitis include controlling infection, reducing tissue edema, facilitating drainage, and maintaining the patency of the sinus ostia.

What Is Your Treatment Plan?

Pharmacologic

- Analgesic as needed[15–16]
- Antibiotic treatment[15–16]
  - Amoxicillin/clavulanate as first-line treatment 5–14 days based on severity and recurrence
  - In patients who are allergic to penicillin (PCN), may use doxycycline or respiratory fluoroquinolones[15–16]
- Intranasal and systemic corticosteroids

Nonpharmacologic

- Moisture
- Saline nasal drops, sprays, or irrigations
- Heated mist
- Increased fluid intake[15–16]

Avoid common causes of sinusitis:

- Allergies
- Complication of acute or chronic rhinitis
- Environmental irritants
- Nasal polyposis
- Viral infection

Education/Counseling

- Return for evaluation if symptoms don't improve within 48 hours.
- Return if there is swelling in the periorbital area.
- Humidify the air and increase fluid intake.
- Avoid allergens.
- Avoid swimming during the acute phase.
- Avoid antihistamines.
- Avoid smoking.[15–16]

SOAP Note

S: Susan is a 54-year-old post-menopausal white female with a 2-week history nasal congestion, facial pain, facial pressure, and dental pain that worsens when bending forward. Reports intermittent nasal fullness and facial pain approximately one to two times per year that have been treated successfully with antibiotics in the past. States she usually uses over-the-counter nasal spray when she starts to feel congestion. Reports 20-pack-year history of tobacco use and coughing intermittently throughout the day. States she usually has straw-colored sputum but has noticed it is a brownish green "for about a week." States she has not been to see a healthcare provider other than at urgent care centers for antibiotics "in about ten years." Childhood immunizations complete. PMH of varicella, rubella, rubeola, and mumps diseases in childhood. NKDA. Alcohol use of about eight drinks per week, no illicit drug use. Lives with husband no children. Denies illness in close contacts.

O: *Vital Signs:* BP 110/76, HR 80, RR 12, T 99.1, Ht 5'6", Wt 160 lbs

GEN: No acute distress

HEENT: Normocephalic, PERRLA, sclera and conjunctiva clear without redness or injection. Ear canal slightly reddened, no discharge. TM clear, pearly, bony landmarks visible. Posterior pharynx slightly erythematous without exudate. No lymphadenopathy. Maxillary and frontal sinuses tender to palpation. Toothache increases with percussion. Dull transillumination of right maxillary sinus, left opaque. Frontal sinuses show dull transillumination. Nares erythematous and edematous bilaterally. Inferior and middle turbinates patent bilaterally. Mucopurulent mucus visible bilaterally. Neck: Supple. Thyroid without nodules or prominence noted.

CV: PMI located at 5th ICS MCL, S_1 and S_2, RRR, no murmurs, no gallops, no rubs. Pedal pulses 2+, no peripheral edema noted, no JVD noted.

Lungs: Coarse crackles that clear with coughing noted throughout. No wheeze, no stridor, no tactile fremitus.

Abdomen: Soft, nontender, nondistended, bowel sounds present × 4 quadrants, no organomegaly

Skin turgor normal, mucous membranes moist.

A: Acute bacterial rhinosinusitis

P: Begin treatment for ABRS with amoxicillin-clavulanate 875/125 mg PO BID × 7 days. Instructions provided for increased oral hydration, warm mist vaporizer, and acetaminophen or ibuprofen OTC for analgesia as needed. S/S of worsening and improvement reviewed. Discussed the relationship of smoking and upper respiratory infections, encouraged smoking cessation, well-woman exam, mammogram, colonoscopy, and immunizations. Discussed ETOH use. Susan verbalized understanding and is "open" to further discussion at future visit. Recheck in two weeks or sooner as needed.

Health Promotion Issues

- Assess motivation for smoking cessation and discuss strategies[8]
- Recommend tetanus booster, annual influenza vaccine[9]

- CAGE assessment—discuss potential side effects of alcohol (ETOH) use[8]
- Schedule well-woman exam[8]
- Schedule mammogram[8]
- Schedule colonoscopy[8]

Guidelines to Direct Care

Centers for Disease Control and Prevention. Recommended adult immunization schedule, by vaccine and age group. 2014. http://www.cdc.gov/vaccines/schedules/hcp/imz/adult.html. Accessed September 2, 2015.

Chow AW, Benninger MS, Brook I, et al. IDSA clinical practice guideline for acute bacterial rhinosinusitis in children and adults. *Clin Infect Dis.* 2012;54(8):e72–e112. http://www.guideline.gov/content.aspx?id=36681. Accessed September 2, 2015.

US Preventive Services Task Force. Recommendations for primary care practice: published recommendations. http://www.uspreventiveservicestaskforce.org/BrowseRec/Index/browse-recommendations. Accessed September 2, 2015.

University of Michigan Health System. Acute rhinosinusitis in adults. Ann Arbor, MI: University of Michigan Health System; 2011. http://www.guideline.gov/content.aspx?id=34408. Accessed September 2, 2015.

Case 5

Tom is an 18-year-old white male who reports he had just returned from a trip with his basketball team when he experienced sudden onset of severe sore throat pain, fever, headache, muscle pain, and malaise. Reports "a few" of his teammates became sick on the trip and were not able to play in the final game. States the teammates had played in the first two games of the tournament. Reports they "try" to not share water bottles when on the bench, but if they come out of the game and quickly need a drink they "just grab whatever bottle is laying there." States he felt ill yesterday, and came in for evaluation because he is feeling worse. Tom states that today he is unable to eat because of his severe sore throat and that is concerning to him. Denies cough, nausea, vomiting, sneezing, and nasal discharge. Childhood immunizations completed, tetanus booster given 2 years ago.

Physical Exam

Vital Signs: BP 112/70, HR 86, RR 14, T 101.5, Ht 6'0", Wt 152 lbs

GEN: Ill-appearing male

HEENT: Normocephalic, PERRLA, sclera and conjunctiva clear without redness or injection. Ear canal without redness or discharge, TM clear, pearly, bony landmarks visible. Oropharynx reddened, tonsillar exudates noted, anterior cervical lymph node (LN) swollen and tender

CV: S_1 and S_2, RRR, no murmurs, no gallops, no rubs

Lungs: Clear to auscultation

Abdomen: Soft, nontender, nondistended, bowel sounds present × 4 quadrants, no organomegaly

What additional assessments/diagnostics do you need?

What is the differential diagnoses list?

What is your working diagnosis?

Additional Assessments/Diagnostics Needed

ROS

Differentiation of group A beta-hemolytic streptococcal (GABHS) infection from viral pharyngitis may be accomplished utilizing clinical symptomatology, epidemiology, and throat culture.[17–19] Proper diagnosis is important to decrease overuse of antibiotics in cases of viral pharyngitis while allowing for treatment of GABHS to reduce suppurative complications and sequelae of infection such as poststreptococcal glomerulonephritis and rheumatic fever.

The Centor criteria stratifies risk based on known epidemiological data and exam findings to arrive at a total score to predict the likelihood of GABHS. While the Infectious Disease Society of America (IDSA) recommends rapid antigen detection testing (RADT) for all patients with clinical symptomatology that is suspicious of GABHS, the Centers for Disease Control and Prevention (CDC), the American Academy of Family Physicians (AAFP), and the American College of Physicians (ACP) recommend RADT testing for adults with a Centor score of 2–3.

Per the CDC, AAFP, and ACP guidelines, a total score of 0–1 allows for exclusion of GABHS infection without further testing in adults. The exception is a score of 1 with a recent family contact of GABHS. A total score of 2–3 necessitates a throat culture or RADT, and a score of 4 or greater suggests the need for empiric antibiotic treatment for presumptive GABHS infection. The Centor criteria assigns one point for each of the following:

- Absence of cough
- Swollen and tender anterior cervical nodes
- Temperature >100.4°F (38°C)
- Tonsillar exudates or swelling
- Ages 3–14 years

The Centor criteria awards zero points for 15–44 years of age and deducts one point for age 45 years and older.

Physical Exam

The examination for this patient should include:

- Detailed history of the onset of symptoms, pattern of illness, chronicity, and sick contacts
- Careful examination of the EENT system and utilization of the Centor criteria to help direct care
- A complete respiratory examination, focusing on any signs or symptoms of respiratory compromise

Routine Labs/Diagnostics

Labs to consider when evaluating the possibility of GABHS infection could include:[17–19]

- RADT testing, as previously discussed
- Throat culture for negative RADT is not recommended in the adult patient but would be recommended in the pediatric population
- CBC with differential may be considered if suppurative symptoms are noted

Differential Diagnoses List

Upper respiratory infection
Viral influenza
Peritonsilar abscess
Viral pharyngitis
GABHS pharyngitis

Working Diagnosis

GABHS pharyngitis

Pathophysiology

GABHS pharyngitis is caused by group A beta-hemolytic *Streptococcus* bacteria.[17–19] GABHS pharyngitis occurs in 5% to 15% of adult cases of acute pharyngitis and 25% of cases of pediatric pharyngitis. In homes with one case of GABHS, approximately 43% will experience GABHS in a second household member. Most infections occur in late winter or early spring, are spread via respiratory secretions, and have an incubation period of 24 to 72 hours. Proper, rapid diagnosis of GABHS can decrease morbidity, lower risk of spread to close contacts, and lessen the appearance of suppurative and poststreptococcal sequelae.

What Is Your Treatment Plan?

Pharmacologic

Antibiotic therapy should be initiated immediately upon diagnosis of GABHS pharyngitis. First-line therapy for adults is penicillin or amoxicillin. For adults allergic to penicillin, erythromycin is recommended. Extended spectrum macrolides and fluoroquinolones are not recommended for treatment of uncomplicated GABHS pharyngitis. Analgesics are utilized as needed.

Nonpharmacologic

- Warm saltwater gargles and soft, soothing foods to increase comfort
- Analgesics as needed for comfort
- Attention to patient education and counseling

Education/Counseling

- Patient instructions to not share utensils, drinks, or food to avoid spread of infection to household contacts
- Medication counseling to ensure adherence to antibiotic treatment
- Drink plenty of fluids
- Get plenty of rest
- May use warm drinks or frozen treats such as sherbet and fruit pops to soothe the throat
- Avoid spicy foods and crunchy, difficult-to-swallow foods
- May use warm saltwater gargles for comfort

SOAP Note

S: Tom is an 18-year-old white male with a 1-day history of sudden onset of severe sore throat pain, fever, headache, muscle pain, malaise, and unable to eat related to throat pain. Reports similar illness in close contacts. Denies cough, nausea, vomiting, sneezing, and nasal discharge. Childhood immunizations completed, tetanus booster given 2 years ago. No annual influenza.

O: *Vital Signs:* BP 112/70, HR 86, RR 14, T 101.5, Height 6'0", Wt 152 lbs

GEN: Ill-appearing male.

HEENT: Normocephalic, PERRLA, sclera and conjunctiva clear without redness or injection. Ear canal without redness or discharge, TM clear, pearly, bony landmarks visible. Oropharynx reddened, tonsillar exudates noted, anterior cervical LN swollen and tender.

CV: S_1 and S_2, RRR, no murmurs, no gallops, no rubs

Lungs: Clear to auscultation

Abdomen: Soft, nontender, nondistended, bowel sounds present $\times$ 4 quadrants, no organomegaly

A: Centor Score = 4 (+ LN, fever, tonsillar exudates, no cough, age 15–44 years); GABHS pharyngitis

P: Patient instructed to begin amoxicillin 500 mg by mouth every 12 hours $\times$ 10 days, use warm saltwater gargles, eat soothing foods, avoid sharing of utensils and food. Off school and out of sports until symptoms improved. Return to clinic as needed or if condition worsens. Schedule appointment for meningitis and influenza vaccinations.

Health Promotion Issues

▶ Discussion of STI prevention, depression, alcohol/drug use, skin cancer prevention/screening, safety[8]

▶ Meningitis vaccine

▶ Annual influenza vaccine[9]

Guidelines to Direct Care

Centers for Disease Control. Acute pharyngitis in adults: physician information sheet. http://www.cdc.gov/getsmart/community/materials-references/print-materials/hcp/adult-acute-pharyngitis.html. Accessed September 2, 2015.

Centers for Disease Control and Prevention. Recommended adult immunization schedule, by vaccine and age group. 2014. http://www.cdc.gov/vaccines/schedules/hcp/imz/adult.html. Accessed September 2, 2015.

Choby BA. Diagnosis and treatment of streptococcal pharyngitis. American Academy of Family Physicians; 2009. http://www.aafp.org/afp/2009/0301/p383.pdf. Accessed September 2, 2015.

Shulman ST, Bisno AL, Clegg HW, et al. Clinical practice guideline for the diagnosis and management of group A streptococcal pharyngitis: 2012 update by the Infectious Diseases Society of America. *Clin Infect Dis*. September 9, 2012. doi:10.1093/cid/cis629.

US Preventive Services Task Force. Recommendations for primary care practice: published recommendations. http://www.uspreventiveservicestaskforce.org/BrowseRec/Index/browse-recommendations. Accessed September 2, 2015.

REFERENCES

1. Rosenfeld RM, Schwartz SR, Cannon CR, et al. Clinical practice guideline: acute otitis externa. *Otolaryngol Head Neck Surg*. 2014;150(1 suppl):S1–S24. doi:10.1177/0194599813517083 .

2. Rosenfeld RM, Schwartz SR, Cannon CR, et al. Clinical practice guideline: acute otitis externa executive summary. *Otolaryngol Head Neck Surg*. 2014;150(2):161–168. doi:10.1177/0194599813517659.

3. Rosenfeld RM, Brown L, Cannon CR, et al; American Academy of Otolaryngology—Head and Neck Surgery Foundation. Clinical practice guideline: acute otitis externa. *Otolaryngol Head Neck Surg*. 2006;134(4 suppl):S4–23.

4. Grandis JR, Curtin HD, Yu VL. Necrotizing (malignant) external otitis: prospective comparison of CT and MR imaging in diagnosis and follow-up. *Radiology*. August 1995;196(2):499–504.

5. Hegde AN, Mohan S, Pandya A, Shah GV. Imaging in infections of the head and neck. *Neuroimaging Clin N Am*. November 2012;22(4):727–754.

6. McAuley D. Ciprofloxacin and hydrocortisone otic. 2014. http://www.globalrph.com/otic.htm#Ciprofloxacin_and_hydrocortisone. Accessed September 2, 2015.

7. Heidelbaugh J, Tortorello M. The adult well male examination. *Am Fam Physician*. May 15, 2012;85(10):964–971. http://www.aafp.org/afp/2012/0515/p964.html. Accessed September 2, 2015.

8. US Preventive Services Task Force. Recommendations for primary care practice: published recommendations. http://www.uspreventiveservicestaskforce.org/BrowseRec/Index/browse-recommendations. Accessed September 2, 2015.

9. Centers for Disease Control and Prevention. 2015 recommended immunizations for adults. http://www.cdc.gov/vaccines/schedules/downloads/adult/adult-schedule-easy-read.pdf. Accessed September 2, 2015.

10. Wallace D, Dykewicz M, Bernstein D, et al. The diagnosis and management of rhinitis: an updated practice parameter. *J Clin Immunol*. 2008;122(2). http://www.aaaai.org/Aaaai/media/MediaLibrary/PDF%20Documents/Practice%20and%20Parameters/rhinitis2008-diagnosis-management.pdf. Accessed September 2, 2015.

11. American Academy of Allergy Asthma and Immunology. AAAAI allergy and asthma medication guide. March 2015. http://www.aaaai.org/conditions-and-treatments/drug-guide/nasal-medication.aspx. Accessed September 2, 2015.

12. American Academy of Ophthalmology. Policy statement: referral of persons with possible eye diseases or injury. 2014. http://www.aao.org/clinical-statement/guidelines-appropriate-referral-of-persons-with-po. Accessed September 2, 2015.

13. Cronau H, Kankanala R, Mauger T. Diagnosis and management of red eye in primary care. *Am Fam Physician*. January 15, 2010; 81(2):137–144. http://www.aafp.org/afp/2010/0115/p137.html#afp20100115p137-t3. Accessed September 2, 2015.

14. Hutnik C, Mohammad-Shahi MH. Bacterial conjunctivitis. *Clin Ophthalmol*. 2010;4:1451–1457. http://www.ncbi.nlm.nih.gov/pmc/articles/PMC3000772/. Accessed September 2, 2015.

15. Chow AW, Benninger MS, Brook I, et al. IDSA clinical practice guideline for acute bacterial rhinosinusitis in children and adults. *Clin Infect Dis*. April 2012;54(8):e72–e112. http://www.guideline.gov/content.aspx?id=36681. Accessed September 2, 2015.

16. University of Michigan Health System. *Acute rhinosinusitis in adults*. Ann Arbor: University of Michigan Health System; August 9, 2011.

17. Shulman ST, Bisno AL, Clegg HW, et al. Clinical practice guideline for the diagnosis and management of group A streptococcal pharyngitis: 2012 update by the Infectious Diseases Society of America. *Clin Infect Dis*. November 2012;55(10):e86–e102.

18. Choby B. Diagnosis and treatment of streptococcal pharyngitis. *Am Fam Physician*. March 1, 2009;79(5):383–390.

19. Centers for Disease Control. Acute pharyngitis in adults: physician information sheet. http://www.cdc.gov/getsmart/community/materials-references/print-materials/hcp/adult-acute-pharyngitis.html. Accessed September 2, 2015.

Common Cardiovascular Disorders in Primary Care

Joanne L. Thanavaro

Chapter Outline

Learning Objectives

Using a case-based approach, the learner will be able to:

1. Identify key history and physical examination parameters for common cardiac disorders seen in primary care, including hypertension, dyslipidemia, chest pain, heart failure, and atrial fibrillation.

2. Summarize recommended laboratory and diagnostic studies indicated for the evaluation of common cardiac disorders seen in primary care.

3. State pathophysiology of common cardiac disorders.

4. Document a clear, concise SOAP note for patients with common cardiac disorders.

5. Identify relevant education and counseling strategies for patients with common cardiac disorders.

6. Develop a treatment plan for common cardiac disorders utilizing current evidence-based guidelines.

Case 1

Mr. Smith is a 40-year-old man who seeks a routine checkup. He reports that he has not seen a healthcare provider in 10 years and thought it was time he had a physical exam. He has no complaints. His past medical history is unremarkable, and he takes no regular medications. He is a construction worker who drinks 4–5 beers after work a few nights a week and who has smoked one-half pack of cigarettes per day for the last 20 years. He denies the use of illicit drugs. His family history is notable for heart disease and hypertension.

Physical Exam

Vital Signs: Blood pressure (BP) 156/96, heart rate (HR) 78, respiratory rate (RR) 12, temperature (T) 98.6, 12, height (Ht) 5'11", weight (Wt) 215 lbs

Head, eyes, ears, nose, and throat (HEENT): Unremarkable

Cardiovascular (CV): S_1 and S_2 regular rate and rhythm (RRR), no murmurs, gallops, or rubs

Lungs: Clear to auscultation

Abdomen: Soft, nontender, + bowel sounds, no organomegaly

Neuro: Unremarkable

What additional assessments/diagnostics do you need?
What is the differential diagnoses list?
What is your working diagnosis?

Additional Assessments/Diagnostics Needed

Evaluation of patients with documented hypertension (HTN) has three objectives:

1. To assess lifestyle and identify other cardiovascular (CV) risk factors or concomitant disorders that may affect prognosis and guide treatment.
   - Evaluate for all major CV risk factors, including:
     - HTN—Mr. Smith has one elevated BP measurement.
     - Cigarette smoking—Mr. Smith is a smoker.

- Obesity—Mr. Smith has a body mass index (BMI) of 30.
- Physical inactivity—Mr. Smith does not exercise.
- Dyslipidemia—You will need to order labs.
- Diabetes mellitus
- Microalbuminuria or estimated glomerular filtration rate (GFR)—You will need to order urine analysis and labs.
- Age—Mr. Smith is 40 years old. This is not a significant risk factor for him.
- Family history—This is a significant risk factor. Father has both HTN and coronary artery disease (CAD) with a myocardial infarction (MI) at age 52.

2. To reveal identifiable causes of HTN, including:
   - Sleep apnea
   - Drug-induced or related causes
   - Chronic kidney disease (CKD)
   - Primary aldosteronism
   - Chronic steroid therapy and Cushing syndrome
   - Pheochromocytoma
   - Coarctation of the aorta
   - Thyroid or parathyroid disease

3. To assess for the presence or absence of target organ damage and cardiovascular disease (CVD), including:
   - Heart
   - Brain
   - CKD
   - Peripheral artery disease (PAD)
   - Retinopathy

   Ask focused review of systems (ROS) questions:

   Especially chest pain, palpitations, shortness of breath (SOB), dyspnea on exertion (DOE), orthopnea, or paroxysmal nocturnal dyspnea (PND)

   Consider CAGE assessment based on his alcohol consumption

Physical Exam

The physical exam for this patient should include:

- Appropriate measurement of BP with verification in the contralateral arm
- Exam of optic fundus
- Calculation of BMI
- Auscultation for carotid, abdominal, and femoral bruits
- Palpation of the thyroid gland
- Thorough examination of the heart and lungs
- Examination of the abdomen for enlarged kidneys, masses, and abnormal aortic pulsations
- Palpation of the lower extremities for edema and pulses
- Neuro assessment

Routine Labs/Diagnostics

Routine labs recommended before initiating therapy include (patient results are in parentheses):

- Electrocardiogram (ECG) (normal sinus rhythm, no ectopy, no ST-T wave changes, normal R wave progression, no left ventricular hypertrophy [LVH])
- Urine analysis (negative)
- Blood glucose (96)
- Hemoglobin and hematocrit (14 + 42.8)
- Serum K (4.0)
- Creatinine (0.8)
- Fasting lipid panel (total cholesterol [TC] 168, low-density lipoproteins [LDL] 100, high-density lipoproteins [HDL] 50, triglycerides [Tri] 140)

Optional tests (not done on Mr. Smith):

- Urine albumin excretion of albumin/creatinine ratio.
- More extensive testing for identifiable causes of HTN is not indicated unless BP control is not achieved. Keep this in mind for cost-effective management.

Working Diagnosis

Elevated BP (subsequently verified with two additional BP measurements)

Tobacco use

Obesity

Alcohol use

Physical inactivity

Pathophysiology

Hypertension is one of the most common cardiovascular problems seen in the primary care setting. It is a major risk factor for stroke, myocardial infarction, vascular disease, and chronic kidney failure. According to the Centers for Disease Control and Prevention (CDC),[1] 67 million American adults have high blood pressure;

only about half have their condition under control. Nearly 1 in 3 American adults has prehypertension, which means their blood pressure is higher than normal, but not yet in the high blood pressure range. Despite many years of research, the cause of most adult hypertension is still unknown and likely multifactorial. Possible factors contributing to hypertension include a genetic predisposition, excess salt intake, and increased adrenergic tone. Growing evidence suggests that HTN may have an immunologic basis. Primary HTN may develop because of environmental or genetic factors. Secondary hypertension has many etiologies, including renovascular, renal parenchymal, and endocrine causes. The majority of adult cases of hypertension are primary (also called essential).[2]

The diagnosis of hypertension has continued to be revised over the last 50 years. The first Joint National Commission on Prevention, Detection, Evaluation, and Treatment of Blood Pressure (JNC) was published in 1976. Since that time, seven more guidelines have been issued through the National Heart, Lung, and Blood Institute, the most recent one being in February 2014. JNC 7 and JNC 8 outline the most recent evidence-based practice guidelines that inform the evaluation and treatment of hypertension.[3,4]

According to JNC 7, blood pressure categories include normal, prehypertension, Stage 1 HTN, and Stage 2 HTN. See Table 1. Key concepts in the JNC 7 guideline include:

- The need for at least two BP readings, 5 minutes apart, while sitting in a chair. Any elevated BP readings should be confirmed in the contralateral arm.
- An appropriate-sized cuff to ensure accuracy.
- Providing patients, verbally and in writing, specific BP numbers and goals.
- JNC 7 also provided information on compelling reasons to choose a specific type of antihypertensive medication.

TABLE 1 JNC 7 Blood Pressure Categories

BP Classification	Systolic BP (mm Hg)	Diastolic BP (mm Hg)
Normal	<120	<80
Prehypertension	120–139	80–89
Stage 1 hypertension	140–159	90–99
Stage 2 hypertension	≥160	≥100

Reproduced from National Heart, Lung, and Blood Institute. The Seventh Report of the Joint National Committee on Prevention, Detection, Evaluation, and Treatment of High Blood Pressure. National High Blood Pressure Education Program. Bethesda, MD: Author; 2004 Aug. http://www.ncbi.nlm.nih.gov/books/NBK9630/pdf/Bookshelf_NBK9630.pdf.

Much of the information in JNC 7 is still clinically appropriate to guide detection and evaluation of hypertension. However, JNC 8 provided updated information on BP goals as well as which medications should be used for the treatment of high blood pressure. JNC 8 guidelines used primarily randomized controlled trials (RCTs) to confirm their recommendations. See the following box.

JNC 8 Recommendations

Recommendation 1

In the general population aged ≥60 years, initiate pharmacologic treatment to lower blood pressure (BP) at systolic blood pressure (SBP) ≥150 mm Hg or diastolic blood pressure (DBP) ≥90 mm Hg and treat to a goal SBP <150 mm Hg and goal DBP <90 mm Hg. (Strong Recommendation—Grade A)

Corollary Recommendation

In the general population aged ≥60 years, if pharmacologic treatment for high BP results in lower achieved SBP (e.g., <140 mm Hg) and treatment is well tolerated and without adverse effects on health or quality of life, treatment does not need to be adjusted. (Expert Opinion—Grade E)

Recommendation 2

In the general population <60 years, initiate pharmacologic treatment to lower BP at DBP ≥90 mm Hg and treat to a goal DBP <90 mm Hg. (For ages 30–59 years, Strong Recommendation—Grade A; for ages 18–29 years, Expert Opinion—Grade E)

Recommendation 3

In the general population <60 years, initiate pharmacologic treatment to lower BP at SBP ≥140 mm Hg and treat to a goal SBP <140 mm Hg. (Expert Opinion—Grade E)

Recommendation 4

In the population aged ≥18 years with chronic kidney disease (CKD), initiate pharmacologic treatment to lower BP at SBP ≥140 mm Hg or DBP ≥90 mm Hg and treat to goal SBP <140 mm Hg and goal DBP <90 mm Hg. (Expert Opinion—Grade E)

Recommendation 5

In the population aged ≥18 years with diabetes, initiate pharmacologic treatment to lower BP at SBP ≥140 mm Hg or DBP ≥90 mm Hg and treat to a goal SBP <140 mm Hg and goal DBP <90 mm Hg. (Expert Opinion—Grade E)

Recommendation 6

In the general nonblack population, including those with diabetes, initial antihypertensive treatment should include a thiazide-type diuretic, calcium channel blocker (CCB), angiotensin-converting enzyme inhibitor (ACEI), or angiotensin receptor blocker (ARB). (Moderate Recommendation—Grade B)

Recommendation 7

In the general black population, including those with diabetes, initial antihypertensive treatment should include a thiazide-type diuretic or CCB. (For general black population: Moderate Recommendation—Grade B; for black patients with diabetes: Weak Recommendation—Grade C)

Recommendation 8

In the population aged ≥18 years with CKD, initial (or add-on) antihypertensive treatment should include an ACEI or ARB to improve kidney outcomes. This applies to all CKD patients with hypertension regardless of race or diabetes status. (Moderate Recommendation—Grade B)

Recommendation 9

The main objective of hypertension treatment is to attain and maintain goal BP. If goal BP is not reached within a month of treatment, increase the dose of the initial drug or add a second drug from one of the classes in recommendation 6 (thiazide-type diuretic, CCB, ACEI, or ARB). The clinician should continue to assess BP and adjust the treatment regimen until goal BP is reached. If goal BP cannot be reached with two drugs, add and titrate a third drug from the list provided. Do not use an ACEI and an ARB together in the same patient. If goal BP cannot be reached using only the drugs in recommendation 6 because of a contraindication or the need to use more than three drugs to reach goal BP, antihypertensive drugs from other classes can be used. Referral to a hypertension specialist may be indicated for patients in whom goal BP cannot be attained using the above strategy or for the management of complicated patients for whom additional clinical consultation is needed. (Expert Opinion—Grade E)

Reproduced from James PA, Oparil S, Carter BL, et al. 2014 Evidence-Based Guideline for the Management of High Blood Pressure in Adults. Report from the Panel Members Appointed to the Eigth Joint National Committee (JNC 8). JAMA. 2014;311(5): 507–520. doi:10.1001/jama.2013.284427.

▌ *What Is Your Treatment Plan?*

▌ Pharmacologic

According to JNC 8 guidelines, we should treat this patient with medication because he is younger than 60 years of age with a systolic BP >150 and a diastolic BP >90 (recommendations 2 and 3). First-line medications should be limited to four classes of medications, including thiazide diuretics (TTDs), calcium channel blockers (CCBs), ACE inhibitors (ACEIs), or angiotensin receptor blockers (ARBs). It's a reasonable approach to discuss these drug categories with the patient and make a decision based on patient preference and cost.

Additional recommendations from JNC 8 guidelines include:

▶ When initiating therapy in African American patients without CKD, use CCBs or TTDs instead of ACEIs because of concerns about higher risk for angioedema.

- Use of ACEIs and ARBs is recommended in all patients with CKD regardless of ethnic background.
- Select one of the following drug treatment strategies:
  - Maximize the dose of the first medication before adding a second drug.
  - Add a second medication before reaching the maximum dose of the first medication.
  - Start with two medication classes separately or as fixed-dose combinations.
- Second- and third-line alternatives to treatment may include higher doses or combinations of first-line agents.
- The following drug categories are recommended as later-line alternatives in JNC 8 based on results of RCTs:
  - Beta blockers
  - Alpha blockers
  - Alpha-1/beta blockers
  - Vasodilating beta blockers
  - Central adrenergic agonists
  - Direct vasodilators
  - Loop diuretics
  - Aldosterone antagonist

Some of these drug categories were not recommended for initial treatment because of a higher composite rate of cardiovascular death, MI, or stroke; others have no good or fair quality RCTs comparing them to the four recommended classes.

Nonpharmacologic

The ultimate goal for this patient with HTN and CAD risk factors is reduction of cardiovascular morbidity and mortality. A variety of therapeutic lifestyle changes are indicated to help control these risk factors. Recommended changes include:

- Weight reduction to a BMI <25. Weight reduction will reduce SBP by approximately 5–20 mm Hg.[3]
- Following the low-sodium DASH diet, which can reduce BP by 8–14 mm Hg.[5]
- Moderation of alcohol consumption, which will reduce BP by 2–4 mm Hg. The American Heart Association recommendation for men is no more than 24 ounces of beer, 10 ounces of wine, or 3 ounces of 80-proof whiskey daily. The recommendation for women is half that of men.[6]

Education/Counseling

- Provide this patient with a written handout on an 1,800-calorie diet plan. If he likes technology, a free app that helps with logging daily food intake is called myfitnesspal.
- Demonstrate how to use the app. Plan a goal of 2 lbs of weight loss weekly. Consider a referral to a dietician to provide additional support.
- Provide written instructions for the DASH diet.

- Assess willingness to decrease alcohol consumption as well as the need for counseling/support.
- Follow the 5 A's and 5 R's for assessing and implementing strategies for smoking cessation.[7,8]
  - The 5 A's approach is a brief, goal-directed way to address tobacco use with patients to help assess for readiness to quit.[22]
    - Ask—about tobacco use at every visit.
    - Advise—or urge the patient to quit in a clear, strong, and personalized manner.
    - Assess—how ready the patient currently is to quit tobacco.
    - Assist—provide help by listening, discussing challenges, providing information on support groups, and offering medications as needed.
    - Arrange—follow-up contact. This may include either a phone call or an office visit. Follow-up is most helpful within the first few weeks of a quit date.
- Patients who are not ready to make a quit attempt may be helped by motivational interviewing.
  - Relevance—encourage the patient to indicate why quitting is personally relevant.
  - Risks—ask the patient to identify potential negative consequences of tobacco use.
  - Rewards—ask the patient to consider potential benefits of smoking cessation.
  - Roadblocks—ask the patient to identify barriers to quitting.
  - Repetition—repeat the 5 R's with every follow-up visit.

SOAP Note

S: Here today for an annual wellness exam. Not seen by a healthcare provider (HCP) for the last 10 years. No complaints. Diet high in processed foods. Snacks frequently on chips and cookies. No routine exercise program. Walks occasionally. 10-pack-year smoking history. Not motivated to make quit attempt at this time. Tried to quit once (10 years ago) cold turkey. Drinks 4–5 beers several times weekly. Denies chest pain, palpitations, SOB, DOE, orthopnea, or PND. CAGE assessment: One positive response (felt the need to cut down on drinking).

O: *Vital Signs:* BP 156/96, HR 78, RR 22, T 98.6, Ht 5'11", Wt 215

GEN: No acute distress.

Skin: No rash, good skin turgor.

ENT: PERRLA, extraocular movements intact (EOMI). No fundoscopic changes. Tympanic membranes (TMs) normal.

Pharynx: No redness or exudates.

Neck: Supple, no thyroid enlargement, no carotid bruits.

Heart: Normal S$_1$ and S$_2$, no thrills, heaves, murmurs, gallops, or rubs. Point of maximal impact (PMI) nondisplaced.

Lungs: Lungs clear to auscultation (CTA) anterior and posterior (A & P), lung expansion equal, no crackles or wheezes.

Abdomen: Soft, nontender, active bowel sounds (BS) × 4, no hepatosplenomegaly, masses, bruit, or herniation.

Extremities: Femoral, dorsalis pedis (DP), and posterior tibial (PT) pulses normal. No edema.

A: Stage 1 HTN

Tobacco use

Obesity

Alcohol use

Physical inactivity

P: *HTN:* Discussed importance of therapeutic lifestyle changes to decrease risk of cardiovascular events. Start hydrochlorothiazide (HCTZ) 12.5 mg daily. Reviewed DASH diet and written guidelines provided.

Tobacco use: Strongly encouraged to stop smoking. Discussed long-term effects of smoking. Not willing to make a quit attempt at this time, but would like to consider possible strategies for smoking cessation. Provided information on support groups. Reviewed how medications work to help with urges. Will discuss at each follow-up visit.

Obesity: Discussed importance of maintaining normal weight. Reviewed DASH diet. Given instructions for following 1,800-calorie DASH diet. Keep daily food log.

Alcohol use: Reviewed American Heart Association (AHA) guidelines for alcohol intake. Agrees to try and limit consumption to one drink daily.

Physical inactivity: Discussed importance of daily activity. After discussion, patient has set goal of 30 minutes of walking daily.

Follow-up: 6 weeks.

Health Promotion Issues

Because this patient presents today with HTN, the primary emphasis should be on methods to control BP and reduce risk factors for heart disease.

Guidelines to Direct Care

Chobanian AV, Bakris GL, Black HR; Joint National Committee on Prevention, Detection, Evaluation, and Treatment of High Blood Pressure. National Heart, Lung, and Blood Institute; National High Blood Pressure Education Program Coordinating Committee. Seventh report of the Joint National Committee on Prevention, Detection, Evaluation, and Treatment of High Blood Pressure. *Hypertension.* 2003;42(6):1206–1252.

Fihn SD, Gardin JM, Abrams J; American College of Cardiology Foundation/American Heart Association Task Force. 2012 ACCF/AHA/ACP/AATS/PCNA/SCAI/STS guideline for the diagnosis and management of patients with stable ischemic heart disease. *Circulation.* April 22, 2014;129(16):e463.

James PA, Oparil S, Carter BL, et al. 2014 evidence-based guideline for the management of high blood pressure in adults: report from the panel members appointed to the Eighth Joint National Committee (JNC 8). *JAMA.* 2014;311(5):507–520.

Jensen MD, Ryan DH, Apovian CM, Ard JD, Comuzzie AG, Donato KA, et al. American College of Cardiology/American Heart Association Task Force on Practice Guidelines; Obesity Society. 2013 AHA/ACC/TOS guideline for the management of overweight and obesity in adults: a report of the American College of Cardiology/American Heart Association Task Force on Practice Guidelines and The Obesity Society. *Circulation.* June 24, 2014;129(25 suppl 2):S102–138.

Case 2

Mrs. Janeway is a 56-year-old female who comes to your office today for follow-up on her blood pressure. She is 4 years postmenopausal and has occasional hot flashes. She is currently using soy products, which seem to be somewhat helpful in relieving her symptoms. She works full time as an administrative assistant and reports high stress levels related to work as well as her daughter's upcoming wedding.

Physical

Past medical history (PMH): Migraines and HTN

Past surgical history (PSH): Cholecystectomy 10 years ago

Family history (FH): + HTN

Social history (SH): Prior smoker. Quit 10 years ago. Denies alcohol use

Current medications: 12.5 mg hydrochlorothiazide

Vital Signs: BP 162/102, HR 80 (regular), RR 14, Ht 5'2", Wt 125, BMI 28.2

Labs today: Total cholesterol 290, triglycerides 280, LDL-C 196, HDL-C 38, hemoglobin A1c (HbA1c) = 5.4

What additional assessments/diagnostics do you need?

What is the differential diagnoses list?

What is your working diagnosis?

Additional Assessments/Diagnostics Needed

History

You need to inquire about any cardiac symptoms, including chest pain, SOB, or palpitations. Inquire about her diet, exercise regimen, and coping strategies for stress. Explore whether she is aware of prior elevated lipid levels and whether she has tried to reduce her levels in the past.

Physical Exam

A physical exam for this patient should include an evaluation for clinical forms of atherosclerotic diseases, including peripheral arterial disease and carotid artery disease, as well as diabetes. Mrs. Janeway's exam was normal.

Routine Labs/Diagnostics

Routine labs recommended before initiating therapy include (patient results are in parentheses):

- Liver function tests (LFTs) (alanine transaminase [ALT] 20; aspartate aminotransferase [AST] 26)
- Thyroid-stimulating hormone (TSH) (2.0)
- Fasting blood sugar (FBS) (96)
- Blood urea nitrogen (BUN)/creatinine (Cr) (18/1.0)
- ECG (normal sinus rhythm, no ectopy, no ST-T wave changes, normal R wave progression, no left ventricular hypertrophy)
- Carotid duplex—only if there is evidence of carotid artery disease, that is, carotid bruits (not performed)

Working Diagnosis

Dyslipidemia

Uncontrolled HTN (stage 2)

Vasomotor symptoms

Stress related to employment and family issues

Pathophysiology

Hypercholesterolemia is an established major cardiovascular risk factor. Atherogenic dyslipidemia is characterized by three lipid abnormalities: elevated small low-density lipoproteins (LDLs), lowered high-density lipoproteins (HDLs), and elevated triglycerides (Tri).[9]

What Is Your Treatment Plan?

Pharmacologic

Dyslipidemia

According to the new National Heart, Lung, and Blood Institute (NHLBI) Adult Treatment Panel (ATP) IV guidelines,[10] the focus is now on atherosclerotic coronary vascular disease (ASCVD) risk reduction. Therapy with HMG-CoA reductase inhibitors (statin drugs) has the best evidence from multiple randomized

controlled trials to be the treatment of choice for dyslipidemia. Four major statin benefit groups have been identified, including:

- Individuals with clinical ASCVD
- Individuals with primary elevations of LDL-C ≥190 mg/dL
- Individuals with diabetes, ages 40–75, with LDL-C 70–189 mg/dL without clinical ASCVD
- Individuals without clinical ASCVD or diabetes who are 40 to 75 years of age with LDL-C 70–189 mg/dL and an estimated 10-year ASCVD risk of 7.5% or higher

To determine ASCVD risk, variables including gender, age, race, total cholesterol, HDL, systolic BP, diabetes, smoking, and a systolic BP >120 are documented into a pooled cohort equation. The free app for the risk calculator is available on both iTunes (iPhones, iPads) and Google Play (Galaxy, Nexus, and other Android devices) and also at the American Heart Association's website (http://myamericanheart.org/cvriskcalculator).

For patients not taking drug therapy for high cholesterol, an ASCVD risk score should be calculated every 4–6 years in patients between the ages of 40 and 70 years who do not have clinical ASCVD or DM and who have an LDL-C range of 70 to 189 mg/dL.

The intensity of statin therapy is used to determine statin use for both primary and secondary prevention. The intensity of the statin drug is based on the average expected LDL-C response to a specific statin and dose:

- *High-intensity statin therapy:* Lowers LDL-C on an average of approximately ≥50%
  - Recommended drugs (daily dose) include atorvastatin 40–80 mg and rosuvastatin 20–40 mg
- *Moderate-intensity statin therapy:* Lowers LDL-C on average 30–50%
  - Recommended drugs (daily dose) include atorvastatin 10–20 mg, rosuvastatin 5–20 mg, simvastatin 20–40 mg, pravastatin 40–80 mg, lovastatin 40 mg, fluvastatin XL 80 mg, fluvastatin 40 mg bid, and pitavastatin 2–4 mg
- *Low-intensity statin therapy:* Lowers LDL-C on average by <30%
  - Recommended drugs (daily dose) include simvastatin 10 mg, pravastatin 10–20 mg, lovastatin 20 mg, fluvastatin 20–40 mg, and pitavastatin 1 mg

Mrs. Janeway falls into a major statin benefit group because she has a primary elevation of LDL-C ≥190. If you put her risk factors into the ASCVD app, her risk is calculated as 9.3%, and she should be on a moderate- to high-intensity statin.

Other key concepts from ATP IV include reinforcing statin adherence and lifestyle changes and checking for secondary causes of dyslipidemia before adding a nonstatin drug. You should add on a nonstatin drug if triglyceride levels are ≥500 mg/dL. Choices include omega-3 fatty acids, niacin, or a fenofibrate. There is no proof that adding a nonstatin to a statin further reduces cardiovascular risk. Nonstatin medications can also be used for patients who cannot tolerate the recommended statin dose or who do not

[handwritten margin note: Use MD calc to determine the app will recommend which intensity statin to treat patient c̄]

achieve the expected statin response and are high risk (LDL-C >190, DM, clinical ASCVD).

▌ Hypertension

Mrs. Janeway's BP is not at goal. Because she has Stage 2 HTN, the addition of a CCB, ACE1, or ARB is recommended.

▌ Nonpharmacologic

Encourage a healthy heart diet. The nutrient composition of the TLC diet includes:[11]

- ▶ Saturated fat < 7% of total calories
- ▶ Polyunsaturated fat up to 10% of calories
- ▶ Monounsaturated fat up to 20% of calories
- ▶ Total fat: 25–30% of calories
- ▶ Carbohydrates: 50–60% of total calories
- ▶ Fiber: 20–30 g/day
- ▶ Cholesterol: <200 mg/day
- ▶ Total calories: 2,000–2,200 for weight maintenance. Because her BMI is above 25, an 1,800-calorie diet should be recommended to help facilitate weight loss.

You can encourage Mrs. Janeway to start an exercise program—the AHA recommends at least 30 minutes 5 days weekly.

▌ Education/Counseling

- ▶ Stress reduction—discuss possible strategies for stress modification. Counseling may be indicated.
- ▶ Vasomotor symptoms—because soy products seem effective, recommend continued use and discuss layering of clothing to help with symptoms.
- ▶ Pharmacologic side effects—discuss proper administration and side effects of statins.

▌ SOAP Note

S: Here today for follow-up on hypertension. No problems taking HCTZ regularly. Admits to high stress levels related to work and preparation for daughter's wedding. Has not been exercising routinely or watching diet. Reports frequent "fast foods" for dinner to save time. Vasomotor symptoms fairly well controlled with use of soy products. Denies chest pain, palpitations, lightheadedness, SOB, or leg cramps.

O: *Vital Signs:* BP 162/102, HR 80 (regular), RR 14, Ht 5'2", Wt 125, BMI 28.2

GEN: No acute distress.

Skin: No rash, good skin turgor.

ENT: PERRLA, EOMI. No fundoscopic changes.

Neck: Supple, no thyroid enlargement, no carotid bruits.

Heart: Normal S_1 and S_2, no thrills, heaves, murmurs, gallops, or rubs. PMI nondisplaced.

Lungs: CTA A & P, equal expansion, no crackles or wheezes.

Abdomen: Soft, nontender, active BS × 4, no hepatosplenomegaly, masses, bruit, or herniation.

Extremities: Femoral, DP, and PT pulses normal. No edema.

A: Uncontrolled HTN (Stage 2)

Dyslipidemia

Vasomotor symptoms

Stress

P: *HTN:* Discussed importance of therapeutic lifestyle changes to decrease risk of cardiovascular events. Continue HCTZ 12.5 and start lisinopril 10 mg PO daily. Reviewed DASH diet and written guidelines provided. Encouraged walking for 30 minutes daily.

Dyslipidemia: Reviewed the potential consequences of untreated dyslipidemia. Explained that she has a lifetime risk of atherosclerotic cardiovascular disease of 50%. Reviewed a heart healthy diet and handouts provided. Encouraged to limit food intake to 1,800 calories daily. Reviewed action, potential side effects, and proper administration of statin drug. Start atorvastatin 20 mg daily.

Vasomotor symptoms: Encouraged continuation of soy products and layering clothing to relieve symptoms.

Stress: Discussed stress-relieving strategies, including deep breathing and relaxation techniques, healthy diet, exercise, and routine sleep pattern.

Follow-up: 6 weeks. Check BP and lipid panel at that time.

▌ Health Promotion Issues

Ask about routine preventive screening, including well-woman exams, mammograms, annual eye exams, and colonoscopy.

▌ *Guidelines to Direct Care*

James PA, Oparil S, Carter BL, et al. 2014 evidence-based guideline for the management of high blood pressure in adults report from the panel members appointed to the Eighth Joint National Committee (JNC 8). *JAMA.* 2014;311(5):507–520. doi:10.1001/jama.2013.284427.

Jensen MD, Ryan DH, Apovian CM, et al; American College of Cardiology/American Heart Association Task Force on Practice Guidelines; Obesity Society. 2013 AHA/ACC/TOS guideline for the management of overweight and obesity in adults: a report of the American College of Cardiology/American Heart Association Task Force on Practice Guidelines and The Obesity Society. *Circulation.* 2014;129(25 suppl 2):S102–S138. doi:10.1161/01.cir.0000437739.71477.ee.

Stone NJ, Robinson JG, Lichtenstein AH, et al; American College of Cardiology/American Heart Association Task Force on Practice Guidelines. 2013 ACC/AHA guideline on the treatment of blood cholesterol to reduce atherosclerotic cardiovascular risk in adults: a report of the American College of Cardiology/American Heart Association Task Force on Practice Guidelines. *J Am Coll Cardiol.* 2014;63(25 Pt B):2889–2934. doi:10.1016/j.jacc.2013.11.002.

Case 3

Mr. Reynolds is a 48-year-old firefighter who you have been treating for HTN and dyslipidemia. He calls your office to speak to you and states that he has been having some very mild chest pain on and off for about 3 months. He's certain that this is not a cardiac problem, but his wife is concerned. He initially noticed chest discomfort when he was at work dressing for a "fire call." One evening last week he had a short "episode" while watching TV. He hasn't had any further symptoms since then.

Physical Exam

PMH: HTN × 5 years—well controlled on Diovan (valsartan) HCTZ 160/12.5 mg PO OD. Dyslipidemia × 3 years, on Vytorin (ezetimibe and simvastatin) 40/10 mg PO OD.

FH: Significant for CAD, HTN, and dyslipidemia.

What additional assessments/diagnostics do you need?
What is the differential diagnoses list?
What is your working diagnosis?

Additional Assessments/Diagnostics Needed

Because this patient is currently asymptomatic, he is given an appointment to be seen in the office today. On arrival he is still pain free.

History

You need a detailed symptom history, including quality, quantity, frequency, duration, chronology, and location of chest pain and any associated symptoms. Precipitating and alleviating factors should be ascertained.

(The chest discomfort is described as a substernal dull aching sensation that started 3 months ago and is gradually increasing in frequency [about 3× weekly]. Usually, it lasts 2–3 minutes and is graded 3 out of 10 on the pain scale. It is precipitated by activity/stress [preparing to go out on a fire call], but one recent episode during rest. No associated SOB, palpitations, nausea, or diaphoresis.)

Physical Exam

A focused physical assessment is needed for this patient, including evaluation of:

1. Vital signs (VS) (BP 138/68, heart rate [HR] 82 and reg, RR 12)
2. Heart (S_1 and S_2 RRR, no murmurs, gallops, or rubs. No carotid bruits)
3. Lungs (clear to auscultation [CTA] without wheeze, crackles, or abnormal breath sounds)
4. Extremities (no peripheral edema)

Routine Labs/Diagnostics

An ECG should be taken within the first 10 minutes of the appointment. This patient's ECG showed a normal sinus rhythm (NSR), without ectopy, and nonspecific ST-T wave changes.

Directed Risk Stratification

Review cardiovascular risk factors. This patient is an intermediate risk because he has classic symptoms of CAD, is <60 years old, and has 3+ risk factors for CAD (HTN, dyslipidemia, and family hx of CAD). The purpose of risk stratification is to determine the likelihood of CAD. Risk stratification should include:

1. Detailed symptom history
2. Focused physical assessment
3. Directed risk factor assessment[12]

A. *High-risk patients:* Those with known CAD, men 60 years or older, women 70 years or older, and patients with ECG changes indicative of ischemia
B. *Intermediate-risk patients:* Those with classic symptoms of CAD in men younger than 60 years or women younger than 70 years; atypical symptoms in diabetics or patients with two or more traditional risk factors; less specific ECG changes
C. *Low-risk patients:* Those whose symptoms are probably not angina, with one or less risk factors and a normal ECG

Differential Diagnoses List

Stable angina

Unstable angina

Acute myocardial infarction

Costrochondritis

Gastroesophageal reflux disease (GERD)

Anxiety

Pulmonary embolism

Pneumothorax

Working Diagnosis

Unstable angina

HTN

Dyslipidemia

Pathophysiology

Chest pain is a common complaint of patients, and the range of possible diagnoses causing chest pain is wide. Only 10% to 34% stem from a cardiac origin. Angina pectoris is the result of myocardial ischemia caused by an imbalance between myocardial blood supply and oxygen demand. Approximately 9.8 million Americans are estimated to experience angina annually, with 500,000 new cases of angina occurring every year.[13] Ischemic chest pain can be due to stable angina, unstable angina, or acute MI. Unique features associated with ischemic chest pain include:

Stable angina: Substernal chest pain with a predictable pattern of frequency; brought on by exertion or meals; brief duration; prompt relief with nitroglycerin

Unstable angina: Less predictable pattern of chest pain; new onset or a change in pattern of angina; more intense; occurs at rest, awakens patient; may or may not be relieved with TNG

Acute MI: Prodromal symptoms are common; pain lasting more than 1 hour; more instability; more associated symptoms; not relieved with TNG

Common nonischemic causes of acute chest pain include gastrointestinal disease (GERD, esophageal spasm), musculoskeletal disorder (costrochondritis), respiratory disease (pneumonia, pleurisy), anxiety, mitral valve prolapse, and acute pericarditis.

What Is Your Treatment Plan?

The main goal is to rule out ischemic heart disease.

This patient was scheduled for a cardiolyte stress test the following day, which turned out to be abnormal. The need for a stress test is not an automatic decision to hospitalize this patient. As long as you can get the test done in a reasonable amount of time, it is appropriate to administer the test on an outpatient basis as long as the patient is currently pain free. Instruct the patient to go to the emergency department (ED) if pain occurs again before the stress test.

This patient subsequently underwent cardiac catheterization, which showed a 98% block in the proximal left anterior descending (LAD) artery (also known as the "widow maker") and 80% blocks in the circumflex and right coronary arteries. He had coronary artery bypass grafting (CABG) × 4 and was seen back in the primary care setting weeks later.

Pharmacologic

Primary care responsibilities include monitoring all cardiovascular risk factors.

HTN: Beta blocker Toprol XL (metoprolol) 25 mg PO in addition to his Diovan HCTZ (valsartan; JNC 7 guidelines state CAD is a compelling reason for beta blockade)

Dyslipidemia: High-intensity statin (rosuvastatin 20 mg)

Angina: Nitroglycerin spray PRN for chest pain; 81 mg of aspirin (ASA) for cardioprotection

Nonpharmacologic

Diet: Instructed on a heart healthy diet. Encouraged to maintain BMI 25.

Exercise: Encouraged to exercise at least 30 minutes daily on most days. Consider referral for cardiac rehabilitation.

Education/Counseling

Discuss signs/symptoms of ischemic chest pain.

Review proper administration of NTG spray.

Stress importance of adherence to medication and TLC.

Provide support. Consider strategies to help cope with stress of cardiac surgery. Assess for possible depression.

SOAP Note (3 weeks after surgery)

S: Here today for follow-up after CABG surgery 3 weeks ago. "Feels pretty good." Is having no problems taking his medications. Denies low moods. Has felt more tired than usual, but this is improving. He is looking forward to returning to work. Walking every day 30 minutes without difficulty. Denies chest pain, SOB, or palpitations. Appetite is good. Trying to avoid snack foods. Denies nausea, vomiting, or diarrhea. Minimal pain associated with suture lines in sternum and leg. Well controlled with Tylenol (acetaminophen) prn.

O: *Vital Signs:* BP 126/82, HR 70 and regular, RR 12, afebrile, Wt 198 lbs, BMI 28.9. No acute distress.

Skin: Sternal and left leg suture lines well approximated with granulation tissue and minimal redness. No drainage from suture lines.

ENT: PERRLA, EOMI. No fundoscopic changes.

Neck: Supple, no thyroid enlargement, no carotid bruits.

Heart: Normal S_1 and S_2, no thrills, heaves, murmurs, gallops, or rubs. PMI nondisplaced.

Lungs: CTA A & P, equal expansion, no crackles or wheezes.

Abdomen: Soft, nontender, active BS × 4, no hepatosplenomegaly, masses, bruit, or herniation.

Extremities: Trace edema, left leg. Femoral, DP, and PT pulses normal.

Psych: Appears calm and is able to discuss surgery and postoperative care without hesitation.

Labs: Lipid panel: TC 170, Tri 146, LDL 80, HDL 45. Comprehensive metabolic panel (CMP): within normal limits. Hemoglobin and hematocrit (H&H) 10/30.

A: Status post-CABG 3 weeks ago: Good healing. No new ischemic episodes.

HTN: At goal

Dyslipidemia: At goal. Watching diet carefully.

P: *CAD:* Discussed importance of lifestyle modification to control all cardiovascular risk factors

HTN: Continue current medications. Encouraged daily walking. Reviewed DASH diet.

Dyslipidemia: At goal. Continue current medications. Reviewed possible side effects of statin medications. Reviewed heart healthy diet. Set goal to lose 10 lbs over next 2 months.

Health Promotion Issues

Should focus on strict adherence to lifestyle modifications to control cardiac risk factors.

Guidelines to Direct Care

Fihn SD, Gardin JM, Abrams J; American College of Cardiology Foundation/American Heart Association Task Force. 2012 ACCF/AHA/ACP/AATS/PCNA/SCAI/STS guideline for the diagnosis and management of patients with stable ischemic heart disease. *Circulation*. April 22, 2014;129(16):e463.

James PA, Oparil S, Carter BL, et al. 2014 Evidence-based guideline for the management of high blood pressure in adults: report from the panel members appointed to the Eighth Joint National Committee (JNC 8). *JAMA*. 2014;311(5):507–520.

Jensen MD, Ryan DH, Apovian CM, Ard JD, Comuzzie AG, Donato KA, et al.; American College of Cardiology/American Heart Association Task Force on Practice Guidelines; Obesity Society. 2013 AHA/ACC/TOS guideline for the management of overweight and obesity in adults: a report of the American College of Cardiology/American Heart Association Task Force on Practice Guidelines and The Obesity Society. *Circulation*. June 24, 2014;129(25 suppl 2):S102–138.

Stone NJ, Robinson JG, Lichtenstein AH, et al; American College of Cardiology/American Heart Association Task Force on Practice Guidelines. 2013 ACC/AHA guideline on the treatment of blood cholesterol to reduce atherosclerotic cardiovascular risk in adults: a report of the American College of Cardiology/American Heart Association Task Force on Practice Guidelines. *J Am Coll Cardiol*. 2014;63(25 Pt B):2889–2934. doi:10.1016/j.jacc.2013.11.002.

Isolated Systolic HTN R/T DM, hyperthyroidism, artery stiffness

Isolated Diastolic HTN us >90mmHg → but causes Systolic HTN

Case 4

Mrs. Porter is a 72-year-old white female who presents to the office complaining of several weeks of worsening exertional dyspnea. Previously, she had been able to work in her garden and mow the lawn, but now she feels short of breath after walking 100 feet. She does not have chest pain when she walks, although in the past, she has had episodes of retrosternal chest pressure with strenuous exertion. Once she felt lightheaded, as if she were about to faint, while climbing a flight of stairs, but the symptom passed after she sat down. Recently, she also has been having some difficulty sleeping at night and has to prop herself up with two pillows. Occasionally, she wakes up at night feeling quite short of breath, which is relieved within minutes by sitting upright and dangling her legs over the bed. She has also noticed that her feet have become swollen, especially by the end of the day.

PMH: Denies any significant past medical history. No rheumatic fever. Takes no medication. No allergies.

PSH: No surgeries.

Past family history (PFH): Unknown.

SH: She doesn't smoke or drink alcohol and prides herself on the fact that she hasn't seen a healthcare provider in years.

Physical Exam

Vital Signs: BP 112/92, HR 86 (regular), RR 16, afebrile.

HEENT: Pink mucosa without pallor, normal thyroid gland, distended neck veins.

CV: Normal S_1, second heart sound that splits during expiration (reverse splitting), + S4 at the apex, nondisplaced apical impulse, and a systolic murmur at the right upper sternal border that radiates to her carotids. The carotid upstrokes have diminished amplitude.

Lungs: Bibasilar inspiratory crackles

What additional assessments/diagnostics do you need?

What is the differential diagnoses list?

What is your working diagnosis?

Additional Information/Diagnostics Needed

ACC/AHA Guidelines for initial evaluation of heart failure recommendations include:[14]

1. Thorough history and physical exam to identify cardiac and noncardiac disorders or behaviors that might cause heart failure or accelerate its development or progression. Obtain a careful history focusing on:

   ▶ Potential clues suggesting etiology of heart failure (HF), including family history.

   ▶ Severity and triggers of dyspnea, fatigue, presence of chest pain, exercise capacity, physical activity, and sexual activity; to determine New York Heart Association (NYHA) class and identify potential symptoms of coronary ischemia.

   ▶ Anorexia and early satiety, weight loss. Gastrointestinal (GI) symptoms are common.

   ▶ Weight gain. Rapid weight gain suggests volume overload.

   ▶ Palpitations and (pre)syncope may indicate paroxysmal atrial fibrillation or ventricular tachycardia.

- Symptoms suggesting transient ischemic attacks (TIAs) or thromboembolism, which affect consideration of need for anticoagulation.
- Development of peripheral edema or ascites suggests volume overload.
- Disordered breathing, sleep problems. Treatment for sleep apnea may improve cardiac function.
- Recent/frequent prior hospitalizations for HF.
- History of discontinuation of medications for HF.
- Medications that may exacerbate HF.
- Diet. Assess for awareness and restriction of sodium and fluid intake (if indicated).
- Adherence to medical regimen.

2. Initial exam should include assessment of volume status, orthostatic BP changes, measurement of height and weight, and calculation of BMI. Patient results: BP 126/76, no orthostatic changes, HR 80 and regular, Ht 62', Wt 110 lbs, BMI 20.

3. Initial labs should include:
   - Complete blood count (CBC) (hemoglobin [Hg] 10.5, hematocrit [HCT] 31, white blood cells [WBCs], 7,500)
   - Urine analysis (negative)
   - Serum lytes (Na 145, K 4.0, Cl 110, Ca 9, Mg 2.9)
   - BUN/CR (22, 1.4)
   - Brain natriuretic peptide (BNP) (350)
   - Fasting blood sugar (FBS) (110)
   - Lipid profile (TC 200, LDL 105, HDL 44, Tri 150)
   - LFTs (ALT 22, AST 34)
   - TSH (2.86)

4. Diagnostics
   - Initial 12-lead ECG and chest X-ray (CXR) ECG results: NSR, mild intraventricular conduction delay (IVCD), LVH, left atrial enlargement (LAE) with ST-T wave abnormalities; CXR results: cardiomegaly, no infiltrates, no pulmonary congestion.
   - Initial 2D echo with Doppler to assess ventricular size, ejection fraction (EF), wall thickness, and valve function (left ventricular 2D echo results: [LV] enlargement with diffuse moderate hypokinesis; EF = 45%, LAE, calcified aortic valve with decreased aortic cusp separation. Aortic gradient 65. Valve area 7 cm^2 right atrium and right ventricle unremarkable). Mild tricuspid and mitral regurgitation. No pulmonary HTN.

Differential Diagnoses List

Heart failure due to:

Myocardial injury
- Alcohol use
- Cocaine
- Ischemic cardiomyopathy (atherosclerotic CAD)
- Rheumatic fever
- Viral myocarditis

Chronic pressure overload
- Aortic stenosis
- Hypertension

Chronic volume overload
- Mitral regurgitation

Infiltrative disease
- Amyloidosis
- Hemochromatosis

Working Diagnosis—Heart failure due to aortic stenosis (based on echo results and cardiac exam)

Pathophysiology

Heart failure is a clinical syndrome that results when the heart cannot provide sufficient blood flow to meet metabolic needs or accommodate systemic venous return. Heart failure results from injury to the myocardium from a variety of causes, including ischemic heart disease, hypertension, and diabetes. Less common etiologies include cardiomyopathies, valvular disease, myocarditis, infections, systemic toxins, and cardiotoxic drugs. Several compensatory mechanisms occur as the failing heart attempts to maintain adequate function. These include increasing cardiac output via the Frank-Starling mechanism, increasing ventricular volume and wall thickness through ventricular remodeling, and maintaining tissue perfusion with augmented mean arterial pressure through activation of neurohormonal systems. Although initially beneficial in the early stages of heart failure, all of these compensatory mechanisms eventually lead to a vicious cycle of worsening heart failure. This common condition affects over 5 million people in the United States at a cost of $10 billion to $38 billion per year.[15]

What Is Your Treatment Plan?

The major goal of acute heart failure is to try to identify an underlying treatable or reversible cause of the disease. The two major treatment goals for patients with chronic heart failure are relief of symptoms and reduction in mortality risk. Heart failure therapies are recommended according to stage. (See Table 2.) Institute pharmacologic treatment based on clinical staging.

Pharmacologic

Stage A Recommendations

1. HTN and lipid disorders should be controlled using contemporary guidelines.

2. Other conditions that may lead to or contribute to HF, such as obesity, diabetes, tobacco use, and cardiotoxic agents, should be controlled or avoided.[14]

TABLE   2 Comparison of ACCF/AHA Stages of HF and NYHA Functional Classification

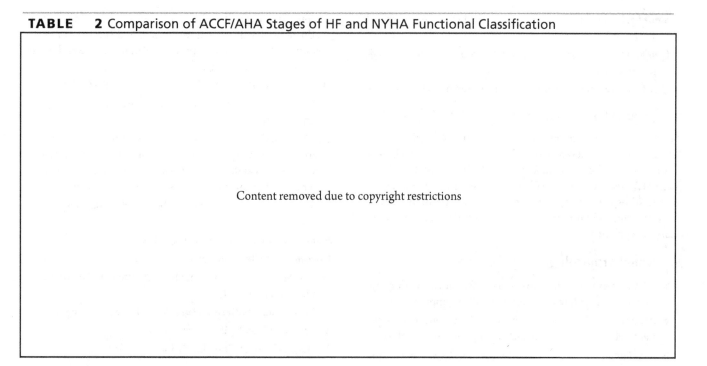

Content removed due to copyright restrictions

Stage B Recommendations

1. In patients with a history of MI and reduced EF, ACE (ACEI) or ARBs should be used to prevent HF.

2. In patients with MI and reduced EF, evidence-based beta blockers (BBs) should be used to prevent HF.

3. In patients with MI, statins should be used to prevent HF.

4. Blood pressure should be controlled to prevent symptomatic HF.

5. ACEIs should be used in all patients with a reduced EF to prevent HF.

6. BBs should be used in all patients with a reduced EF.

7. An implantable cardiodefibrillator (ICD) is reasonable in patients with asymptomatic ischemic cardiomyopathy who are at least 40 days post-MI, have an LVEF <35%, and are on guideline-directed medical therapy (GDMT).

8. Nondihydropyridine calcium channel blockers (CCBs) may be harmful in patients with low LVEF.[13]

Stage C Recommendations

Diuretics: Recommended in patients with fluid retention (to reduce edema by reduction of blood volume and venous pressures)

ACE inhibitors: Recommended for all patients (for neurohormonal modification, vasodilation, improvement in LVEF, and survival benefit)

ARBs: Recommended in patients who are ACEI intolerant; ARBs are reasonable as alternative to ACEIs as first-line therapy; addition of an ARB may be considered in persistently symptomatic patients on GDMT (for neurohormonal modification, vasodilatation, improvement in LVEF, and survival benefit). Routine combined use of an ACEI, ARB, and aldosterone antagonist is potentially harmful.

BBs: Use of one of three BBs proven to reduce mortality (bisoprolol, carvedilol, and metoprolol succinate) is recommended for all stable patients. (In addition to reduced mortality, BBs help with neurohormonal modification, improvement in symptoms and LVEF, arrhythmia prevention, and control of ventricular rate.)

Aldosterone receptor antagonists: Recommended in patients with NYHA classes II–IV who have LVEF ≤35%; recommended in patients following acute myocardial infarction (AMI) who have LVEF ≤40 with symptoms of HF or diabetes mellitus (DM) (for additive diuresis, symptom control, improved heart rate variability, decreased ventricular arrhythmias, reduced cardiac workload, improved LVEF, and increased survival).

Hydralazine and isosorbide dinitrate: Combination recommended for African Americans with NYHA classes III–IV HF on GDMT (to improve symptoms, ventricular function, exercise capacity, and survival).

Digoxin: Can be beneficial in patients with HF (by small increases in cardiac output, improvement in symptoms, and decreased rate of hospitalizations).

Anticoagulation: Patients with chronic HF with permanent/persistent/paroxysmal atrial fibrillation (AF) and an additional risk factor for cardioembolic stroke should receive chronic anticoagulation therapy; anticoagulation is not recommended in chronic HF, without AF, a prior thromboembolic event, or cardioembolic source.

Statins: Not beneficial as adjunctive therapy when prescribed solely for HF.

Omega-3 fatty acids: Supplementation is reasonable to use as adjunctive therapy.

CCBs: Not recommended as routine treatment in HF.[14]

Stage D Recommendations

Some patients with chronic HF will continue to deteriorate and develop persistent severe symptoms despite maximum GDMT. Terms to describe these patients include "advanced HF," "end-stage HF," and "refractory HF." Care of these patients frequently includes hospitalization, continuous inotropic infusions, device management, and hospice care and falls outside the scope of primary care practice.

Nonpharmacologic

▶ *Diet:* Sodium restriction is reasonable for patients with symptomatic heart failure to reduce congestive symptoms.

▶ *Activity:* Regular physical activity is safe and effective for patients who are able to participate to improve functional status.

▶ *Rehabilitation:* Cardiac rehabilitation can be useful in clinically stable patients.

Education/Counseling

▶ All patients should receive specific education to facilitate heart failure self-care.

▶ Discuss signs/symptoms of heart failure.

▶ Review proper administration of all medications.

▶ Stress importance of adherence to medication and TLC.

▶ Encourage daily weights and to call office for a weight gain of 5 lbs over 2 days or increasing SOB, paroxsymal nocturnal dyspnea (PND), and orthopnea.

▶ Describe rationale for cardiology referral.

▶ Assess for possible depression.

Care of the patient with heart failure is generally shared between the cardiologist and the primary care provider. Stable patients may only see their cardiologist one to two times yearly, so the NP needs to know how to carefully monitor these patients and when to consult the specialist.

SOAP Note

S: 72-year-old female comes to the office today complaining of several weeks of worsening SOB with exercise. She is unable to work in her yard and becomes SOB after walking 100 feet. One episode of lightheadedness while climbing one flight of stairs, which resolves with rest. Occasional nighttime awakening with SOB, which improves within minutes by sitting upright. Three to four episodes of retrosternal chest pressure with strenuous exertion over the last 2 months that last 3–4 minutes and are relieved by rest; accompanied by SOB.

Appetite is poor lately, but denies nausea, vomiting, or constipation. Her diet has not changed, and she tries to avoid foods high in sodium. Reports swollen feet at the end of the day and increased fatigued.

O: *Vital Signs:* BP 112/92, HR 86 (regular), RR 16, afebrile.

EENT: Pink mucosa without pallor, normal thyroid gland, distended neck veins.

CV: Normal S_1, second heart sound that splits during expiration, + S4 at the apex, nondisplaced apical impulse, and a systolic murmur at the right upper sternal border that radiates to her carotids. Carotid upstrokes have diminished amplitude.

Lungs: Respiratory pattern unlabored. Bibasilar inspiratory crackles.

Abdomen: Soft, nontender with good bowel sounds.

Extremities: Bilateral pretibial edema + 2.

Labs: CMP, TSH wnl. Baseline BNP elevated at 350. Mild anemia (H&H 10.5/31).

ECG: consistent with LVH, LAE, and ST-T wave changes.

2D echo consistent with aortic stenosis.

A: Stage 2C heart failure due to aortic stenosis

Angina

ASCVD risk—9.4%

P: Discussed pathophysiology of aortic stenosis and heart failure. Anticipatory guidance that surgery is likely indicated. Reviewed low-sodium diet—written guidelines provided. Limit exercise until seen by cardiology. Medications: furosemide 20 mg, lisinopril 10 mg. Referral to cardiology (due to significant aortic stenosis and anginal symptoms).

▶ Precaution needs to be taken to avoid hypotension with medical treatment for congestive heart failure (CHF) in severe AS.

▶ Don't order a stress test; this is dangerous and may precipitate a serious cardiac event.

▶ Patient should be seen by cardiology within 1 week.

Health Promotion Issues

A focus on health promotion is not a priority concern at this visit. However, be sure to discuss vaccinations (Pneumovac, influenza, Zostavax), annual vision exams, and screening mammograms and colonoscopy at follow-up visits.

Guidelines to Direct Care

Yancy CW, Jessup M, Bozkurt B, et al; American College of Cardiology Foundation; American Heart Association Task Force on Practice Guidelines. 2013 ACCF/AHA guideline for the management of heart failure: a report of the American College of Cardiology Foundation/American Heart Association Task Force on Practice Guidelines. *J Am Coll Cardiol.* 2013;62(16):e147–239. doi:10.1016/j.jacc.2013.05.019.

Case 5

Mr. Wilson is a 70-year-old white male who presents to the office with palpitations, SOB, and pedal edema. His symptoms started 1 week ago.

PMH: ST segment elevation myocardial infarction (STEMI) (2 years ago), dyslipidemia, HTN, and HF

FH: + CAD, DM

SH: Nonsmoker. Drinks 1–2 beers daily

Meds: Furosemide 40 mg, enalapril 10 mg, rosuvastatin 20 mg, metoprolol XL 50 mg, spironalactone 25 mg, ASA 81 mg, fish oil 1,000 mg

Physical Exam

Vital Signs: BP 115/76, HR 110 (irregularly irregular), RR 14, afebrile

Normal physical exam

ECG: Atrial fibrillation with rapid ventricular response (RVR)

What additional assessments/diagnostics do you need?

What is the differential diagnoses list?

What is your working diagnosis?

Additional Assessments/Diagnostics Needed

Key concepts for the history of a patient with new-onset atrial fibrillation include:[18]

Presence and nature of symptoms associated with AF

Clinical type of AF

Onset of the first symptomatic episode or date of discovery of AF

Frequency, duration, precipitating factors, and mode of termination

Response to pharmacologic agents

Presence of underlying heart disease. Look for reversible conditions

Diagnostics

ECG should be evaluated to identify:

Rhythm (verify AF)

LV hypertrophy

P-wave duration and shape or fibrillatory wave

Pre-excitation

Bundle branch block (BBB)

Prior MI

Other atrial arrhythmias

Transthoracic echocardiogram to identify:

▶ Valvular heart disease

▶ Left atrium (LA) and right atrium (RA) size

▶ Left ventricle (LV) and right ventricle (RV) size

▶ Peak RV pressure (pulmonary hypertension)

▶ LA thrombus (low sensitivity)

▶ Pericardial disease[18–20]

Labs

For first episode of AF or when ventricular rate is difficult to control, test for TSH, renal function, and hepatic function.

Additional testing may be ordered as follows:

▶ Six-minute walk test—to evaluate for the adequacy of rate control

▶ Exercise testing—to evaluate for the adequacy of rate control and to reproduce exercise-induced AF or to exclude ischemia before treatment

▶ Holter or event monitor—to confirm type of arrhythmia if not present on initial ECG

▶ Transesophageal echocardiogram—to identify LA thrombus and guide cardioversion

▶ Electrophysiological (EP) study—to clarify the mechanism of tachycardia, identify predisposing arrhythmias, and seek sites for possible ablation

▶ CXR—to evaluate lung parenchyma or pulmonary vasculature when clinical findings suggest an abnormality[18–20]

Differential Diagnoses List

Arrhythmia

Working Diagnosis

Atrial fibrillation

CAD

Dyslipidemia

HTN

HF

Pathophysiology

Atrial fibrillation is a supraventricular tachyarrhythmia characterized by uncoordinated atrial activation and consequent deterioration of atrial function. Atrial fibrillation is the most common sustained arrhythmia in the United States. The prevalence of AF is on the rise, and women account for over 50% of cases in daily practice. In the United States, AF affects approximately 2.2 million adults, and in the past 20 years there has been a 66% increase in hospital admissions for this arrhythmia. The clinical manifestations may be self-limited or require intervention and may be immediately recognized (palpations, hemodynamic or thromboembolic consequences) or asymptomatic for a period of unknown duration. In some patients, AF may exacerbate CHF or cause chest pain, dyspnea, fatigue, lightheadedness, or syncope.[19] The risks associated with AF include thromboembolic events (stroke and infarction of other organs), increased risk of dementia, reduced left ventricular failure (LVF), clinical heart failure, and risk for MI and renal dysfunction.[19,20]

What Is Your Treatment Plan?

Treatment considerations include decisions regarding rate or rhythm control, direct cardioversion, and assessment for preventing thromboembolism.

Recommendations for Rate Control

▶ To control ventricular rate, a BB or a nondihydropyridines CCB can be used.[19]

▶ A resting heart rate of <80 is reasonable for symptomatic management of atrial fibrillation.

▶ Lenient rate control (resting HR of <110) may be appropriate for asymptomatic patients with preserved LF function.

▶ Oral amiodarone may be useful for rate control when other measures don't work or are contraindicated.

▶ Digoxin is no longer considered a first-line therapy for rapid AF and is best used in combination with other agents.

Recommendations for Maintenance of Sinus Rhythm

▶ Before initiating antiarrhythmic drug therapy, treat precipitating or reversible causes.[19]

▶ Antiarrhythmic drugs are recommended in patients with AF to maintain SR depending on underlying heart disease with comorbidities.

▶ Recommended drugs include amiodarone, dofetilide, dronedarone, flecanide, propafenone, and sotalol.

▶ In general, most NPs refer to a cardiologist for initiation of these medications.

Recommendations for Direct Cardioversion

▶ Direct cardioversion can be used for AF or atrial flutter, and, if unsuccessful, repeated attempts can be made.[19]

▶ In general, direct cardioversion is used for AF or atrial flutter that is not responsive to medications or for patients with hemodynamic instability.

▶ For patients with rapid AF, the NP should admit the patient to the hospital where intravenous (IV) medications can be given.

Recommendations for Preventing Thromboembolism

▶ Antithrombotic treatment should be based on shared decision making, discussion of risk of stroke and bleeding, and patient preference.[19]

▶ Antithrombotic therapy selection should be based on the risk of thromboembolism.

▶ CHA_2DS_2-VASc score is recommended to assess stroke risk.

▶ Warfarin is recommended for patients with mechanical heart valves.

▶ With prior stroke, TIA, or CHA_2DS_2-VASc score ≥2, oral anticoagulant options include warfarin, dabigatran, rivaroxaban, or apixaban.

▶ With nonvalvular AF and a CHA_2DS_2-VASc score of 1, no antithrombotic therapy, treatment with an oral anticoagulant, or ASA may be considered.

Nonpharmacologic

▶ *Diet:* Encourage a heart healthy diet, low in cholesterol and fat.

▶ *Activity:* Encourage at least 30 minutes of daily exercise.

Education/Counseling

▶ Discuss the nature of atrial fibrillation and possible symptoms.

▶ Describe how to safely take all medications prescribed.

▶ Discuss monitoring needs (if on warfarin).

▶ Instruct patient on when to call (new symptoms, bleeding).

▶ Teach patient how to take heart rate and to call if heart rate exceeds 110.

▶ Review cardiovascular risk factor modification strategies.

SOAP Note

S: Mr. Wilson is a 70-year-old white male who presents today with new symptoms of palpitations, SOB, and ankle swelling. Onset of symptoms started 1 week ago. He has been taking all his routine medications daily. Initial onset of palpitations started at rest and has been occurring, on and off, all week. He feels "more winded" than usual. He denies chest pain, syncope, or lightheadedness. Appetite has been good. Denies nausea, vomiting, or diarrhea. No headaches.

TABLE 3 Assessment of Stroke Risk: CHA₂DS₂-VASc Score[22]

Risk Factor	Score	Mr. Wilson's Score
Stroke/TIA/TE	2	
Age	2	
AGE	1	1
HTN	1	1
DM	1	
CHF/LV dysfunction	1	1
Vascular disease	1	1
Female gender	1	
		4
		Stroke risk (%/year) 2.2–15.2%
		Should receive oral anticoagulation

Data from ClinCalc.com. CHA2DS2-VASc calculator for atrial fibrillation. http://clincalc.com/Cardiology/Stroke/CHADSVASC.aspx. Updated October 24, 2015. Accessed September 4, 2015.

O: *Vital Signs:* BP 115/76, HR 110 (irregularly irregular), RR 14, afebrile.

No acute distress.

HEENT: PERRLA, EOMs intact. Normal fundoscopic exam. Neck: Supple, no thyroid enlargement, jugular vein distention (JVD), or carotid bruits.

CV: HR irregularly irregular, no murmurs, gallops, or rubs.

Resp: No labored breathing. LCTA, equal expansion, no crackles, wheezes, or egophony.

Abdomen: Soft, nontender, good bowel sounds, no organomegaly.

Extremities: DP and PT pulses +2, trace pedal edema.

Labs: CMP, TSH, CBC wnl. Lipids: TC 150, Tri 190, LDL 72, HDL 40

ECG: Atrial fibrillation, VR 115

2D Echo: LVEF 45%, no evidence of thrombus or LVH

A: Atrial fibrillation—new onset, CHA₂DS₂-VASc score = 4 (Table 3)

CAD: Stable

Dyslipidemia: Well controlled

HTN: At JNC 8 goals

HF: Stable

P: Atrial fibrillation—increase metoprolol to 100 mg for better HR control. Start rivaroxaban 20 mg daily

Dyslipidemia: Continue rosuvastatin and fish oil. Low-cholesterol, low-fat diet encouraged

HTN: DASH diet, reviewed AHA guidelines for alcohol (ETOH) consumption

HF: Continue furosemide, enalapril, and spironalactone. Daily weights

Follow-up: 2 weeks

Health Promotion Issues

Should focus on strict adherence to lifestyle modifications to control cardiac risk factors.

Guidelines to Direct Care

January CT, Wann LS, Alpert JS, et al. 2014 AHA/ACC/HRS guideline for the management of patients with atrial fibrillation: executive summary. *J Am Coll Cardiol.* 2014;64(21):2246–2280. http://content.onlinejacc.org/article.aspx?articleid=1854231. Accessed September 4, 2015.

REFERENCES

1. Centers for Disease Control and Prevention. Vital signs: awareness and treatment of uncontrolled hypertension among adults—United States, 2003–2010. *MMWR.* 2012;61(35):703–709.

2. Meena S. Hypertension. 2014. http://emedicine.medscape.com/article/241381-overview#aw/2aab6b2b4. Accessed September 4, 2015.

3. http://www.nhlbi.nih.gov/health-pro/guidelines/current/hypertension-jnc-7

4. James PA, Oparil S, Carter BL, et al. 2014 evidence-based guideline for the management of high blood pressure in adults: report from the panel members appointed to the Eighth Joint National Committee (JNC 8). *JAMA.* 2014;311(5):507–520. http://jama.jamanetwork.com/article.aspx?articleid=1791497. Accessed September 4, 2015.

5. American Heart Association. The American Heart Association's diet and lifestyle recommendations. August 12, 2015. http://www.heart.org/HEARTORG/GettingHealthy/NutritionCenter/HealthyEating/The-American-Heart-Associations-Diet-and-Lifestyle-Recommendations_UCM_305855_Article.jsp. Accessed September 4, 2015.

6. American Heart Association. Alcohol and heart health. January 12, 2015. http://www.heart.org/HEARTORG/GettingHealthy/NutritionCenter/HealthyEating/Alcohol-and-Heart-Disease_UCM_305173_Article.jsp. Accessed September 4, 2015.

7. Fiore MC, Jaen CR, Baker TB. A clinical practice guideline for treating tobacco use and dependence: 2008 update. A U.S. public health service report. *Am J Prev Med.* 2008;35(2):158–176.

8. Larzelere MM, Williams DE. Promoting smoking cessation. *Am Fam Physician.* 2012;85:591–598.

9. Lee M, Saver JL, Towfighi A, Chow J, Ovbiagle B. *Atherosclerosis.* 2011;217:492–498.

10. Stone NJ, Robinson J, Lichenstein AH, et al. 2013 ACC/AHA guideline on the treatment of blood cholesterol to reduce atherosclerotic cardiovascular risk in adults: a report of the American College of Cardiology/American Heart Association Task Force on Practice Guidelines. *J Am Coll Cardiol.* July 1, 2014;63(25 Pt B):2889–2934. doi:10.1016/j.jacc.2013.11.002.

11. US Dept of Health and Human Services, National Institutes of Health, National Heart, Lung, and Blood Institute. *Your guide to*

lowering your cholesterol with TLC (therapeutic lifestyle changes). December 2005. http://www.nhlbi.nih.gov/health/public/heart/chol/chol_tlc.pdf. Accessed September 4, 2015. NIH Publication No. 06–5235. Accessed September 4, 2015.

12. Goff DC Jr, Lloyd-Jones DM, Bennett G, et al. 2013 ACC/AHA guideline on the assessment of cardiovascular risk. A report of the American College of Cardiology/American Heart Association Task Force on Practice Guidelines. *Circulation.* 2014;129:549–573.

13. Alaeddini A, Shirani J. Angina pectoris. Medscape. 2013. http://emedicine.medscape.com/article/150215-overview. Accessed September 4, 2015.

14. Yancy CW, Jessup M, Bozkurt B, et al. ACCF/AHA Practice Guideline: 2013 ACCF/AHA guideline for the management of heart failure: a report of the American College of Cardiology Foundation/American Heart Association Task Force on Practice Guidelines. *Circulation.* 2013;128:e240–e327. https://circ.ahajournals.org/content/128/16/e240.full#sec-8. Accessed September 4, 2015.

15. Kemp CD, Conte JV. The pathophysiology of heart failure. *Cardiovasc Pathol.* September–October 2012;21(5):365–371. doi:10.1016/j.carpath.2011.11.007.

16. Kane GC, Karon BL, Mahoney DW, et al. Progression of left ventricular diastolic dysfunction and risk of heart failure. *JAMA.* 2011;306:856–863.

17. Criteria Committee of the New York Heart Association. *Nomenclature and criteria for diagnosis of diseases of the heart and great vessels.* 9th ed. Boston, MA: Little, Brown; 1994.

18. Gutierrez C, Blanchard DG. Atrial fibrillation: diagnosis and treatment. *Am Fam Physician.* 2011;83:61–68.

19. January CT, Wann LS, Alpert JS, et al. 2014 AHA/ACC/HRS guideline for the management of patients with atrial fibrillation: executive summary. *J Am Coll Cardiol.* 2014;64(21):2246–2280. http://content.onlinejacc.org/article.aspx?articleid=1854231. Accessed September 4, 2015.

20. Rosenberg MA, Gottdiener JS, Heckbert SR, Mukamal KJ. Echocardiographic diastolic parameters and risk of atrial fibrillation: the Cardiovascular Health Study. *Eur Heart J.* 2012;33(7):904–912.

21. Piccini JP, Stevens SR, Chang Y, et al. Renal dysfunction as a predictor of stroke and systemic embolism in patients with nonvalvular atrial fibrillation. *Circulation.* 2013;127(2):224–232.

22. ClinCalc.com. CHA$_2$DS$_2$-VASc calculator for atrial fibrillation. http://clincalc.com/Cardiology/Stroke/CHADSVASC.aspx. Accessed September 4, 2015.

Common Respiratory Disorders in Primary Care

Joanne L. Thanavaro

Chapter Outline

Learning Objectives

Using a case-based approach, the learner will be able to:

1. Identify key history and physical examination parameters for common pulmonary disorders seen in primary care including influenza, acute bronchitis, asthma, COPD, and CAP.

2. Summarize recommended laboratory and diagnostic studies indicated for the evaluation of common pulmonary disorders seen in primary care.

3. State pathophysiology of common pulmonary disorders.

4. Document a clear, concise SOAP note for patients with common pulmonary disorders.

5. Identify relevant education and counseling strategies for patients with common pulmonary disorders.

6. Develop a treatment plan for common pulmonary disorders utilizing current evidence-based guidelines.

Case 1

Mrs. Cleaver is a 48-year-old female who comes to the office accompanied by her husband. She's complaining of fatigue, fever, and chills for the last 2 days. She recently returned home from California where she was taking care of her three grandchildren for the last 3 weeks. She reports that the kids all had "colds" but got better without treatment. Her past medical history (PMH) is remarkable for idiopathic cardiomyopathy, diabetes mellitus type 2, and hypertension. She is a non-smoker and nondrinker. She has not been able to exercise since she returned home because of her extreme tiredness. Her medications include: carvedilol 6.25 BID, lisinopril 20 mg, and aldactone 25 mg daily. She planned to get her influenza vaccine sometime next week.

Physical Exam

Vital Signs: Blood pressure (BP) 126/76, heart rate (HR) 65, respiratory rate (RR) 12, temperature (T) 99.8.

General (GEN): No acute distress

Eyes, ears, nose, and throat (EENT): Pharyngeal redness without exudates. Tympanic membranes (TMs) without bulging or fluid lines

Heart: S_1 and S_2 regular rate and rhythm (RRR) with pansystolic murmur along the left sternal border

Lungs: Clear to auscultation

Abdomen: Soft, nontender with good bowel sounds

What additional assessments/diagnostics do you need?

What is the differential diagnoses list?

What is your working diagnosis?

Additional Assessments/Diagnostics Needed

Review of Systems (ROS)

Ask about common signs and symptoms of influenza, including:

Fever/chills

Cough

Sore throat

Runny nose

Nasal congestion

Muscle or body aches

Headaches

Fatigue

Vomiting and diarrhea (more common in children)

Physical Exam

For patients with comorbid conditions, be sure to evaluate for any worsening of underlying conditions. In this patient, it is important not only to rule out pneumonia but also to evaluate for heart failure and uncontrolled diabetes.

Routine Labs/Diagnostics

▶ The Centers for Disease Control and Prevention (CDC), World Health organization (WHO), and Infectious Disease Society of America recommend that healthcare providers diagnose influenza clinically.

▶ Testing is recommended for:
  ▶ Hospitalized patients with influenza-like illnesses
  ▶ Patients who died of an influenza-like illness (to clarify etiology)
  ▶ Patients for whom decisions about infection control and treatment of close contacts is a concern[1-3]

▶ Sensitivities of rapid diagnostic tests are approximately 50–70% when compared with viral culture or reverse transcription polymerase chain reaction (RT-PCR); specificities of rapid diagnostic tests for influenza are appropriately 90–95%.

▶ False-positive (and true-negative) results occur more frequently when disease prevalence in the community is low, usually at the beginning and end of the flu season.

▶ False-negative (and true-positive) results occur more frequently when disease prevalence is high in the community, which is usually at the height of the flu season.[4]

Differential Diagnoses List

Upper respiratory tract infection
Influenza

Working Diagnosis—Influenza

Pathophysiology

Influenza is a contagious respiratory illness caused by the influenza viruses that infect the nose, throat, and lungs. Viruses spread mainly by droplets when people cough, sneeze, or talk. Contagiousness of influenza occurs 1 day before symptoms to 5–7 days after illness. These viruses are unpredictable, and their severity can vary widely from season to season. Older people; children; pregnant women; people with asthma, chronic obstructive pulmonary disease (COPD), diabetes, or heart, kidney, or neurologic disease; and people with weakened immune systems (HIV, AIDS, cancer, or chronic steroid use) are at greater risk for serious complications. Complications of flu include bacterial pneumonia, sinus infections, dehydration, worsening of chronic medical conditions, and death.[5]

What Is Your Treatment Plan?

Pharmacologic

- Annual flu vaccines
- Trivalent flu vaccine—protects against two influenza A viruses (an H1N1 and an H3N2) and an influenza B virus. Available vaccines include:
  - Standard-dose trivalent shots (IIV3) that are manufactured using virus grown in eggs
  - Intradermal trivalent shot—approved for people 18 through 64 years of age
  - High-dose trivalent shot—approved for people 65 years and older
  - Trivalent shot containing virus grown in cell culture—approved for people 18 years and older
  - Recombinant trivalent shot that is egg free—approved for people 18 years and older
- Quadrivalent flu vaccine—protects against two influenza A viruses and two influenza B viruses. Available vaccines include:
  - Quadrivalent flu shot
  - Quadrivalent nasal spray—approved for people 2 through 49 years of age
- Antiviral drugs
  - Two antiviral drugs recommended by the CDC
    - Oseltamivir (Tamiflu) and Zanamir (Relenza)
  - If used, should be started within 2 days of initial symptoms and taken for at least 5 days
    - Can lessen symptoms and reduce duration of symptoms by 1–2 days
    - Can prevent serious flu-related complications for people with high-risk health conditions
    - Side effects include nausea, vomiting, diarrhea, dizziness, cough, and headache[6]

Nonpharmacologic

- Drink plenty of liquids—choose water, juice, and warm soups to prevent dehydration. Drink enough liquid so that your urine is pale yellow or clear.
- Rest.
- Consider pain relievers such as Tylenol (acetaminophen) or ibuprofen to help with body aches.[7]

Education/Counseling

- The best way to prevent influenza is to get a flu vaccine every season.
- Yearly flu vaccination is ideally by October.
- It takes 2 weeks after vaccination for antibodies to develop that protect against infection.
- Everyone 6 months of age and older should get a flu vaccine every year.
- Reinforce that you can't get the flu from a flu shot.
- Side effects that can occur include soreness, redness, or swelling at the injection site, low-grade fever, and body aches. Life-threatening allergic reactions are very rare and may include breathing problems, hoarseness, wheezing, hives, tachycardia, or dizziness. These reactions occur among persons with a severe allergy to eggs and usually occur within a few minutes to a few hours after administration.[7]

SOAP Note

S: Mrs. Cleaver presents today with a 2-day history of fatigue, fever, and chills. She recently returned home from babysitting her grandchildren, who all had "colds." She has a sore throat, nasal congestion, and a mild headache. She denies cough, vomiting, diarrhea, chest pain, shortness of breath (SOB), ankle swelling, or lightheadedness. Her blood sugars have been slightly elevated from her normal fasting blood sugar (FBS) range of 130–140, and she continues to eat and drink without difficulty. She has continued all her regular medications. She has not had her annual flu vaccine yet.

O: *Vital Signs:* BP 126/76, HR 65, RR 12, T 99.8

GEN: No acute distress

EENT: No redness or crusting of eyes. TMs without bulging or fluid lines in bilateral ears. Pharyngeal redness without exudates. No thyromegaly or carotid bruits

Heart: S_1 and S_2 RRR with pansystolic murmur along the left sternal border unchanged from previous exam. Point of maximal impact (PMI) minimally displaced laterally

Lungs: Clear to auscultation. No crackles, fremitus, or egophony. No dullness to palpation

Abdomen: Soft, nontender with good bowel sounds

Extremities: Full range of motion of all extremities. No leg edema. Dorsalis pedis and posterior tibialis pulses +2. No open lesions on feet

Neuro: Alert and oriented × 3

Recent Labs (1 month ago): Blood urea nitrogen (BUN) 10, creatinine (Cr) 0.8, potassium (K) 4.0, hemoglobin A1c 6.0

A: *Likely influenza:* Day 2

Cardiomyopathy: Stable

Diabetes mellitus type 2: Controlled

Hypertension (HTN): At Eighth Joint National Committee (JNC 8) goals

P: Discussed rationale for use of antivirals, given her PMH of cardiomyopathy and diabetes mellitus (DM). Oseltamivir 75 mg BID × 5 days. Quadrivalent influenza vaccine today for both patient and husband. Reviewed possible side effects of antiviral drug and influenza vaccine. Discussed measures to prevent spread of virus (hand washing, covering sneezes).

Drink plenty of fluids. Tylenol (acetaminophen) for muscle aches. Monitor blood sugars daily. Continue all other medications as before. Call back if symptoms don't gradually improve over the next week or if she develops SOB or chest pain or is unable to eat or drink.

Health Promotion Issues

▶ Annual influenza vaccination

Guidelines to Direct Care

Advisory Committee for Immunization Practices (ACIP). ACIP vaccine recommendations. http://www.cdc.gov/vaccines/hcp/acip-recs/. Accessed September 16, 2015.

Grohskopf LA, Olsen SJ, Sokolow LZ, et al. Prevention and control of seasonal influenza with vaccines: recommendations of the Advisory Committee on Immunization Practices (ACIP)—United States, 2014–15 influenza season. *MMWR.* 2014;63(32):691–697. http://www.cdc.gov/mmwr/preview/mmwrhtml/mm6332a3.htm. Accessed September 16, 2015.

Case 2

Mr. Gretsky is a 60-year-old engineer who comes to the clinic stating he has been feeling terrible for the last 4 days. He reports having cold symptoms, including a sore throat, runny nose, body aches, and fatigue. His cough was initially dry, but now he has some yellowish sputum. His cough is making it difficult for him to speak and is interfering with his ability to work. Last evening he developed pain in the left side of his chest when he coughs. His PMH is significant only for hypertension. He takes lisinopril 20 mg daily. He denies alcohol use and quit smoking 20 years ago.

Physical Exam

Vital Signs: BP 140/88, HR 88, RR 14, T 98.1

HEENT: Mild pharyngeal erythema

Heart: S_1 and S_2 RRR without gallops, murmurs, or rubs

Lungs: Clear to auscultation. No dullness to percussion

Abdomen: Soft, nontender with good bowel sounds (BS)

What additional assessments/diagnostics do you need?

What is the differential diagnoses list?

What is your working diagnosis?

Additional Assessments/Diagnostics Needed

Acute bronchitis may be suspected in patients with an acute respiratory infection with cough, and the diagnosis can be made clinically. Sputum cytology may be helpful if the cough is persistent. Chest X-ray (CXR) should be performed only in patients whose physical examination is suggestive of pneumonia.

Differential Diagnosis:

Acute bronchitis

Allergic rhinitis

Asthma

COPD

Common cold

Influenza

Congestive heart failure exacerbation

Gastroesophageal reflux disease

Occupational exposures

Malignancy

Working Diagnosis—Acute bronchitis

Pathophysiology

Cough is the most common symptom compelling patients to come to the office for treatment. Acute bronchitis is an acute respiratory infection with a normal chest radiograph that is manifested by cough with or without phlegm production that lasts for up to 3 weeks. Because many illnesses also present with a cough, this diagnosis can be difficult to distinguish from other illnesses.

The evaluation of adults with an acute cough illness, or with presumptive diagnosis of uncomplicated acute bronchitis, should focus on ruling out pneumonia.

Chronic bronchitis is defined by a productive cough that lasts at least 3 months per year for at least 2 consecutive years. The presence of purulent sputum is not predictive of bacterial infection. Gastroesophageal reflux disease also causes a cough but is usually associated with increased symptoms at night, heartburn, and a sour taste in the mouth. More than 90% of cases of acute cough illness are nonbacterial. Viral etiologies include influenza, parainfluenza, respiratory syncytial virus (RSV), and adenovirus; bacterial agents include *Bordetella*, pertussis, *Mycoplasma pneumoniae*, and *Chlamydophila pneumonia*.[8]

What Is Your Treatment Plan?

Treatment of acute bronchitis is divided into prescribing antibiotics and symptom management.

[handwritten: try to avoid anbx. 2° to likely Viral]

Pharmacologic

Antibiotics:[9]

- ▶ Not routinely indicated and should be avoided to minimize antibiotic resistance and *Clostridium difficile* infection.
- ▶ Guidelines suggest a trial of an antitussive medication (such as codeine, dextromethorphan, or hydrocodone) (American College of Chest Physician [ACCP] Guidelines).[10]
- ▶ Although commonly used, expectorants and inhaler medications are not recommended for routine use.
- ▶ Beta-agonist inhalers may be beneficial for patients with wheezing.
- ▶ There are no data to support the use of oral corticosteroids.
- ▶ *Pelargonium* (also known as kalwerbossie, South African geranium, or rabassam) was shown to improve return to work in patients (2 days earlier) compared to those taking placebo.[10, 11]

Nonpharmacologic

- ▶ Drink plenty of fluids
- ▶ Dark honey for symptom relief

Education/Counseling

- ▶ Many healthcare providers are reluctant to not prescribe antibiotics because it is difficult convincing patients that antibiotics are usually ineffective against acute bronchitis.
- ▶ Methods for managing patient expectations for medication to treat acute bronchitis include:
  - ▶ Define the illness as a "chest cold" or "viral upper respiratory infection."
  - ▶ Instruct patients that symptoms may last about 3 weeks.
  - ▶ Explain that antibiotics don't reduce duration of symptoms and may cause side effects or antibiotic resistance.

- ▶ Consider a delayed "wait-and-see prescription" for antibiotics. Instruct patients to not fill prescription until at least 7–10 days, when symptoms are likely to subside without treatment.
- ▶ Provide information sheets for symptom management, viral infections and antibiotics, and ensuring close follow-up by phone or a scheduled follow-up visit.[9]

SOAP Note

S: Mr. Gretsky is a 60-year-old patient who reports having cold symptoms, including a sore throat, runny nose, body aches, and fatigue for the last 4 days. He developed a cough, which now is occasionally productive of yellowish sputum. Cough is his worse symptom, and it's making it difficult for him to work. His cough was initially dry, but now he has some yellowish sputum. He also has left-sided chest pain when he coughs. He had his flu vaccine 1 month ago at his work health clinic.

O: *Vital Signs:* BP 140/88, HR 88, RR 14, T 98.1

GEN: No acute distress. Coughing frequently with occasional yellowish sputum.

EENT: Eyes without redness or crusting. Ears no redness, TMs normal without bulging or fluid line. Nasal turbinates mildly red with serous drainage. Pharynx red with +1 tonsils without exudates.

Heart: S_1 and S_2 RRR without murmurs, gallops, or rubs

Lungs: Clear to auscultation. No egophony or fremitus. No dullness to percussion. No wheezing

Abdomen: Soft, nontender with good bowel sounds

Extremities: No edema

A: Acute bronchitis

HTN: At JNC 8 guideline goals

Prior smoker

P: Discussed the nature of acute bronchitis. Explained that antibiotics are not indicated for bronchitis even with discolored sputum. Given CDC patient handout on avoidance of antibiotics for viral conditions. Drink plenty of fluids and rest. Tylenol for chest wall pain. Try dark honey for symptom relief. *Pelargonium* may also be used. Congratulate patient for his continued smoking cessation. Given anticipatory guidance regarding likelihood of cough lasting for another 7–10 days. Call back if symptoms don't gradually decrease.

Health Promotion Issues

- ▶ Discuss importance of annual influenza vaccine.
- ▶ Wash hands frequently and practice good hygiene.

Guidelines to Direct Care

Braman SS. Chronic cough due to acute bronchitis: ACCP evidence-based clinical practice guidelines. *Chest.* 2006; 129(1 suppl):95S–103S. http://journal.publications.chestnet .org/data/Journals/CHEST/22039/95S.pdf

Centers for Disease Control and Prevention. Acute cough illness (acute bronchitis) physician information sheet (adults). http://www.cdc.gov/getsmart/community/materials-references/print-materials/hcp/adult-acute-cough-illness.html. Accessed September 16, 2015. http://www.cdc.gov/getsmart/campaign-materials/info-sheets/adult-acute-cough-illness.pdf

Case 3

Jennifer is a 27-year-old slender white female who presents today with a complaint of a chronic cough of more than 2 months and shortness of breath. Sometimes the cough produces clear phlegm. Her episodes of SOB are occurring more often, up to several times a week, and it seems to take longer for her to recover. She has difficulty breathing at night and can sometimes hear a "wheezing sound." It occasionally feels like there is "a band around my chest and it's frightening." She has also been very tired lately and has a decreased appetite. Jennifer smokes 2 packs of cigarettes a day, a habit she began at 15 years of age.

Physical Exam

Vital Signs: BP 104/64, HR 94 (regular), RR 20, T 97.6

EENT: Visual fields and extraocular movements (EOMs) intact. TMs translucent, gray, light reflex and landmarks visible, no fluid. Nose: Mucosa pink, clear discharge, no polyps. Mouth: No pharyngeal edema, exudates, or lymphadenopathy. No frontal/maxillary sinus tenderness. Negative transillumination

Lungs: Resonant to percussion, lung expansion equal. No increase in anteroposterior (AP)/lateral diameter. Diffuse expiratory wheezes bilaterally. No voice sounds or tactile fremitus

CV: S_1, S_2 RRR, no murmurs, rubs, or gallops

Abdomen: Nontender, no masses or guarding. BS+

Neuro: No tremors, strength 5/5. Tender paracervical muscles to palpation

Extremities: No edema, pulses 2+

What additional assessments/diagnostics do you need?

What is the differential diagnoses list?

What is your working diagnosis?

Additional Assessments/Diagnostics Needed

ROS

ROS that focuses on the following key indicators for a diagnosis (dx) of asthma:

- ▶ Wheezing
- ▶ History of any of the following: cough, worse particularly at night, recurrent wheeze, recurrent difficulty in breathing, recurrent chest tightness

- ▶ Symptoms occur or worsen in the presence of exercise, viral infection, animals with fur or hair, house dust mites (in mattresses, pillows, etc.), mold, smoke (tobacco/wood), pollen, changes in weather, strong emotional expression (laughing or crying), airborne chemicals or dusts, menstrual cycles
- ▶ Symptoms occur or worsen at night, awakening the patient

Classify asthma severity. See Table 1.[12]

Physical Exam

Physical exam (PE) given is adequate to start dx list and treatment (tx) plan

Routine Labs/Diagnostics Needed

- ▶ Pulmonary function test was done after bronchodilation with albuterol

    Ratio of forced expiratory volume in 1 second to forced vital capacity (FEV_1/FVC) <70% of predicted

    FEV_1 56% of predicted

- ▶ Allergy tests—used to document specific allergens suggested by clinical history or to reinforce need for environmental control (not done in this patient)

Differential Diagnoses List

COPD

Asthma

CHF

Pulmonary embolism

Mechanical obstruction of the airways (benign and malignant tumors)

Pulmonary infiltration with eosinophilia

Cough secondary to drugs

Vocal cord dysfunction

Working Diagnosis

Moderate persistent asthma

Pathophysiology

Asthma is a chronic inflammatory disorder of the airways that involves the interaction of airflow obstruction, bronchial hyperresponsiveness, and underlying inflammation. The interaction of these

TABLE 1 Classification of Asthma Severity

Components of Severity		Classification of Asthma Severity (patients age 12 years or older)			
				Persistent	
		Intermittent	**Mild**	**Moderate**	**Severe**
Impairment Normal FEV$_1$/ FVC: 8–9 y 85%, 20–39 y 80%, 40–59 y 75%, 60–80 y 70%	Symptoms	<2 days/week	>2 days/week but not daily	Daily	Throughout the day
	Nighttime awakenings	≤2 times/month	3–4 times/month	>1 time/week, but not nightly	Often 7 times/week
	SABA use for symptom control	≤2 days/week	>2 days/week, but not daily and not >1 time/day	Daily	Several times per day
	Interference with normal activity	None	Minor limitation	Some limitation	Extreme limitation
	Lung function	Normal FEV$_1$ between exacerbations	FEV$_1$ >80% of predicted FEV$_1$/FVC normal	FEV$_1$ >60% but <80% of predicted FEV$_1$/FVC reduced 5%	FEV$_1$ <60% of predicted FEV$_1$/FVC reduced >5%
Risk	Exacerbations requiring oral systemic corticosteroids	0–1/y[a]	>2/y[a]		
		Consider severity and interval since last exacerbation. Frequency and severity may fluctuate over time for patients in any severity category. Relative annual risks of exacerbations may be related to FEV$_1$.			

Reproduced from National Asthma Education and Prevention Program, Third Expert Panel on the Diagnosis and Management of Asthma. Expert Panel Report 3: Guidelines for the Diagnosis and Management of Asthma. Bethesda, MD: National Heart, Lung, and Blood Institute; 2007 Aug.

features determines the clinical presentation and the severity of the disease, including variable and recurring symptoms such as coughing, wheezing, shortness of breath, and chest tightness.[12, 13]

Although asthma usually presents in children, it is common among persons over the age of 65 and is an important cause of illness and death among older adults. When asthma does occur in advanced age, the symptoms are similar to those of young adults. However, asthma can be more dangerous in older adults because they are more likely to develop respiratory failure even with mild attacks.[12–14]

What Is Your Treatment Plan?

Pharmacologic

After you determine disease severity, the National Asthma Education and Prevention Program (NAEPP) guidelines recommend a stepwise approach to the pharmacologic management of asthma for ages 12 and older.[12]

Step 1: Preferred: Short-acting beta-2-agonist (SABA) prn

Step 2: Preferred: Low-dose inhaled corticosteroids (ICS)

Alternative: Cromolyn, leukotriene receptor antagonists (LTRA), nedocromil, or theophylline

Step 3: Preferred: Low-dose ICS and long-acting beta-2-agonist (LABA) or medium-dose ICS

Alternative: Low-dose ICS and either LTRA, theophylline, or zileuton

Step 4: Preferred: Medium-dose ICS and LABA

Alternative: Medium-dose ICS and LTRA or theophylline or zilueton

Step 5: Preferred: High-dose ICS and LABA and oral corticosteroid and consider omalizumab for patients who have allergies

Step 6: Preferred: High-dose ICS and LABA and oral corticosteroid and consider omalizumab for patients who have allergies

An important component of this stepwise treatment strategy is reevaluation of treatment within 2 to 6 weeks of diagnosis so medications can be adjusted.

Nonpharmacologic

▶ Follow up in 1 month to develop action treatment plan based on peak flow measurements[15]

▶ Evaluate symptom control on routine follow-up using one of the following:

▸ Asthma Therapy Assessment Questionnaire (https://evidencebasedpractice.osumc.edu/Documents/Guidelines/ATAQChecklist.pdf)

▸ Asthma Control Questionnaire (http://aafa.org/pdfs/SWP%20final%20questionnaire.pdf)

▸ Asthma Control Test (http://www.asthmacontrol.com)

Education/Counseling

▶ Discuss and demonstrate correct device technique.

▶ Discuss importance of annual influenza vaccine.

▶ Provide peak flow meter and instructions to take peak flow measurement daily × 1 month.

▶ Smoking cessation: Make a strong recommendation to quit, discuss motivation to attempt smoking cessation, and offer strategies for smoking cessation.[12]

SOAP Note

S: Jennifer presents today with a complaint of a chronic cough of more than 2 months and shortness of breath. She has daily symptoms and awakens with nighttime symptoms 2–3 times a week. Sometimes the cough produces clear phlegm. She reports wheezing and chest tightness that worsen when she goes to the gym. She has stopped going to the gym because of the SOB. She is trying to cut down her smoking habit; now down to 1 pack daily. No other environmental exposures except her pet cat, which she has slept with nightly for the last 4 years. She reports her cousin has asthma.

O: *Vital Signs:* BP 104/64, HR 94 (regular), RR 20, T 97.6

EENT: Visual fields and EOM intact. TMs translucent, gray, light reflex and landmarks visible, no fluid. Nose: Mucosa pink, clear discharge, no polyps. Mouth: No pharyngeal edema, exudates, or lymphadenopathy. No frontal/maxillary sinus tenderness. Negative transillumination.

Lungs: Resonant to percussion, lung expansion equal. No increase in AP/lateral diameter. Diffuse expiratory wheezes bilaterally. No voice sounds or tactile fremitus.

CV: S_1, S_2 RRR, no murmurs, rubs, or gallops

Abdomen: Nontender, no masses or guarding. BS+

PFTs taken 10 minutes after 2 puffs of albuterol: FEV_1/FVC <70% of predicted; FEV_1 56% of predicted

A: Moderate persistent asthma

Tobacco use

P: Discussed etiology and pathophysiology of asthma, signs of deterioration, and when to contact healthcare provider. Discussed the purpose of inhaled SABA, LABA, and inhaled corticosteroid. Start albuterol 1–2 puffs prn for SOB and wheezing and 100/50 fluticasone propionate/salmeterol diskus, 1 puff twice daily. Demonstrated use of inhalers; returned demonstration without difficulty. Emphasized importance of rinsing mouth after inhaler use to minimize chance of developing candidiasis. Recommended having cat sleep in another room, which she is reluctant to do. Described how smoking affects asthma. She would like to try to titrate her cigarette smoking down gradually. Plan is to decrease daily cigarettes down to 15 daily within the next month. She is strongly motivated to stop smoking because symptoms are interfering with sleep and ability to exercise. Ordered and demonstrated proper use of peak flow meter. Take daily measurement for 1 month and bring these values to 1-month follow-up visit. Evaluate symptoms and develop asthma action plan at that time.

Health Promotion Issues

▶ Annual influenza vaccine

▶ Use nonsteroidal anti-inflammatory drugs (NSAIDs) sparingly because they may exacerbate symptoms

Guidelines to Direct Care

Global Initiative for Asthma. *Pocket Guide for Asthma Management and Prevention.* http://www.ginasthma.org/local/uploads/files/GINA_Pocket_April20_1.pdf. Accessed September 16, 2015.

National Heart, Lung, and Blood Institute. Expert Panel Report 3: guidelines for the diagnosis and management of asthma. http://www.nhlbi.nih.gov/health-pro/guidelines/current/asthma-guidelines. Accessed September 16, 2015.

Case 4

Mr. Lucas is a 65-year-old man complaining of increasing shortness of breath over the last few months. He reports that he is used to being SOB with physical exertion but has started to feel SOB when performing basic daily activities. He denies fever, sick contact, or weight loss. He does report a chronic cough that is occasionally productive of whitish sputum but has not noticed any recent change in the frequency or character of his cough. He doesn't take any regular medication. He has a 65-pack-year history of cigarette smoking.

Physical Exam

Vital Signs: BP 138/88, HR 88 (regular), RR 18, T 98.8

GEN: Thin and mildly dyspneic

Lungs: No evidence of consolidation or focal abnormality, fairly diffuse mild end-expiratory wheezing. Breathing through pursed lips and has a prolonged expiratory phase during quiet breathing.

CV: S_1 and S_2 RRR, faint heart sounds with no murmurs

Abdomen: Soft, nontender with good bowel sounds. No bruits

Extremities: Full range of motion of all extremities. No cyanosis or edema

What additional assessments/diagnostics do you need?

What is the differential diagnoses list?

What is your working diagnosis?

Additional Assessments/Diagnostics Needed

ROS

Key indicators for considering a COPD diagnosis include:

- Chronic cough
- Chronic sputum production
- Repeated episodes of acute bronchitis
- Dyspnea that is progressive, persistent, worse on exercise, and worse with respiratory infections
- History of exposure to risk factors, including tobacco smoke, occupational dust and chemicals, smoke from home cooking and heating fuels
- Three tools helpful for assessing COPD include:
  - *COPD Assessment Test (CAT):* Measures health status impairment in COPD[16]
  - *Clinical COPD Questionnaire (CCQ):* Measures clinical control in COPD[17]
  - *Modified British Medical Research Council (MMRC) dyspnea scale:* Measures health status and predicts future mortality risk[18]
- To assess for risk of exacerbations, use the history of exacerbations and spirometry. High-risk patients are those with two or more exacerbations within the last year, those with an FEV_1 <50% of predicted values, or patients with one or more hospitalizations for COPD[19]
- Assess for comorbid conditions—these may influence mortality and hospitalizations and should be evaluated routinely:
  - Cardiovascular diseases
  - Osteoporosis
  - Respiratory infections
  - Anxiety and depression
  - Diabetes
  - Lung cancer
  - Bronchiectasis

Physical Exam

This patient has some classic findings, including expiratory wheezing, pursed-lip breathing, and a prolonged expiratory phase. Other notable findings to look for include an increased anteroposterior (AP) diameter, use of accessory muscles of respiration, hyperresonace to percussion, hypoxemia, cyanosis, and signs of right heart failure in advanced cases.

Routine Labs/Diagnostics

1. Spirometry is required to establish the diagnosis and severity of disease

   Gold Staging System for COPD Severity[19]

   Description Findings (based on postbronchodilator FEV_1)

   0 At risk for COPD—risk factors and chronic symptoms but normal spirometry

   1 Mild COPD
   FEV_1/FVC ratio <0.70
   FEV_1 ≥80% of predicted value

   0 Moderate COPD
   FEV_1/FVC ratio <0.70
   FEV_1 50% to <80% of predicted value
   May have chronic symptoms

   0 Severe COPD
   FEV_1/FVC ratio <70%
   FEV_1 <30% of predicted value
   May have chronic symptoms

   0 Very severe COPD
   FEV_1/FVC ratio <70%
   FEV_1 <30% of predicted value OR
   FEV_1 <50% of predicted value plus severe chronic symptoms

2. Chest X-ray—pulmonary hyperinflation, flattening of the diaphragm, and increased retrosternal clear space on the later view are all classic findings for COPD. Valuable to exclude alternative diagnoses

3. Alpha-1 antitrypsin deficiency screening for alpha-1 antitrypsin deficiency, which is a rare autosomal cause of emphysema in young patients with no smoking history. Not indicated for this patient. Perform when COPD develops in patients of Caucasian descent younger than the age of 45 or with a strong family history of COPD

4. Complete blood count (CBC) to evaluate for elevated hemoglobin and hematocrit (H&H) (common in COPD) and for elevated white blood cell count due to infection

5. Pulse oximetry to evaluate for oxygen saturation and need for supplemental oxygen therapy

6. Electrocardiogram (ECG) to evaluate for right ventricular hypertrophy

Arterial blood gases are not indicated in the primary care setting.

Differential Diagnoses List

Asthma
Congestive heart failure
Bronchiectasis
Tuberculosis
Diffuse panbronchiolitis

Working Diagnosis COPD

Pathophysiology

COPD is a common preventable and treatable disease. COPD is the third leading cause of death in the United States and has continued to increase in incidence. The burden of this disease will likely increase in the future because of continued exposure to COPD risk factors and the aging population.

COPD is characterized by persistent airflow limitation involving both small airway disease and parenchymal destruction. In the small airways, flow limitation is due to airway inflammation, airway fibrosis, luminal plugs, and increased airway resistance. Parenchymal destruction occurs because of loss of alveolar attachments and a decrease in elastic recoil.[19–21]

What Is Your Treatment Plan?

[handwritten: LABA's- B2-agonist ex: Salmeterol + Formoterol; anticholinergics: tiotropium]

Pharmacologic

Bronchodilators:

- ▶ Principal agents include beta-2 agonists, anticholinergics, theophylline, or combination therapy
- ▶ May be prescribed as needed or on a schedule to prevent or reduce symptoms
- ▶ Long-acting agents reduce exacerbations and hospitalization and improve symptoms
- ▶ Combining bronchodilators from different pharmacologic classes instead of increasing the dose of a single agent may improve efficacy and decrease the risk of side effects[19]

Inhaled corticosteroids: *[handwritten: ie, Qvar, pulmicort, Symbicort, Flovent]*

- ▶ Scheduled treatment with these medications improves symptoms, lung function, and quality of life and reduces frequency of exacerbations in patients with an FEV_1 <60% of predicted.
- ▶ These drugs may increase risk of pneumonia.[19]

Combination therapy:

- ▶ Combining a long-acting beta-2 agonist with an inhaled corticosteroid is more effective in improving lung function and reducing exacerbations in patients with moderate to very severe COPD.
- ▶ Adding a third agent (anticholinergic) to the drug regimen appears to provide additional benefit.
- ▶ Phosphodiesterase-4 inhibitors are indicated for patients in GOLD 3 and GOLD 4 stages to reduce exacerbations.[19]

Theophylline:

- ▶ Less effective and less well tolerated than inhaled long-acting bronchodilators; not recommended if those drugs are available and affordable.
- ▶ Low-dose theophylline reduces exacerbations but doesn't improve postbronchodilator lung function.[19]

Antibiotics:

- ▶ Only should be used for treating infectious exacerbations of COPD and other bacterial infections.
- ▶ Chronic treatment with systemic corticosteroids should be avoided because of an unfavorable benefit-to-risk ratio.[19]

Nonpharmacologic

- ▶ *Oxygen therapy:* Long-term administration of oxygen (>15 hours daily) has been shown to increase survival in patients with severe resting hypoxemia.
- ▶ *Ventilatory support:* A combination of noninvasive ventilation with long-term oxygen therapy may be helpful in patients with pronounced daytime hypercapnia.
- ▶ *Surgery:* Surgical treatment options include lung volume reduction surgery and lung transplantation in appropriately selected patients.[19]

Education/Counseling

Education and counseling are important to help prevent exacerbations. Exacerbations negatively affect quality of life, accelerate the rate of decline of lung function, are associated with significant mortality, and have a high socioeconomic cost.[19]

- ▶ Smoking cessation has the greatest capacity to influence the progression of COPD. Encourage all patients who smoke to quit. Pharmacotherapy and nicotine replacement increase long-term smoking abstinence. Use the 5 A's and 5 R's.
- ▶ Encourage regular physical activity. Recommend pulmonary rehabilitation program.

SOAP Note

S: Mr. Lucas is a 65-year-old man complaining of increasing shortness of breath over the last few months. He recently has noticed increasing SOB while performing basic daily activities. In the past he has had dyspnea on exertion (DOE). He has a chronic cough that is occasionally productive of whitish sputum; no recent change in the character of his cough. He takes no regular medication. Significant 65-pack-year smoking history.

O: *Vital Signs:* BP 142/86, HR 76, RR 18, afebrile. O_2 saturation 94%

GEN: Thin, mildly dyspneic

HEENT: PERRLA, EOMs intact. Normal fundoscopic exam. No sinus tenderness on palpation. TMs normal, turbinates without redness or bogginess, pharynx without exudates. Neck: Supple, no lymphadenopathy, thyroid enlargement, jugular vein distention (JVD), or carotid bruits

Cardiovascular (CV): S_1 and S_2 regular rate and rhythm without murmurs, gallops, or rubs

Resp: No labored breathing. Lungs: Increased AP diameter, no dullness to palpation, decreased breath sounds throughout with mild expiratory wheezing

Abdomen: Soft, nontender, good bowel sounds, no organomegaly

Extremities: Dorsalis pedis (DP) and posterior tibial (PT) pulses +2, trace pedal edema

CXR: Pulmonary hyperinflation, flattening of the diaphragm

Pulmonary function test (after bronchodilation with 2 puffs albuterol) FEV_1/FVC ratio 0.60; FEV_1 60% of predicted value

CBC: H&H 16/48, white blood cells (WBCs) 3.8

CAT test = 25

MRRC score = 3

Clinical COPD questionnaire—deferred until after therapy is initiated

A: COPD (moderate, stage 2)

Tobacco use disorder

P: Discussed the nature of COPD. Albuterol, 1–2 puffs q 4–6 hours as needed for shortness of breath. Fluticasone propionate/salmeterol inhaled 250/50, 1 puff inhaled every 12 hours. Demonstrated proper use of inhalers. Returned demonstration without difficulty. Referral for pulmonary rehabilitation exercise program. Discussed importance of risk reduction, including smoking cessation, and offered medication to assist with smoking cessation. Declines at this time but has strong motivation to quit. Wants to try slow taper of cigarettes. Avoid vigorous outdoor exertion or stay inside on high-pollution days. Will evaluate for home oxygen on a routine basis. Discussed strategies for minimizing dyspnea, including pursed-lip breathing. Influenza and pneumococcal vaccine today.

Follow-up: 1 month

Health Promotion Issues

▸ Influenza vaccines yearly

▸ Pneumococcal polysaccharide vaccine is recommended for COPD patients 65 years and older and for COPD patients younger than age 65 with an FEV_1 <40% of predicted

Guidelines to Direct Care

Global Initiative for Chronic Obstructive Lung Disease. http://www.goldcopd.org/. Accessed September 16, 2015.

Centers for Disease Control and Prevention. Prevention and control of seasonal influenza with vaccines: recommendations of the Advisory Committee on Immunization Practices (ACIP)—United States, 2014–15 influenza season. *MMWR.* 2014;63(32):691–697. http://www.cdc.gov/mmwr/preview/mmwrhtml/mm6332a3.htm. Accessed September 16, 2015.

Case 5

Mr. Roos is a 57-year-old man who comes to the office complaining of fever and a cough. He states that he felt completely healthy 4 days ago, but on the following day started feeling feverish and coughed up yellowish-green phlegm the next morning. His symptoms have progressively worsened. He also mentions that his chest hurts on the right side when he takes a deep breath. He reports that his wife was sick with milder but similar symptoms a week or two ago.

PMH: Includes hypertension and arthritis. His medications include metoprolol and celecoxib. He smokes roughly a pack of cigarettes per day but does not drink alcohol or use other drugs. No drug allergies.

Physical Exam

Vital Signs: BP 128/86, HR 101 (regular), RR 18, T 37.4°C

GEN: Appears mildly tachypneic, but is not in distress

What additional assessments/diagnostics do you need?

What is the differential diagnoses list?

What is your working diagnosis?

Additional Assessments/Diagnostics Needed

ROS

Evaluate for presence of comorbidities (to direct antibiotic tx), including chronic heart, lung, liver, or renal disease; DM; alcoholism; malignancies; asplenia; immunosuppressing conditions or use of immunosuppressing drugs; use of antimicrobials within the previous 3 months (in which case an alternative from a different class should be selected); or other risks for drug-resistant *Streptococcus pneumoniae* (DRSP) infection.

Physical Exam

▸ The physical exam should include a respiratory, cardiovascular, abdominal, skin, and mental health assessment

▸ Physical exam for this patient revealed decreased breath sounds, dullness to percussion, and increased tactile fremitus in the right lower lobe. All other systems were within normal limits

▸ Assess for criteria for clinical stability including:[22]

  ▸ Temp ≤37.8°C

  ▸ HR ≤100 bpm

  ▸ RR ≤24 breaths/min

  ▸ Systolic blood pressure (SBP) ≥90 mm Hg

  ▸ Arterial oxygen sat ≥90%

  ▸ Ability to maintain oral intake

  ▸ Normal mental status

▸ Assess for severity of illness

  ▸ CURB-65 criteria help determine hospital admission decision (confusion, uremia, respiratory rate, low blood pressure, age 65 or greater) (Curb-65 Pneumonia Severity Score).[23]

[Handwritten annotations:] Place hands on Chest Say "99" Anterior + Posterior. Tactile fremitus normal ↑ Anterior just below clavicle + posterior between Scapula and Should ↓ as you go lower down back. If increases Suggests consolidation or pneumonia

▶ Pneumonia Severity Index (PSI) can be used to identify patients with CAP who may be candidates for outpatient treatment versus inpatient treatment (Pneumonia Severity Index Calculator).[24]

General

The information below (general, PMH, physical exam, and lab and radiology findings) all relate to the pneumonia severity index.

1. Age in years: *Add* 1 point per year
2. Gender: *Subtract* 10 points for women
3. Nursing home resident: *Add* 10 points

Past Medical History

1. Cancer: *Add* 30 points
2. Liver disease: *Add* 20 points
3. CHF: *Add* 10 points
4. CVA: *Add* 10 points
5. Chronic kidney disease: *Add* 10 points

Examination Findings

1. Altered level of consciousness: *Add* 20 points
2. Breathing rate >30 rpm: *Add* 20 points
3. Systolic BP <90 mm Hg: *Add* 20 points
4. Temperature not 95–104°F (35–40°C): *Add* 15 points
5. Heart rate >125 bpm: *Add* 10 points

Labs

Arterial blood gas (ABG):

1. Arterial pH <7.35: *Add* 30 points
2. PaO$_2$ <60 mm Hg (<90% O$_2$ sat): *Add* 10 points

Keep in mind that arterial blood gases (ABGs) are not usually ordered in the primary care setting. This parameter limits the ability to use this scoring system in the office. However, its use is helpful for patients presenting to the emergency department (ED) where an ABG can be obtained.

Labs: Serum chemistry:

1. Serum sodium <130 mEq/L: *Add* 20 points
2. Blood urea nitrogen (BUN) >64 mg/dL: *Add* 20 points
3. Serum glucose >250 mg/dL: *Add* 10 points
4. Blood count—hematocrit <30%: *Add* 10 points
5. Chest X-ray—pleural effusion: *Add* 10 points

Scoring

1. Class 1: Points 0: Mortality 0.1% (low risk)
2. Class 2: Points <70: Mortality 0.6% (low risk)
3. Class 3: Points 71–90: Mortality 2.8% (low risk)
4. Class 4: Points 91–130: Mortality 8.2% (moderate risk)

(handwritten margin notes: Relate to PSI Scale)

(handwritten margin notes: PSI Scale generally not used in primary care setting as ABG's are not typically ordered (unless in patient or ER))

5. Class 5: Points >130: Mortality 29.2% (high risk)

Interpretation

1. Classes 1–2: Outpatient management
2. Class 3: Consider short observation hospital stay
3. Classes 4–5: Inpatient management

Additional Diagnostics Needed

CBC (WBC = 14,900, neutrophils = 87%, platelets = 310,000/uL, Hgb = 16, Hct = 48)

Basic metabolic panel (BMP) (Na = 137, K = 4.1, BUN = 15, Cr = 1.0, BG = 148)

Pulse oximetry (98%)

Chest X-ray (consolidation of right midlobe. No pleural effusion noted)

Pulmonary function tests (PFTs) (not really helpful in this situation, i.e., we expect them to be abnormal)

Sputum/blood cultures: The overall yield and infrequent positive impact on clinical care argue against the routine use of blood and sputum cultures. Therefore, the guidelines suggest empirical treatment for patients in the outpatient setting (as long as you have risk stratified appropriately).

Differential Diagnoses List

Community-acquired pneumonia (CAP)

COPD

Lung abscess

Pulmonary embolism

Congestive heart failure (CHF)

Neoplasms

Sarcoidosis

Working Diagnosis

Community-acquired pneumonia

Tobacco use disorder

Pathophysiology

CAP is one of the most common infectious diseases. *Streptococcus pneumoniae, Haemophilus influenzae,* and *Moraxella catarrhalis* are the pathogens that account for approximately 85% of CAP. CAP usually occurs as a result of inhalation or aspiration of the pathogen into a lung segment or lobe; it may also occur from a distant source or from bacteremia. Morbidity and mortality are highest in elderly patients and immunocompromised hosts.[25]

What Is Your Treatment Plan?

CURB-65 score indicates that this patient can be treated in the outpatient setting. PSI score was not calculated because of unavailability of ABGs.

Pharmacologic

Basic concepts:

- ▶ Patients with pneumonia should be treated with antibiotics for at least 5 days.
- ▶ Antibiotics should not be stopped until the patient has been afebrile for at least 48 to 72 hours.
- ▶ The most common causes of CAP in outpatients are *S. pneumoniae, Mycoplasma pneumoniae,* and *H. influenzae;* patient history, clinical findings, and epidemiology may suggest a cause that could alter therapy. See Table 2.

Nonpharmacologic

- ▶ Drink fluids to avoid dehydration.
- ▶ Take deep breaths and cough hourly.
- ▶ Use a humidifier to make air warm and moist.
- ▶ Rest.
- ▶ Take acetaminophen, ibuprofen, or naproxen for fever or pain.[25]

Education/Counseling

- ▶ Emphasize importance of taking the antibiotic until gone, even if symptoms improve.
- ▶ Call back if you develop new or worsening shortness of breath, chest pain, or confusion or cough up bloody or rust-colored mucus.

- ▶ For smokers, patients must have repeat CXR in 6 months to verify that pneumonia was not caused by underlying mass.[25]

SOAP Note

S: Mr. Roos is a 57-year-old man who reports fever and productive sputum, which began 3 days ago. His symptoms have progressively worsened. He denies SOB, DOE, palpitations, lightheadedness, or headaches. He reports that his chest hurts on the right side when he takes a deep breath. He is currently able to drink fluids without difficulty, but his appetite is poor. He denies nausea, vomiting, diarrhea, or abdominal pain. His wife was sick with milder symptoms a week or two ago but got better without treatment. He smokes 1 pack of cigarettes daily but does not drink alcohol. He has not taken any antibiotics for the last several years. PMH is significant for HTN and arthritis. Had influenza vaccine this year but never got pneumococcal vaccine.

O: *Vital Signs:* T 37.4°C, BP 128/86, RR 18, HR 101 (regular), pulse oximetry 98%

GEN: Appears mildly tachypneic, but is not in distress

Skin: Warm and dry, good skin turgor

HEENT: No sinus tenderness. PERRLA, EOMs intact. Normal fundoscopic exam. TMs normal, turbinates mildly reddened, but no discharge. Pharynx without exudate, cobblestoning, or enlargement. Neck: Supple, no thyroid enlargement, JVD, or carotid bruits. No lymphadenopathy

---

TABLE 2 Clinical Characteristics and Possible Antibiotic Choices

Patient Characteristics	Outpatient Oral Antibiotic Regimen
Previously healthy; no risk factors for drug-resistant *S. pneumoniae*	Macrolide • Azithromycin • Clarithromycin • Erythromycin OR • Doxycycline

Comorbidity or risk factor for drug-resistant *S. pneumoniae*, including:
• Use of a broad spectrum antibiotic in the previous 3 months
• Age older than 65 years
• Alcoholism
• Chronic disease (e.g., heart, lung, liver, or kidney disease; diabetes)
• Cancer
• Asplenia
• Exposure to a child in day care
• Immunosuppression
 	
Note: If the patient has received an antibiotic within the previous 3 months, pick an option from a different class.
	Macrolide PLUS beta-lactam:
	• High-dose amoxicillin
	• Alternative to macrolide-doxycycline
	Alternative to oral beta-lactams:
	• PO cefpodoxime or cefuroxime IM ceftriaxone
	OR
	• Respiratory fluoroquinolone:
	  • Moxifloxacin
	  • Levofloxacin
	  • Gemifloxacin

Lives in a region with >25% or higher rate of infection with high-level (MIC ≥16 mcg/mL) macrolide-resistant *S. pneumoniae*	As above

Courtesy of *Prescriber's Letter.*

CV: HR RRR without murmurs, gallops, or rubs

Resp: No labored breathing. Decreased breath sounds, dullness to percussion, and increased tactile fremitus in the right lower lobe (RLL). Mild crackles in the RLL without wheezes or egophony

Abdomen: Soft, nontender, good bowel sounds, no organomegaly

Extremities: DP and PT pulses +2, trace pedal edema

Mental Status: Awake and oriented × 3

Labs: CBC (WBC = 14,900, neutrophils = 87%, platelets = 310,000/uL, Hgb = 16, Hct = 48)

BMP (Na = 137, K = 4.1, BUN = 15, Cr = 1.0, BG = 148)

CXR: Consolidation of right midlobe. No pleural effusion noted

CURB-65 Pneumonia Severity Score = 1 point (age) low risk

A: *CAP:* Clinically stable

HTN: At JNC 8 goals

Tobacco use: Poor motivation to try quit attempt at this time

P: *CAP:* Azithromycin 500 mg daily × 3 days. Discussed importance of taking antibiotic until gone. Drink fluids, rest, take deep breaths and cough hourly, use humidifier. May use acetaminophen for fever or pain. Pneumococcal vaccine today.

HTN: Continue metoprolol. Encouraged heart healthy lifestyle.

Tobacco use: Advised regarding the importance of smoking cessation. Stressed that smoking may contribute to development of pneumonia. Patient is willing to discuss smoking cessation strategies at follow-up visit. Handouts provided on possible smoking cessation interventions.

Health Promotion Issues

▶ Recommend yearly influenza vaccine.

▶ Recommend pneumococcal vaccine now.

▶ Wash hands frequently and practice good hygiene.

▶ Strongly recommend smoking cessation and offer treatment options.

Guidelines to Direct Care

Mandell LA, Wunderink RG, Anzueto A, et al. Infectious Diseases Society of America/American Thoracic Society Consensus guidelines on the management of community-acquired pneumonia in adults. *Clin Infect Dis.* 2007;44:S27–72.

REFERENCES

1. World Health Organization. WHO recommendations on the use of rapid testing for influenza diagnosis. http://www.who.int/influenza/resources/documents/RapidTestInfluenza_WebVersion.pdf. Accessed September 4, 2014.

2. Harper SA, Bradley JS, Englund JA, et al. Expert Panel of the Infectious Diseases Society of America: Seasonal influenza in adults and children—diagnosis, treatment, chemoprophylaxis and institutional outbreak management: clinical practice guideline. *Clin Infect Dis.* 2009;48(8):1003–1032. Accessed September 4, 2014.

3. Centers for Disease Control and Prevention. Guidance for clinicians on the use of rapid influenza diagnostic tests. http://www.cdc.gov/flu/professionals/diagnosis/clinician_guidance_ridt.htm. Accessed September 4, 2014.

4. Lab Tests Online. Influenza tests. http://labtestsonline.org/understanding/analytes/flu/. Accessed September 4, 2014.

5. Erlikh IV, Abraham S, Kondamudi VK. Management of influenza. *Am Fam Physician.* 2010;82(9):1087–1095.

6. Centers for Disease Control and Prevention. Vaccine recommendations of the ACIP. http://www.cdc.gov/vaccines/hcp/acip-recs/recs-by-date.html. Accessed September 4, 2014.

7. Centers for Disease Control and Prevention. Flu treatment and what to do if you get sick. http://www.cdc.gov/flu/faq/what-to-do.htm. Accessed September 4, 2014.

8. Wenzel RP, Fowler AA. Clinical practice—acute bronchitis. *N Engl J Med.* 2006;355(20):2125–2130.

9. Albert RH. Diagnosis and treatment of acute bronchitis. *Am Fam Physician.* 2010;82(11):1345–1350.

10. Braman SS. Chronic cough due to acute bronchitis: ACCP evidence-based clinical practice guidelines. *Chest.* 2006;129(I suppl):95S–103S. http://www.ncbi.nlm.nih.gov/pubmed/16428698

11. Matthys H, Eisebitt R, Seith B, Heger M. Efficacy and safety of an extract of *Pelargonium sidoides* (EPs 7630) in adults with acute bronchitis. A randomized, double-blind, place-controlled trial. *Phytomedicine.* 2003;10(suppl 4):7–17.

12. National Heart, Lung, and Blood Institute. Guidelines for the diagnosis and management of asthma (EPR-3). http://www.nhlbi.nih.gov/health-pro/guidelines/current/asthma-guidelines. Accessed September 4, 2014.

13. US Census Bureau. 2008 national population projections: percent distribution of the projected population by selected age groups and sex for the United States: 2010 to 2050. https://www.census.gov/population/projections/data/national/2008/summarytables.html. Accessed September 4, 2014.

14. Older–Adults and Asthma https://www.aafa.org/display.cfm?id=8&sub=17&cont=173. Accessed September 30, 2015.

15. National Heart, Lung, and Blood Institute. Asthma action plan. http://www.nhlbi.nih.gov/health/resources/lung/asthma-action-plan-html. Accessed September 4, 2014.

16. COPD Assessment Test. COPD assessment test. http://catestonline.org. Accessed September 4, 2014.

17. CCQ. Clinical COPD questionnaire. http://www.ccq.nl. Accessed September 4, 2014.

18. Spiromics. Modified Medical Research Council dyspnea scale (mMRC questionnaire). http://www.cscc.unc.edu/spir/public/

UNLICOMMMRCModifiedMedicalResearchCouncilDyspnea Scale08252011.pdf. Accessed September 4, 2014.

19. Global Initiative for Chronic Obstructive Lung Disease. Home page. http://www.goldcopd.org. Accessed September 4, 2014.

20. Miniño AM, Xu J, Kochanek KD; Division of Vital Statistics. Deaths: preliminary data for 2008. *Natl Vital Stat Rep.* 2010;59(2):1–52. http://www.cdc.gov/nchs/data/nvsr/nvsr59/nvsr59_02.pdf. Accessed September 4, 2014.

21. Murphy SL, Xu J, Kochanek KD; Division of Vital Statistics. Deaths: preliminary data for 2010. *Natl Vital Stat Rep.* 2012;60(4):1–51. http://www.cdc.gov/nchs/data/nvsr/nvsr60/nvsr60_04.pdf. Accessed September 4, 2014.

22. Mandell LA, Wunderink RG, Anzueto A, et al. Infectious Diseases Society of America/American Thoracic Society consensus guidelines on the management of community-acquired pneumonia in adults. *Clin Infect Dis.* 2007;44(suppl 2):S27–72. https://www.thoracic.org/statements/resources/mtpi/idsaats-cap.pdf. Accessed September 4, 2014.

23. Medscape. CURB-65 pneumonia severity score. http://reference.medscape.com/calculator/curb-65-pneumonia-severity-score. Accessed September 4, 2014.

24. The Ohio State University College of Medicine. Pneumonia Severity Index (PSI) calculator. http://internalmedicine.osu.edu/pulmonary/cap/10849.cfm. Accessed September 4, 2014.

25. Cunha BA. Community-acquired pneumonia. Medscape. 2014. http://emedicine.medscape.com/article/234240-overview#a1. Accessed September 4, 2014.

Common Gastrointestinal Disorders in Primary Care

Joanne L. Thanavaro

Chapter Outline

Learning Objectives

Using a case-based approach, the learner will be able to:

1. Identify key history and physical examination parameters for common gastrointestinal disorders seen in primary care, including GERD, abdominal pain, diverticulitis, IBS, and infectious diarrhea.

2. Summarize recommended laboratory and diagnostic studies indicated for the evaluation of common gastrointestinal disorders seen in primary care.

3. State pathophysiology of common gastrointestinal disorders.

4. Document a clear, concise SOAP note for patients with common gastrointestinal disorders.

5. Identify relevant education and counseling strategies for patients with common gastrointestinal disorders.

6. Develop a treatment plan for common gastrointestinal disorders utilizing current evidence-based guidelines.

Case 1

Mr. Martin, a 38-year-old patient known to this practice, presents today with concern about epigastric and substernal pain that has progressively worsened over the past 3 to 4 months. He admits to mild "heartburn" after eating a large meal for at least the last 2 years. He has used over-the-counter (OTC) products sporadically with relatively good response. Three months ago, after a large meal and several drinks, he awoke with severe burning discomfort that extended from his midchest to his jaw. This episode lasted 30 minutes before he was able to fall back to sleep. Now he is experiencing the same type of attacks 2–3 times weekly. He's tried to avoid large meals and is now sleeping on two pillows at night; these measures have mildly improved the pain. He also reports onset of generalized abdominal pain, this time occurring in the daytime. The pain occurs both after meals and at random times during the day. He has been taking antacids with each meal, but his pain persists. His past medical history is remarkable for depression, which was diagnosed 4 months ago. He was started on nortriptyline 75 mg at bedtime, and that has helped his mood significantly. He is a nonsmoker and drinks 2–3 alcoholic beverages a week.

Physical Exam

Vital Signs: Blood pressure (BP) 138/72, heart rate (HR) 80 (regular), respiratory rate (RR) 18, temperature (T) 98.6, height (Ht) 72 inches, weight (Wt) 280 lbs

General (GEN): No acute distress. Sitting comfortably in chair. Cooperative

Heart: S_1 and S_2 regular rate and rhythm (RRR) without murmurs, rubs, or gallops

Lungs: Clear to auscultation (CTA)

Abdomen: Convex with good bowel sounds. No bruits. Soft with no palpable masses. Moderate palpation creates discomfort in the upper abdomen in the midline.

No hepatomegaly. No evidence of hernia. Rectal exam reveals soft brown stool that tests negative for occult blood.

What additional assessments/diagnostics do you need?

What is the differential diagnoses list?

What is your working diagnosis?

Additional Assessments/Diagnostics Needed

Review of Systems (ROS)

Be sure to inquire about alarm and atypical signs of gastroesophageal reflux disease (GERD).[1]

Atypical signs of GERD include:

► Chronic cough
► Asthma
► Recurrent sore throat
► Recurrent laryngitis
► Dental enamel loss
► Subglottic stenosis
► Globus sensation
► Chest pain
► Onset of symptoms at age >50 years

Alarm/warning signs suggesting complicated GERD include:

► Dysphagia
► Odynophagia
► Gastrointestinal bleeding
► Iron-deficiency anemia
► Weight loss

- ▶ Early satiety
- ▶ Vomiting

Labs

Labs obtained today:

Hemoglobin (HGB) 14.1, white blood cells (WBCs) 8.0, prothrombin time (PT) and International Normalized Ratio (INR) within normal limits (WNL)

Alanine aminotransferase (ALT) 31, aspartate aminotransferase (AST) 47

Amylase 44, lipase 62

Cholesterol 360

Urinalysis (UA) normal

Electrocardiogram (ECG): normal sinus rhythm (NSR), HR 84, axis –30. No ectopy. No evidence of left ventricular hypertrophy (LVH) or ST-T wave changes

Establishing the Diagnosis of GERD

- ▶ A presumptive diagnosis can be established if the patient presents with typical symptoms of heartburn and regurgitation.
- ▶ Patients with noncardiac chest pain suspected to be caused by GERD should have a diagnostic evaluation before institution of therapy.[2]

Imaging → *not indicated see unless... below*

- ▶ Barium radiographs should not be performed to diagnose GERD.
- ▶ Upper endoscopy is not required in the presence of typical GERD symptoms; it is indicated only in the presence of alarm symptoms and for screening patients at high risk for complications.
- ▶ Routine biopsies from the distal esophagus are not recommended.
- ▶ Esophageal manometry is recommended only for preoperative evaluation, but not for diagnostic purposes.
- ▶ Screening for *Helicobacter pylori* infection is not recommended, and treatment of *H. pylori* is not routinely required as part of antireflux therapy.[2]

Differential Diagnoses List

Gastric or duodenal ulcer

Bleeding secondary to peptic ulcer disease

Dyspepsia

Neoplasia

Cardiovascular disease (atypical chest pain)

Hiatal hernia

GERD

Working Diagnosis—GERD

Pathophysiology

The Montreal consensus defines gastroesophageal reflux as a condition that occurs when the reflux of stomach contents causes frequent troublesome symptoms that have an adverse effect on the patient's well-being. The true prevalence of GERD is hard to determine because symptoms are subjective and many patients treat these symptoms without seeing a healthcare provider. Several mechanisms contribute to reflux, all of which result in the failure of the gastroesophageal junction to prevent gastric contents from entering the esophagus. Generally, GERD symptoms occur as a result of transient inappropriate relaxation of the lower esophageal sphincter (LES), but the gastroesophageal junction may be mechanically compromised related to decreased LES resting tone, hiatal hernia, or both. Risk factors for GERD include alcohol and caffeine intake, obesity, and smoking.[3]

What Is Your Treatment Plan?

Pharmacologic

- ▶ An 8-week course of proton pump inhibitor (PPI) therapy is the treatment of choice for symptom relief and healing of erosive esophagitis.
- ▶ There are no major differences in efficacy of PPIs currently available.
- ▶ Delayed-release PPIs should be administered 30 to 60 minutes before meals.
- ▶ Initiate PPI therapy once daily before breakfast. Consider twice daily dosing for patients with only partial response to medication or those with nighttime symptoms.
- ▶ Consider switching to another PPI for patients who get only partial symptom relief.
- ▶ Maintenance of PPI therapy should be administered to patients who continue to have symptoms after discontinuing medication and to patients with complications, including erosive esophagitis and Barrett's esophagus.
- ▶ Patients requiring long-term PPI use should be prescribed the lowest possible dose that achieves symptom relief; intermittent or "on demand" therapy is a viable option.
- ▶ H_2- receptor antagonist therapy can be used as a maintenance option in patients without erosive disease for symptom relief; bedtime H_2RA therapy can be used in addition to daytime PPI therapy in selected patients with objective evidence of nighttime reflux. This combination may cause the development of tachyphylaxis with several weeks of therapy.
- ▶ Therapy for GERD other than acid suppression (including prokinetics and/or baclofen) should not be used without diagnostic evaluation.[2]

Nonpharmacologic

▶ Elevate head of bed 6 to 8 inches.

▶ Avoid recumbency <u>and</u> sleeping for 3–4 hours post-prandially.

▶ Stop smoking.

▶ Avoid large meals.

▶ Decrease fatty meals.

▶ Consider avoiding certain foods that can trigger reflux, such as chocolate, caffeine, alcohol, and acidic and/or spicy food.

▶ Lose weight.

▶ Avoid medications that can aggravate potential symptoms.[1]

Surgery

▶ Potential surgical options include laparoscopic fundoplication or bariatric surgery in obese patients.

▶ Reasons for surgical referral may include patient desire to discontinue medications, nonadherence to medication, intolerable side effects of medications, refractory or persistent symptoms despite maximal medical therapy, and the presence of a large hiatal hernia.[1]

Education/Counseling

▶ Discuss lifestyle interventions.

▶ Consider referral to dietician for weight loss guidance.

▶ Give instructions for proper administration of medications.

SOAP Note

S: Mr. Martin presents today with progressively worsening epigastric and substernal chest pain for the last 3–4 months. He reports heartburn after eating large meals for the last 2 years. One episode awakened him at night after eating a large meal and having several alcoholic drinks; he had severe burning from midchest extending up to his jaw. That episode lasted 30 minutes, and since then he has been limiting his portion sizes and sleeping on two pillows. These measures have resulted in some mild improvement, but he still has symptoms 2–3 times weekly. Antacids provide mild relief. He is a nonsmoker and drinks 2–3 beverages weekly. Except for one nighttime occurrence, he denies any alarm symptoms, including dysphagia, odynophagia, bleeding, weight loss, or early satiety.

O: *Vital Signs:* BP 138/72, HR 80 (regular), RR 18, T 98.6, body mass index (BMI) 43

GEN: No acute distress

Ears, eyes, nose, and throat (EENT): Eyes with pink conjunctivae, no yellowish tint to sclera, normal fundoscopic exam.

Ears: Normal tympanic membranes (TMs) without bulging or fluid lines. Nose: No bogginess of turbinates. No thyromegaly or carotid bruits

Heart: S_1 and S_2 RRR without murmurs, gallops, or rubs

Lungs: CTA

Abdomen: Soft, mild tenderness to palpation in epigastric area. No hepatomegaly or splenomegaly. No masses or rebound

Extremities: No edema. Bilateral dorsalis pedis and posterior tibialis pulses +2. No varicosities

Labs: HGB 14.1, WBCs 8.0, PT and INR normal. ALT 31, AST 47, amylase 44, lipase 62, cholesterol 360

ECG: NSR without ectopy, left ventricular hypertrophy (LVH), or ST-T wave changes

A: GERD

Obesity

Dyslipidemia

P: Discussed possible risk factors for GERD, including obesity and alcoholic beverages. Start omeprazole 40 mg PO daily 30 minutes before breakfast. Stressed importance of taking medication daily and 30 minutes before breakfast. Reviewed 1,800-calorie diet for weight reduction. Written guidelines provided. Referral to dietitian for weight management. Exercise (walking) 30 minutes daily to help with weight loss. Avoid any foods that trigger symptoms, avoid large fatty meals, avoid alcohol, and refrain from eating after 8 p.m. Elevate head of bed with shock blocks.

Follow-up in 1 month to evaluate efficacy of medication for symptom management. Will also get full lipid panel at that time and discuss need for statin therapy at that time.

Health Promotion Issues

▶ Weight maintenance

▶ Smoking cessation

▶ Healthy diet with avoidance of food triggers

Guidelines to Direct Care

Katz PO, Gerson LB, Vela MF. Diagnosis and management of gastroesophageal reflux disease. *Am J Gastroenterol.* 2013;108:308–328. http://gi.org/guideline/diagnosis-and-managemen-of-gastroesophageal-reflux-disease. Accessed September 16, 2015.

University of Michigan Health System. Gastroesophageal reflux disease (GERD). Ann Arbor: University of Michigan Health System; May 2012. http://www.guideline.gov/content.aspx?id=37564. Accessed September 16, 2015.

Case 2

Sandy is a 19-year-old college freshman with abdominal pain and diarrhea. She presents today, stating, "I feel terrible. My stomach hurts and I have diarrhea." For the last 3 days she has not felt well and reports decreased energy and mild to moderate abdominal discomfort. The abdominal discomfort is worse after eating. This morning she woke up at 5 a.m. with generalized abdominal pain that was dull and aching in character. The pain was moderately severe and was associated with several watery bowel movements and nausea. She vomited at 6 a.m., and her roommate brought her over to the student healthcare clinic. Sandy denies cough, fever, dysuria, bloody stools, or mucus in her stools. She has never had an episode like this before. She denies traveling outside of the country in the last 5 years. Her past medical history (PMH) is unremarkable. Last menstrual period was 2 weeks ago.

Physical Exam

Vital Signs: BP 100/70, HR 70 and regular, RR 18 and even, T 100.3

GEN: Alert and lying quietly on the exam table on left side with hips flexed

CV: S_1 and S_2 RRR without murmurs, rubs, or clicks

Lungs: CTA

Abdomen: Bowel sounds slightly increased throughout the abdomen. Abdomen soft with mild tenderness to palpation especially at the umbilicus. No rebound tenderness. No masses or organomegaly. Rectal exam deferred

What additional assessments/diagnostics do you need?

What is the differential diagnoses list?

What is your working diagnosis?

Additional Assessments/Diagnostics Needed

ROS

Identification of location of pain can help with narrowing down etiology.[4] See Table 1.

Scoring Systems

The Alvarado score combines clinical and lab findings to assign a score from 1 to 10, with higher scores associated with increased likelihood of appendicitis. See Table 2. This scoring system does not inform the provider regarding the need for computed tomography (CT) scanning, and imaging is recommended even with low scores.[4]

Labs

Urine: Human chorionic gonadotropin (HCG) negative, negative for chlamydia/gonorrhea, complete blood count (CBC) consistent with leukocytosis, C-reactive protein (CRP) = 40

TABLE 1 Perceived Location of Pain

Content removed due to copyright restrictions

TABLE 2 Alvarado Scoring

Content removed due to copyright restrictions

Imaging: The American College of Radiology provides guidance for appropriate imaging for patients with abdominal pain.[5] For patients with fever, leukocytosis, and possible appendicitis, CT of the abdomen and pelvis is recommended. Oral or rectal contrast may not be needed depending on institutional preference. However, in the primary care setting the goal is to get this patient to the emergency department where imaging and definitive treatment can be provided.

Differential Diagnoses List

Early appendicitis—first few hours it mimics gastroenteritis, especially in this age group

Influenza/gastroenteritis

Urinary tract infection (UTI)

Ovarian cysts

Diabetes mellitus (DM)

Pelvic inflammatory disease (PID)

Ectopic pregnancy

Hepatitis

Working Diagnosis—Acute appendicitis

Pathophysiology

Abdominal pain is a common complaint that prompts a patient to be evaluated by both primary care providers and gastroenterologists. Noxious stimuli can result in pain within the abdomen by various mechanisms. The two principal mechanisms of pain are parietal pain and visceral pain; parietal pain occurs with irritation of the parietal peritoneum and usually presents as a sharp, well-localized discomfort, whereas visceral pain, affecting the abdominal viscera, can result from traction on the peritoneum, distention of a hollow viscus, or muscular traction. Because pain fibers innervating the visceral structures are bilateral, pain is often perceived in the midline and can be dull and poorly localized. Visceral pain is often felt at a distant site from the actual location of the abnormality. Referred pain is felt in areas distant to the diseased organ.[6]

Pharmacologic

Appendectomy remains the only curative management for patients with appendicitis. However, antibiotic coverage prior to surgery is recommended and should provide both aerobic and anaerobic coverage. The duration of antibiotic treatment also depends on the stage of appendicitis when diagnosed, findings during surgery, and postoperative course.[7]

Surgery

Appendectomy is the most common form of urgent gastrointestinal surgery. The appendix can be removed either laparoscopically (LA) or through an open surgical procedure (OA). Abscesses, if present, will also be drained. Wound infections are more likely after LA compared to the open technique, but the incidence of intra-abdominal abscess is increased with laparoscopy. Surgical stay is shortened and pain is lessened with LA, but the procedure is more costly than OA.[8]

Education/Counseling

For this patient, anticipatory guidance regarding the nature of your suspicions that this may be appendicitis and assistance with transportation to the closest emergency department are essential. Prepare the patient for the likelihood of surgery and offer to call family and give update.

SOAP Note

S: This 19-year-old college freshman presents today with her roommate. She reports abdominal pain with diarrhea that started 3 days ago and has progressively worsened. Pain is worse after eating and rated 6/10 today. She woke up this morning with generalized abdominal pain that is dull and aching in character. She has watery bowel movements and nausea and vomited once. Her pain now seems to be around her umbilicus. Her appetite has been poor since the onset of symptoms. Sandy denies cough, fever, dysuria, bloody stools, or mucus in her stools. She has never had an episode like this before. She denies traveling outside of the country in the last 5 years. Her PMH is unremarkable. Last menstrual period was 2 weeks ago.

O: *Vital Signs:* BP 100/70, HR 70 (regular), RR 18, T 100.3

GEN: Alert and lying quietly on the exam table on left side with hips flexed

Skin: Slightly diaphoretic

CV: S_1 and S_2 RRR without murmurs, rubs, or clicks

Lungs: Clear to auscultation

Abdomen: Abdomen symmetric without distention. No scars or visible pulsations. Bowel sounds slightly increased throughout the abdomen. No bruits. Abdomen soft with moderate tenderness to percussion and at the umbilicus and at McBurney's point. No rebound tenderness. No rigidity. No masses or organomegaly. No costovertebral angle (CVA) tenderness. Pelvic exam normal. Rectal exam deferred

Labs: Urine HCG negative, negative for chlamydia/gonorrhea, no ketones

CBC: WBCs 16,000 cells/mm³ with left shift, CRP 40

Imaging: Will need CT of the abdomen and pelvis

A: Abdominal pain of unknown etiology. Suspect appendicitis (Alvarado score of 7); vital signs (VS) stable

P: Roommate here and agrees to driving Sandy to nearby hospital, which is 5 minutes away. Called Mom and she is on her way to the hospital. Called emergency department (ED) and discussed clinical presentation with Dr. Baker, who agrees to schedule imaging on arrival. Instructed Sandy to call for 1-week follow-up here after discharge from hospital.

Health Promotion Issues

▶ Schedule a follow-up visit 1 week after discharge to evaluate the post-operative course and to discuss health promotion issues.

Guidelines to Direct Care

Howell JM, Eddy OL, Lukens TW, Thiessen ME, Weingart SD, Decker WW. (2010). Clinical policy: critical issues in the evaluation and management of emergency department patients with suspected appendicitis. *Ann Emerg Med.* 2010;55:71–116. http://www.guideline.gov/content.aspx?id=15598. Accessed September 16, 2015.

Case 3

Ms. Hawkins is a 78-year-old retired musician. She was in generally good health until 5 a.m. this morning. She awoke with mild abdominal cramping and the need to defecate. She went to the bathroom and passed bright red blood mixed with stool. Over the next 2 hours she had four bowel movements, each with only bright red blood. No more stools or bleeding for the last 4 hours. She reports a good appetite with no recent weight loss until this episode. She eats a healthy diet with lots of fruits and vegetables. She denies epigastric pain, nausea, and vomiting and has no history of peptic ulcer disease or gastrointestinal bleeding (GI) bleeding. She has a remote memory of hemorrhoids, manifested by streaks of bright red blood on the toilet tissue. She denies the use of laxatives. Her PMH includes hypertension (HTN) for 20 years that is well controlled with 50 mg atenolol daily. She also has degenerative joint disease that was well controlled with Tylenol (acetaminophen) until recently. She feels her pain is getting worse and would like to try a new medication. Denies taking any OTC medications.

Physical Examination

Vital Signs: BP 120/70 supine, 108/62 standing, HR 104 (regular), RR 14, T 100

GEN: Mildly obese, pleasant, no acute distress

Head, eyes, ears, nose, and throat (HEENT): Fundi with arteriovenous (AV) nicking. Oropharynx clear. Neck: Supple without adenopathy or thyromegaly. Carotids +2 without bruits

CV: S_1 and S_2 RRR, no murmurs, gallops, or rubs. Point of maximal impact (PMI) 5th intercostal space (ICS), midclavicular line (MCL)

Resp: Lungs clear to auscultation

Abdomen: Soft with active bowel sounds. No bruits. Moderate tenderness to palpation in left lower quadrant. No organomegaly

Rectal: No masses or tenderness. Stool bloody

Neuro: Oriented × 3, cognition intact

What additional assessments/diagnostics do you need?

What is the differential diagnoses list?

What is your working diagnosis?

Additional Assessments/Diagnostics Needed

ROS

▶ Determine whether patient has ever had a colonoscopy.

▶ Determine amount of blood with each stool.

Routine Labs/Imaging

▶ CBC, comprehensive metabolic panel (CMP).

▶ Imaging may be needed to determine cause of bleeding.

Differential Diagnoses List

Hemorrhoids

Anal fissure

Rectal varices

Diverticular disease

Infectious colitis

Ischemic colitis

Inflammatory bowel disease (IBD)

Colon cancer

Working Diagnosis—Lower GI bleeding—likely diverticular disease

Pathophysiology

Acute gastrointestinal bleeding (GIB) is a common medical emergency and involves a spectrum of clinical presentations depending on the cause and the site of bleeding. Most GIB episodes are self-limited and require only supportive therapy, although GIB accounts for almost 20,000 deaths annually. Lower GIB increases with age, and there is a higher incidence in males. Diverticular disease refers to symptomatic and asymptomatic disease due to colonic diverticula, which result from mucosal outpouching through the wall of the colon. Use of nonsteroidal anti-inflammatory drugs, corticosteroids, and opiate analgesics and low-fiber diets are associated with an increased risk. Colonic diverticular bleeding is the most common cause of overt lower GI bleeding in adults; bleeding stops spontaneously in 75% of patients.[9-11]

What Is Your Treatment Plan?

Criteria for outpatient management:

▶ Reliability to return for medical reevaluation if condition worsens

▶ Compliance with outpatient treatment plan

▶ Abdominal pain is not severe

▶ No higher than a low-grade fever

▶ Can tolerate oral intake

▶ No or minimal comorbid illnesses

▶ Available support system[12]

Pharmacologic

▶ In acute uncomplicated diverticulitis, antibiotic treatment for 10–14 days is recommended.

- Antibiotics should be based on the usual bacteria, which include Gram-negative rods and anaerobes.
- Reasonable choices include a quinolone with metronidazole, amoxicillin and clavulanate, or trimethoprim-sulfamethoxazole with metronidazole.
- The use of anti-inflammatory agents such as mesalamine seems promising, but randomized controlled trials are required to obtain efficacy and safety data.[11,13]

Nonpharmacologic

Dietary recommendations:

- Avoid red meat and foods that are high in fat.
- Increase dietary fiber.
- Avoidance of seeds, nuts, popcorn, and other similar foods is unnecessary.[11]

Education/Counseling

- Explain etiology of diverticular disease and discuss need for hospitalization in light of bleeding, orthostatic blood pressure changes, fever, and lack of support systems if symptoms worsen.
- Anticipatory guidance for hospitalization should include likelihood of intravenous fluids, antibiotics, lab work, and imaging, or colonoscopy if bleeding continues.
- If bleeding can't be controlled with endoscopic or angiographic therapy, surgery may be required.[11]

SOAP Note

S: Ms. Hawkins was in generally good health until 5 a.m. this morning when she awoke with mild abdominal cramping and the need to defecate. She reports passing bright red blood mixed with stool 5 times early this morning, but no further episodes for the last 4 hours. She believes the bleeding was "a lot" because it filled the toilet bowl each time. She recalls having some streaks of blood on her stool many years ago related to hemorrhoids. She denies abdominal pain, nausea, vomiting, tenesmus, or lightheadedness and has no history of peptic ulcer disease or GI bleeding. She denies the use of laxatives. Her last colonoscopy was 4 years ago and was normal. Daily medications include atenolol for HTN and Tylenol for degenerative joint disease (DJD).

O: *Vital Signs:* BP 120/70 supine, 108/62 standing, HR 104 (regular), RR 14, T 100

GEN: Mildly obese, pleasant, no acute distress

Skin: Warm, dry, pink, good turgor

HEENT: Fundi with AV nicking. Oropharynx clear. Neck: Supple without adenopathy or thyromegaly. Carotids +2 without bruits

CV: S_1 and S_2 RRR, no murmurs, gallops, or rubs. PMI 5th ICS, MCL

Resp: LCTA

Abdomen: Soft with active bowel sounds. No bruits. Moderate tenderness to palpation in left lower quadrant. No guarding or organomegaly

Rectal: No masses, tenderness, hemorrhoids, or anal fissure. Stool bloody

Extremities: No edema

Neuro: Oriented × 3 with cognition intact

A: Lower GI bleeding—suspect diverticular disease

P: Admit to hospital. Discussed case presentation with hospitalist and requested GI referral.

Church friend (Sophie) called and will transport Ms. Hawkins to the nearby hospital. Follow-up 1 week after hospital discharge. Will discuss any further issues associated with GIB and her request to change DJD medication at that time.

Health Promotion Issues

- Discuss at follow-up visit.

Guidelines to Direct Care

Zuccaro G. Management of the adult patient with acute lower gastrointestinal bleeding. *Am J Gastroenterol.* 1998;93: 1202–1208. http://gi.org/guideline/management-of-the-adult-patient-with-acute-lower-gastrointestinal-bleeding. Accessed September 15, 2015.

Feingold D, Steele SR, Lee S, et al. Practice parameters for the treatment of sigmoid diverticulitis. *Dis Colon Rectum.* 2014;57:284–294. https://www.fascrs.org/sites/default/files/downloads/publication/practice_parameters_for_the_treatment_of_sigmoid.2.pdf. Accessed September 15, 2015.

Case 4

Sally, a 26-year-old recruiting specialist, presents today with complaints of abdominal bloating and increased flatus. She's had diarrhea daily for the last week and has stopped eating during the day in order to reduce the diarrhea while working. When she eats in the evening, she gets diarrhea during the night. She denies heartburn, abdominal pain, and bloody or mucous stools. Weight fluctuates 5 pounds with her menstrual cycle. She reports abdominal bloating and alternating constipation and diarrhea since high school. Defecation improves the symptoms. Sally tries to manage her diarrhea by not eating much and drinks lots of water when she's constipated.

Her weight has remained stable despite these symptoms. She admits to feeling tired, fatigued, and stressed; she is a single mother who has two young children to support and finds the demands of her job overwhelming. She is a perfectionist and believes that her personality contributes to the problem. Significant family history includes her mother, who had a gastric ulcer at age 41.

Physical Exam

Vital Signs: BP 138/76, HR 76 and regular, RR 14, T. 99

GEN: Appears slightly anxious but pleasant and cooperative

CV: S_1 and S_2 RRR without murmurs, gallops, or rubs

Resp: LCTA

Abdomen: Normal bowel sounds in all 4 quadrants. No bruits. Soft with mild tenderness in the right and left lower quadrants. No masses. Percussion reveals normal liver borders. No splenomegaly.

Rectal: Nontender. Normal vault with no masses. Small amount of formed stool, brown, negative for fecal occult blood

What additional assessments/diagnostics do you need?

What is the differential diagnoses list?

What is your working diagnosis?

Additional Assessments/Diagnostics Needed

ROS

Assess for Rome III irritable bowel syndrome (IBS) criteria:

▶ Recurrent abdominal pain or discomfort at least 3 days per month in the last 3 months with two or more of the following:
   ▶ Improvement with defecation
   ▶ Onset associated with a change in frequency of stools
   ▶ Onset associated with a change in form of stools[14]

The Bristol Stool Scale can be used to describe stool consistency to differentiate constipation from diarrhea and monitor treatment responses.[15]

Determine IBS subtype:

▶ *IBS—Diarrhea (IBS-D):* 25% of the time patient has frequent loose stools that are small and medium volumes, and 75% of the time they are not accompanied by abdominal discomfort. Stools are 6–7 on the Bristol Scale.

▶ *IBS—Constipation (IBS-C):* Stool is hard and pellet-like 25% of the time and is 1–2 on the Bristol Scale. Loose or watery stools occur less than 25% of the time.

▶ *IBS—Mixed (IBS-M):* Stools are hard and lumpy 25% of the time, loose and mushy 25% of the time, and normal 50% of the time.

▶ *Unsubtyped IBS:* The patient has insufficient abnormality of stool consistency to fit any category.[16]

Ask about alarm features, including:

▶ Anemia
▶ Rectal bleeding
▶ Nocturnal symptoms
▶ Weight loss
▶ Recent antibiotic use
▶ Onset after 50 years of age
▶ Family history of colorectal cancer, IBD, or celiac disease

Colonoscopy is the diagnostic study of choice when alarm symptoms are present.[17]

Routine Labs

Labs and invasive testing should be kept to a minimum because they are expensive, generally low yield, and may reinforce illness behaviors. Recommended initial screening includes a complete blood count, sedimentation rate, and fecal occult blood test. Screening for celiac disease should be considered in all IBS patients, especially those with IBS-D and IBS-M. A complete metabolic profile, stool cultures, and *Clostridium* toxin may be ordered if clinically indicated but are generally low-yield studies.[14]

Differential Diagnoses List

IBD

IBS

Celiac disease

Lactose intolerance

Hyperthyroidism or hypothyroidism

Gastroenteritis

Intestinal infection

Diverticular disease

Working Diagnosis—Irritable bowel disease

Pathophysiology

No single pathophysiologic abnormality has been found to adequately explain the symptomatology of IBS, and the etiology is likely to be multifactorial, including abnormalities of GI motility, visceral hypersensitivity, GI inflammation, disturbances along the brain–gut axis, and psychological factors. The role of small intestinal overgrowth (SIBO) has been recently proposed as a contributing factor in IBS.[14]

What Is Your Treatment Plan?

Pharmacologic

▶ *Antibiotics:* There is moderate evidence that the poorly absorbable antibiotic rifaximin is effective in reducing total IBS symptoms and bloating in IBS-D. The guidelines still give a weak recommendation for this agent.

- *Antispasmodics:* Certain antispasmodics (otilonium, hyoscyamine cimetropium, pinaverium, and dicyclomine) provide symptomatic short-term relief in IBS.
- *Loperamide:* Although loperamide is an effective antidiarrheal, there is no evidence supporting its use for relief of global IBS symptoms.
- *Antidepressants:*
  - Tricyclic antidepressants and selective serotonin reuptake inhibitors are effective for symptom relief in IBS.
  - Side effects are common and may limit patient tolerance.
- *Serotonergic agents:* Serotonin (5-hydroxytryptamine [5-HT]) plays a role in gastrointestinal secretion, motility, and sensation; alosteron is effective in female IBS-D.
- *Prosecretory agents:* Linaclotide is superior to placebo for the treatment of IBS-C.[18]

Nonpharmacologic

- *Diet and dietary manipulation:* Very few patients can accurately identify presumed offending food, and there is little research supporting any specific diet that helps with IBS symptoms. In general, patients should avoid foods they believe trigger symptoms.
- *Fiber:*
  - Increased intake of dietary fiber is frequently recommended to improve bowel function for IBS; insoluble fibers can cause bloating and abdominal discomfort.
  - Soluble fibers and psyllium provide relief in IBS.
- *Probiotics, prebiotics:*
  - Probiotics and prebiotics have been used for decades based on the theory that small intestinal bacterial overgrowth (SIBO) may exacerbate IBS symptoms.
  - There is insufficient evidence to recommend these for IBS at this time.
- *Peppermint:* Peppermint oil can be found in various preparations. Limited evidence suggests that it can help relax smooth muscle by attenuation of visceral reactivity and modulation of pain in IBS. Peppermint is superior to placebo and is a low-risk therapy that may help in some patients.
- *Psychological therapies:* Cognitive behavior therapy, hypnotherapy, multicomponent psychology therapy via telephone conversations, and dynamic psychotherapy have all been explored and have been shown to be effective in IBS. Availability of skilled therapists remains a barrier to this type of intervention.[18]

Education/Counseling

- Establishing a therapeutic relationship is one of the most important components of managing a patient with IBS.
- Explain the proposed mechanism of IBS.
- Discuss the nature of the illness and address any concerns. Assure patients that although symptoms are real, they are not life-threatening.

- Be sure the patient is aware of the chronic nature of IBS and that a normal life span is expected.
- Develop realistic expectations and involve the patient in treatment decisions.[16]

SOAP Note

S: Sally presents today with abdominal symptoms that began over 10 years ago. She has abdominal pain that waxes and wanes and is accompanied by diarrhea alternating with constipation, abdominal bloating, and flatulence. Her symptoms improve with defecation but are present almost daily. She denies anemia, weight loss, fever or chills, nocturnal symptoms, or recent antibiotic use but reports frequent fatigue. Her weight has been stable, with no more than a 5-lb variance for the last year. She limits her food intake when she has diarrhea and increases her water intake to about eight 8-oz glasses of water daily when she's constipated. She denies a family history of colon cancer, celiac disease, or IBD. She admits to high stress levels related to a job with overwhelming demands, being a single mom with two small children, and "being a perfectionist." Denies low mood but admits to feeling anxious frequently; no insomnia, anhedonia, or panic. Stress increases her gastrointestinal symptoms.

O: *Vital Signs:* BP 138/76, HR 76 and regular, RR 14, T 99

GEN: Appears slightly anxious but pleasant and cooperative

Skin: Warm, dry, pink without lesions, good turgor

CV: S_1 and S_2 RRR without murmurs, gallops, or rubs

Resp: LCTA

Abdomen: Normal bowel sounds in all 4 quadrants. No bruits. Soft with mild tenderness in the right and left lower quadrants. No masses. Percussion reveals normal liver borders. No splenomegaly

Rectal: Nontender. Normal vault with no masses. Small amount of formed stool, brown, negative for fecal occult blood

Psych: Discusses symptoms without hesitation. Good eye contact. Brief tearfulness when describing her stress levels; responded quickly to reassurance and acknowledgment of symptoms

CBC: Red blood cells (RBCs) 4.5, hemoglobin and hematocrit (H&H) 14/42

Erythrocyte sedimentation rate (ESR): 4

Immunoglobulin A (IgA) anti-tissue transglutaminase (TTG) pending

A: IBS-M

Anxiety

P: Long discussion regarding the likelihood of IBS. Explained proposed etiology, chronic nature, and possible strategies for reducing symptoms. Reviewed labs and gave assurance that these are normal. Provided guidance for methods of limiting stress, including realistic expectations for job goals, parenting, and symptom management. Reviewed diet and recommended avoiding any foods that seem to trigger symptoms. Will discuss gluten-free diet if IgATTG is positive. Recommended psyllium, which may help with symptoms. Try peppermint. Hyoscyamine 0.125 mg every 4 hours prn for abdominal cramping. Use loperamide sparingly for diarrhea symptoms. Citalopram 10 mg daily. Explained how selective serotonin reuptake inhibitor (SSRI) drugs may help with IBS symptoms. Offered counseling, but she declines at this time. She would like to see if medications improve symptoms. Close and frequent follow-up visits. Next appointment in 2 weeks.

Health Promotion Issues

▶ Discuss the importance of exercise and good sleep habits to help with stress levels.

▶ Recommend stress management techniques and/or counseling.

Guidelines to Direct Care

Ford AC, Moayyedi P, Lacy BD, et al. American College of Gastroenterology monograph on the management of irritable bowel syndrome and chronic idiopathic constipation. *Am J Gastroenterol.* 2014;109:S2–S26. http://gi.org/wp-content/uploads/2014/08/IBS_CIC_Monograph_AJG_Aug_2014.pdf. Accessed September 16, 2015.

Case 5

Mr. Jacobs is a 68-year-old male who was discharged 14 days ago for community-acquired pneumonia (CAP). He has a past history of chronic obstructive pulmonary disease (COPD) and cigarette smoking. He was recovering well from his CAP and reports minimal shortness of breath (SOB) and cough. He denies wheezing. He received both his influenza and pneumococcal vaccines in the hospital. Today he is concerned about new-onset diarrhea that began 3 days ago and generally feeling ill. He denies nausea and vomiting but has abdominal pain and bloating. He is drinking plenty of fluids and taking OTC Imodium (loperamide) with little improvement in his diarrhea. He is a former smoker and drinks no alcohol.

Physical Exam

Vital Signs: BP supine 136/78, HR 78 (regular), RR 16, T 98.4

GEN: Thin, frail-looking male with mild dyspnea

HEENT: Normal fundoscopic exam. Nasal turbinates pink and moist. Ears without redness or discharge. Pharynx no exudates or postnasal drip. Neck: Supple without adenopathy or thyromegaly. Carotids +2 without bruits

CV: S_1 and S_2 RRR, no murmurs, gallops, or rubs. PMI 5th ICS, MCL

Resp: Decreased lung sounds throughout all lungs fields. No crackles or wheezes

Abdomen: Soft with hyperactive bowel sounds in all 4 quadrants. No organomegaly. Mild diffuse tenderness to palpation

Rectal: No masses or tenderness. Stool guaiac negative

Neuro: Oriented × 3, cognition intact

What additional assessments/diagnostics do you need?
What is the differential diagnoses list?
What is your working diagnosis?

Additional Assessments/Diagnostics Needed

ROS

▶ Ask about the stool character (watery, bloody, mucus-filled, purulent, bilious).

▶ Evaluate for signs of dehydration, including decreased urine output, thirst, dizziness, or change in mental status.

▶ A food and travel history is important to evaluate for potential exposures.

▶ Inquire about recent antibiotic use.

Physical Exam

▶ Ill appearance, dry mucous membranes, delayed capillary refill, tachycardia, and orthostatic vital signs can signal severe dehydration.[19]

Routine Labs

▶ Most watery diarrhea is self-limited, and testing is not usually indicated.

▶ Specific diagnostic testing should be reserved for patients with severe dehydration, persistent fever, bloody stool, or immunosuppression.

▶ Occult blood should be done and is moderately sensitive and specific for inflammatory diarrhea.

▶ Stool cultures—because of cost, cultures should be obtained only in the presence of grossly bloody stool, severe dehydration, signs of inflammatory disease, symptoms lasting 3 to 7 days, or immunosuppression. Testing stool for leukocytes is no longer recommended because of the wide variability in sensitivity and specificity.

- *Clostridium difficile* (CD) testing is recommended for:
  - Patients who develop unexplained diarrhea after 3 days of hospitalization
  - Patients who develop unexplained diarrhea while using antibiotics or within 3 months of discontinuing antibiotics
- Ova and parasites testing is recommended only for:
  - Persistent diarrhea lasting more than 7 days, especially if associated with:
    - Travel to mountainous regions
    - Diarrhea in persons with AIDS or men who have sex with men
    - Community waterborne outbreaks[19]

Differential Diagnoses List

Infectious: Noninflammatory:

- Viruses: Norwalk virus, rotavirus, adenovirus, astrovirus, coronavirus
- Preformed toxin (food poisoning): *Staphylococcus aureus*, *Bacillus cereus*, *Clostridium perfringens*
- Toxin production: Enterotoxigenic *Escherichia coli*, *Vibrio cholerae*, *Vibrio parahaemolyticus*
- Protozoa: *Giardia lamblia*, *Cryptosporidium*, *Cyclspora*, *Isopora*[19]

Infectious: Invasive or inflammatory:

- *Shigella*, *Salmonella*, *Campylobacter*, enteroinvasive *E. coli*, *Yersinia enterocolitica*, *Clostridium difficile* (pseudomembranous colitis), *Entamoeba histolytica*, *Neisseria gonorrhoeae*, *Listeria monocytogenes*[19]

Noninfectious:

- Drug reaction
- Ulcerative colitis, Crohn's disease
- Ischemic colitis
- Fecal impaction
- Laxative abuse
- Emotional stress[19]

Working Diagnosis—Acute diarrhea likely due to Clostridium difficile

Pathophysiology

CD colitis is inflammation of the colon due to infection from CD, which is a spore-forming bacteria.[20] Colitis occurs when these bacteria replace the normal gut bacteria usually following antibiotic treatment. In the past decade, a strain with increased virulence has been responsible for outbreaks in Canada, Europe, and the United States. This strain (NAP1/B1/027) produces 15- to 20-fold more toxin than previous strains and is associated with more severe disease and mortality rates of 7% or greater. Risk factors for CD diarrhea include: (1) antibiotic use—all antibiotics have been implicated, but increased risk with clindamycin, cephalosporins, penicillins, and fluoroquinones; (2) antineoplastic agents; (3) hospital or nursing care, but outpatient disease is becoming more common; (4) advanced age; (5) comorbid disease, including malignancy, renal failure, and generalized debility; (6) gastrointestinal manipulation with surgery or tube placement; and (7) use of histamine-2 blockers and proton-pump inhibitors.[21]

What Is Your Treatment Plan?

Pharmacologic

- If a patient has a strong pretest suspicion for CD infection (CDI), empiric therapy should be considered regardless of the laboratory testing results.
- Discontinue any inciting antimicrobial agent(s) if possible.
- Patients with mild-to-moderate CDI should be treated with metronidazole 500 mg orally three times per day for 10 days.
- Patients with severe CDI should be treated with vancomycin 125 mg four times daily for 10 days.
- Failure to respond to metronidazole therapy within 5–7 days should prompt consideration of a change in therapy to vancomycin at standard dosing.
- For mild-to-moderate CDI in patients who are intolerant or allergic to metronidazole and for pregnant and breastfeeding women, vancomycin should be used at standard dosing.
- The use of antiperistaltic agents to control diarrhea from confirmed or suspected CDI should be limited or avoided because they may obscure symptoms and precipitate complicated disease. Use of antiperistaltic agents in the setting of CDI must always be accompanied by medical therapy for CDI.
- Management of severe and complicated CDI should include intravenous fluid resuscitation, electrolyte replacement, and pharmacologic venous thromboembolism prophylaxis. In the absence of ileus or significant abdominal distention, oral or enteral feeding should be continued.
- Vancomycin delivered orally (125 mg four times per day) plus intravenous metronidazole (500 mg three times a day) is the treatment of choice in patients with severe and complicated CDI who have no significant abdominal distention.
- Vancomycin delivered orally (500 mg four times per day) and per rectum (500 mg in a volume of 500 mL four times a day) plus intravenous metronidazole (500 mg three times a day) is the treatment of choice for patients with complicated CDI with ileus or toxic colon and/or significant abdominal distention.
- The first recurrence of CDI can be treated with the same regimen that was used for the initial episode. If severe, however, vancomycin should be used. The second recurrence should be treated with a pulsed vancomycin regimen.

- If there is a third recurrence after a pulsed vancomycin regimen, fecal microbiota transplant (FMT) should be considered.
- There is limited evidence for the use of adjunct probiotics to decrease recurrences in patients with recurrent CDI (RCDI).
- No effective immunotherapy is currently available.
- Any diarrheal illness in women who are pregnant or postpartum should prompt testing for *C. difficile*.[20]

Nonpharmacologic

- Surgical consult should be obtained in all patients with complicated CDI, especially patients with CDI and hypotension requiring vasopressor therapy; clinical signs of sepsis and organ dysfunction (renal and pulmonary); mental status changes; white blood cell count ≥50,000 cells/μL; lactate ≥5 mmol/L; or failure to improve on medical therapy after 5 days.[20]

Education/Counseling

- Take your medication exactly as prescribed. Don't take half doses or skip doses.
- Wash your hands often, especially after going to the bathroom and before preparing food.
- People who live with you should also wash their hand frequently.

SOAP Note

S: Mr. Jacobs was discharged 14 days ago for CAP. He reports taking 10 days of levofloxacin. He was recovering well from his CAP and taking his regular medications for COPD. He denies wheezing and is SOB only with increased exertion. He received both his influenza and pneumococcal vaccines in the hospital. Today he is concerned about new-onset diarrhea, which began 3 days ago, and feeling very tired. He denies nausea or vomiting but has diffuse abdominal pain rated 5/10. He reports 6–8 episodes of profuse watery diarrhea daily. He is drinking plenty of fluids and denies thirst or decreased urine output. OTC Imodium is not decreasing his diarrhea.

O: *Vital Signs:* BP supine 136/78 (no orthostatic changes), HR 78 (regular), RR 16, T 98.4

GEN: Thin, frail-looking male with mild dyspnea

Skin: Warm, dry, pink, good turgor

HEENT: Normal fundoscopic exam. Nasal turbinates pink and moist. Ears without redness or discharge. Pharynx: No exudates or postnasal drip. Neck: Supple without adenopathy or thyromegaly. Carotids +2 without bruits

CV: S_1 and S_2 RRR, no murmurs, gallops, or rubs. PMI 5th ICS, MCL

Resp: Barrel chest. No dullness to percussion. Decreased lung sounds throughout all lungs fields. No crackles or wheezes

Abdomen: Soft with hyperactive bowel sounds in all 4 quadrants. No organomegaly. Moderate tenderness to palpation in left lower quadrant

Rectal: No masses or tenderness. Stool guaiac negative

Neuro: Oriented × 3, cognition intact

A: Acute diarrhea: Likely CDI related to antibiotic use during hospitalization for CAP

COPD: Stable

CAP: Resolving

P: Stools for CDI but will treat empirically given recent hospitalization and antibiotic use.

Metronidazole 500 mg orally three times per day for 10 days. Avoid all alcohol while taking this medication.

Discontinue Imodium.

Drink at least six 8-oz glasses of fluid daily. Suggest Gatorade for electrolyte replacement.

Continue all inhalers. Encouraged to remain smoke free.

Check BMP today to check for electrolyte imbalance.

Call for medical records to review labs and imaging done during hospitalization.

Follow-up: 2 weeks. Call back if diarrhea doesn't improve. Get CXR at that time in light of recent CAP in a smoker.

Health Promotion Issues

- Discuss prevention measures that should be used by all healthcare providers, including washing their hands with soap and water or an alcohol-based hand solution before and after caring for every patient. Encourage patient to confirm that all HCPs wash their hands before taking care of him.
- Only take antibiotics prescribed by your HCP.[22]

Guidelines to Direct Care

Centers for Disease Control and Prevention. Frequently asked questions about *Clostridium difficile*. http://www.cdc.gov/HAI/pdfs/cdiff/Cdiff_tagged.pdf. Accessed September 16, 2015.

Cohen SH, Gerding DN, Johnson S, et al. Clinical practice guidelines for *Clostridium difficile* infection in adults: update by the Society for Healthcare Epidemiology of America (SHEA) and the Infectious Diseases Society of America (IDSA). 2010. http://www.idsociety.org/uploadedFiles/IDSA/Guidelines-Patient_Care/PDF_Library/cdiff2010a.pdf. Accessed September 16, 2015.

Surawicz CM, Brandt LJ, Binion DG, et al. Guidelines for diagnosis, treatment and prevention of *Clostridium difficile* infections. *Am J Gastroenterol.* 2013;108:478–498. http://www.guideline.gov/content.aspx?id=45139. Accessed September 16, 2015.

REFERENCES

1. Agency for Healthcare Research and Quality. Gastroesophageal reflux disease (GERD). http://www.guideline.gov/content.aspx?id=37564. Accessed September 4, 2015.

2. Katz PO, Gerson LB, Vela MF. Diagnosis and management of gastroesophageal reflux disease. *Am J Gastroenterol*. 2013;108:308–328. http://gi.org/guideline/diagnosis-and-managemen-of-gastroesophageal-reflux-disease/. Accessed September 4, 2015.

3. Seccombe J, Gyawali CP. Gastroesophageal reflux disease. In: Gyawali CP, ed. *Gastroenterology Subspecialty Consult*. 3rd ed. Philadelphia, PA: Wolters Kluwer; 2012:108–109. *Washington Manual Subspecialty Consult*.

4. Armstrong C. ACEP releases guidelines on evaluation of suspected acute appendicitis. *Am Fam Physician*. 2010;15:1043–1044.

5. American College of Radiology. ACR appropriateness criteria. 2013. https://acsearch.acr.org/docs/69357/Narrative/. Accessed September 4, 2015.

6. Asomban AW. Abdominal pain. In: Gyawali CP, ed. *Gastroenterology Subspecialty Consult*. 3rd ed. Philadelphia, PA: Wolters Kluwer; 2012:108–109. *Washington Manual Subspecialty Consult*.

7. Craig S. Appendicitis treatment and management. 2014. http://emedicine.medscape.com/article/773895-treatment. Accessed September 4, 2015.

8. Sauerland S, Jaschinski E, Neugebauer AM. Laparoscopic versus open surgery for suspected appendicitis. *Cochrane Database Syst Rev*. 2010;(10):CD001546. doi:10.1002/14651858.CD001546.pub3.

9. Humes D, Smith JK, Spiller RC. Colonic diverticular disease. *Am Fam Physician*. 2011;84:1163–1164.

10. Gray DM. Acute gastrointestinal bleeding. In: Gyawali CP, ed. *Gastroenterology Subspecialty Consult*. 3rd ed. Philadelphia, PA: Wolters Kluwer; 2012:48–61. *Washington Manual Subspecialty Consult*.

11. Salzman H, Dustin L. Diverticular disease: diagnosis and treatment. *Am Fam Physician*. 2005;72:1229–1234.

12. World Gastroenterology Organization. Practice guidelines. http://www.worldgastroenterology.org/guidelines/global-guidelines/diverticular-disease/diverticular-disease-english. Accessed September 4, 2015.

13. Boynton W, Floch M. New strategies for the management of diverticular disease—insights for the clinician. *Ther Adv Gastroenterol*. 2013;6:205–213.

14. Cassell BE, Sayuk GS. Irritable bowel syndrome. In: Gyawali CP, ed. *Gastroenterology Subspecialty Consult*. 3rd ed. Philadelphia, PA: Wolters Kluwer; 2012:190–198. *Washington Manual Subspecialty Consult*.

15. Bristol stool chart. http://mcathcart.squarespace.com/storage/bristol_stool_chart.pdf. Accessed September 4, 2015.

16. Wadlund DL. Meeting the challenge of IBS. *Nurse Pract*. 2012;37:23–30.

17. Wilkins T, Pepitone C, Alex B, Schade RR. Diagnosis and management of IBS in adults. *Am Fam Physician*. 2012;86:419–425.

18. Ford AC, Moayyedi P, Lacy BD, et al. American College of Gastroenterology monograph on the management of irritable bowel syndrome and chronic idiopathic constipation. *Am J Gastroenterol*. 2014;109(suppl 1):S2–S26.

19. Barr W, Smith A. Acute diarrhea. *Am Fam Physician*. 2014;89:180–189.

20. Surawicz CM, Brandt LJ, Binion DG, et al. Guidelines for diagnosis, treatment, and prevention of *Clostridium difficile* infections. *Am J Gastroenterol*. 2013;108:478–498.

21. Hessen MT. In the clinic. *Clostridium difficile* infection. *Ann Intern Med*. 2010;153(7):ITC41-15.

22. Centers for Disease Control and Prevention. Frequently asked questions about *Clostridium difficile*. http://www.cdc.gov/HAI/pdfs/cdiff/Cdiff_tagged.pdf. Accessed September 4, 2015.

Common Hematologic Disorders in Primary Care

Karen S. Moore

Learning Objectives

Using a case-based approach, the learner will be able to:

1. Identify key history and physical examination parameters for common hematologic disorders seen in primary care, including anemia and thalassemia.

2. Summarize recommended laboratory and diagnostic studies indicated for the evaluation of common hematologic disorders seen in primary care.

3. State pathophysiology of common hematologic disorders.

4. Document a clear, concise SOAP note for patients with common hematologic disorders.

5. Identify relevant education and counseling strategies for patients with common hematologic disorders.

6. Develop a treatment plan for common hematologic disorders utilizing current evidence-based guidelines.

Case 1

Mr. Frederick is a 66-year-old African American male who presents with complaints of (c/o) fatigue, increased shortness of breath that worsens with walking or activity, and "just feeling bad." Mr. Frederick has not been to a primary care provider in "about 10 years." States he went to the emergency room (ER) "about a month ago" and was diagnosed with hypertension (HTN) and kidney disease. States he was started on medications to decrease fluid retention and treat his HTN and referred to your office for follow-up. Unsure of last tetanus vaccination date, does not get annual influenza vaccines. States he had "regular childhood" immunizations. Denies significant illness prior to recent diagnoses. Denies chest pain, coughing, dizziness, vomiting. When queried further, Mr. Frederick reports some nausea and itching skin that has gotten progressively worse over the last few months. Denies surgeries or prior hospitalizations. Denies alcohol use, illicit drug use, tobacco use. No known drug allergies (NKDA). Current medications: furosemide 10 mg QD and lisinopril 5 mg QD.

Physical Exam

Vital Signs: Blood pressure (BP) 168/94, heart rate (HR) 116, respiratory rate (RR) 20, temperature (T) 98.8, height (Ht) 6'2", weight (Wt) 325 lbs

General (GEN): Progressive fatigue. Denies fever, chills, or night sweats. No acute distress

Head, eyes, ears, nose, and throat (HEENT): Head normocephalic without evidence of masses or trauma. Pupils equal, round, react to light, accommodation (PERRLA), extraocular movements (EOMs) full to confrontation. Noninjected. Fundoscopic exam unremarkable with exception of pale retinal background. Palpebral conjunctiva pale. Ear canal without redness or irritation, tympanic membranes (TMs) clear, pearly, bony landmarks visible. No discharge, no pain noted. Pale nasal mucosa. Posterior pharynx pale. Neck: Supple without masses. No thyromegaly. No jugular vein distention (JVD) noted.

Skin: Dry skin with pruritus, no discoloration, no open areas noted

Cardiovascular (CV): S_1 and S_2 regular rate and rhythm (RRR), no murmurs, no rubs. 2+ edema noted to bilateral mid-pretibial region of lower extremities

Lungs: Clear to auscultation

Abdomen: Soft, nontender, nondistended, bowel sounds present × 4 quadrants, no organomegaly, no bruits

Rectal: Normal vault, good tone, heme-negative stool

Neuro: Cranial nerves (CN) II–XII intact. Rhine/Weber normal, Romberg negative. Sensation intact, deep tendon reflexes (DTR) 2+

What additional assessments do you need?

What is the differential diagnoses list?

What is your working diagnosis?

Additional Assessments/Diagnostics Needed

Mr. Frederick presents with symptoms of anemia and chronic kidney disease.[1–8] Anemia is characterized by decreased hemoglobin and hematocrit identified on lab testing but may have multiple causes requiring different interventions to correct underlying disease pathology. It is important to identify the underlying cause of Mr. Frederick's anemia.

His diagnosis of HTN and his fluid retention dictate that a more careful evaluation be completed to evaluate for cardiovascular disease. It is important to remember that HTN can be a complication of kidney disease, or it may have been a causative factor. Because Mr. Frederick has not been evaluated in 10 years, it is difficult to determine whether his HTN preceded the kidney failure or the elevated blood pressure is a result of worsening kidney function. Regardless, evaluation of complications of HTN and kidney disease should be undertaken as well as identification of the cause of his anemia.

Evaluation for patients with suspected anemia should include:

- Risk factors for anemia:
  - Anemia risk increases with age. Although the exact etiology of anemia in elderly persons may be multifactorial, advancing age is a known risk factor for anemia.
  - A diet that is deficient in quality protein sources and B vitamins is a known risk factor for anemia. Hematopoiesis requires healthy levels of macronutrients and micronutrients to carry out cell production and maturation.
  - Intestinal disorders such as malabsorptive disorders, parasitism, lack of intrinsic factor, gastric bypass surgery, Crohn's disease, and ulcerative colitis increase the risk of anemia.
  - Chronic diseases such as thyroid, liver, kidney, or autoimmune diseases as well as HIV/AIDS and cancer increase the risk of anemia. Mr. Frederick has a recent diagnosis of chronic kidney disease, so you need to investigate whether his kidney disease is the cause of his anemia.
  - Pregnancy, childbirth, and dysfunctional uterine bleeding predispose women to anemia.
  - Inherited diseases such as sickle cell disease or trait as well as the thalassemias can interfere with production and maturation of red blood cells.
  - Bone marrow dysfunction such as myelodysplastic syndrome, blood or bone cancers, and marrow suppression by medications, toxins, or disease increase the risk of anemia.
- Identifiable causes of anemia:
  - *Bleeding:* Either chronic or acute blood loss can be the cause of anemia. In the case of Mr. Frederick, he denies any signs or symptoms of upper gastrointestinal blood loss, he is male, which precludes menstrual abnormalities as the cause of his anemia, and his stool was negative for blood during exam, which lessens the likelihood that his anemia is related to lower gastrointestinal loss. Depending on his laboratory testing, this cause of anemia may need to be explored in addition to other more likely causes.
  - *Diminished red blood cell (RBC) production:* For Mr. Frederick, his diagnosis of kidney disease should increase suspicion of the potential cause of his anemia. Chronic kidney disease is associated with a decreased level of erythropoietin, which is a hormone secreted by the kidneys that is necessary for RBC production. This probable etiology for Mr. Frederick's anemia should be further explored with laboratory testing.
  - *Rapid rates of red blood cell destruction:* Inherited or acquired diseases that cause an increased rate of RBC destruction can lead to anemia. Mr. Frederick's medical history does not suggest any of these potential causes nor does his physical examination reveal enlargement or abnormality of his spleen. If suspected, laboratory studies to rule out sickle cell disease and thalassemia should be performed. If other causes are ruled out, further studies for causative agents of hemolytic anemia may be undertaken.

- Presence or absence of complications of anemia:
  - Arrhythmia
  - Congestive heart failure
  - End organ damage such as liver and kidney failure

ROS

Focus additional questions on assessment of the impact that his anemia symptoms are having on his activities of daily living as well as potential clues to the cause of his anemia, including:

- Fatigue (Mr. Frederick reports fatigue)
- Chest pain (denies)
- Palpitations (denies)
- Shortness of breath (SOB) (Mr. Frederick reports SOB)
- Dyspnea on exertion (DOE) (Mr. Frederick reports DOE)
- Dizziness (denies)
- Headache (denies)
- Coolness in hands and feet or paresthesias (denies)
- Nausea/vomiting—patients with chronic kidney disease often report nausea (Mr. Frederick reports nausea)
- Worsening of these symptoms with activity can provide an estimate of the severity of anemia

Further discussion of cardiovascular risk factors should also be explored, including:

- HTN—Mr. Frederick has been diagnosed with HTN
- Cigarette smoking—Mr. Frederick is a nonsmoker
- Obesity—Mr. Frederick has a body mass index of 41.7
- Physical inactivity—Mr. Frederick does not exercise
- Dyslipidemia—you will need to order labs
- Diabetes mellitus—you will need to order labs
- Microalbuminuria or estimated glomerular filtration rate (GFR)—you will need to order urine analysis and labs. This will be in addition to other kidney-related evaluations
- Age—Mr. Frederick is 66 years old
- Family history—when queried further, he reports his mother and father both had HTN, diabetes mellitus (DM), and chronic kidney disease (CKD). These are significant risk factors

Physical Exam

The physical examination for this patient should include:

- A thorough assessment of the heart and lungs for signs and symptoms (s/s) of cardiac complications of anemia and kidney disease (arrhythmias, extracardiac sounds, murmurs or rubs, auscultation of lungs)
- Evaluation for fluid overload (peripheral edema, JVD, cardiac and lung evaluation)

- Appropriate measurement of blood pressure with verification in the contralateral arm
- Palpation of the lower extremities for edema and peripheral pulses
- Examination of the abdomen for enlarged spleen, liver, changes in kidneys (either enlarged or smaller than anticipated), masses, and abnormal aortic pulsations
- Examination of the skin and nails for complications of anemia and kidney disease (pruritus, spoon nails [koilonychias])
- Examination of the mucous membranes for s/s of anemia (pallor, glossitis of the tongue, angular cheilitis of the mouth)

▌ Routine Labs

Routine labs for Mr. Frederick should include those directed at assessing his kidney function as well as his anemia and end organ function.

Baseline studies:

- Comprehensive metabolic panel, including:
  - Albumin (normal)
  - Alkaline phosphatase (normal)
  - ALT (alanine aminotransferase) (normal)
  - AST (aspartate aminotransferase) (normal)
  - Blood urea nitrogen (BUN) (elevated)
  - Creatinine (elevated)
  - Calcium (normal)
  - Chloride (normal)
  - Carbon dioxide (normal)
  - Glucose (normal)
  - Potassium (high normal range)
  - Sodium (normal)
  - Total bilirubin (normal)
  - Total protein (normal)
- Complete blood count, including:
  - RBC (low)
  - Hemoglobin (Hgb) 11% (low)
  - Hematocrit (Hct) 33% (low)
  - MCV mean corpuscular volume (normal)
  - MCH mean corpuscular hemoglobin (normal)
  - MCHC mean corpuscular hemoglobin concentration (normal)
  - Platelets (normal)
  - White blood cells (WBCs) (basophils, eosinophils, lymphocytes, monocytes, neutrophils) (normal)

Additional kidney function studies:

- Urinalysis (UA) (protein ++)
- 24-hour urine (A 24-hour urine is completed to assess for sedimentation and creatinine clearance to provide information on kidney function)

- Glomerular filtration rate (GFR) 40 (mL/min per 1.73 m²)—GFR of 30–59 is considered Stage 3 CKD[7]

Additional anemia studies:

- Serum iron (low)
- Serum ferritin (low)
- Total iron-binding capacity (TIBC) (low)
- Vitamin B_{12} (may be abnormal in some anemias, but in the case of Mr. Frederick it is normal)
- Folate (may be abnormal in some anemias, but in the case of Mr. Frederick it is normal)
- Reticulocyte count (low)
- Red cell distribution width (RDW) (variable but within normal range)
- Peripheral blood smear (poikilocytosis)

Additional labs:

- *Liver function tests:* Done as baseline study related to possible causes of anemia and potential for cholesterol management (normal)
- *Cholesterol panel:* Advised to assess for cardiovascular disease (CVD). Done as baseline study related to Mr. Frederick's age and years since last primary care evaluation (Mr. Frederick's cholesterol and low-density lipoprotein [LDL]/high-density lipoprotein [HDL] ratio results suggest the need for further intervention)
- *Thyroid studies:* If thyroid disease is suspected (not done for Mr. Frederick)
- *EPO:* Erythropoietin (EPO) studies may be ordered to determine whether CKD and resultant erythropoietin deficiency is the cause of anemia (Mr. Frederick's EPO is low)

Potential diagnostic studies:

- Renal ultrasound—to determine size, shape, and density of kidneys
- Renal biopsy—to determine precise etiology of kidney disease

▌ *Differential Diagnoses List*

Chronic kidney disease
Anemia of chronic disease
Anemia of B_{12} deficiency
Anemia of folate deficiency
Hypertension
Cardiovascular disease
Congestive heart failure
Diabetes mellitus
Obesity

▌ *Working Diagnoses*

Chronic kidney disease—Stage 3
Anemia of chronic disease

Hypertension

Obesity

Pathophysiology

Anemia is defined as a hemoglobin level of less than 12.0 mg/dL in adult females and less than 13.5 mg/dL in adult males.[1-8] Anemia is the most common blood disorder in the United States and affects nearly 3 million persons annually. Anemia of chronic disease (ACD), as in the case of chronic kidney disease, is caused primarily by decreased erythropoietin leading to a decreased reticulocyte count. ACD is diagnosed by careful observation of the lab values. ACD is referred to as a normocytic, normochromic anemia. This means that the MCV is normal, and MCHC is normal. The reticulocyte count is low, with variability in the size of the RBCs, but the RDW is still within normal limits. The RBCs may demonstrate abnormal shapes on the smear, known as poikilocytosis. The serum iron and TIBC will be low.

Although other forms of anemia may also be present and co-exist in a patient with chronic kidney disease or other chronic illnesses, Mr. Frederick's lab results suggest an anemia caused by erythropoietin insufficiency leading to lowered RBC production by the bone marrow.

What Is Your Treatment Plan?

Pharmacologic

Continue Mr. Frederick on his current dosage of furosemide and lisinopril.[1-8] This medication regimen may need to be adjusted once evaluated by a renal specialist, but at the current dosage it should be well tolerated by Mr. Frederick. Remember that anemia is treated by identifying the root cause and then treating that disease process. In the case of chronic kidney disease, erythropoietin deficiency is the cause of the anemia so that is where you should focus your treatment. Erythropoietin-stimulating agents (ESAs) are given via injection and could be a consideration for Mr. Frederick. ESAs should be initiated and managed by the renal specialist because this medication is not without risk. Mr. Frederick's Hgb is 11%, which is the target Hgb for persons with chronic kidney disease. For that reason, it is unlikely that ESAs would be initiated. Iron supplementation will generally be initiated whether or not ESAs are included in Mr. Frederick's treatment plan. Oral iron may not be effective in patients with CKD related to decreased absorption of iron from the gastrointestinal (GI) tract. Intravenous (IV) iron may be an acceptable alternative if iron stores do not improve with oral iron dosing regimens but should be managed by the renal specialist.

Nonpharmacologic

- Referral to a renal specialist.
- Consider RBC transfusion if Hgb is below target based upon patient's s/s and comorbid conditions. This is not indicated in Mr. Frederick
- Renal ultrasound—to be ordered by renal specialist
- Renal biopsy—to be ordered by renal specialist

- Lifestyle modifications to decrease CVD risk
  - Dietary modifications for weight loss, chronic kidney disease, CVD
  - Increase activity
- Dietary consultation
- Electrocardiogram (ECG) in office
- Consider cardiology consultation for further evaluation of CVD with exercise tolerance test (ETT)

Education/Counseling

- Lifestyle modifications
  - Dietary modifications
  - Sodium restriction
  - Weight loss
- Dietary consultation
- Signs and symptoms of worsening anemia/CKD
- Living well with CKD

SOAP Note

S: Mr. Frederick is a 66-year-old African American male who presents with c/o fatigue, DOE, and malaise as well as nausea and itching. Mr. Frederick has not been to a primary care provider in "about 10 years." Mr. Frederick was diagnosed with HTN and renal disease at the emergency room one month ago, started on medications for treatment, and referred for primary care follow-up. Unsure of last tetanus vaccination date, does not get annual influenza vaccines. States he had "regular childhood" immunizations. Denies significant illness prior to recent diagnoses. Denies chest pain, coughing, dizziness, vomiting. Denies surgeries or prior hospitalizations. Denies alcohol use, illicit drug use, tobacco use. NKDA. Current medications: furosemide 10 mg QD and lisinopril 5 mg QD.

O: *Vital Signs:* BP 168/94, P 116, RR 20, T 98.8, Ht 6'2", Wt 325 lbs

GEN: Progressive fatigue. Denies fever, chills, or night sweats. No acute distress

HEENT: Head normocephalic without evidence of masses or trauma. PERRLA, EOMs full to confrontation. Noninjected. Fundoscopic exam unremarkable with exception of pale retinal background. Palpebral conjunctiva pale. Ear canal without redness or irritation, TM clear, pearly, bony landmarks visible. No discharge, no pain noted. Pale nasal mucosa. Posterior pharynx pale. Neck supple without masses. No thyromegaly. No JVD noted

Skin: Dry skin with pruritus, no discoloration, no open areas noted

CV: S_1 and S_2 RRR, no murmurs, no rubs. 2+ edema noted to bilateral mid-pretibial region of lower extremities

Lungs: Clear to auscultation

Abdomen: Soft, nontender, nondistended, bowel sounds present × 4 quadrants, no organomegaly, no bruits

Rectal: Normal vault, good tone, heme-negative stool

Neuro: CN II–XII intact. Rhine/Weber normal, Romberg negative. Sensation intact, DTR 2+.

Lab Results: RBC, Hgb, Hct, retic, serum Fe, TIBC decreased, RDW, MCV, MCHC normal

A: Chronic kidney disease—Stage 3

   Anemia of chronic disease

   Hypertension

   Obesity

P: Refer to renal specialist for further evaluation and management of renal disease and recommendations for anemia of chronic disease. Recommend lifestyle and dietary modifications for renal, CVD, and weight loss. Refer to dietitian. Continue lisinopril and furosemide. Vaccinations recommended: hepatitis A, hepatitis B, pneumonia, shingles, and annual influenza. Schedule colonoscopy. Follow-up in 2 weeks to assess medication tolerance, verify referral appointments, and review plan of care.

■ Health Promotion Issues[7–8]

▶ Vaccinations: Hepatitis A, hepatitis B, pneumonia, shingles, annual influenza

▶ Schedule colonoscopy

■ Guidelines to Direct Care

Centers for Disease Control and Prevention. Recommended adult immunization schedule, by vaccine and age group. 2015. http://www.cdc.gov/vaccines/schedules/hcp/imz/adult.html. Accessed September 16, 2015.

Kidney Disease: Improving Global Outcomes (KDIGO) Anemia Work Group. KDIGO clinical practice guideline for anemia in chronic kidney disease. *Kidney Int Suppl.* 2012; 2(4):279–335. http://www.kdigo.org/clinical_practice_guidelines/pdf/KDIGO-Anemia%20GL.pdf. Accessed September 16, 2015.

Kidney Disease: Improving Global Outcomes (KDIGO) Anemia Work Group. KDIGO 2012 clinical practice guideline for the evaluation and management of chronic kidney disease. *Kidney Int Suppl.* 2013(3):1. http://www.kdigo.org/clinical_practice_guidelines/pdf/CKD/KDIGO_2012_CKD_GL.pdf. Accessed September 16, 2015.

US Preventive Services Task Force. Published recommendations. http://www.uspreventiveservicestaskforce.org/BrowseRec/Index/browse-recommendations. Accessed September 16, 2015.

World Health Organization. *Haemogolobin concentrations for the diagnosis of anaemia and assessment of severity.* Vitamin and Mineral Nutrition Information System. Geneva: World Health Organization; 2011. http://www.who.int/vmnis/indicators/haemoglobin.pdf. Accessed September 16, 2015.

■ Case 2

Mrs. Williams is a 68-year-old white female who presents with a complaint of fatigue that has gradually worsened over the last 6 months. The fatigue is not associated with chest pain, SOB, diaphoresis, or palpitations. She also recently noticed coldness as well as numbness and tingling in her lower extremities and intermittent dizziness when moving quickly from a seated to a standing position. Denies changes in bowel/bladder habits, denies appetite changes. Past medical history (PMH) of measles, mumps, rubella, and chickenpox in childhood. Denies significant medical conditions. Uses occasional ibuprofen as needed for arthralgia. No surgeries or hospitalization. NKDA. Reports immunizations up-to-date, tetanus booster vaccination 3 years ago, shingles and pneumonia vaccination 2 years ago, influenza vaccination annually. Mrs. Williams's last mammogram and well-woman exam were 3 years ago, and both were normal. Natural menopause and last menstrual period 15 years ago. Denies tobacco use, alcohol consumption, illicit drug use.

■ Physical Exam

Vital Signs: BP 126/80 supine, 118/76 sitting, 110/68 standing with reported mild dizziness, HR 82 regular, RR 14, T 98.7, Ht 5'5", Wt 135 lbs

GEN: Progressive fatigue that is causing her to cut down on her normal activities. Denies fever, chills, or night sweats. No acute distress

HEENT: Head normocephalic without evidence of masses or trauma. PERRLA, EOMs full to confrontation. Noninjected. Fundoscopic exam unremarkable with exception of pale retinal background. Palpebral conjunctiva pale. Ear canal without redness or irritation, TM clear, pearly, bony landmarks visible. No discharge, no pain noted. Pale nasal mucosa. Posterior pharynx pale with beefy red tongue. Neck: Supple without masses. No thyromegaly. No JVD

CV: S_1 and S_2 RRR, no murmurs, no gallops, no rubs

Lungs: Clear to auscultation

Abdomen: Soft, nontender, nondistended, bowel sounds present × 4 quadrants, no organomegaly, no bruits

Back: Nontender to palpation. No pain with forward flexion of low back but reports some mild dizziness with touching toes. No costovertebral angle (CVA) tenderness

GU: Normal pelvic exam

Rectal: Normal vault, good tone, heme-negative stool

Neuro: CN II–XII intact. Rhine/Weber normal, Romberg positive. Some difficulty with tandem walking. Paresthesias noted with monofilament testing of bilateral feet, DTR 1+

What additional assessments/diagnostics do you need?

What is the differential diagnoses list?

What is your working diagnosis?

▉ *Additional Assessments/Diagnostics Needed*

Mrs. Williams presents with symptoms of anemia that are suspicious for a vitamin-deficient cause.[1–4,7–10] Further exploration of her medical history, including family history, as well as laboratory and diagnostic studies will be important to help narrow the potential cause. Her symptoms of coolness, numbness, and tingling in her extremities as well as dizziness and swelling of her tongue need to be evaluated further to determine whether these could be attributed to her anemia or another cause.

Evaluation for Mrs. Williams's suspected anemia should include:

▶ Risk factors for anemia:
  ▸ Anemia risk increases with age. Although the exact etiology of anemia in elderly persons may be multifactorial, advancing age is a known risk factor for anemia.
  ▸ A diet that is deficient in quality protein sources and B vitamins is a known risk factor for anemia. Because you suspect a vitamin-deficient cause in the case of Mrs. Williams, a careful dietary assessment should be conducted.
  ▸ Intestinal disorders such as malabsorptive disorders, parasitism, lack of intrinsic factor, gastric bypass surgery, Crohn's disease, and ulcerative colitis increase the risk of anemia. Mrs. Williams denies a personal history of intestinal disorders but does report a family history of pernicious anemia in her mother.
  ▸ Chronic diseases such as thyroid, liver, kidney, or autoimmune diseases as well as HIV/AIDS and cancer increase the risk of anemia. Mrs. Williams denies personal history of chronic disease, reports history of autoimmune disorder in her mother.
  ▸ Pregnancy, childbirth, and dysfunctional uterine bleeding predispose women to anemia. Mrs. Williams is postmenopausal and denies any abnormal bleeding.
  ▸ Inherited diseases such as sickle cell disease or trait as well as the thalassemias can interfere with production and maturation of red blood cells. Mrs. Williams has no history of inherited blood disorders.
  ▸ Bone marrow dysfunction such as myelodysplastic syndrome, blood or bone cancers, and marrow suppression by medications, toxins, or disease increase the risk of anemia. Mrs. Williams denies history of these diseases.

▶ Identifiable causes of anemia:
  ▸ *Bleeding:* Either chronic or acute blood loss can be the cause of anemia. In the case of Mrs. Williams, she denies any signs or symptoms of upper gastrointestinal blood loss, she denies any postmenopausal bleeding, and her stool was negative for blood during exam, which lessens the likelihood that her anemia is related to lower gastrointestinal loss. Depending on her laboratory testing, this cause of anemia may need to be explored in addition to other more likely causes.
  ▸ *Diminished red blood cell (RBC) production:* Laboratory testing will determine whether a vitamin deficiency is the cause for Mrs. Williams's diminished blood counts.
  ▸ *Rapid rates of red blood cell destruction:* Inherited or acquired diseases that cause an increased rate of RBC destruction can lead to anemia. Mrs. Williams's medical history does not suggest any of these potential causes nor does her physical examination reveal enlargement or abnormality of the spleen. If other causes are ruled out, further studies for causative agents of hemolytic anemia may be undertaken.

▶ Presence or absence of complications of anemia:
  ▸ Arrhythmia
  ▸ Congestive heart failure
  ▸ End organ damage such as liver and kidney failure

▉ ROS

Focus additional questions on assessment of the impact that her anemia symptoms are having on her activities of daily living as well as potential clues to the cause of her anemia, including:

▶ Fatigue (Mrs. Williams reports fatigue)
▶ Chest pain (denies)
▶ Palpitations (denies)
▶ Shortness of breath (SOB) (denies)
▶ Dyspnea on exertion (DOE) (denies)
▶ Dizziness (Mrs. Williams reports dizziness)
▶ Headache (denies)
▶ Coolness in hands and feet or paresthesias (Mrs. Williams reports this symptom)
▶ Worsening of these symptoms with activity can provide an estimate of the severity of the anemia (Mrs. Williams reports worsening with activity)

Explore her health history further, making note of hints to what the vitamin deficiency may be:

▶ Alcohol (ETOH) use (denies)
▶ Medications that may interfere with absorption such as hormones, anticonvulsants, antineoplastic agents (denies)
▶ Diet recall (vegetarian, low intake of B vitamins)

- Additional risk factors: Women of northern European ancestry who are prematurely gray with blue eyes, living in a northern cold climate, have an increased risk of pernicious anemia

Physical Exam

The physical examination for this patient should include:

- A thorough assessment of the heart and lungs for s/s of cardiac complications of anemia (arrhythmias, extracardiac sounds, murmurs or rubs, auscultation of lungs)
- Evaluation for fluid overload (peripheral edema, JVD, cardiac and lung evaluation)
- Appropriate measurement of blood pressure with verification in the contralateral arm and in various positions (orthostatic)
- Palpation of the lower extremities for edema and peripheral pulses
- Examination of the abdomen for enlarged spleen, liver, changes in kidneys, masses, and abnormal aortic pulsations
- Examination of the skin and nails for complications of anemia (spoon nails [koilonychias])
- Examination of the mucous membranes for s/s of anemia (pallor, glossitis of the tongue, angular cheilitis of the mouth)

Routine Labs

Routine labs for Mrs. Williams should include those directed at assessing her anemia.

Baseline studies:

- Comprehensive metabolic panel, including:
  - Albumin (normal)
  - Alkaline phosphatase (normal)
  - ALT (alanine aminotransferase) (elevated)
  - AST (aspartate aminotransferase) (normal)
  - BUN (normal)
  - Creatinine (normal)
  - Calcium (normal)
  - Chloride (normal)
  - Carbon dioxide (normal)
  - Glucose (normal)
  - Potassium (normal)
  - Sodium (normal)
  - Total bilirubin (normal)
  - Total protein (normal)
- Complete blood count, including:
  - RBC (low)
  - Hgb (low)
  - Hct (low)
  - MCV (elevated)
  - MCH (normal)
  - MCHC (normal)
  - Platelets (low)
  - WBCs (basophils, eosinophils, lymphocytes, monocytes, neutrophils) (low)
- Urinalysis (normal)

Additional anemia studies:

- Serum iron (normal)
- Serum ferritin (normal)
- Total iron-binding capacity (TIBC) (normal)
- B_{12} (low)
- Folate (normal)
- Reticulocyte count (normal)
- RDW (elevated)
- Peripheral blood smear (macrocytosis, hyperpigmented neutrophils, and giant platelets)
- Schilling's test (positive)

Additional Labs and Diagnostic Testing

- *Liver function tests:* Done as baseline study related to possible causes of anemia and potential for cholesterol management. Lactate dehydrogenase (LDH) is elevated.
- *Cholesterol panel:* Advised to assess for CVD. Done as baseline study related to Mrs. Williams's age and years since last primary care evaluation. Mrs. Williams's cholesterol panel is normal.
- *Thyroid studies:* If thyroid disease is suspected. This was completed and was normal for Mrs. Williams.
- *EPO:* Erythropoietin studies may be ordered to determine whether erythropoietin deficiency is the cause of anemia. Not done in this case.
- *KOH test:* Potassium hydroxide (KOH) test on scraping from tongue to determine whether fungal infection is responsible for the glossitis observed on Mrs. Williams's examination. The test was negative for fungal infection.
- *Schilling's test:* The Schilling's test is helpful in differentiating vitamin B_{12}–deficiency anemia from folic acid–deficiency anemia. Mrs. Williams's Schilling's test is positive, which is diagnostic for vitamin B_{12} deficiency.

Potential Diagnostic Studies

- Colonoscopy for wellness and to rule out (r/o) occult GI bleed

Differential Diagnoses

Anemia of vitamin B_{12} deficiency

Anemia of folate deficiency

Iron-deficiency anemia—related to (r/t) malignancy, GI blood loss

Postural hypotension

Glossitis—can be r/t B_{12} or folate deficiency

Peripheral vascular disease (PVD)

Working Diagnosis

Hypoproliferative macrocytic anemia secondary to vitamin B_{12} deficiency

Peripheral neuropathy related to vitamin B_{12} deficiency

Leukopenia secondary to vitamin B_{12} deficiency

Thrombocytopenia secondary to vitamin B_{12} deficiency

Elevated LDH and ALT secondary to vitamin B_{12} deficiency

Glossitis due to vitamin B_{12} deficiency

Pathophysiology

Vitamin B_{12} deficiency leads to decreased production of RBC and resultant anemia.[9] This deficiency can be caused by a lack of intrinsic factor and is commonly known as pernicious anemia. Pernicious anemia occurs when cells in the stomach that synthesize intrinsic factor are damaged by disease or surgical disruption, as with gastric bypass. Pernicious anemia occurs more often in women than in men, especially those of northern European descent with fair skin and blue eyes who reside in cool northern regions. Another cause of vitamin B_{12} deficiency is damage to the intestine leading to an inability of the GI track to absorb vitamin B_{12}. This occurs in disease processes such as celiac disease, Crohn's disease, or parasitism. Vitamin B_{12} deficiency may occur simultaneously with other forms of anemia such as folate-deficiency and iron-deficiency anemia.

What Is Your Treatment Plan?

Mrs. Williams is not acutely ill and has had progressive generalized fatigue for 6 months.[9] Her lab work clearly demonstrates vitamin B_{12} deficiency, and she is complaining of neurologic problems (coolness in extremities, gait disorder, dizziness) consistent with her vitamin B_{12}–deficiency anemia.

Her BP is stable, but she does have BP changes with position. She is not tachycardic, not febrile, and not actively bleeding. She needs treatment for her vitamin deficiency and a colonoscopy screening to rule out any GI blood loss and as a general health maintenance recommendation.

Pharmacologic

▶ Start on 1,000 mcg of vitamin B_{12} daily for 14 days and then every week for 12 weeks. Then titrate down to monthly. This monthly regimen will probably be required for life. Nasal vitamin B_{12} is fairly expensive. Patients can use oral vitamin B_{12} as long as absorption is not the issue causing the deficiency, but many patients still come in monthly for a vitamin B_{12} injection.

Nonpharmacologic

▶ Transfusion is not necessary for this patient. With supplementation, her anemia should improve.

▶ Plan a colonoscopy within the next day or so. She may also need an upper GI work-up. Her results of the colonoscopy will dictate how soon a follow-up colonoscopy is needed. If polyps are found, she will need screening every 3 years.

Education/Counseling

▶ Review diet with Mrs. Williams to identify areas of concern.

▶ Schedule a formal dietary consultation to educate Mrs. Williams about ways to increase foods rich in vitamin B_{12}.

▶ Encourage this patient to increase her fluids. This should help with the orthostatic hypotension she is experiencing.

SOAP Note

S: Mrs. Williams is a 68-year-old postmenopausal white female who presents with a complaint of fatigue, dizziness with position changes, and coolness and numbness in extremities that has gradually worsened over the last 6 months. She denies chest pain, SOB, diaphoresis, or palpitations, changes in bowel/bladder habits, appetite changes. PMH of measles, mumps, rubella, and chickenpox in childhood. Uses occasional ibuprofen as needed for arthralgia. NKDA. She reports her immunizations are up-to-date. Mrs. Williams's last mammogram and well-woman exam were 3 years ago, and both were normal. No tobacco use, alcohol consumption, illicit drug use.

O: *Vital Signs:* BP 126/80 supine, 118/76 sitting, 110/68 standing with reported mild dizziness, HR 82 regular, RR 14, T 98.7, Ht 5'5", Wt 135 lbs

GEN: Progressive fatigue that is causing her to cut down on her normal activities. Denies fever, chills, or night sweats. No acute distress

HEENT: Head normocephalic without evidence of masses or trauma. PERRLA, EOMs full to confrontation. Noninjected. Fundoscopic exam unremarkable with exception of pale retinal background. Palpebral conjunctiva pale. Ear canal without redness or irritation, TM clear, pearly, bony landmarks visible. No discharge, no pain noted. Pale nasal mucosa. Posterior pharynx pale with beefy red tongue. Neck supple without masses. No thyromegaly. No JVD

CV: S_1 and S_2 RRR, no murmurs, no gallops, no rubs

Lungs: Clear to auscultation

Abdomen: Soft, nontender, nondistended, bowel sounds present × 4 quadrants, no organomegaly, no bruits

Back: Nontender to palpation. No pain with forward flexion of low back but reports some mild dizziness with touching toes. No CVA tenderness

GU: Normal pelvic exam

Rectal: Normal vault, good tone, heme-negative stool

Neuro: CN II–XII intact. Rhine/Weber normal, Romberg positive. Some difficulty with tandem walking. Paresthesias noted with monofilament testing of bilateral feet, DTR 1+

Lab results:

▶ RBC, Hgb, Hct, WBC, B_{12} decreased

▶ LDH, ALT, MCV, RDW elevated

▶ Peripheral blood smear (macrocytosis, hyperpigmented neutrophils, and giant platelets)

▶ Schilling's test (positive)

A: Hypoproliferative macrocytic anemia secondary to vitamin B_{12} deficiency

Peripheral neuropathy related to vitamin B_{12} deficiency

Leukopenia secondary to vitamin B_{12} deficiency

Thrombocytopenia secondary to vitamin B_{12} deficiency

Elevated LDH and ALT secondary to vitamin B_{12} deficiency

Glossitis due to vitamin B_{12} deficiency

P: Begin vitamin B_{12} supplementation. Refer for dietary consultation to increase vitamin B_{12}–rich foods. Schedule colonoscopy, mammogram, and well-woman exam. Recheck in 1 month.

■ Health Promotion Issues[7–8]

▶ Schedule for a mammogram once her anemia is stable.

▶ Vaccinations are up-to-date.

▶ Schedule well-woman exam

▶ Schedule colonoscopy.

Remember that anemia is never normal, and the history and physical exam are key in narrowing down the diagnosis. Be certain to carefully review medications for a cause of anemia. Vitamin B_{12} deficiency usually occurs over 3 or more years, and by the time you make the diagnosis, neurologic manifestations may be present. Also, iron-deficiency anemia (IDA) occurs in about a third of patients with pernicious anemia, which may be a cause for incomplete response to therapy.

■ Guidelines to Direct Care

Centers for Disease Control and Prevention. Recommended adult immunization schedule, by vaccine and age group. 2015. http://www.cdc.gov/vaccines/schedules/hcp/imz/adult.html. Accessed September 16, 2015.

US Preventive Services Task Force: Published recommendations. http://www.uspreventiveservicestaskforce.org/BrowseRec/Index/browse-recommendations. Accessed September 16, 2015.

World Health Organization. Haemogolobin concentrations for the diagnosis of anaemia and assessment of severity. Vitamin and Mineral Nutrition Information System. Geneva: World Health Organization; 2011. http://www.who.int/vmnis/indicators/haemoglobin.pdf. Accessed September 16, 2015.

■ Case 3

Mrs. Smith is a 63-year-old African American female who recently had a blood count done at her local health fair. She was told to see her healthcare provider because she had a "low blood count." Mrs. Smith is in generally good health with a history of degenerative joint disease (DJD) of the hips, which necessitated right hip replacement 2 years ago. She takes no daily medications, uses aspirin (ASA) occasionally for "aches and pains," and has NKDA. She donates blood about every 6 months and has never been told she has anemia. Mrs. Smith has been married for the past 43 years and has three grown children who are alive and well. She and her husband are retired and live in an isolated area about 90 miles from the health clinic. Vaccinations up-to-date, including tetanus, Pneumovax, shingles, and an annual flu shot. Well-woman exam and mammogram completed last year and all normal. Feels well and denies fatigue, weight loss, or easy bruising. Denies chest pain, SOB, palpitations, lightheadedness, orthopnea, or paroxysmal nocturnal dyspnea (PND). Denies recent upper respiratory infections. No chronic cough or sputum production. No abdominal pain, weight loss, nausea, vomiting, or diarrhea. Denies bloody stools or mucus in stools. Denies illicit drug use, denies tobacco use, reports drinks approximately four cocktails per night.

■ Physical Exam

Vital Signs: BP 138/88, P 96 regular, RR 16, T 97.6, Ht 5′6″, Wt 150 lbs

GEN: Healthy-appearing, enthusiastic woman, very cooperative

Skin: Several scattered seborrheic keratoses

HEENT: PERRLA, EOMs full to confrontation. Normal pharynx without exudates. No JVD or thyromegaly

CV: S_1 and S_2 RRR, no murmurs, gallops, or rubs

Resp: Clear to auscultation

Breasts: No masses

Abdomen: Soft, nontender, nondistended. Bowel sounds present × 4 quadrants. No masses or organomegaly

Rectal: Normal vault, good tone. No hemorrhoids. Fecal occult blood testing negative

Neuro: Normal cerebral functioning. Cranial nerves II–XII intact. Normal sensory and motor exam, Romberg-normal

What additional assessments/diagnostics do you need?

What is the differential diagnoses list?

What is your working diagnosis?

■ Additional Assessments/Diagnostics Needed

Mrs. Smith presents without symptoms of anemia but with suspicion that anemia may be present.[1–4,7–8,10–13] Detailed exploration of her medical history, including family history, and laboratory and diagnostic studies will be important to help narrow the potential cause. She is asymptomatic at this time, which would suggest that the anemia is not severe and has not been a longstanding issue.

Evaluation for Mrs. Smith's suspected anemia should include:

- ▶ Risk factors for anemia:
  - ▶ *Age*
  - ▶ *Diet:* Exploration of Mrs. Smith's diet would be necessary to determine dietary intake of vitamin B_{12}, folate, and iron
  - ▶ *Intestinal disorders:* Mrs. Smith denies a history of intestinal disorders.
  - ▶ *Chronic diseases:* Mrs. Smith denies personal history of chronic disease.
  - ▶ *Females:* Pregnancy, childbirth, and dysfunctional uterine bleeding predispose women to anemia. Mrs. Smith is postmenopausal and denies any abnormal bleeding.
  - ▶ *Inherited:* Mrs. Smith has no history of inherited blood disorders.
  - ▶ *Bone marrow dysfunction such as myelodysplastic syndrome, blood or bone cancers, and marrow suppression by medications, toxins, or disease:* Drugs that can decrease folic acid measurements include alcohol, aminosalicylic acid (ASA), birth control pills, estrogens, tetracyclines, ampicillin, chloramphenicol, erythromycin, methotrexate, penicillin, aminopterin, phenobarbital, phenytoin, and drugs to treat malaria.
- ▶ Identifiable causes of anemia:
  - ▶ *Bleeding:* Either chronic or acute blood loss can be the cause of anemia. In the case of Mrs. Smith, she denies any signs or symptoms of upper gastrointestinal blood loss, she denies any postmenopausal bleeding, and her stool was negative for blood during exam, which lessens the likelihood that her anemia is related to lower gastrointestinal loss. Depending on her laboratory testing, this cause of anemia may need to be explored in addition to other more likely causes.
  - ▶ *Diminished red blood cell (RBC) production:* Laboratory testing will determine whether a vitamin deficiency is the cause for Mrs. Smith's diminished blood counts.
  - ▶ *Rapid rates of red blood cell destruction:* Inherited or acquired diseases that cause an increased rate of RBC destruction can lead to anemia. Mrs. Smith's medical history does not suggest any of these potential causes nor does her physical examination reveal enlargement or abnormality of the spleen. If other causes are ruled out, further studies for causative agents of hemolytic anemia may be undertaken.
- ▶ Presence or absence of complications of anemia:
  - ▶ Arrhythmia (not present)
  - ▶ Congestive heart failure (not present)
  - ▶ End organ damage such as liver and kidney failure (not present)

ROS

Focus additional questions on assessment of the impact that her anemia symptoms are having on her activities of daily living as well as potential clues to the cause of her anemia, including:

- ▶ Fatigue (denies)
- ▶ Chest pain (denies)
- ▶ Palpitations (denies)
- ▶ Shortness of breath (SOB) (denies)
- ▶ Dyspnea on exertion (DOE) (denies)
- ▶ Dizziness (denies)
- ▶ Headache (denies)
- ▶ Coolness in hands and feet or paresthesias (denies)
- ▶ Worsening of these symptoms with activity can provide an estimate of the severity of her anemia (denies)

Explore her health history further, making note of hints to what the cause of anemia may be:

- ▶ ETOH use. Administer CAGE questionnaire (Mrs. Smith reports drinking 4 cocktails per night)
- ▶ Medications that may interfere with absorption such as hormones, anticonvulsants, antineoplastic agents (Mrs. Smith reports using ASA for her DJD)
- ▶ Diet recall (vegetarian, low intake of B vitamins) (denies)

Physical Exam

The physical examination for this patient should include:

- ▶ A thorough assessment of the heart and lungs for s/s of cardiac complications of anemia (arrhythmias, extracardiac sounds, murmurs or rubs, auscultation of lungs)
- ▶ Evaluation for fluid overload (peripheral edema, JVD, cardiac and lung evaluation)
- ▶ Appropriate measurement of blood pressure with verification in the contralateral arm
- ▶ Palpation of the lower extremities for edema and peripheral pulses
- ▶ Examination of the abdomen for enlarged spleen, liver, changes in kidneys, masses, and abnormal aortic pulsations
- ▶ Examination of the skin and nails for complications of anemia (spoon nails [koilonychias])
- ▶ Examination of the mucous membranes for s/s of anemia (pallor, glossitis of the tongue, angular cheilitis of the mouth)

Routine Labs

Routine labs for Mrs. Smith should include those directed at assessing her anemia.

Baseline studies:

- ▶ Comprehensive metabolic panel, including:
  - ▶ Albumin (normal)
  - ▶ Alkaline phosphatase (normal)

- ALT (alanine aminotransferase) (elevated)
- AST (aspartate aminotransferase) (elevated)
- BUN (normal)
- Creatinine (normal)
- Calcium (normal)
- Chloride (normal)
- Carbon dioxide (normal)
- Glucose (normal)
- Potassium (normal)
- Sodium (normal)
- Total bilirubin (normal)
- Total protein (normal)
- Complete blood count, including:
  - RBC (low)
  - Hgb (low)
  - Hct (low)
  - MCV (elevated)
  - MCH (normal)
  - MCHC (normal)
  - Platelets (low)
  - WBC (basophils, eosinophils, lymphocytes, monocytes, neutrophils) (low)
- Urinalysis (normal)

Additional anemia studies:

- Serum iron (normal)
- Serum ferritin (normal)
- Total iron-binding capacity (TIBC) (normal)
- Vitamin B_{12} (normal)
- Folate (low)
- Reticulocyte count (normal)
- RDW (elevated)
- Peripheral blood smear (abnormally large RBC—megaloblasts)
- Schilling's test (negative)

Additional Labs and Diagnostic Testing

- *Liver function tests:* Done as baseline study related to possible causes of anemia and potential for alcohol-related changes (elevated)
- *Cholesterol panel:* Advised to assess for CVD. Done as baseline study related to Mrs. Smith's age (normal)
- *Thyroid studies:* If thyroid disease is suspected. Not done in this case

- *EPO:* Erythropoietin studies may be ordered to determine whether erythropoietin deficiency is the cause of anemia. Not done in this case
- *Schilling's test:* The Schilling's test is helpful in differentiating vitamin B_{12}–deficiency anemia from folic acid–deficiency anemia. Mrs. Smith's Schilling's test is negative.

Potential diagnostic studies:

- Colonoscopy for wellness and to r/o occult GI bleed

Differential Diagnoses List

Folic acid deficiency

Vitamin B_{12} deficiency

Iron-deficiency anemia

Anemia of blood loss

Alcohol abuse

Working Diagnoses

Anemia due to frequent blood donations

Occult GI malignancy (ruled out by colonoscopy)

Alcohol abuse

Folate deficiency

Pathophysiology[12,13,20]

Folate deficiency leads to decreased production of RBCs and resultant anemia. This deficiency can be caused by a diet lacking in folic acid, alcoholism, use of certain medications, and pregnancy. Mrs. Smith's alcohol consumption would be defined as heavy drinking and would be a substantial risk factor for folic acid deficiency. Folate deficiency may occur simultaneously with other forms of anemia such as vitamin B_{12}–deficiency and iron-deficiency anemia.

What Is Your Treatment Plan?

Pharmacologic

- Begin oral iron therapy. FeSO4 325mg QD. Include client education about the drug
- Discuss proper administration (on empty stomach), possibility of constipation, dark-colored stools.
- Start folic acid 0.4 mg PO QD.

Nonpharmacologic

- Discuss diet to increase foods with iron and folic acid.
- Follow-up in 3 months to check complete blood count (CBC), folic acid, and BP. Don't expect return to normal folic acid for 2–3 months.

Education/Counseling[12,13,19,20]

▶ Encourage no more than two blood donations per year (three blood donations per year is roughly equivalent to the blood loss of normal menses in one year). The American Red Cross suggests waiting about 56 days between donations.

▶ Review other healthy lifestyle issues with her: exercise, stress management, diet

▶ Discuss ETOH use. According to the American Heart Association (AHA), women should drink no more than 4 oz of wine, 12 oz of beer, or 1 oz of hard liquor daily. Discuss risk of falls with Mrs. Smith related to ETOH use. When considering referral for ETOH-related issues, consider that the primary care provider (PCP) is likely to have the best working and trusting relationship with the patient. Discuss the ETOH issue and the impact ETOH is having on her health. Refer only when the patient is in agreement with the need for this. Without buy-in from the patient, she may not follow through or may be reluctant to share other concerns with you.

SOAP Note

S: Mrs. Smith is a 63-year-old African American female who reports a low blood count was identified at a local health fair. She reports a history of degenerative joint disease in her hips that necessitated a right hip replacement 2 years ago. She takes no daily medications currently, but she uses aspirin as needed for joint pain. NKDA. She donates blood about every 6 months and has never been told she has anemia. Mrs. Smith is retired, has been married for the past 43 years, and has three grown children who are alive and well. Vaccinations up-to-date; well-woman exam and mammogram completed last year were normal. Feels well and denies fatigue, weight loss, or easy bruising. Denies chest pain, SOB, palpitations, lightheadedness, orthopnea, or PND. No abdominal pain, weight loss, nausea, vomiting, diarrhea, bloody stools, or mucus in stools. Reports she drinks approximately four cocktails per night, but denies tobacco use or illicit drug use.

O: *Vital Signs:* BP 138/88, P 96 regular, RR 16, T 97.6, Ht 5'6", Wt 150 lbs

GEN: Healthy-appearing, enthusiastic woman, very cooperative

Skin: Several scattered seborrheic keratoses

HEENT: PERRLA, EOMs full to confrontation. Normal pharynx without exudates. No JVD or thyromegaly

CV: S_1 and S_2 RRR, no murmurs, gallops, or rubs

Resp: Clear to auscultation

Breasts: No masses

Abdomen: Soft, nontender, nondistended. Bowel sounds present × 4 quadrants. No masses or organomegaly

Rectal: Normal vault, good tone. No hemorrhoids. Fecal occult blood testing negative

Neuro: Normal cerebral functioning. Cranial nerves II–XII intact. Normal sensory and motor exam, Romberg-normal

A: Anemia due to frequent blood donations

Occult GI malignancy (ruled out by colonoscopy)

Alcohol abuse

Folate deficiency

P: Colonoscopy to r/o GI malignancy. Begin folate 0.4 mg PO QD and iron 325 mg PO QD. Encourage reevaluation of alcohol consumption and referral to appropriate support/treatment as she is willing. Encourage diet rich in folic acid.

Health Promotion Issues[7–8]

▶ Colonoscopy

▶ Vaccinations are up-to-date

Guidelines to Direct Care

American Heart Association. Alcohol and heart health. http://www.heart.org/HEARTORG/GettingHealthy/NutritionCenter/HealthyEating/Alcohol-and-Heart-Health_UCM_305173_Article.jsp. Accessed September 16, 2015.

American Red Cross. Donating blood: eligibility guidelines. http://www.redcrossblood.org/donating-blood/eligibility-requirements. Accessed September 16, 2015.

Centers for Disease Control and Prevention. Recommended adult immunization schedule, by vaccine and age group. 2015. http://www.cdc.gov/vaccines/schedules/hcp/imz/adult.html. Accessed September 16, 2015.

National Institutes of Health, National Institute on Alcohol Abuse and Alcoholism. Alcohol use disorder guideline. http://www.niaaa.nih.gov/alcohol-health/overview-alcohol-consumption/alcohol-use-disorders. Accessed September 16, 2015.

US Dept of Agriculture, US Dept of Health and Human Services. *Dietary Guidelines for Americans, 2010.* 7th ed. Washington, DC: US Government Printing Office; December 2010. http://health.gov/dietaryguidelines/dga2010/dietaryguidelines2010.pdf. Accessed September 16, 2015.

US Preventive Services Task Force. Published recommendations. http://www.uspreventiveservicestaskforce.org/BrowseRec/Index/browse-recommendations. Accessed September 16, 2015.

Case 4

Mr. Snow is a 65-year-old male with progressively increasing SOB over the last 2 months. His SOB sometimes occurs at rest and often prevents him from shopping and walking up an incline. Admitted to the hospital 6 months ago with an episode of unstable angina that did not progress to acute myocardial infarction (AMI). Takes 325 mg ASA, 50 mg atenolol, and 40 mg simvastatin since his recent admission. Denies any other chronic medical problems or surgeries. NKDA. Smoked 20 cigarettes daily × 30 years. Stopped "cold turkey" after recent hospital admission. Rarely sees a healthcare provider. Does not believe in immunizations. Denies fever or rashes. No pruritus or skin color changes. Denies chest pain (CP), palpitations, or dizziness. Reports progressively increasing SOB both at rest and with exertion. Denies cough, sputum production, wheezing, orthopnea, or PND. Denies weight change. No abdominal pain, nausea, or vomiting. Denies bloody or mucous stools.

Physical Exam

Vital Signs: BP 120/70, HR 56 regular, RR 14, T 98.5, Ht 6'0", Wt 165 lbs

GEN: Alert and cooperative. In no apparent distress.

HEENT: Head normocephalic without evidence of masses or trauma. PERRLA, EOMs full to confrontation. Noninjected. Fundoscopic exam unremarkable with exception of pale retinal background. Palpebral conjunctiva pale. Ear canal without redness or irritation, TM clear, pearly, bony landmarks visible. No discharge, no pain noted. Pale nasal mucosa. Posterior pharynx pale. Neck: Supple without masses. No thyromegaly. No JVD noted

Skin: No discoloration, no open areas or abnormalities noted

CV: S_1 and S_2 regular with a soft aortic ejection murmur in the aortic area. No radiation to carotids or axilla. No JVD. No peripheral edema

Lungs: Minimal scattered rhonchi that resolve with coughing

Abdomen: Bowel sounds present in all quads. Abdomen soft with no organomegaly

Rectal: Normal vault, good tone, heme-positive stool

Neuro: Normal cerebral functioning. CN II–XII intact. Normal sensory and motor exam, Romberg negative

What additional assessments/diagnostics do you need?
What is the differential diagnoses list?
What is your working diagnosis?

Additional Assessments/Diagnostics Needed

Mr. Snow presents with symptoms that are troubling and may be attributable to respiratory disease, cardiac causes, or anemia.[1–4,7–8,10,14–18] Mr. Snow's history suggests that any of the aforementioned causes are plausible. Further exploration, laboratory testing, and diagnostics will need to be completed to provide clarity and direct treatment.

ROS

Focus additional questions on assessment of the impact that his anemia symptoms are having on his activities of daily living as well as potential clues to the cause of his anemia, including:

- Chest pain (denies)
- Palpitations (denies)
- Shortness of breath (SOB) (Mr. Snow reports SOB)
- Dyspnea on exertion (DOE) (Mr. Snow reports DOE)
- Dizziness (denies)
- Headache (denies)
- Coolness in hands and feet or paresthesias (denies)
- Nausea/vomiting (denies)
- Worsening of these symptoms with activity can provide an estimate of the severity of his anemia

Further discussion of cardiovascular risk factors should also be explored, including:

- *HTN:* None noted
- *Cigarette smoking:* Mr. Snow is a former smoker but is not currently
- *Obesity:* Mr. Snow has a normal body mass index
- *Physical inactivity:* Mr. Snow does not exercise
- *Dyslipidemia:* Present but under treatment by cardiologist
- *Diabetes mellitus:* You will need to order labs
- *Age:* Mr. Snow is 65 years old
- *Family history:* When queried further he reports his mother and father both had HTN and CVD. This is a significant risk factor

Evaluation for Suspected Anemia

- Risk factors for anemia:
  - Anemia risk increases with age. Although the exact etiology of anemia in elderly persons may be multifactorial, advancing age is a known risk factor for anemia.
  - A diet that is deficient in quality protein sources and B vitamins is a known risk factor for anemia. Hematopoiesis requires healthy levels of macronutrients and micronutrients in order to carry out cell production and maturation.
  - Intestinal disorders such as malabsorptive disorders, parasitism, lack of intrinsic factor, gastric bypass surgery, Crohn's disease, and ulcerative colitis increase the risk of anemia.

- Chronic diseases such as thyroid, liver, kidney, or autoimmune diseases as well as HIV/AIDS and cancer increase the risk of anemia.
- Pregnancy, childbirth, and dysfunctional uterine bleeding predispose women to anemia.
- Inherited diseases such as sickle cell disease or trait as well as the thalassemias can interfere with production and maturation of red blood cells.
- Bone marrow dysfunction such as myelodysplastic syndrome, blood or bone cancers, and marrow suppression by medications, toxins, or disease increase the risk for anemia.
- Identifiable causes of anemia:
  - *Bleeding:* Either chronic or acute blood loss can be the cause of anemia. In the case of Mr. Snow, he does have symptoms of lower gastrointestinal blood loss because his stool was positive for blood during examination today. This potential cause of his anemia will need to be explored with further diagnostic studies.
  - *Diminished red blood cell (RBC) production:* Mr. Snow's history does not suggest this as a potential cause of his anemia. If other causes are ruled out, further studies may need to be completed.
  - *Rapid rates of red blood cell destruction:* Inherited or acquired diseases that cause an increased rate of RBC destruction can lead to anemia. Mr. Snow's medical history does not suggest any of these potential causes nor does his physical examination reveal enlargement or abnormality of his spleen. If suspected, laboratory studies to rule out sickle cell disease and thalassemia should be performed. If other causes are ruled out, further studies for causative agents of hemolytic anemia may be undertaken.
- Presence or absence of complications of anemia:
  - Arrhythmia
  - Congestive heart failure
  - End organ damage such as liver and kidney failure

Physical Exam

The physical examination for this patient should include:

- A thorough assessment of the heart and lungs for s/s of cardiac complications of anemia and kidney disease (arrhythmias, extracardiac sounds, murmurs or rubs, auscultation of lungs). Mr. Snow has an ejection murmur.
- Evaluation for fluid overload (peripheral edema, JVD, cardiac and lung evaluation). None noted.
- Appropriate measurement of blood pressure with verification in the contralateral arm. Mr. Snow has a normal BP bilaterally.
- Palpation of the lower extremities for edema and peripheral pulses. None noted.

- Examination of the abdomen for enlarged spleen, liver, changes in kidneys (either enlarged or smaller than anticipated), masses, and abnormal aortic pulsations. None noted.
- Examination of the skin and nails for complications of anemia and kidney disease (pruritus, spoon nails [koilonychias]). None noted.
- Examination of the mucous membranes for s/s of anemia (pallor, glossitis of the tongue, angular cheilitis of the mouth). Pallor noted.

Labs

Mr. Snow is under the care of a cardiologist since his hospital admission 6 months ago, when his cholesterol panels were completed and a medication regimen initiated. Laboratory evaluation at this visit should focus on those issues that may be contributing to his increasing SOB.

- *D-dimer:* D-dimer may be completed if a pulmonary embolism (PE) is suspected. Mr. Snow is not acutely SOB and is in no apparent distress, so this cause is unlikely. The D-dimer may be elevated with inflammation from a number of causes, so false positives are possible. This evaluation was not done for this patient at this visit.
- *WBC:* Will be completed as part of CBC to evaluate for potential of infection

Routine Labs

Routine labs for Mr. Snow should include those directed at assessing for anemia, infection, and end organ function.

Baseline studies:
- Comprehensive metabolic panel, including:
  - Albumin (normal)
  - Alkaline phosphatase (normal)
  - ALT (alanine aminotransferase) (normal)
  - AST (aspartate aminotransferase) (normal)
  - BUN (normal)
  - Creatinine (normal)
  - Calcium (normal)
  - Chloride (normal)
  - Carbon dioxide (normal)
  - Glucose (normal)
  - Potassium (normal)
  - Sodium (normal)
  - Total bilirubin (normal)
  - Total protein (normal)
- Complete blood count, including:
  - RBC (low)
  - Hgb 11.9% (low)
  - Hct 38% (low)

- ▸ MCV (low normal)
- ▸ MCH (normal)
- ▸ MCHC (normal)
- ▸ Platelets (normal)
- ▸ WBCs (basophils, eosinophils, lymphocytes, monocytes, neutrophils) (normal)

Additional kidney function studies:

- ▸ Urinalysis (UA) (normal)

Additional anemia studies:

- ▸ Serum iron (low)
- ▸ Serum ferritin (low)
- ▸ Total iron-binding capacity (TIBC) (high)
- ▸ Vitamin B_{12} (Not completed for Mr. Snow)
- ▸ Folate (Not completed for Mr. Snow)
- ▸ Reticulocyte count (elevated)
- ▸ RDW (elevated)
- ▸ Peripheral blood smear (variably sized with some abnormally shaped and some hypochromic RBC noted)

Additional Labs

- ▸ Cholesterol panel—completed at prior hospitalization. Medications managed by cardiologist
- ▸ Thyroid studies—not completed for Mr. Snow
- ▸ EPO—not completed for Mr. Snow

Diagnostics should include:

- ▸ In-office EKG—unchanged from prior studies
- ▸ Chest X-ray to rule out pneumonia and evaluate cardiac size and anatomical structures of lungs—negative for pneumonia, cardiac silhouette normal, lung with changes noted consistent with COPD
- ▸ Colonoscopy—Mr. Snow has blood in his stool per the test during the examination. Further evaluation is necessary to rule out malignancy, determine extent of ongoing blood loss.

Differential Diagnoses

Chronic obstructive pulmonary disease (COPD)—smoker, rhonchi

Cardiac failure—left sided, angina

Anemia—ASA, diet, pallor, ejection murmur

Poor physical conditioning

Asthma

Pneumonia

PE—may occur in the absence of coughing up blood

GI bleeding—subclinical bleeding, has been taking ASA for past 6 months

Ejection murmur

Working Diagnosis

Anemia related to subclinical bleeding due to ASA use

COPD

Hyperlipidemia

Ejection murmur

Pathophysiology

Iron-deficiency anemia can be caused by a low-iron diet, loss of blood, impaired iron absorption, or loss of body stores of iron that have been depleted by disease states.[18] Early iron-deficiency anemia (IDA) is characterized by a normocytic, possibly hypochromic anemia with progression to a microcytic hypochromic anemia in later phases. In the case of Mr. Snow, his anemia has been precipitated by ASA use and a subclinical GI bleed and is in an early phase, according to his lab values. With correction of the underlying disease process and iron supplementation, his anemia should correct.

What Is Your Treatment Plan?

Pharmacologic

- ▸ Begin iron supplementation with FeSO4 at 325 mg PO QD.
- ▸ Modify ASA regimen to 81 mg QD. ASA would be recommended in this patient r/t his murmur and for CVD, but if the bleeding continues, further consultation with the cardiologist would need to be initiated to determine risk/benefit of continued therapy. Simply reducing the ASA is the easiest and most cost-effective plan. Proton pump inhibitor therapy is not indicated because of lack of GI symptoms.[7–8,15,17–18]

Nonpharmacologic

- ▸ Consider pulmonary function testing to determine whether further treatment is indicated for his COPD.
- ▸ Keep normal follow-ups with cardiology.
- ▸ Congratulate him on decision to quit smoking and encourage him to stay the course.
- ▸ Continue follow-up (f/u) with cardiologist.

Education/Counseling[10,12,14–16]

- ▸ Diet education with an emphasis on iron-rich foods
- ▸ Education regarding s/s of worsening
- ▸ Medication education—when and how to take, side effects (constipation). Change in color of stool, nausea
- ▸ Educate patient on pursed-lip breathing and COPD management goals

SOAP Note

S: Mr. Snow is a 65-year-old male with a 2-month history of progressively increasing SOB at rest and worsening dyspnea on exertion. Mr. Snow was hospitalized for unstable angina without MI 6 months ago and was started on ASA

325 mg, atenolol 50 mg, and simvastatin 40 mg daily. NKDA. 30-pack-year history of tobacco use but stopped "cold turkey" after recent hospital admission. Rarely sees a healthcare provider. Does not believe in immunizations. Denies fever or rashes. No pruritus or skin color changes. Denies CP, palpitations, or dizziness. Denies cough, sputum production, wheezing, orthopnea, or PND. Denies weight change, abdominal pain, nausea, vomiting, or bloody or mucous stools.

O: *Vital Signs:* BP 120/70, P 56 regular, RR 14, T 98.5, Ht 6'0", Wt 165 lbs

GEN: Alert and cooperative. In NAD

HEENT: Head normocephalic without evidence of masses or trauma. PERRLA, EOMs full to confrontation. Noninjected. Fundoscopic exam unremarkable with exception of pale retinal background. Palpebral conjunctiva pale. Ear canal without redness or irritation, TM clear, pearly, bony landmarks visible. No discharge, no pain noted. Pale nasal mucosa. Posterior pharynx pale. Neck supple without masses. No thyromegaly. No JVD noted

Skin: No discoloration, no open areas or abnormalities noted

CV: S_1 and S_2 regular with a soft aortic ejection murmur in the aortic area. No radiation to carotids or axilla. No JVD. No peripheral edema

Lungs: Minimal scattered rhonchi that resolve with coughing

Abdomen: Bowel sounds present in all quads. Abdomen soft with no organomegaly

Rectal: Normal vault, good tone, heme-positive stool

Neuro: Normal cerebral functioning. CN II–XII intact. Normal sensory and motor exam, Romberg negative

ECG: Unchanged

Labs: Normocytic, hypochromic anemia consistent with IDA

A: Anemia related to subclinical bleeding due to ASA use

COPD

Hyperlipidemia

Ejection murmur

P: Mr. Snow presents today with subclinical lower GI bleeding secondary to ASA therapy resulting in IDA. Mr. Snow's history and physical examination are also significant for hyperlipidemia, ejection murmur, and COPD. Cardiology is already involved

and following lipid management and ejection murmur. Will start Mr. Snow on FeSo4 325 mg PO QD today, continue on atenolol and simvastatin ordered by cardiologist. Education provided regarding COPD management, health management, and immunization recommendations today. Mr. Snow verbalized understanding of topics discussed but currently refuses vaccination for prevention of shingles, pneumonia, influenza, tetanus.

▌ Health Promotion Issues[7–8,12]

▶ Encourage routine follow-ups for health maintenance.

▶ Encourage routine cardiology follow-up.

▶ Immunizations recommended: shingles, pneumonia, influenza, tetanus.

▌ *Guidelines to Direct Care*

Centers for Disease Control and Prevention. Recommended adult immunization schedule, by vaccine and age group. 2015. http://www.cdc.gov/vaccines/schedules/hcp/imz/adult.html. Accessed September 16, 2015.

Qaseem A, Humphrey LL, Fitterman N, et al. Treatment of anemia in patients with heart disease: a clinical practice guideline from the American College of Physicians. *Ann Intern Med.* December 3, 2013;159(11):770–779.

US Dept of Agriculture, US Dept of Health and Human Services. *Dietary Guidelines for Americans, 2010.* 7th ed. Washington, DC: US Government Printing Office; December 2010. http://health.gov/dietaryguidelines/dga2010/dietary guidelines2010.pdf. Accessed September 16, 2015.

US Preventive Services Task Force. Published recommendations. http://www.uspreventiveservicestaskforce.org/Browse Rec/Index/browse-recommendations. Accessed September 16, 2015.

Vestbo J, Hurd SS, Agustí AG, et al. Global strategy for the diagnosis, management, and prevention of chronic obstructive pulmonary disease. 2013. http://www.goldcopd.org/uploads/users/files/GOLD_Report_2013_Feb20.pdf

World Health Organization. Haemogolobin concentrations for the diagnosis of anaemia and assessment of severity. Vitamin and Mineral Nutrition Information System. Geneva: World Health Organization; 2011. http://www.who.int/vmnis/indicators/haemoglobin.pdf. Accessed September 16, 2015.

▌ Case 5

Latisha is a 38-year-old African American woman who presents to the clinic for a new patient physical examination. Latisha is concerned about persistent mild fatigue, which she reports has been gradually worsening for the last 6 months. She has noted a gradual decrease in her work tolerance and feels "washed out" at the end of the workday. She reports no changes in her diet. She denies nausea, vomiting, or diarrhea. She has not noted any dark stools or blood in her stools but admits to an occasional mild nosebleed. She also mentions that her menstrual flow has been a little heavier than usual for the past several months. She denies cold intolerance, muscle weakness, fever, chills, or joint pain. She began to take over-the-counter vitamins, one tablet a day, 2 weeks ago. She reports feeling a bit better since she started her vitamins.

Past Medical History

Allergies: NKDA

Medical illnesses: HTN, hx of depression treated 5 years ago with no reoccurrences

Hospitalizations: Normal vaginal delivery 10 years ago

S/P laparoscopic tubal ligation at the age of 33

Medications: Vasotec 10 mg daily

Multivitamin with iron daily

ASA 1 tablet 325 mg daily

Family History

Latisha was born in the United States. Her parents are natives of Algeria. No family history of sickle cell disease, diabetes, kidney disease, HTN, cancer, or thyroid disease.

Social History

Her parents are college professors. Latisha has one brother who is alive and well and attends a local high school. Latisha is employed at a local insurance company. She denies any changes in her work, home, or social life. She is a nonsmoker and a nondrinker. She denies illicit drug use.

Health Promotion History

Latisha's immunizations are up-to-date, including tetanus. She has never had a mammogram. She does SBE occasionally. She only sees her healthcare provider when she has a problem.

Focused ROS

General: Denies weight loss, night sweats, muscle aches, joint pain, lymphadenopathy, or fever

HEENT: Occasional mild nosebleed

CV: Denies chest pain, leg swelling, and palpitations

Resp: Denies SOB, DOE, or orthopnea. No cough or recent respiratory tract infections

GI: Denies nausea, vomiting, diarrhea, melena, or blood in her stools

GU: Denies polydipsia, polyuria, or polyphagia. Increase in menstrual flow for the past several months

Physical Exam

Vital Signs: BP 110/88, P 82 (regular), RR 14, T 99, Ht 5'2", Wt 135 lbs

GEN: Alert, oriented × 3, well nourished, in no acute distress

Skin: Normal distribution, normal skin turgor, no rashes

HEENT: Palpebral conjunctivae are pale bilaterally. No lymphadenopathy

CV: S_1 and S_2 RRR, no murmurs, gallops, or rubs

Lungs: Clear to auscultation

Breasts: No masses or tenderness

Abdomen: Soft, nontender, no organomegaly

Neuro: Unremarkable

Extremities: Unremarkable

Pelvic: Normal

Rectal: Normal vault, no hemorrhoids, stool negative for occult blood

What additional assessments/diagnostics do you need?

What is the differential diagnoses list?

What is your working diagnosis?

Additional Assessments/Diagnostics Needed

Further exploration of Latisha's history should include exploration of the following:[1–4,7,8,18,19]

▶ What is the reason for taking ASA (Latisha reports she takes ASA for "heart health," but it was not ordered by another healthcare provider.)

▶ More info regarding her nosebleeds, diet, menstrual flow, headache, palpitations, fever, or sore throat (Latisha denies headache, palpitations, fever, or sore throat)

The following lab studies should be completed:

Baseline studies:

▶ Comprehensive metabolic panel, including:
  ▶ Albumin (normal)
  ▶ Alkaline phosphatase (normal)
  ▶ ALT (alanine aminotransferase) (normal)
  ▶ AST (aspartate aminotransferase) (normal)
  ▶ BUN (normal)
  ▶ Creatinine (normal)
  ▶ Calcium (normal)
  ▶ Chloride (normal)
  ▶ Carbon dioxide (normal)
  ▶ Glucose (normal)
  ▶ Potassium (normal)
  ▶ Sodium (normal)
  ▶ Total bilirubin (normal)
  ▶ Total protein (normal)
▶ Complete blood count, including:
  ▶ RBC (normal)
  ▶ Hgb (low)

- ▸ Hct (low)
- ▸ MCV (low)
- ▸ MCH (low)
- ▸ MCHC (low)
- ▸ Platelets (normal)
- ▸ WBC (basophils, eosinophils, lymphocytes, monocytes, neutrophils) (normal)

Additional kidney function studies:

- ▸ Urinalysis (UA) (normal)

Additional anemia studies:

- ▸ Serum iron (normal)
- ▸ Serum ferritin (normal)
- ▸ Total iron-binding capacity (TIBC) (normal)
- ▸ Reticulocyte count (normal)
- ▸ RDW (normal)
- ▸ Peripheral blood smear (nucleated target cells, poikilocytosis, microcytic, hypochromic RBC)

Additional labs:

- ▸ Thyroid studies—if thyroid disease is suspected. Not done for Latisha
- ▸ Hemoglobin electrophoresis—this test will determine whether thalassemia is present. Latisha's results were elevated A2 level and increased levels of Hgb F consistent with alpha thalassemia

Differential Diagnoses

Iron-deficiency anemia—Latisha is of reproductive age with monthly blood loss, making iron-deficiency anemia the most likely cause. Because of the microcytic hypochromic indices, the megaloblastic anemias can be ruled out.

Thalassemia—Latisha's parents are from the "thalassemia belt," so this diagnosis needs to be considered during the evaluation process.

Lead exposure—there are no apparent risk factors, but with the information you currently have from your evaluation it is a possibility.

Anemia of chronic disease—not likely based upon current information.

Hypertension—well controlled on current regimen.

Working Diagnoses

Alpha thalassemia

Hypertension

Pathophysiology

Thalassemia is a group of hereditary anemias caused by abnormalities on the protein chains that make up hemoglobin.[19]

Symptoms range from asymptomatic carrier states to fatal illness. Adult hemoglobin is made up primarily of alpha and beta chains. Thalassemia is most often seen in persons of African, Asian, Mediterranean, or Middle Eastern descent. The thalassemias are among the most common inherited disorders. Problems result from ineffective erythropoiesis. Thalassemia minor usually goes unrecognized until adulthood and is found on routine lab evaluation. It is a hypochromic and microcytic anemia and is most easily confirmed by hemoglobin electrophoresis, which would demonstrate an elevated A2 level, increased levels of hemoglobin F, or both. In some patients, the diagnosis can be confirmed by a family tree showing the presence of anemia, microcytosis, or splenomegaly.

▮ What Is Your Treatment Plan?

▮ Pharmacologic

- ▸ Discontinue the multivitamin (MVI). MVI with iron is not indicated for Latisha's alpha thalassemia.
- ▸ Continue vasotec.
- ▸ Discontinue ASA. Not indicated for this patient.[1–4,7–8,19]

▮ Nonpharmacologic

- ▸ Refer to hematology. Latisha should be referred to hematology for development of a monitoring plan and possible genetic counseling. Thalassemia is dependent on the ethnic origins of the client. B-thalassemia is seen in clients of Greek and Italian descent most commonly, and A-thalassemia is seen most commonly in African Americans, American Indians, and Asians.

▮ Education/Counseling

The importance of diagnosing thalassemia minor lies in the genetic information obtained because it does not require therapy. Sometimes lab data may indicate IDA, but iron is not needed unless there is excessive blood loss. In fact, iron therapy is harmful because iron overload may cause organ damage. It is very important that this patient is educated to avoid all iron (FE) supplements and foods high in FE.

▮ SOAP Note

S: Latisha is a 38-year-old African American woman of Algerian descent who presents to the clinic for a new patient physical examination. Latisha is concerned about persistent worsening fatigue. Latisha denies nausea, vomiting, diarrhea, dark stools, or blood in her stools but admits to an occasional mild nosebleed and heavier than usual menstrual periods. She denies cold intolerance, muscle weakness, fever, chills, or joint pain. She began to take an over-the-counter MVI, one tablet a day, 2 weeks ago. She reports feeling a bit better since she started taking the MVI.

O: *Vital Signs:* BP 110/88, P 82 (regular), RR 14, T 99, Ht 5'2", Wt 135 lbs

GEN: Alert, oriented × 3, well nourished, in no acute distress

Skin: Normal distribution, normal skin turgor, no rashes

HEENT: Palpebral conjunctivae are pale bilaterally. No lymphadenopathy

CV: S_1 and S_2 RRR, no murmurs, gallops, or rubs

Lungs: LCTA

Breasts: No masses or tenderness

Abdomen: Soft, nontender, no organomegaly

Neuro: Unremarkable

Extremities: Unremarkable

Pelvic: Normal

Rectal: Normal vault, no hemorrhoids, stool negative for occult blood

Labs: Nucleated target cells, poikilocytosis on smear. Microcytic, hypochromic anemia. Hgb electrophoresis consistent with alpha thalassemia

A: Alpha thalassemia — *microcytic hypochromic anemia*

Hypertension

P: Patient presents with alpha thalassemia. Refer to hematology for further evaluation. Continue vasotec. Discontinue ASA and MVI. Follow up in 6 months to reevaluate HTN and discuss results and understanding of information from hematology consultation.

Health Promotion Issues

▶ Emphasize importance of health maintenance and routine follow-up.

▶ Discuss alpha thalassemia and provide basic education prior to hematology consultation.

Guidelines to Direct Care

Centers for Disease Control and Prevention. Recommended adult immunization schedule, by vaccine and age group. 2015. http://www.cdc.gov/vaccines/schedules/hcp/imz/adult.html. Accessed September 16, 2015.

US Preventive Services Task Force. Published recommendations. http://www.uspreventiveservicestaskforce.org/BrowseRec/Index/browse-recommendations. Accessed September 16, 2015.

World Health Organization. Haemogolobin concentrations for the diagnosis of anaemia and assessment of severity. Vitamin and Mineral Nutrition Information System. Geneva: World Health Organization; 2011. http://www.who.int/vmnis/indicators/haemoglobin.pdf. Accessed September 16, 2015.

Conclusion

Keep in mind that the signs and symptoms of anemia are caused by decreased delivery of oxygen to peripheral tissues. Anemia is a common problem in primary care with dietary issues as a frequent causation. The leading cause of anemia in the United States is iron deficiency, followed by folate deficiency and vitamin B_{12} deficiency. You should suspect anemia if your patient complains of dizziness, exertional dyspnea, fatigue, headaches, loss of libido, mood changes, sleep problems, tinnitus, weakness, glossitis, jaundice, neuropathy, pallor, peripheral edema, splenomegaly, tachycardia, hemic murmur, or pica.

REFERENCES

1. American Society of Hematology. For patients: anemia. 2010. http://www.hematology.org/Patients/Anemia/. Accessed September 8, 2015.

2. Makipopur S, Kanapuru B, Ershler WB. Unexplained anemia in the elderly. *Semin Hematol.* October 2008;45(4):250–254. doi:10.1053/j.seminhematol.2008.06.003.

3. National Heart, Lung, and Blood Institute. What is anemia? 2012. http://www.nhlbi.nih.gov/health/health-topics/topics/anemia/.

4. World Health Organization. Haemogolobin concentrations for the diagnosis of anaemia and assessment of severity. 2011. http://www.who.int/vmnis/indicators/haemoglobin.pdf.

5. Kidney Disease: Improving Global Outcomes (KDIGO) Anemia Work Group. KDIGO clinical practice guideline for anemia in chronic kidney disease. *Kidney Int Suppl.* August 2012;2(4):279–335. http://www.kdigo.org/clinical_practice_guidelines/pdf/KDIGO-Anemia%20GL.pdf.

6. Kidney Disease: Improving Global Outcomes (KDIGO) Anemia Work Group. KDIGO 2012 clinical practice guideline for the evaluation and management of chronic kidney disease. *Kidney Int Suppl.* 2013;(3):1 http://www.kdigo.org/clinical_practice_guidelines/pdf/CKD/KDIGO_2012_CKD_GL.pdf.

7. US Preventive Services Task Force. Screening recommendations. http://www.uspreventiveservicestaskforce.org/BrowseRec/Index/browse-recommendations.

8. Centers for Disease Control and Prevention. Recommended adult immunization schedule, by vaccine and age group. 2014. http://www.cdc.gov/vaccines/schedules/hcp/imz/adult.html.

9. Langan R, Zawistoski K. Update on vitamin B_{12} deficiency. *Am Fam Physician*. 2011;83(12):1425–1430. http://www.aafp.org/afp/2011/0615/p1425.html.

10. US Dept of Agriculture and US Dept of Health and Human Services. *Dietary Guidelines for Americans, 2010*. 7th ed. Washington, DC: US Government Printing Office; 2010.

11. Ghadban R, Almourani R. Folate (folic acid). 2014. http://emedicine.medscape.com/article/2085523-overview.

12. American Heart Association. Alcohol and heart health. January 12, 2015. http://www.heart.org/HEARTORG/GettingHealthy/NutritionCenter/HealthyEating/Alcohol-and-Heart-Health_UCM_305173_Article.jsp.

13. National Institutes of Health, National Institute on Alcohol Abuse and Alcoholism. Alcohol use disorder. http://www.niaaa.nih.gov/alcohol-health/overview-alcohol-consumption/alcohol-use-disorders.

14. Qaseem A, Humphrey LL, Fitterman N, et al. Treatment of anemia in patients with heart disease: a clinical practice guideline from the American College of Physicians. *Ann Intern Med*. December 3, 2013;159(11):770–779.

15. Vestbo J, Hurd SS, Agustí AG, et al. Global strategy for the diagnosis, management, and prevention of chronic obstructive pulmonary disease. 2013. http://www.goldcopd.org/uploads/users/files/GOLD_Report_2013_Feb20.pdf.

16. Johnson-Wimbley TD. Diagnosis and management of iron deficiency anemia in the 21st century. *Therap Adv Gastroenterol*. May 2011;4(3):177–184. http://www.ncbi.nlm.nih.gov/pmc/articles/PMC3105608/.

17. Short MW, Domagalski JE. Iron deficiency anemia: evaluation and management. *Am Fam Physician*. 2013;87(2):98–104. http://www.aafp.org/afp/2013/0115/p98.

18. Piel FB, Weatherall DJ. The a-thalassemias. *N Engl J Med*. 2014;371(20):1908–1916.

19. American Red Cross. Eligibility requirements. February, 2015. http://www.redcrossblood.org/donating-blood/eligibility-requirements.

20. National Institutes of Health, National Institute on Alcohol Abuse and Alcoholism. Alcohol use disorder guideline. February, 2015. http://www.niaaa.nih.gov/alcohol-health/overview-alcohol-consumption/alcohol-use-disordersConclusion

Common Endocrine Disorders in Primary Care

Karen S. Moore

Chapter Outline

Learning Objectives

Using a case-based approach, the learner will be able to:

1. Identify key history and physical examination parameters for common endocrine disorders seen in primary care.

2. Summarize recommended laboratory and diagnostic studies indicated for the evaluation of common endocrine disorders seen in primary care.

3. State pathophysiology of common endocrine disorders.

4. Document a clear, concise SOAP note for patients with common endocrine disorders.

5. Identify relevant education and counseling strategies for patients with common endocrine disorders.

6. Develop a treatment plan for common endocrine disorders utilizing current evidence-based guidelines.

Case 1

Rudolph is a 14-year-old male who presents with complaints of (c/o) a sudden increase in thirst and urination as well as recent 5-lb unintentional weight loss. Rudolph's mother accompanies him to this appointment and states he has been doing usual activities and eating normally, but "he just seems off." Mother reports that Rudolph is normally an A student but has lately been sleeping more and "daydreaming" in class, according to reports from his teachers. Denies significant past medical history, denies recent known illness, denies known illness in close contacts. Denies headaches, chest pain, coughing, dizziness, nausea, vomiting. Denies surgeries or prior hospitalizations. No known drug allergies (NKDA). Reports all childhood immunizations were completed. States he does not normally receive the annual influenza vaccine because he does not think he needs it. Family history is significant for maternal grandmother with diabetes mellitus (DM), hypertension (HTN), and coronary artery disease (CAD) as well as paternal grandfather with DM and CAD. After mother leaves the examination room, Rudolph denies sexual activity and denies alcohol use, illicit drug use, tobacco use. Rudolph further states that he is feeling more drowsy during the daytime but feels he is sleeping well at night, so he is unsure why he is dozing in class. States he feels frustrated with his current state of health because it is interfering with his ability to "hang out" with friends.

Physical Exam

Vital Signs (VS): Blood pressure (BP) 96/54, heart rate (HR) 60 regular, respiratory rate (RR) 12, temperature (T) 98.5, height (Ht) 5'6", weight (Wt) 120 lbs

General (GEN): Well-appearing young male in no acute distress

Head, eyes, ears, nose, and throat (HEENT): Head normocephalic without evidence of masses or trauma. Pupils equal, round, react to light, accommodation (PERRLA), extraocular movements (EOMs) full to confrontation. Noninjected. Fundoscopic exam unremarkable. Ear canal without redness or irritation, tympanic membranes (TMs) clear, pearly, bony landmarks visible. No discharge, no pain noted. Oropharynx without redness, mucous membranes dry with thickened saliva noted. Neck supple without masses. No thyromegaly. No jugular vein distention (JVD) noted. No abnormalities along hairline. Skin: No lesions, no vesicles, no masses, no redness or erythema noted. Slight pruritus noted during examination.

Cardiovascular (CV): S_1 and S_2 regular rate and rhythm (RRR), no murmurs, no rubs

Lungs: Clear to auscultation (CTA)

Abdomen: Soft, nontender, nondistended, bowel sounds present × 4 quadrants, no organomegaly, no bruits

Genitourinary (GU): Tanner stage IV. No herniations, no masses, no discharge noted. No pain noted during examination.

What additional assessments/diagnostics do you need?

What is the differential diagnoses list?

What is your working diagnosis?

Additional Assessments/Diagnostics Needed

Ask focused review of systems (ROS) questions:[1-8]

▶ Nutritional assessment such as a 24-hour diet recall to assess for eating disorders and obvious nutritional deficits

▶ Ask Rudolph about any changes in urination quality, color, burning or irritation

▶ Inquire with Rudolph about any psychosocial issues such as bullying or depression

Exam

Rudolph's examination was relatively benign and vague in presentation, which is often the case with new-onset diabetes in younger patients. The differential diagnosis list is therefore broad and nonspecific prior to further in-office diagnostics.

Routine Labs/Diagnostics

A urinalysis (UA) was performed in the clinic and demonstrated very high levels of glucose and ketones. A fingerstick blood glucose was then taken, and the results displayed as HIGH ALERT. Rudolph and his mother were instructed to immediately proceed to the emergency room for admission and treatment, which they did. It would be anticipated that an arterial blood gas would be performed as soon as he arrived at the hospital to manage his presumptive ketoacidosis one would anticipate given his degree of hyperglycemia and ketosis. As part of the diagnostic workup for Rudolph, a C-peptide and autoantibodies may also be drawn and sent.

Differential Diagnoses List

Mononucleosis
Eating disorder
Depression
Diabetes mellitus

Working Diagnosis—Diabetes mellitus, type 1

Pathophysiology

Diabetes mellitus type 1 is believed to be an autoimmune response that causes the destruction of the insulin-producing beta cells within the islets of Langerhans in the pancreas. The destruction of the beta cells renders the patient unable to make insulin. For that reason, patients with type 1 DM cannot be managed on oral hypoglycemic agents but rather must receive exogenous insulin via injection or continuous infusion.

What Is Your Treatment Plan?

Immediate hospitalization for initial treatment of new-onset diabetes mellitus type 1 is necessary for this patient.[1-8] Rudolph is a young man who, based upon his Tanner staging, will continue to grow, causing his metabolic demands to vary. As such, once he is discharged from the hospital, referral to an endocrinologist would be anticipated related to the need for aggressive management of insulin therapy. Many young patients are managed quite well with an insulin pump, tight control of hyper-/hypoglycemia, and frequent monitoring. If a pump is not preferred, frequent monitoring and multiple daily injections of insulin would be utilized. Education for Rudolph, his mother, and other close family members and friends on the signs and symptoms (s/s) of hypo-/hyperglycemia and emergency protocols is very important.

Pharmacologic

Once Rudolph is stabilized, he will be managed on an insulin therapy regimen delivered via multiple daily injections or an infusion pump. The goal of insulin therapy is always to provide for the most stable blood sugar throughout the day and night while minimizing interventions by the patient when possible. Starting doses of insulin are based on weight, with a typical range of 0.4–0.5 u/kg/day. For many older insulin-dependent patients, long-acting insulin is given as a baseline dosage with sliding scale at mealtime monitoring. In young diabetic patients, more frequent monitoring with alteration in daily dosage is necessary to account for pubertal changes, menstruation, and changing body mass.

Nonpharmacologic

▶ Diabetes education:

  ▸ Diet management and its effect on diabetes

  ▸ Activity and how it relates to blood sugar control

  ▸ Sick-day management and how to modify insulin therapy when he is unable to eat or drink

  ▸ s/s of hypo-/hyperglycemia

  ▸ Blood sugar monitoring

  ▸ Emergency action plans

Education/Counseling

▶ Support groups can be very helpful to young people experiencing a life-altering illness.

▶ Parents and siblings may also benefit from a support group directed at their specific needs.

▶ Diabetes education for patient and close contacts should be encouraged. For Rudolph, this should include teachers, close peers, and coaches.[1-8]

SOAP Note

S: Rudolph is a 14-year-old male who presents with c/o a sudden increase in thirst and urination as well as recent 5-lb unintentional weight loss. Rudolph's mother accompanies him to this appointment and states he has been doing usual activities and eating normally, but "he just seems off." Mother reports that Rudolph is normally an A student but has lately been sleeping more and "daydreaming" in class, according to reports from his teachers. Denies significant past medical history, denies recent known illness, denies known illness in close contacts. Denies headaches, chest pain, coughing, dizziness, nausea, vomiting. Denies surgeries or prior hospitalizations. NKDA. Reports all childhood immunizations were completed. States he does not normally receive the annual influenza vaccine because he does not think he needs it. Family history is significant for maternal grandmother with DM, HTN, and CAD as well as paternal grandfather with DM and CAD. After mother leaves the examination room, Rudolph denies sexual activity and denies alcohol use, illicit drug use, tobacco use. Rudolph further states that he is feeling more drowsy during the daytime but feels he is sleeping well at night, so he is unsure why he is dozing in class. States he feels frustrated with his current state of health because it is interfering with his ability to "hang out" with friends.

O: *VS:* BP 96/54, HR 60 regular, RR 12, T 98.5, Ht 5'6", Wt 120 lbs

GEN: Well-appearing young male in no acute distress

HEENT: Head normocephalic without evidence of masses or trauma. PERRLA, EOMs full to confrontation. Noninjected. Fundoscopic exam unremarkable. Ear canal without redness or irritation, TMs clear, pearly, bony landmarks visible. No discharge, no pain noted. Oropharynx without redness, mucous membranes dry with thickened saliva noted. Neck supple without masses. No thyromegaly. No JVD noted. No abnormalities along hairline. Skin: No lesions, no vesicles, no masses, no redness or erythema noted. Slight pruritus noted during examination.

CV: S_1 and S_2 RRR, no murmurs, no rubs

Lungs: Clear to auscultation

Abdomen: Soft, nontender, nondistended, bowel sounds present × 4 quadrants, no organomegaly, no bruits

GU: Tanner stage IV. No herniations, no masses, no discharge noted. No pain noted during examination

A: Diabetes mellitus, type 1

P: Rudolph presents today with his mother and is found to have elevated blood sugar and urine ketones. Immediate hospitalization is ordered with follow-up at endocrinologist for management. Return follow-up at this office upon discharge from the hospital. Instructions provided to patient, hospital notified of need for immediate admission and endocrinology consultation. Patient, mother, and hospital triage registered nurse (RN) verbalized understanding of instructions and agreed to plan of care.

▮ Health Promotion

▶ Influenza vaccination annually

▶ Reassess post-hospitalization

▮ Guidelines to Direct Care

American Association of Clinical Endocrinologists. AACE/ACE comprehensive diabetes management algorithm. *Endocr Pract.* 2015;21(4):e1–e10. https://www.aace.com/files/aace_algorithm.pdf. Accessed September 22, 2015.

Centers for Disease Control and Prevention. Recommended adult immunization schedule, by vaccine and age group. 2014. http://www.cdc.gov/vaccines/schedules/hcp/imz/adult.html. Accessed September 2, 2015.

Handelsman Y, Bloomgarden ZT, Grunberger G, et al. American Association of Clinical Endocrinologists and American College of Endocrinology—clinical practice guidelines for developing a diabetes mellitus comprehensive care plan. *Endocr Pract.* 2015;21(4 suppl 1):1–87.

US Dept of Agriculture and US Dept of Health and Human Services. *Dietary Guidelines for Americans, 2010.* 7th ed. Washington, DC: US Government Printing Office; 2010.

US Preventive Services Task Force. Recommendations for primary care practice: published recommendations. http://www.uspreventiveservicestaskforce.org/BrowseRec/Index/browse-recommendations. Accessed September 22, 2015.

▮ Case 2

Mrs. Nelson is a 58-year-old female who presents for her annual physical examination. At her last visit, Mrs. Nelson was noted to be 50 lbs overweight, and she was advised to begin lifestyle modifications to include dietary changes and increased activity. She now reports she has been walking for "about a half hour" daily but states she is so tired and thirsty that she is finding it difficult to "go any longer than that." When queried, she reports increased hunger, thirst, and urination, but states she is not sure if it is just related to her lifestyle changes "or something else." Denies any pain, fever, cough, night sweats, shortness of breath, orthopnea, or chest pain. Denies abdominal pain, nausea, vomiting, or changes in bowel habits. States she does have increased urination, but denies dysuria, discharge, hesitancy, or sensation of incomplete voiding. Reports natural menopause 6 years ago with no spotting or abnormal bleeding since that time. Well-woman exam and mammogram last year were normal. Reports childhood history of measles, mumps, rubella, and chickenpox. States she receives her annual influenza vaccination, has not received Pneumovax nor shingles vaccination. A review of her chart reveals her tetanus was updated 2 years ago. Denies tobacco use, denies alcohol (ETOH), denies illicit drug use. Lives with her husband of 35 years and reports they are in a mutually monogamous relationship. They have three children and one grandchild who live nearby.

▮ Physical Exam

VS: BP 145/90, HR 100 (regular), T 98.7, Ht 5'1", Wt 200 lbs

GEN: Well-appearing, obese female in no apparent distress

HEENT: Head normocephalic without evidence of masses or trauma. PERRLA, EOMs full to confrontation. Noninjected. Fundoscopic exam unremarkable. Ear canal without redness or irritation, TMs clear, pearly, bony landmarks visible. No discharge, no pain noted. Oropharynx pink, mucous membranes dry. Neck supple without masses. No thyromegaly. No JVD noted.

CV: S_1 and S_2 RRR, no murmurs, no rubs

Lungs: Clear to auscultation

Abdomen: Soft, round, nontender, nondistended, bowel sounds present × 4 quadrants, no organomegaly, no bruits

What additional assessments/diagnostics do you need?

What is the differential diagnoses list?

What is your working diagnosis?

Additional Assessments/Diagnostics Needed

For Mrs. Nelson, you want to focus on her objective findings on examination (weight, age) and her chief complaints (inability to lose weight, increased hunger, increased thirst, and increased urination) as well as her pertinent negatives (no orthopnea, no chest pain, lungs clear on examination, CV normal) to determine what to explore with lab and diagnostic evaluation.[1-6,9] In anticipation of the addition of medications, and because this is her annual examination, cholesterol and liver function tests (LFTs) will be ordered. Thyroid panel and complete blood count (CBC) will look for potential cause of her fatigue, but the most telling labs by far will be her complete metabolic panel (CMP) and UA.

Routine Labs/Diagnostics

▶ CBC—normal

▶ UA—moderately elevated glucose, slightly elevated protein, no ketones

▶ CMP—blood urea nitrogen (BUN)/creatinine (Cr) elevated, glucose 325 mg/dL

▶ Hemoglobin A1c (HbA1c)—12.2%

▶ Thyroid panel—normal

▶ LFTs—normal

▶ Cholesterol—total cholesterol elevated (210), low-density lipoproteins (LDL) high, high-density lipoproteins (HDL) low (28)

▶ Electrocardiogram (ECG)—normal

Differential Diagnoses List

Diabetes mellitus type 1

Diabetes mellitus type 2

Thyroid dysfunction

CAD/congestive heart failure (CHF)

HTN

Hyperlipidemia

Working Diagnosis

Diabetes mellitus type 2

Hyperlipidemia

HTN

Pathophysiology

Type 2 diabetes mellitus (DM) occurs when the body either stops making enough insulin to meet metabolic demands or the cells of the body become resistant to the insulin produced. Oral agents used for the management of type 2 DM are directed primarily at decreasing insulin resistance, encouraging pancreatic secretion of insulin or blocking the reabsorption of glucose by the kidneys. Some patients with type 2 DM need insulin injections for management of their disease either intermittently, during times of illness and hospitalizations, or permanently, as their disease progresses.

What Is Your Treatment Plan?

Mrs. Nelson's urinalysis and laboratory results demonstrate a clear picture of type 2 diabetes mellitus.[1-6,9] A urinalysis with elevated blood sugar and absence of ketones coupled with elevations in serum glucose and HgbA1C are typical in type 2 DM. Based on Mrs. Nelson's glucose levels, the findings of elevated BUN/Cr and proteinuria are not unanticipated related to the stress that elevated glucose places on the kidneys. Mrs. Nelson's cholesterol panel and continued struggles with obesity support the need for more aggressive dietary and lifestyle modifications.

Pharmacologic

▶ Glucophage 850 mg PO BID. Glucophage, in addition to its hypoglycemic effect, causes a decrease in appetite, which can assist with weight loss in obese, diabetic patients.

▶ Angiotensin-converting enzyme (ACE) inhibitor such as quinapril 10 mg PO QD as starting dose for management of her blood pressure and for the added benefits of delaying the onset of nephropathy and retinopathy. Begin blood pressure (BP) medication for her today based on prior attempts at lifestyle management that have not had the desired impact on her BP and her new diagnosis of DM, which will benefit from this medication class.

▶ Atorvastatin 20 mg PO QD for management of her dyslipidemia.

Nonpharmacologic

▶ Diabetic education referral
  ▸ Diet management and its effect on diabetes
  ▸ Activity and how it relates to blood sugar control
  ▸ Sick-day management and how to modify medication therapy when she is unable to eat or drink
  ▸ s/s of hypo-/hyperglycemia
  ▸ Blood sugar monitoring
  ▸ Emergency action plans

Education/Counseling

▶ Dietary consult and comprehensive weight reduction program recommended

▶ Diabetes education

SOAP Note

S: Mrs. Nelson is a 58-year-old female who presents for her annual physical examination. At her last visit, Mrs. Nelson was noted to be 50 lbs overweight, and she was advised to begin lifestyle modifications to include dietary changes and increased activity. She now reports she has been walking for "about a half hour" daily but states she is so tired and thirsty that she is finding it difficult to "go any longer than that." When queried, she reports increased hunger, thirst, and urination, but states she is not sure if it is just related to her lifestyle changes. Denies any pain, fever, cough, night sweats, shortness of breath, orthopnea, or chest pain. Denies abdominal pain, nausea, vomiting, or changes in bowel habits. States she does have increased urination, but denies dysuria, discharge, hesitancy, or sensation of incomplete voiding. Reports natural menopause 6 years ago with no spotting or abnormal bleeding since that time. Well-woman exam and mammogram last year were normal. Reports childhood history of measles, mumps, rubella, and chickenpox. States she receives her annual influenza vaccination, has not received Pneumovax nor shingles vaccination. A review of her chart reveals her tetanus was updated 2 years prior. Denies tobacco use, denies ETOH, denies illicit drug use. Lives with her husband of 35 years and reports they are in a mutually monogamous relationship. They have three children and one grandchild who live nearby

O: *VS:* BP 145/90, HR 100 (regular), T 98.7, Ht 5'1", Wt 200 lbs

GEN: Well-appearing, obese female in no apparent distress

HEENT: Head normocephalic without evidence of masses or trauma. PERRLA, EOMs full to confrontation. Noninjected. Fundoscopic exam unremarkable. Ear canal without redness or irritation, TMs clear, pearly, bony landmarks visible. No discharge, no pain noted. Oropharynx pink, mucous membranes dry. Neck supple without masses. No thyromegaly. No JVD noted.

CV: S_1 and S_2 RRR, no murmurs, no rubs

Lungs: Clear to auscultation

Abdomen: Soft, round, nontender, nondistended, bowel sounds present × 4 quadrants, no organomegaly, no bruits

A:

1. Diabetes mellitus type 2

2. Hyperlipidemia

3. HTN

P: Mrs. Nelson's labs were reviewed with her at this visit. She agrees to medications and referrals to diabetes educator and structured weight loss program. Prescriptions provided at this visit: Glucophage 850 mg BID, atorvastatin 20 mg PO QD, quinapril 10 mg PO QD. Patient verbalizes understanding of the need for glucose monitoring and blood pressure monitoring at home to allow for adjustment of medication dosages. Follow-up in 2 weeks.

Health Promotion

▶ Healthy lifestyle (diet, activity)

▶ Referral to structured weight loss program

▶ Continue annual influenza vaccine

Guidelines to Direct Care

American Association of Clinical Endocrinologists. AACE/ACE comprehensive diabetes management algorithm. *Endocr Pract.* 2015;21(4):e1–e10. https://www.aace.com/files/aace_algorithm.pdf. Accessed September 22, 2015.

Centers for Disease Control and Prevention. Recommended adult immunization schedule, by vaccine and age group. 2014. http://www.cdc.gov/vaccines/schedules/hcp/imz/adult.html. Accessed September 2, 2015.

Centers for Disease Control and Prevention. Vaccine recommendations of the ACIP. http://www.cdc.gov/vaccines/hcp/acip-recs/. Accessed September 22, 2015.

Handelsman Y, Bloomgarden ZT, Grunberger G, et al. American Association of Clinical Endocrinologists and American College of Endocrinology—clinical practice guidelines for developing a diabetes mellitus comprehensive care plan. *Endocr Pract.* 2015;21(4 suppl 1):1–87.

Stone NJ, Robinson JG, Lichtenstein AH, et al; American College of Cardiology/American Heart Association Task Force on Practice Guidelines. 2013 ACC/AHA guideline on the treatment of blood cholesterol to reduce atherosclerotic cardiovascular risk in adults: a report of the American College of Cardiology/American Heart Association Task Force on Practice Guidelines. *J Am Coll Cardiol.* 2014;63(25 Pt B):2889–2934.

US Dept of Agriculture and US Dept of Health and Human Services. *Dietary Guidelines for Americans, 2010.* 7th ed. Washington, DC: US Government Printing Office; 2010.

US Preventive Services Task Force. Recommendations for primary care practice: published recommendations. http://www.uspreventiveservicestaskforce.org/BrowseRec/Index/browse-recommendations. Accessed September 2, 2015.

Case 3

Mrs. Smith is a 52-year-old female who comes today with c/o weight gain in spite of 1400-calorie restricted diet, fatigue, and "mental fogginess." States she noticed weight gain and a feeling of being sluggish a few years ago but attributed this to "the change of life." States she had her last menstrual period over 1 year ago and thought she would feel better once her very heavy periods ceased, but states she does not. When queried, reports she has some constipation, "always feels cold," has noticed thinning hair, aching muscles, and stiff joints. Denies any fever, cough, night sweats, shortness of breath, or chest pain. Denies abdominal pain, nausea, vomiting, or diarrhea. Denies increased urination, dysuria, discharge, hesitancy, or sensation of incomplete voiding. Reports childhood history of measles, mumps, and chickenpox. States she does not receive annual influenza vaccination and "avoids vaccination" because she is "afraid of needles." Unsure of the date of her last tetanus vaccination. Well-woman exam and mammogram last year were normal. Has not had a colonoscopy. Denies tobacco use, denies ETOH, denies illicit drug use. Lives alone since the sudden death of her spouse last year and is not sexually active. States she has two sons who live nearby and have been a source of support for her since her husband's death.

Physical Exam

VS: BP 130/84, HR 64 (regular), RR 12, T 98.4, Ht 5'6", Wt 220 lbs

GEN: Well-appearing obese female in no apparent distress

HEENT: Head normocephalic without evidence of masses or trauma. PERRLA, EOMs full to confrontation. Noninjected. Fundoscopic exam unremarkable. Ear canal without redness or irritation, TMs clear, pearly, bony landmarks visible. No discharge, no pain noted. Neck supple without masses. Thyroid noted to be enlarged and with multiple nodules palpable on examination. No JVD noted. Hair with marked thinning noted on scalp, forearms, and legs. No palpable lymph nodes (LN)

Skin: Skin without lesions but appears dry and thinning over forearms and legs. Pruritus noted intermittently throughout examination.

CV: S_1 and S_2 RRR, no murmurs, no rubs

Lungs: Clear to auscultation

Abdomen: Soft, round, nontender, nondistended, bowel sounds present × 4 quadrants, no organomegaly, no bruits

What additional assessments/diagnostics do you need?

What is the differential diagnoses list?

What is your working diagnosis?

Additional Assessments/Diagnostics Needed

Ask focused ROS questions. In the case of Mrs. Smith, a few compelling issues need to be explored through further evaluation and exploration during the history and physical examination.

▶ Explore family history for autoimmune disease or thyroid disease in first-degree relative, which would place Mrs. Smith at a greater risk of autoimmune thyroiditis. Mrs. Smith reports her father had Hashimoto's thyroiditis (a form of autoimmune thyroiditis) as well as rheumatoid arthritis, and her sister had Hashimoto's thyroiditis and papillary thyroid cancer. Mrs. Smith is from a country that routinely utilizes iodine supplementation (i.e., iodized salt), which makes iodine deficiency as the cause for her potential hypothyroidism highly unlikely.

▶ Explore depression utilizing a screening tool such as the Patient Health Questionnaire (PHQ-9). Mrs. Smith's PHQ-9 score was 3, which correlates to an interpretation of minimal depression. This suggests that although the mental fogginess and history that could correlate to depression may be a comorbid or related factor, depression does not seem to be a significant cause of her current issues.

▶ Derive more detail about her heavy periods, when the fatigue began, and whether it has gotten better or worse in the time since her periods ceased to determine what role anemia may play in her current complaints. In Mrs. Smith, anemia is not thought to be the causative factor because her complaints persisted after her heavy periods ceased and did not improve over time, but rather worsened. If there is anemia present, it would be thought to be related to an anemia of chronic disease and not blood loss. A colonoscopy would be recommended for her age and would certainly help to differentiate another potential source of occult blood loss.

Exam[1–4,10,11]

Mrs. Smith's thyroid examination was abnormal, with both enlargement and nodularity noted in examination findings.[1–4,10,11] This examination coupled with symptoms of hypothyroidism such as weight gain, skin and hair changes, fatigue/malaise, constipation, and cold intolerance point us in the direction of the need for a thyroid evaluation.

Routine Labs/Diagnostics

Routine screening for thyroid disease is recommended in patients who present with diagnoses of:

- Autoimmune diseases (i.e., type 1 diabetes mellitus, Addison's disease, rheumatoid arthritis [RA])
- Constitutional symptoms (constipation, malaise, fatigue, weight gain, dysmenorrhea)
- Changes in skin, hair, or nails (alopecia, textural changes, vitiligo)
- Lipidemia (hypercholesterolemia, mixed hyperlipidemia)
- Cardiac diseases (hypertension, dysrhythmia, congestive heart failure)
- Dementia
- Anemia

Currently, the US Preventive Services Task Force (USPSTF) has concluded that the evidence is insufficient to recommend for or against routine thyroid screening in asymptomatic, nonpregnant adults.

In the case of Mrs. Smith, she has a family history of thyroid disease, including autoimmune thyroiditis and papillary cancer of the thyroid as well as history and physical (H&P) consistent with thyroid disease.

Laboratory Testing

Her workup will include the following:

- CBC
- UA
- CMP
- Thyroid panel (thyroid-stimulating hormone [TSH], free T4, free T3, total T3, calcitonin, thyroglobulin, anti-thyroid antibody titers—TgAb, TPOAb, TRAb)
- LFTs
- Cholesterol panel
- Vitamin D

Diagnostic Testing

In addition to laboratory testing, a fine-needle aspiration (FNA) of the thyroid nodules would be recommended based on her family history of thyroid cancer and clinical presentation.[10,11] A FNA can help definitively diagnose autoimmune thyroiditis as well as help to exclude malignancy. Although thyroid scans and ultrasounds may help identify whether a nodule is suspicious for malignancy, only biopsy can definitively determine whether malignancy is present. The variability of thyroid nodules from one nodule to another in the same thyroid and even across varying regions of the same nodule make definitive diagnosis with FNA biopsy improbable for all cases of malignancy. If cancer is suspected and the FNA is indeterminate, a partial or completed thyroidectomy with pathology of the suspicious nodule would be needed for a final diagnosis.

Differential Diagnoses List

Hypothyroidism
Autoimmune thyroiditis
Thyroid cancer
Anemia
Depression
Obesity
Hypercholesterolemia
Vitamin D deficiency

Working Diagnosis

Hypothyroidism
Autoimmune thyroiditis
Vitamin D deficiency
Hypercholesterolemia
Obesity

Pathophysiology

The thyroid is a butterfly-shaped gland that rests at the base of the anterior neck and produces thyroid hormones.[10,11] Hypothyroidism is a decreased amount of circulating thyroid hormones that presents with varying degrees of distress and a variety of symptoms. In its most severe form, untreated hypothyroidism can lead to a life-threatening condition known as myxedema. Hypothyroidism can be caused by a number of factors, including insufficient dietary intake of iodine, autoimmune dysfunction, prior thyroid surgery, treatment with radioactive iodine, radiation to the neck, pituitary gland dysfunction, and medications such as lithium. Autoimmune thyroiditis occurs when the body's immune cells attack the thyroid and infiltrate the thyroid gland. Treatment for hypothyroidism is through thyroid hormone replacement therapy.

What Is Your Treatment Plan?

Mrs. Smith's FNA was negative for malignancy but positive for inflammatory cells consistent with Hashimoto's thyroiditis.[1–4,10,11] Her laboratory results revealed an elevated TSH and a low T4, low T3, and positive thyroid antibody titers. She was started on a thyroid dose to approximate 1.6 mcg/kg of lean body weight to be taken daily on an empty stomach with a full glass of water. Her CBC was normal, cholesterol slightly elevated, and vitamin D level very low at 10 ng/mL.

Pharmacologic

- Levothyroxine 150 mcg PO QD
- Ergocalciferol (vitamin D_2) 50,000 U PO once a week
- TdaP immunization

Nonpharmacologic

- Lifestyle modifications for weight reduction and cholesterol normalization
- Order colonoscopy

Education/Counseling

- Education re: s/s of worsening condition
- Medication education for vitamin D_2 and levothyroxine
- Education re: TdaP complications and adverse reactions
- Dietary counseling for weight reduction and cholesterol reduction
- Discussion of need for health and wellness activities such as immunizations and screening tests
- Discussion of resources for grief support

SOAP Note

S: Mrs. Smith is a 52-year-old female who comes today with c/o weight gain in spite of 1400-calorie restricted diet, fatigue, and "mental fogginess." States she noticed weight gain and a feeling of being sluggish a few years ago but attributed this to "the change of life." States she had her last menstrual period over 1 year ago and thought she would feel better once her very heavy periods ceased, but states she does not. When queried, reports she has some constipation, "always feels cold," has noticed thinning hair, aching muscles, and stiff joints. Denies any fever, cough, night sweats, shortness of breath, or chest pain. Denies abdominal pain, nausea, vomiting, or diarrhea. Denies increased urination, dysuria, discharge, hesitancy, or sensation of incomplete voiding. Reports childhood history of measles, mumps, and chickenpox. States she does not receive annual influenza vaccination and "avoids vaccination" because she is "afraid of needles." Unsure of the date of her last tetanus vaccination. Well-woman exam and mammogram last year were normal. Has not had a colonoscopy. Denies tobacco use, denies ETOH, denies illicit drug use. Mrs. Smith lives alone since the sudden death of her spouse last year and is not sexually active. States she has two sons who live nearby and have been a source of support for her since her husband's death.

O: *VS:* BP 130/84, HR 64 (regular), RR 12, T 98.4, Ht 5'6", Wt 220 lbs

GEN: Well-appearing obese female in no apparent distress

HEENT: Head normocephalic without evidence of masses or trauma. PERRLA, EOMs full to confrontation. Noninjected. Fundoscopic exam unremarkable. Ear canal without redness or irritation, TMs clear, pearly, bony landmarks visible. No discharge, no pain noted. Neck supple without masses. Thyroid noted to be enlarged and with nodularity palpable on examination. No JVD noted. Hair with marked thinning noted on scalp, forearms, and legs

Skin: Skin without lesions but appears dry and thinning over forearms and legs. Pruritus noted intermittently throughout examination

CV: S_1 and S_2 RRR, no murmurs, no rubs

Lungs: Clear to auscultation

Abdomen: Soft, round, nontender, nondistended, bowel sounds present $\times$ 4 quadrants, no organomegaly, no bruits

A:

1. Hypothyroidism
2. Autoimmune thyroiditis
3. Hypercholesterolemia
4. Vitamin D deficiency
5. Obesity
6. Depression, minimal

P: Mrs. Smith returns following laboratory testing and FNA. FNA results discussed that describe no malignancy but Hashimoto's thyroiditis. Laboratory testing results discussed and treatment for hypothyroidism and vitamin D deficiency initiated. Diet and lifestyle modification for weight reduction and cholesterol reduction discussed in some detail. Mrs. Smith declines formal dietary consultation at this time but will consider it if her individual attempts at weight loss are not successful. Grief support again discussed, and patient states she feels she is coping well with the support of her children and friends. Prescriptions provided today: levothyroxine 150 mcg PO QD and ergocalciferol (vitamin D_2) 50,000 U PO once a week. TdaP immunization provided today with review of vaccine information statement (VIS) and s/s of adverse reactions discussed. Verbalized understanding. Follow-up in 4–6 weeks to assess for weight loss, therapeutic response to medications.

Health Promotion

- Influenza vaccination
- Tetanus booster
- Colonoscopy

Guidelines to Direct Care

Centers for Disease Control and Prevention. Recommended adult immunization schedule, by vaccine and age group. 2014. http://www.cdc.gov/vaccines/schedules/hcp/imz/adult.html. Accessed September 2, 2015.

Garber JR, Cobin RH, Gharib H; American Association of Clinical Endocrinologists and American Thyroid Association Taskforce on Hypothyroidism in Adults. Clinical practice guidelines for hypothyroidism in adults: cosponsored by the American Association of Clinical Endocrinologists and the American Thyroid Association. *Thyroid.* 2012;22(12): 1200–1235. doi:10.1089/thy.2012.0205.

Jonklaas J, Bianco AC, Bauer AJ; American Thyroid Association Task Force on Thyroid Hormone Replacement. Guidelines for the treatment of hypothyroidism prepared by the American Thyroid Association Task Force on Thyroid Hormone Replacement. *Thyroid.* 2014;24(12):1670–1751. doi:10.1089/thy.2014.0028.

US Dept of Agriculture and US Dept of Health and Human Services. *Dietary Guidelines for Americans, 2010.* 7th ed. Washington, DC: US Government Printing Office; 2010.

US Preventive Services Task Force. Recommendations for primary care practice: published recommendations. http://www.uspreventiveservicestaskforce.org/BrowseRec/Index/browse-recommendations. Accessed September 2, 2015.

Case 4

Mrs. Pitt is a 35-year-old female who reports that lately she has been having difficulty sleeping and reports feeling anxious and irritable. States she sometimes feels like her heart is "pounding out of [her] chest." When queried, reports she has been experiencing diarrhea with frequent stools that appear more loose than usual for her. States she is "constantly" hungry but cannot seem to gain weight. Denies any fever, cough, night sweats, shortness of breath, or chest pain. Denies abdominal pain, nausea, vomiting, or constipation. Denies increased urination, dysuria, discharge, hesitancy, or sensation of incomplete voiding. Reports childhood immunizations are up-to-date, tetanus booster 4 years ago, receives annual influenza vaccination. Well-woman exam last year was normal. Denies ETOH use, denies illicit drug use. Reports 20-pack-year history of tobacco use. Lives with husband and 2-year-old son. Utilizes intrauterine device for contraception and states she is "done having kids."

Physical Exam

VS: BP 118/78, HR 122 (irregular), RR 16, T 98.3, Ht 5'9", Wt 140 lbs

GEN: Well-appearing female noted to be moving about in the exam room and having difficulty focusing on questions as they are posed to her

HEENT: Head normocephalic without evidence of masses or trauma. PERRLA, EOMs full to confrontation. Exophthalmos with puffy eyelids noted on examination. Fundoscopic exam unremarkable. Ear canal without redness or irritation, TMs clear, pearly, bony landmarks visible. No discharge, no pain noted. Neck supple without masses. Thyroid noted to be enlarged on palpation but without pain or nodularity. No JVD noted. No abnormalities along hairline

Skin: Reddened plaques noted to pretibial region of left lower extremity without pruritus or discharge. Skin noted to be warm and moist to trunk and extremities

CV: S_1 and S_2 with intermittently irregular rhythm, no murmurs, no rubs

Lungs: Clear to auscultation

Abdomen: Soft, nontender, nondistended, bowel sounds hyperactive × 4 quadrants, no organomegaly, no bruits

Musculoskeletal (MS): No pain with palpation of neck, back, upper extremities (UE), lower extremities (LE) no muscle weakness noted. Full range of motion of neck, back, UE, LE without c/o pain

Neuro: Sensation intact to bilateral upper and lower extremities, deep tendon reflexes (DTR) 3+ at biceps, triceps, brachioradialis, patellar, and Achilles bilaterally. Fine tremor in bilateral hands and fingers noted with extension of hands and forearms during examination. Romberg negative, heel/toe walk normal. Bilateral UE/LE strength 5/5

What additional assessments/diagnostics do you need?

What is the differential diagnoses list?

What is your working diagnosis?

Additional Assessments/Diagnostics Needed

Ask focused ROS questions. In the case of Mrs. Pitt, a few compelling issues need to be explored through further evaluation and exploration during the history and physical examination.[1–4,12]

▶ Explore family history for autoimmune disease or thyroid disease in first-degree relatives because this would place her at a greater risk of autoimmune thyroiditis. Mrs. Pitt reports she has no known family history of autoimmune disease but is not fully aware of her paternal health history.

▶ Explore whether there are any issues that would explain the tremor, moist skin, anxiety, and irritability. Denies any prior issues with anxiety, any recent stressful events.

▶ Explore personal and family history of cardiac disease, valvular disease, palpitations, and dysrhythmias. Denies any personal or family history of significant cardiac illness.

Exam

Mrs. Pitt's thyroid examination was abnormal with thyroid enlargement, eye changes, skin changes, and neurologic, and gastrointestinal (GI) symptoms. This examination coupled with irritability, anxiety, rapid heart rate, and hand tremor points in the direction of hyperthyroidism.

Routine Labs/Diagnostics

In the case of Mrs. Pitt, her history and physical examination are suggestive of Graves' disease, a form of autoimmune hyperthyroidism.

Laboratory Testing

In the case of Mrs. Pitt, with her examination findings of Graves' ophthalmology and Graves' dermopathy, the diagnosis can be made on the basis of the physical examination, with laboratory testing utilized to help guide treatment recommendations. Her workup will include the following:

- CBC
- CMP
- LFTs may be performed depending on anticipated treatment regimen
- Quantitative serum human chorionic gonadotropin (hCG)
- Thyroid panel (TSH, free T4, free T3, total T3, calcitonin, thyroglobulin, anti-thyroid antibody titers—TgAb, TPOAb, TRAb)

Diagnostic Testing

In addition to laboratory testing, a radioactive uptake scan may be ordered for:[12]

- Suspected hyperthyroidism without definitive signs or symptoms of Graves' disease
- An enlarged thyroid with multiple thyroid nodules

An in-office ECG was performed to evaluate the heart rhythm irregularity identified during exam with a finding of sinus tachycardia.

Differential Diagnoses List

Hyperthyroidism

Graves' disease

Anxiety

Tachycardia

Skin disorder (Graves' vs. unknown etiology)

Exophthalmos (Graves' vs. other)

Tobacco use

Working Diagnosis

Graves' disease

Tachycardia secondary to hyperthyroidism

Graves' exophthalmos

Graves' dermopathy

Tobacco use

Pathophysiology

The thyroid is a butterfly-shaped gland that rests at the base of the anterior neck and produces thyroid hormones.[12] Hyperthyroidism is defined as an increased amount of circulating thyroid hormones. Circulating thyroid hormones are affected by the thyroid-stimulating and thyroid-suppressing feedback loops that are under the direction of the hypothalamus, pituitary, and thyroid gland. Laboratory testing will frequently show elevated levels of T4 and T3 with very low TSH. Clinically, hyperthyroidism presents with varying degrees of distress and a variety

of symptoms. Hyperthyroidism is commonly caused by an autoimmune condition. Treatment for hyperthyroidism includes treatment of troubling symptoms as well as the underlying hyperthyroidism. Risk factors for Graves' disease include the following:

- Family or personal history of autoimmune disease
- Female
- Younger than 40 years of age
- Recent emotional or physical stressors
- Pregnancy or recent childbirth
- Smoking

What Is Your Treatment Plan?

Pharmacologic

- To treat the inflammation of Graves' dermopathy, a topical hydrocortisone preparation can be used.
- A beta blocker will be prescribed to manage the tachycardia until treatment for her hyperthyroidism can be completed.
- Methimazole can be used to block the production of thyroid hormones for the treatment of hyperthyroidism. This can be temporarily used prior to radioactive iodine ablation of the thyroid gland or surgical removal of the thyroid gland. It can also be used in place of ablation or surgery but is not commonly considered a good long-term treatment because of side effects of the medications.[1-4,12]

Nonpharmacologic

- Radioactive iodine ablation of the thyroid gland
- Surgical removal of the thyroid gland

Education/Counseling

- Education re: s/s of worsening condition
- Medication education for beta blocker, methimazole, hydrocortisone cream

SOAP Note

S: Mrs. Pitt is a 35-year-old female who reports that lately she has been having difficulty sleeping and reports feeling anxious and irritable. States she sometimes feels like her heart is "pounding out of [her] chest." When queried, reports she has been experiencing diarrhea with frequent stools that appear more loose than usual for her. States she is "constantly" hungry but cannot seem to gain weight. Denies any fever, cough, night sweats, shortness of breath, or chest pain. Denies abdominal pain, nausea, vomiting, or constipation. Denies increased urination, dysuria, discharge, hesitancy, or sensation of incomplete voiding. Reports childhood immunizations are up-to-date, tetanus booster 4 years ago, receives annual influenza vaccination. Well-woman exam last year was normal. Denies ETOH use, denies illicit drug use. Reports 20-pack-year history of tobacco use. Lives with husband and 2-year-old son. Utilizes intrauterine device for contraception and states she is "done having kids."

O: *VS:* BP 118/78, HR 122 (irregular), RR 16, T 98.3, Ht 5'9", Wt 140 lbs

GEN: Well-appearing female noted to be moving about in the exam room and having difficulty focusing on questions as they are posed to her

HEENT: Head normocephalic without evidence of masses or trauma. PERRLA, EOMs full to confrontation. Exophthalmos with puffy eyelids noted on examination. Fundoscopic exam unremarkable. Ear canal without redness or irritation, TMs clear, pearly, bony landmarks visible. No discharge, no pain noted. Neck supple without masses. Thyroid noted to be enlarged on palpation but without pain or nodularity. No JVD noted. No abnormalities along hairline

Skin: Reddened plaques noted to pretibial region of left lower extremity without pruritus or discharge. Skin noted to be warm and moist to trunk and extremities

CV: S_1 and S_2 with intermittently irregular rhythm, no murmurs, no rubs

Lungs: Clear to auscultation

Abdomen: Soft, nontender, nondistended, bowel sounds hyperactive × 4 quadrants, no organomegaly, no bruits

MS: No pain with palpation of neck, back, UE, LE. No muscle weakness noted. Full range of motion of neck, back, UE, LE without c/o pain

Neuro: Sensation intact to bilateral upper and lower extremities, DTR 3+ at biceps, triceps, brachioradialis, patellar, and Achilles bilaterally. Fine tremor in bilateral hands and fingers noted with extension of hands and forearms during examination. Romberg negative, heel/toe walk normal. Bilateral UE/ LE strength 5/5

A:

1. Graves' disease
2. Tachycardia secondary to hyperthyroidism
3. Graves' exophthalmos
4. Graves' dermopathy
5. Tobacco use

P: Mrs. Pitt presents with recent onset of symptoms consistent with Graves' disease. ECG demonstrates sinus tachycardia in clinic today. Labs drawn and sent: CBC, CMP, serum hCG, and LFTs in preparation for probable radioactive iodine ablation of thyroid gland, thyroid panel to evaluate status and verify Graves' diagnosis. Prescriptions provided today: metoprolol 25 mg PO QD for tachycardia, hydrocortisone cream for lower extremity dermopathy. Referral to Radiation Oncology center for radioactive iodine ablation evaluation. Discussed the need to avoid pregnancy during this time, s/s of worsening, medication side effects, plan of care, and smoking cessation. Verbalized understanding.

Health Promotion

▶ Smoking cessation

▶ Radioactive iodine safety and precautions

▶ Medication use and monitoring

Guidelines to Direct Care

Bahn Chair RS, Burch HB, Cooper DS; American Thyroid Association; American Association of Clinical Endocrinologists. Hyperthyroidism and other causes of thyrotoxicosis: management guidelines of the American Thyroid Association and American Association of Clinical Endocrinologists. *Thyroid.* 2011;17(3):593–646.

Centers for Disease Control and Prevention. Recommended adult immunization schedule, by vaccine and age group. 2014. http://www.cdc.gov/vaccines/schedules/hcp/imz/adult.html. Accessed September 2, 2015.

US Dept of Agriculture and US Dept of Health and Human Services. *Dietary Guidelines for Americans, 2010.* 7th ed. Washington, DC: US Government Printing Office; 2010.

US Preventive Services Task Force. Recommendations for primary care practice: published recommendations. http://www.uspreventiveservicestaskforce.org/BrowseRec/Index/browse-recommendations. Accessed September 2, 2015.

Case 5

Mrs. Lopez is a 62-year-old female who returns for follow-up of her previously diagnosed hypertension (HTN), obesity, and concerns about her blood sugar. She reports when queried that she has been unable to make substantial lifestyle modifications related to family stressors. States she frequently eats takeout food and, when asked to provide a diet recall, lists only one serving of fruits/vegetables for 2 days and no whole grains. States she does not like the taste of high-fiber whole grain foods, fruits, or vegetables. States she has approximately 3–5 servings of fried foods and drinks approximately a 2-liter bottle of carbonated beverages daily. Denies any fever, cough, night sweats, shortness of breath, or chest pain. Denies abdominal pain, nausea, vomiting, or constipation. Denies increased urination, dysuria, discharge, hesitancy, or sensation of incomplete voiding. Reports childhood immunizations are up-to-date, pneumonia vaccine 2 years ago, shingles vaccination last year, tetanus booster 2 years ago, receives annual influenza vaccination. Well-woman exam and mammogram last year were normal. Natural menopause at the age of 53. Denies ETOH use, denies tobacco use, denies illicit drug use. Lives alone, with no family nearby.

Physical Exam

VS: BP 148/94, HR 72 (regular), RR 12, T 98.5, Ht 5'0", Wt 210 lbs. BMI 41.01. Waist circumference 58 inches

GEN: Well-appearing female in no apparent distress. Morbidly obese body habitus noted

HEENT: Head normocephalic without evidence of masses or trauma. PERRLA, EOMs full to confrontation. Noninjected. Fundoscopic exam unremarkable. Ear canal without redness or irritation, TMs clear, pearly, bony landmarks visible. No discharge, no pain noted. Neck supple without masses. No thyromegaly. No JVD noted. No abnormalities along hairline

Skin: Skin without lesions, pruritus, irritation, or discharge. Hair distribution normal throughout upper extremities and lower extremities

CV: S_1 and S_2 RRR, no murmurs, no rubs

Lungs: Clear to auscultation

Abdomen: Soft, round, nontender, nondistended, bowel sounds present $\times$ 4 quadrants, no organomegaly, no bruits

What additional assessments/diagnostics do you need?
What is the differential diagnoses list?
What is your working diagnosis?

Additional Assessments/Diagnostics Needed

Routine Labs/Diagnostics

▶ CMP—glucose 205 mg/dL
▶ LFTs—elevated
▶ Cholesterol—total cholesterol elevated (250), LDL high, HDL low (28), triglycerides 185 mg/d[1–6,9]

Differential Diagnoses List

Obesity
Diabetes mellitus
Hypertension
Dyslipidemia
Metabolic syndrome
Abnormal liver enzymes

Working Diagnosis

Obesity
Diabetes mellitus

Hypertension
Dyslipidemia
Metabolic syndrome
Abnormal liver enzymes

Pathophysiology

Metabolic syndrome is a phenomenon of increased insulin resistance seen primarily in patients who are obese and sedentary.[1–6,9] Risk factors for metabolic syndrome are:

▶ Age greater than 60 years
▶ Hispanic or Asian
▶ Abdominal obesity
▶ Personal history of gestational diabetes
▶ Family history of diabetes
▶ History of cardiovascular disease (CVD), nonalcoholic fatty liver disease, or polycystic ovary syndrome (PCOS)

A person is said to have metabolic syndrome if he or she has three out of the five following metabolic conditions:

▶ Elevated blood sugar (>100 mg/dL fasting untreated; any treatment for DM)
▶ Elevated blood pressure (>130/85 mm Hg untreated; any level treated for HTN)
▶ Abdominal obesity (>35 inches for women, >40 inches for men)
▶ High triglycerides (>150 mg/dL)
▶ Low HDL (<40 mg/dL in men and <50 mg/dL in women untreated; any treatment for low HDL)

When these conditions occur together, the patient's risk of morbidity and mortality from CVD/CAD is significantly increased. Metabolic syndrome is also known as insulin resistance syndrome, obesity syndrome, syndrome X, dysmetabolic syndrome, and hypertriglyceridemic waist.

What Is Your Treatment Plan?

Pharmacologic

▶ Glucophage 850 mg PO BID—Glucophage, in addition to its hypoglycemic effect, also causes a decrease in appetite that can assist with weight loss in obese, diabetic patients.
▶ ACE inhibitor such as quinapril 10 mg PO QD as starting dose for management of her blood pressure and for the added benefits of delaying the onset of nephropathy and retinopathy.
▶ Atorvastatin 20 mg PO QD for management of her dyslipidemia. This medication would not be started today secondary to elevated liver enzymes until further evaluation of her liver status.[1–6,9]

Nonpharmacologic

▶ Dietary consult
▶ Comprehensive weight reduction program

- ▶ Referral for diabetic education consultation
- ▶ Lifestyle modifications
  - ▶ Exercise
  - ▶ Weight loss
  - ▶ Dietary counseling

Education/Counseling

- ▶ Medication information
- ▶ What to expect during her workup for abnormal liver enzymes
- ▶ In-office diabetes education to include:
  - ▶ Diet management and its effect on diabetes
  - ▶ Activity and how it relates to blood sugar control
  - ▶ Medication
  - ▶ s/s of hypo-/hyperglycemia
  - ▶ Blood sugar monitoring
  - ▶ Emergency action plans[1-6,9]

SOAP Note

S: Mrs. Lopez is a 62-year-old female who returns for follow-up of her previously diagnosed HTN, obesity, and concerns about her blood sugar. She reports when queried that she has been unable to make substantial lifestyle modifications related to family stressors. States she frequently eats takeout food and, when asked to provide a diet recall, lists only one serving of fruits/vegetables for 2 days and no whole grains. States she does not like the taste of high-fiber whole grain foods, fruits, or vegetables. States she has approximately 3–5 servings of fried foods and drinks approximately a 2-liter bottle of carbonated beverages daily. Denies any fever, cough, night sweats, shortness of breath, or chest pain. Denies abdominal pain, nausea, vomiting, or constipation. Denies increased urination, dysuria, discharge, hesitancy, or sensation of incomplete voiding. All immunizations up to date. Well-woman exam and mammogram last year were normal. Natural menopause at the age of 53. Denies ETOH use, denies tobacco use, denies illicit drug use. Lives alone, with no family nearby.

O: *VS:* BP 148/94, HR 72 (regular), RR 12, T 98.5, Ht 5'0", Wt 210 lbs. BMI 41.01. Waist circumference 58 inches

GEN: Well-appearing female in no apparent distress. Morbidly obese body habitus noted

HEENT: Head normocephalic without evidence of masses or trauma. PERRLA, EOMs full to confrontation. Noninjected. Fundoscopic exam unremarkable. Ear canal without redness or irritation, TMs clear, pearly, bony landmarks visible. No discharge, no pain noted. Neck supple without masses. No thyromegaly. No JVD noted. No abnormalities along hairline

Skin: Skin without lesions, pruritus, irritation, or discharge. Hair distribution normal throughout upper extremities and lower extremities

CV: S_1 and S_2 RRR, no murmurs, no rubs

Lungs: Clear to auscultation

Abdomen: Soft, round, nontender, nondistended, bowel sounds present × 4 quadrants, no organomegaly, no bruits

A:

1. Obesity
2. Diabetes mellitus
3. Hypertension
4. Dyslipidemia
5. Metabolic syndrome
6. Abnormal liver enzymes

P: Mrs. Lopez has been attempting weight loss and lifestyle management independently with no improvement. On examination today she is found to meet criteria for metabolic syndrome. Discussed at length the urgency in managing her conditions, lifestyle modification, and weight reduction to prevent further deterioration and modify her risk for CVD/CAD. Verbalized understanding and is now willing to pursue an aggressive, medically managed weight loss plan. Discussed the need for structure and assistance with learning how to appropriately eat for weight loss and eventual management. Discussed the workup anticipated for her abnormal liver enzymes, which you anticipate will be related to fatty liver disease secondary to chronic obesity. Will begin on the following medications today: Glucophage 850 mg PO BID and quinapril 10 mg PO QD. Will hold on prescription for atorvastatin 20 mg PO QD for management of her dyslipidemia until further evaluation of her liver status is completed. Follow-up after completion of liver ultrasound.

Health Promotion

- ▶ Weight loss
- ▶ Healthy diet
- ▶ Increased activity

Guidelines to Direct Care

American Association of Clinical Endocrinologists. AACE/ACE comprehensive diabetes management algorithm. *Endocr Pract.* 2015;21(4):e1–e10. https://www.aace.com/files/aace_algorithm.pdf. Accessed September 22, 2015.

Centers for Disease Control and Prevention. Recommended adult immunization schedule, by vaccine and age group. 2014. http://www.cdc.gov/vaccines/schedules/hcp/imz/adult.html. Accessed September 2, 2015.

Handelsman Y, Bloomgarden ZT, Grunberger G, et al. American Association of Clinical Endocrinologists and American College of Endocrinology—clinical practice guidelines for developing a diabetes mellitus comprehensive care plan. *Endocr Pract.* 2015;21(4 suppl 1):1–87.

Stone NJ, Robinson JG, Lichtenstein AH, et al; American College of Cardiology/American Heart Association Task Force on Practice Guidelines. 2013 ACC/AHA guideline on the treatment of blood cholesterol to reduce atherosclerotic cardiovascular risk in adults: a report of the American College of Cardiology/American Heart Association Task Force on Practice Guidelines. *J Am Coll Cardiol.* 2014;63(25 Pt B): 2889–2934.

US Dept of Agriculture and US Dept of Health and Human Services. *Dietary Guidelines for Americans, 2010.* 7th ed. Washington, DC: US Government Printing Office; 2010.

US Preventive Services Task Force. Recommendations for primary care practice: published recommendations. http://www.uspreventiveservicestaskforce.org/BrowseRec/Index/browse-recommendations. Accessed September 2, 2015.

REFERENCES

1. US Preventive Services Task Force. Recommendations for primary care practice: published recommendations. http://www.uspreventiveservicestaskforce.org/BrowseRec/Index/browse-recommendations. Accessed September 2, 2015.

2. Centers for Disease Control and Prevention. Recommended adult immunization schedule, by vaccine and age group. 2014. http://www.cdc.gov/vaccines/schedules/hcp/imz/adult.html. Accessed September 2, 2015.

3. US Dept of Agriculture and US Dept of Health and Human Services. *Dietary Guidelines for Americans, 2010.* 7th ed. Washington, DC: US Government Printing Office; 2010.

4. National Heart, Lung, and Blood Institute. What is metabolic syndrome? http://www.nhlbi.nih.gov/health/health-topics/topics/ms. Accessed July 12, 2015.

5. American Association of Clinical Endocrinologists. AACE/ACE comprehensive diabetes management algorithm. *Endocr Pract.* 2015;21(4):e1–e10. https://www.aace.com/files/aace_algorithm.pdf. Accessed September 22, 2015.

6. Handelsman Y, Bloomgarden ZT, Grunberger G, et al. American Association of Clinical Endocrinologists and American College of Endocrinology—clinical practice guidelines for developing a diabetes mellitus comprehensive care plan. *Endocr Pract.* 2015;21 (4 suppl 1):1–87.

7. Centers for Disease Control and Prevention Division of Nutrition, Physical Activity, and Obesity. BMI percentile calculator for child and teen. http://nccd.cdc.gov/dnpabmi/Calculator.aspx. Accessed September 24, 2015.

8. World Health Organization. Sexual maturity rating (Tanner staging) in adolescents. http://www.ncbi.nlm.nih.gov/books/NBK138588/. Accessed September 24, 2015.

9. Stone NJ, Robinson JG, Lichtenstein AH, et al; American College of Cardiology/American Heart Association Task Force on Practice Guidelines. 2013 ACC/AHA guideline on the treatment of blood cholesterol to reduce atherosclerotic cardiovascular risk in adults: a report of the American College of Cardiology/American Heart Association Task Force on Practice Guidelines. *J Am Coll Cardiol.* 2014;63(25 Pt B):2889–2934.

10. Garber JR, Cobin RH, Gharib H; American Association of Clinical Endocrinologists and American Thyroid Association Taskforce on Hypothyroidism in Adults. Clinical practice guidelines for hypothyroidism in adults: cosponsored by the American Association of Clinical Endocrinologists and the American Thyroid Association. *Thyroid.* 2012;22(12):1200–1235. doi:10.1089/thy.2012.0205.

11. Jonklaas J, Bianco AC, Bauer AJ; American Thyroid Association Task Force on Thyroid Hormone Replacement. Guidelines for the treatment of hypothyroidism prepared by the American Thyroid Association Task Force on Thyroid Hormone Replacement. *Thyroid.* 2014;24(12):1670–1751. doi:10.1089/thy.2014.0028.

12. Bahn RS, Burch HB, Cooper DS, et al. Hyperthyroidism and other causes of thyrotoxicosis: management guidelines of the American Thyroid Association and American Association of Clinical Endocrinologists. *Endocr Pract.* 2011;17(3). https://www.aace.com/files/hyperguidelinesapril2013.pdf. Accessed September 24, 2015.

Common Women's Health Disorders in Primary Care

Joanne L. Thanavaro and Karen S. Moore

Chapter Outline

Learning Objectives

Using a case-based approach, the learner will be able to:

1. Identify key history and physical examination parameters for common women's health issues seen in primary care, including sexually transmitted illness, contraception, amenorrhea, urinary tract infections, and menopause.

2. Summarize recommended laboratory and diagnostic studies indicated for the evaluation of common women's health disorders seen in primary care.

3. State pathophysiology of common women's health issues.

4. Document a clear, concise SOAP note for patients with common women's health disorders.

5. Identify relevant education and counseling strategies for patients with common women's health issues.

Case 1

Sally is a 26-year-old female who presents today because of an abnormal vaginal discharge and itching and burning around the vagina. She also reports pain with urination. Symptoms began 3 days ago. She has one male sexual partner, takes an oral birth control pill daily, but only occasionally uses condoms. She hasn't discussed her symptoms with her boyfriend. She tried over-the-counter medication for a yeast infection without any improvement. She has never had a sexually transmitted illness before and is very concerned about her symptoms. Her last menstrual period was 2 weeks ago.

Physical Exam

Vital Signs (VS): Blood pressure (BP) 110/68, heart rate (HR) 70 (regular), respiratory rate (RR) 14, temperature (T) 98.6, height (Ht) 5'0", weight (Wt) 110 lbs, body mass index (BMI) 21.5

General (GEN): Appears slightly anxious

Head, eyes, ears, nose, and throat (HEENT): Unremarkable—no pharyngitis or mucous patches

Heart: S_1 and S_2 regular rate and rhythm (RRR) without murmurs, rubs, or gallops

Lungs: Clear to auscultation

Abdomen: Soft, nontender with bowel sounds in all quadrants

Genitourinary (GU): No suprapubic, flank pain, or costovertebral tenderness on palpation

Extremities: Full range of motion (ROM) in upper and lower extremities

Reproductive: Pelvic exam consistent with purulent vaginal discharge and cervical friability. No cervical motion tenderness

Rectal: Digital rectal exam negative for mucosal friability, purulent discharge, or perianal lesions. Small amount of brown stool is guaiac negative

Her urine specimen in the office today is negative for bacteria, white blood cells (WBCs), and blood.

Qualitative human chorionic gonadotropin (hCG) today is negative.

What additional assessments/diagnostics do you need?

What is the differential diagnoses list?

What is your working diagnosis?

Additional Assessments/Diagnostics Needed

Review of Systems (ROS)

Ask about the following items:

▶ Past history of sexually transmitted infections (STIs) (including HIV and viral hepatitis)
▶ Sexual contact with persons known to have STIs
▶ Use of condoms
▶ Number of recent or new sexual partners (past 60 days)
▶ History of sexual assault
▶ Rash
▶ Pain in joints
▶ Fever
▶ Pharyngeal discomfort
▶ Change in odor, amount, quality, or color of vaginal discharge
▶ Dysuria
▶ Lower abdominal or pelvic pain
▶ Date of last menses[1,2]

Exam

Key components of the physical exam include:

▶ Skin examination
▶ Oral examination
▶ Joint examination
▶ Pelvic exam
▶ Rectal exam
▶ Pelvic bimanual examination[1,2]

Routine Labs

▶ Nucleic acid amplification testing
  ▶ Most sensitive tests for detecting chlamydia and gonorrhea infection[3]
  ▶ May be performed on endocervical, urethral, vaginal pharyngeal, rectal, or urine samples[4]

- Consider screening for other STIs, including syphilis and HIV
- Retesting for chlamydia and gonorrhea several months after treatment is useful for detecting repeated infection[9]

Differential Diagnoses List

Chlamydia

Bacterial vaginosis

Trichomoniasis

Candidiasis

Gonorrhea

Mycoplasma genitalium

Reactive arthritis

Septic arthritis

Syphilis

Lyme disease

Pelvic pain due to

- Ovarian cysts
- Ectopic pregnancy
- Endometriosis
- Ovulation

Bacterial endocarditis

Both Gonorrhea + Chlamydia Are State reportable [handwritten annotation]

Working Diagnosis—Genital chlamydia and gonorrhea

Pathophysiology

Chlamydia infection is the most common reportable infection in the United States. Over 1 million cases were reported to the Centers for Disease Control and Prevention (CDC) in 2011. Gonorrhea is the second most reportable infection, with over 300,000 cases reported in 2011. Infections caused by these organisms can result in cervicitis, urethritis, proctitis, and pelvic inflammatory disease and can negatively affect a woman's reproductive functioning; these infections can cause involuntary infertility, ectopic pregnancy, low-birth-weight babies, prematurity, fetal demise, and congenital infection. Chlamydial and gonococcal infections also increase susceptibility to the transmission of HIV.[1,5]

What Is Your Treatment Plan?

Pharmacologic

- Chlamydial infections
  - Azithromycin 1 g orally in a single dose (may be given as an observed dose) OR
  - Doxycycline 100 mg orally twice daily for 7 days
  - Alternative regimens:
    - Erythromycin base 500 mg orally four times daily for 7 days OR
    - Erythromycin ethylsuccinate 800 mg orally four times daily for 7 days OR

- Levofloxacin 500 mg once daily for 7 days OR
- Ofloxacin 300 mg orally twice daily for 7 days
- Gonorrheal infections
  - Ceftriaxone 250 mg IM in a single dose PLUS
  - Azithromycin 1 g orally in a single dose
  - Alternative regimen:
    - Cefixime 400 mg orally in a single dose (only if IM ceftriaxone not available) PLUS
    - Azithromycin 1 g orally in a single dose[6]

Nonpharmacologic

Education/counseling to include:

- Discuss sexual behavior changes to help avoid infection, including abstaining from sex, using condoms, limiting the number of sex partners, and modifying sexual practices.[7]
- Asymptomatic chlamydial infection is common. Annual screening of all sexually active women <25 years of age is recommended.
- Screening of older women is recommended for those at increased risk of infection:
  - Those with a new sex partner
  - More than one sex partner
  - A sex partner with concurrent partners
  - A sex partner who has an STI
- Persons treated for chlamydia should abstain from sexual intercourse for 7 days after a single-dose therapy or until completion of a 7-day treatment course and resolution of symptoms (if present).
- To minimize risk for infection, all sex partners should be treated.

SOAP Note

S: Sally is a 22-year-old female who presents today because of an abnormal vaginal discharge, itching and burning around the vagina, and dysuria. Symptoms began 3 days ago. She tried over-the-counter medication for a yeast infection without any improvement. She reports no prior diagnoses of STIs or sexual assault and denies having sex with persons known to have STIs. She's had one male sexual partner for the last 6 months and occasionally uses condoms.

She denies rash, joint pain, pharyngeal discomfort, or lower abdominal or pelvic pain. Her last menstrual period was 2 weeks ago. Her only medication is an oral contraceptive pill, which she takes daily. She is a nonsmoker and drinks two to four drinks on the weekends.

O: *VS:* BP 110/68, HR 70 (regular), RR 14, T 98.6, Ht 5'0", Wt 110 lbs, BMI 21.5

GEN: Appears slightly anxious

Skin: No rash

HEENT: Unremarkable—no pharyngitis or mucous patches

Heart: S_1 and S_2 RRR without murmurs, rubs, or gallops

Lungs: Clear to auscultation

Abdomen: Soft, nontender with bowel sounds in all quadrants

GU: No suprapubic, flank pain, or costovertebral tenderness on palpation

Extremities: Full ROM without pain in upper and lower extremities

Reproductive: Pelvic exam consistent with purulent vaginal discharge and cervical friability. No cervical motion tenderness

Rectal: Digital rectal exam negative for mucosal friability, purulent discharge, or perianal lesions. Small amount of brown stool is guaiac negative

Urine dip today is negative for bacteria, WBCs, and blood.

Qualitative human chorionic gonadotropin (hCG) is negative.

A: STI—suspect chlamydia

P: Nucleic acid amplification test (NAAT) for chlamydia and gonorrhea. Venereal Disease Research Laboratory (VDRL) test, human immunodeficiency virus (HIV) antibody screening test.

Treat for chlamydia and gonorrhea with azithromycin 1 g orally in a single dose.

Discussed safe sex habits. Encouraged continued use of oral contraception. Informed that sex partner must be treated to avoid reinfection. Avoid sexual intercourse for 7 days. Start first vaccine for human papillomavirus (HPV) today. Follow-up in 1 month for second dose.

▌ Health Promotion Issues

▶ Encourage continued use of oral contraceptives; explain that medications do not prevent sexually transmitted illnesses and condoms should be used for every sexual encounter.

▶ Encourage vaccination for human papillomavirus (HPV).[8]

▌ *Guidelines to Direct Care*

Centers for Disease Control and Prevention. 2015 Sexually transmitted diseases treatment guidelines. http://www.cdc.gov/std/tg2015/default.htm. Accessed September 25, 2015.

▌ Case 2

Remy is an 18-year-old female who presents to the practice today to discuss contraception methods. She has been in a relationship with one male partner for the last 6 months. They have been using condoms, but her partner would like her to get on the pill. He finds the condoms bothersome. She has recently been accepted into college and is looking forward to starting her first semester as a college student. She does not want to become pregnant for at least 10 years and would like to discuss contraceptive strategies; she thinks the pill might be a good option. She has never had an STI. She smokes only occasionally (4–5 cigarettes on the weekend) and does not drink. She is healthy with no past medical history and takes no medication. She reports her last menstrual period (LMP) was about 3 weeks ago, but she isn't really sure.

▌ *Physical Exam*

VS: BP 120/72, HR 76 (regular), RR 14, T 98.6, Ht 5'8", Wt 145 lbs, BMI 22

GEN: Well-developed, well-nourished female. She appears comfortable answering questions during this visit.

HEENT: Unremarkable

Heart: S_1 and S_2 RRR without murmurs, rubs, or gallops

Lungs: Clear to auscultation

Abdomen: Soft, nontender with bowel sounds in all quadrants

GU: No suprapubic, flank pain, or costovertebral tenderness on palpation

Extremities: Full ROM in upper and lower extremities

Qualitative hCG today is negative.

What additional assessments/diagnostics do you need?

What is the differential diagnoses list?

What is your working diagnosis?

▌ *Additional Assessments/Diagnostics Needed*

▌ ROS

▶ Medical history

  ▶ To ensure that method of contraception is safe

  ▶ Last menstrual period

  ▶ Menstrual frequency, length, and amount of bleeding

  ▶ Gynecologic and obstetric history

    ➤ Recent delivery, miscarriage, or termination

  ▶ Contraceptive use

  ▶ Allergies

  ▶ Infectious or chronic health conditions

  ▶ Other characteristics that may affect medical eligibility criteria for contraceptive methods[9]

- Pregnancy intention
  - Are children desired?
  - Desired timing and spacing of children
- Contraceptive experience and preferences
  - What methods are currently being used
  - Methods used in the past
  - Use of emergency contraception
  - Use of contraception at last sex
  - Difficulties with prior methods
  - Specific preferred methods (if known)
  - Have contraception methods been discussed with partner
- Sexual history and risk assessment
  - Sexual practices
  - Partners
  - Past STI history
  - Steps taken to prevent STIs[10]

Exam

- Should be limited to blood pressure evaluation before starting hormonal contraceptives or a pelvic exam before placing an intrauterine device
- Weight measurement for monitoring changes
- Pregnancy testing if needed; history is usually satisfactory
- Requiring prerequisite preventative services, including cervical cytology or breast exam, can introduce unnecessary barriers to contraceptive care[9]

Routine Labs

- Requiring prerequisite evaluation for STIs, diabetes mellitus, dyslipidemia, liver disease, or thrombophilia can introduce unnecessary barriers to contraceptive care.[10]

Working Diagnosis—Contraception counseling

Overview

The CDC has released recommendations regarding family planning services. Contraception should ideally be addressed in five steps, including establishing and maintaining rapport, obtaining clinical and social information, working interactively to select the most effective medically appropriate method, obtaining limited physical assessment, and providing method, instructions, and follow-up plan. Providers should discuss all methods that can safely be used by the patient even if the woman is an adolescent or a nulliparous woman. Counseling should include providing the most effective options first before less effective strategies and providing quality family planning services. Increasing contraceptive counseling in primary care may reduce unintended pregnancy.[9,11]

What Is Your Treatment Plan?

Pharmacologic

- Implant (less than 1 pregnancy per 100 women in a year)
- Injectable (6% of every 100 women experienced an unintended pregnancy in a year)
- Pill, patch, or ring (9% of every 100 women experienced an unintended pregnancy in a year)
- Spermicide (28% of every 100 women experienced an unintended pregnancy in a year)[10]

Nonpharmacologic

- Diaphragm (12% of every 100 women experienced an unintended pregnancy in a year)
- Female condom (21% of every 100 women experienced an unintended pregnancy in a year)
- Withdrawal (22% of every 100 women experienced an unintended pregnancy in a year)
- Sponge (24% of every 100 parous women, 12% of every 100 nulliparous women experienced an unintended pregnancy in a year)
- Fertility-awareness-based methods (24% of every 100 women experienced an unintended pregnancy in a year)[9]

Education/Counseling

- Discuss possible methods of contraception with instructions on effectiveness, proper administration, and possible adverse effects. Use teach-back methods to ensure understanding.
- Discuss instructions for missed doses (with oral or transdermal agents).
- Discuss importance of use of condoms with every sexual encounter to prevent STIs.

SOAP Note

S: Remy is an 18-year-old female who is here today to discuss contraception methods. She has been in a relationship with one male partner for the last 6 months. They have been using condoms, but her partner would like her to get on the pill. He finds the condoms bothersome. Remy has no experience with any other methods of contraception. She has recently been accepted into college and is looking forward to starting her first semester as a college student. She does not want to become pregnant for at least 10 years and would like to discuss contraceptive strategies; she thinks the pill might be a good option. She has never had an STI and has never been pregnant. She has always been healthy, takes no medication except for an occasional Advil for headaches, and exercises about three to four times weekly. She smokes only occasionally (4–5 cigarettes on the weekend) and does not drink. She reports her LMP was about 3 weeks ago, but she really isn't sure.

O: *VS:* BP 120/72, HR 76 (regular), RR 14, T 98.6, Ht 5'8", Wt 145 lbs, BMI 22

GEN: Well-developed, well-nourished female. She appears comfortable answering questions during this visit.

HEENT: Unremarkable

Heart: S_1 and S_2 RRR without murmurs, rubs, or gallops

Lungs: Clear to auscultation

Abdomen: Soft, nontender with bowel sounds in all quadrants

GU: No suprapubic, flank pain, or costovertebral tenderness on palpation

Extremities: Full ROM in upper and lower extremities

Qualitative hCG today is negative.

A: Contraception counseling in a healthy young female

P: All methods of contraception were reviewed with an explanation of effectiveness, how to use the method, and possible side effects. After a long discussion, Remy would like to try an oral contraceptive agent. She does not want any method that requires a procedure and feels she would be very responsible about taking medication daily. It is important to her that she continues to have a monthly menstrual cycle. She is prescribed a 1-year supply of levonorgestrel/ethinyl estradiol 1 mg daily and is started today using the "quick method." Instructions were provided for late or missed pills, and she is counseled to another means of contraception if she needs to take antibiotics. She is counseled to use condoms with every sexual encounter to prevent STIs. She is advised to return at any time to discuss side effects or other

problems; she should return if she wants to change her method of contraception. She is advised to consider HPV vaccination, but she wants to discuss this with her partner. Remy is encouraged to come back for a preventative exam within the next year.

Health Promotion Issues

▶ Recommend HPV vaccination

▶ Recommend complete smoking cessation

▶ Recommend healthy diet, routine exercise, and healthy sleep patterns

▶ Discuss use of seat belts

Guidelines to Direct Care

Division of Reproductive Health, National Center for Chronic Disease Prevention and Health Promotion. US selected practice recommendations (US SPR) for contraceptive use, 2013: adapted from the World Health Organization selected practice recommendations for contraceptive use, 2nd edition. *MMWR.* 2013;62(RR05):1–46. http://www.cdc.gov/mmwr/preview/mmwrhtml/rr6205a1.htm?s_cid=rr6205a1_w. Accessed September 24, 2015.

Gavin L, Moskosky S, Carter M, et al. Providing quality family planning services: recommendations of CDC and the U.S. Office of Population Affairs. *MMWR.* 2014;63(RRo4):1–29. http://www.cdc.gov/mmwr/preview/mmwrhtml/rr6304a1.htm. Accessed September 24, 2015.

Case 3

Casey is a 24-year-old female who reports she has not had a menstrual period for over 3 months. States she is sexually active, in a committed relationship with a male, and uses condoms for birth control any time she has sexual intercourse. States her menstrual periods have always been regular, lasting 5 days and occurring every 28 to 30 days. Denies significant past medical history. Denies any pain, fever, cough, night sweats, shortness of breath, orthopnea, or chest pain. Denies abdominal pain, nausea, vomiting, or changes in bowel habits. Denies dysuria, discharge, hesitancy, or sensation of incomplete voiding. Denies headache, dizziness, vision changes, hearing loss. Well-woman exam 6 months ago was normal. Reports childhood immunizations up-to-date. Last tetanus booster was in her senior year of high school. Does not receive annual influenza vaccine. Denies tobacco use, denies alcohol (ETOH), denies illicit drug use. Denies unsafe living situation, denies violence in her current relationship.

Physical Exam

VS: BP 98/64, HR 54 (regular), RR 12, T 98.5, Ht 5'8", Wt 100 lbs, BMI 15.2

GEN: Cachectic-appearing female in no apparent distress

HEENT: Head normocephalic without evidence of masses or trauma. Pupils equal, round, react to light, accommodation (PERRLA), extraocular movements (EOMs) intact. Noninjected. Fundoscopic exam unremarkable. Ear canal without redness or irritation, tympanic membranes (TMs) clear, pearly, bony landmarks visible. No pain, no discharge noted. Oropharynx without redness, no discharge, no exudate, no pain noted. Neck supple without masses. No thyromegaly. No jugular vein distention (JVD) noted. No abnormalities along hairline

Skin: No redness, no warmth, no pruritus, no discharge noted. Hair distribution is noted to be thinning on scalp and sparse on trunk and extremities but in a normal distribution pattern

Cardiovascular (CV): S_1 and S_2 RRR, no murmurs, no rubs

Lungs: Clear to auscultation

Abdomen: Soft, nontender, nondistended, bowel sounds present × 4 quadrants, no organomegaly, no bruits

GU: No suprapubic, flank pain, or costovertebral tenderness on palpation. Pelvic exam without discharge or abnormality noted. No cervical motion tenderness

Rectal: Digital rectal exam negative for mucosal friability, purulent discharge, or perianal lesions. Small amount of brown stool is guaiac negative

What additional assessments/diagnostics do you need?

What is the differential diagnoses list?

What is your working diagnosis?

Additional Assessments/Diagnostics Needed[15–17]

Evaluation of amenorrhea should be approached in a systematic fashion to appropriately differentiate between the possible etiologies for this condition. Considerations should include:

- Obstruction or congenital anomalies. These would be identifiable on physical examination.
- Physiologic reasons such as pregnancy, menopause, contraception, hormones.
- Pituitary dysfunction, including autoimmune disease, medications that suppress normal function, and tumors.
- Hypothalamic dysfunction, which can include infections such as meningitis, traumatic brain injury, and eating disorders.
- Endocrine gland disorders such as tumor, Cushing syndrome, adrenal disease.

Ask focused ROS questions. On Casey's examination, her BMI is 15.2, which is markedly underweight. It would be important to explore diet and exercise, how she perceives her current weight and level of fitness. Casey reports she is an avid runner, and approximately 6 months ago she increased her miles per day in preparation for a marathon. States she has lost about 10 to 15 pounds during that time of intense training because she has difficulty keeping up with her daily caloric needs.

Exam

Attention should be paid to hair growth and distribution, secondary sexual characteristics, findings that suggest a congenital causation, thyroid examination, central nervous system involvement, and BMI. For Casey, only her BMI was abnormal.

Routine Labs/Diagnostics[15–17]

- Quantitative urine human chorionic gonadotropin (hCG)
- Thyroid panel (thyroid-stimulating hormone [TSH], free T4, free T3, total T3, calcitonin, thyroglobulin, anti-thyroid antibody titers—TgAb, TPOAb, TRAb)
- Serum luteinizing hormone (LH)
- Follicle-stimulating hormone (FSH)
- In some cases, if exogenous androgens or congenital anomalies are suspected, further testing would be indicated.

Diagnostic testing for amenorrhea could include:

- Pelvic ultrasound
- MRI of the pituitary

Differential Diagnoses List

Pregnancy

Eating disorder

Thyroid dysfunction

Functional hypothalamic amenorrhea

Working Diagnosis—Functional hypothalamic amenorrhea

Pathophysiology[15–17]

Amenorrhea can be broadly divided into primary and secondary. Primary amenorrhea is the absence of menarche in a female at least 16 years of age and possessing secondary sexual characteristics. Secondary amenorrhea is the lack of a menstrual period for at least 3 months in a female who was previously experiencing menses. In the case of an adult female with previously normal menstrual periods who reports a history of aggressive exercise, caloric intake insufficient to meet bodily demands leading to weight loss, and cessation of menses, a functional hypothalamic amenorrhea has occurred. Functional hypothalamic amenorrhea occurs when the body is stressed by weight loss, extremes of exercise, or stess and the hypothalamic-pituitary-ovarian axis becomes disrupted, causing loss of gonadotropin-releasing hormone pulsatility. The condition is treated by correcting the underlying cause of the dysfunction.

What Is Your Treatment Plan?[15–17]

Pharmacologic

No medications would be recommended for Casey.

Nonpharmacologic

- Decrease training regimen
- Increase daily caloric intake to meet metabolic demands
- Recommend dietitian familiar with marathon runner training methods to advise on calories needed to meet metabolic demands

Education/Counseling

- Dietary consultation
- Balance of exercise and dietary intake
- Continue use of condoms or other birth control method to prevent pregnancy

SOAP Note

S: Casey is a 24-year-old female who reports she has not had a menstrual period for over 3 months. States she is sexually active, in a committed relationship with a male, and uses condoms for birth control any time she has sexual intercourse. States her menstrual periods have always been regular, lasting 5 days and occurring every 28 to 30 days. Denies significant past medical history. Denies any pain, fever, cough, night sweats, shortness of breath, orthopnea, or chest pain. Denies abdominal pain, nausea, vomiting, or changes in bowel habits. Denies dysuria, discharge, hesitancy, or sensation of incomplete voiding. Well-woman exam 6 months ago was normal. Reports childhood immunizations up-to-date. Last tetanus booster was greater than 6 years ago. Does not receive annual influenza vaccine. Denies tobacco use, denies ETOH, denies illicit drug use. Denies unsafe living situation, denies violence in her current relationship.

O: *VS:* BP 98/64, HR 54 (regular), RR 12, T 98.5, Ht 5'8", Wt 100 lbs, BMI 15.2

GEN: Cachectic-appearing female in no apparent distress

HEENT: Head normocephalic without evidence of masses or trauma. PERRLA, EOMs intact. Noninjected. Fundoscopic exam unremarkable. Ear canal without redness or irritation, TMs clear, pearly, bony landmarks visible. No pain, no discharge noted. Oropharynx without redness, no discharge, no exudate, no pain noted. Neck supple without masses. No thyromegaly. No JVD noted. No abnormalities along hairline

Skin: No redness, no warmth, no pruritus, no discharge noted. Hair distribution is noted to be thinning on scalp and sparse on trunk and extremities but in a normal distribution pattern

CV: S_1 and S_2 RRR, no murmurs, no rubs

Lungs: Clear to auscultation

Abdomen: Soft, nontender, nondistended, bowel sounds present × 4 quadrants, no organomegaly, no bruits

GU: No suprapubic, flank pain, or costovertebral tenderness on palpation. Pelvic exam without discharge or abnormality noted. No cervical motion tenderness

Rectal: Digital rectal exam negative for mucosal friability, purulent discharge, or perianal lesions. Small amount of brown stool is guaiac negative

A: Functional hypothalamic amenorrhea

P: Casey is a thin young female who presents with 3-month history of amenorrhea. Reports increased marathon training, decreased caloric intake, and weight loss in the months preceding the onset of amenorrhea. Labs drawn and sent but will recommend lifestyle changes and refer to dietitian and exercise physiologist to treat presumptive cause of functional hypothalamic amenorrhea. Education regarding running safety reviewed with patient. Annual influenza vaccination recommended, but patient declines at this time. Follow-up in 1 month.

Health Promotion[12–14]

▶ Annual influenza vaccination

▶ Running safety

  ▶ Reflective gear

  ▶ Safe streets

  ▶ Aware of surroundings

  ▶ Run with a partner or group

  ▶ Obey safety rules

Guidelines to Direct Care

American Psychiatric Association. *Practice Guideline for the Treatment of Patients with Eating Disorders.* 3rd ed. Washington, DC: American Psychiatric Association; 2006.

Centers for Disease Control and Prevention. Recommended adult immunization schedule, by vaccine and age group. 2014. http://www.cdc.gov/vaccines/schedules/hcp/imz/adult.html. Accessed September 2, 2015.

US Dept of Agriculture and US Dept of Health and Human Services. *Dietary Guidelines for Americans, 2010.* 7th ed. Washington, DC: US Government Printing Office; 2010.

US Preventive Services Task Force. Recommendations for primary care practice: published recommendations. http://www.uspreventiveservicestaskforce.org/BrowseRec/Index/browse-recommendations. Accessed September 2, 2015.

Case 4

Delilah is a 30-year-old female who presents with complaints of (c/o) dysuria, urgency, and burning on urination. Denies new sexual partner, states she is in a mutually monogamous relationship for the past 5 years. States when queried that she often does not use the restroom after sexual intercourse and "sometimes forgets and wipes back to front." Denies significant past medical history. Denies any pain, fever, cough, night sweats, shortness of breath, orthopnea, or chest pain. Denies abdominal pain, nausea, vomiting, or changes in bowel habits. Denies vaginal discharge, pruritus, or vaginal irritation. Denies headache, dizziness, vision changes, hearing loss. Well-woman exam 6 months ago was normal. Reports childhood immunizations up-to-date. Last tetanus booster was 6 years ago. Receives annual influenza vaccine. Denies tobacco use, denies ETOH, denies illicit drug use. Denies unsafe living situation, sexual assault; denies violence in her current relationship.

Physical Exam

VS: BP 120/76, HR 64 (regular), RR 14, T 98.9, Ht 5'6", Wt 150 lbs

GEN: Well-appearing female in no apparent distress

HEENT: Head normocephalic without evidence of masses or trauma. PERRLA, EOMs intact. Noninjected. Fundoscopic exam unremarkable. Ear canal without redness or irritation, TMs clear, pearly, bony landmarks visible. No discharge, no pain noted. Neck supple without masses. No thyromegaly. No JVD noted. No abnormalities along hairline, no evidence of nits or infestation

Skin: No redness, no warmth, no pruritus, no discharge noted. Hair distribution in normal distribution and pattern

CV: S_1 and S_2 RRR, no murmurs, no rubs

Lungs: Clear to auscultation

Abdomen: Soft, nontender, nondistended, bowel sounds present × 4 quadrants, no organomegaly, no bruits. Reports discomfort and urinary urgency with palpation of bladder

GU: No suprapubic, flank pain, or costovertebral tenderness on palpation. Pelvic exam without discharge or abnormality noted. No cervical motion tenderness

Rectal: Digital rectal exam negative for mucosal friability, purulent discharge, or perianal lesions. Small amount of brown stool is guaiac negative

What additional assessments/diagnostics do you need?

What is the differential diagnoses list?

What is your working diagnosis?

Additional Assessments/Diagnostics Needed[18]

Ask focused ROS questions:

▶ Evaluate for any potential sexual trauma

▶ Evaluate for any potential STI

▶ Consider evaluation for systemic illness such as diabetes mellitus (DM) if symptoms recur after treatment

Routine Labs/Diagnostics

▶ UA—positive for white blood cells (WBCs) and nitrates

▶ If systemic symptoms, a complete blood count (CBC) may be drawn and sent

Differential Diagnoses List

Uncomplicated urinary tract infection (UTI)

Vaginal infection

STI

Working Diagnosis—Uncomplicated UTI

Pathophysiology[18]

UTI in females is often caused by contamination with bacteria from sexual activity or improper cleansing after toileting. Bacteria is able to migrate up the urethra related to the female anatomy and relatively short distance from the orifice to the bladder. Infrequent toileting is also contributory to UTI because the mechanical act of micturition helps to cleanse the urethra.

What Is Your Treatment Plan?[18]

Pharmacologic

▶ In the case of an uncomplicated UTI in non-pregnant females, short course antibiotic treatment can be initiated based on clinical signs and symptoms of UTI without lab confirmation of infective organism.

▶ Trimethoprim-sulfamethozole 160 mg PO BID × 3 days

▶ Alternate treatment with a quinolone such as levaquin or nitrofurantoin could be utilized

▶ Phenazopyridine for urinary tract anesthetic properties

Patients should be instructed to take all of the antibiotic as prescribed. Discussion of medication side effects including possible interference with oral contraceptives should also be addressed.

Nonpharmacologic

▶ Hygiene instruction
  ▸ Postcoital voiding
  ▸ Showers as opposed to bathing to avoid urinary tract contamination
  ▸ Wipe from front to back
  ▸ Phenazopyridine staining of urine, contact lenses, and body fluids

▶ Increase fluids to increase voiding and aid in mechanical cleansing of urethra

Education/Counseling

▶ Hygiene instructions

▶ Medication instruction

▶ Increase oral intake of fluids

▶ Increase frequency of voiding

SOAP Note

S: Delilah is a 30-year-old female who presents with c/o dysuria, urgency, and burning on urination. Denies new sexual partner, states she is in a mutually monogamous relationship for the past 5 years. States when queried that she often does not use the restroom after sexual intercourse and sometimes forgets and wipes back to front. Denies fever, denies significant past medical history. Denies any pain, fever, cough, night sweats, shortness of breath, orthopnea, or chest pain. Denies abdominal pain, nausea, vomiting, or changes in bowel habits. Denies vaginal discharge, pruritus, or vaginal irritation. Well-woman exam 6 months ago was normal. Reports all immunizations are up-to-date. Denies tobacco use, denies ETOH, denies illicit drug use. Denies unsafe living situation, sexual assault; denies violence in her current relationship.

O: *VS:* BP 120/76, HR 64 (regular), RR 14, T 98.9, Ht 5'6", Wt 150 lbs

GEN: Well-appearing female in no apparent distress

HEENT: Head normocephalic without evidence of masses or trauma. PERRLA, EOMs intact. Noninjected. Fundoscopic exam unremarkable. Ear canal without redness or irritation, TMs clear, pearly, bony landmarks visible. No discharge, no pain noted. Neck supple without masses. No thyromegaly. No JVD noted. No abnormalities along hairline, no evidence of nits or infestation

Skin: No redness, no warmth, no pruritus, no discharge noted. Hair distribution in normal distribution and pattern

CV: S_1 and S_2 RRR, no murmurs, no rubs

Lungs: Clear to auscultation

Abdomen: Soft, nontender, nondistended, bowel sounds present × 4 quadrants, no organomegaly, no bruits. Reports discomfort and urinary urgency with palpation of bladder

GU: No suprapubic, flank pain, or costovertebral tenderness on palpation. Pelvic exam without discharge or abnormality noted. No cervical motion tenderness

Rectal: Digital rectal exam negative for mucosal friability, purulent discharge, or perianal lesions. Small amount of brown stool is guaiac negative

A: Uncomplicated UTI

P: Urinalysis (UA) confirms clinical diagnosis of UTI. Begin trimethoprim-sulfamethozole 160mg/800 mg PO BID × 3 days and phenazopyridine. Instruct in medications, urinary tract hygiene, showering instead of bathing, wiping front to back, postcoital voiding, increasing fluids to encourage voiding. Verbalized understanding. Routine follow-up needed, but no urgent follow-up necessary unless symptoms worsen or persist.

Health Promotion[12-14]

▶ Safety

▶ Vaccine schedule

Guidelines to Direct Care

American College of Obstetricians and Gynecologists. *Treatment of Urinary Tract Infections in Nonpregnant Women.* Washington, DC: American College of Obstetricians and Gynecologists; 2008. (ACOG Practice Bulletin no. 91). http://www.guideline.gov/content.aspx?id=12628. Accessed September 25, 2015.

Centers for Disease Control and Prevention. Recommended adult immunization schedule, by vaccine and age group. 2014. http://www.cdc.gov/vaccines/schedules/hcp/imz/adult.html. Accessed September 2, 2015.

US Dept of Agriculture and US Dept of Health and Human Services. *Dietary Guidelines for Americans, 2010.* 7th ed. Washington, DC: US Government Printing Office; 2010.

US Preventive Services Task Force. Recommendations for primary care practice: published recommendations. http://www.uspreventiveservicestaskforce.org/BrowseRec/Index/browse-recommendations. Accessed September 2, 2015.

Case 5

Mrs. Brownlee is a 50-year-old female who presents today with c/o dysfunctional uterine bleeding, night sweats, sleep disturbance, and irritability. She denies vasomotor symptoms during the day and states she is most bothered by the heavy menstrual periods that seem to be coming at "random times." Denies significant past medical history. Denies any pain, fever, cough, shortness of breath, orthopnea, or chest pain. Denies abdominal pain, nausea, vomiting, or changes in bowel habits. Denies dysuria, discharge, hesitancy, or sensation of incomplete voiding. Denies headache, dizziness, vision changes, hearing loss. Well-woman exam and mammogram 1 year ago were normal, but states she was told she was probably entering "the change." Reports childhood immunizations up-to-date. Last tetanus booster was 4 years ago. Does not receive annual influenza vaccine. Denies tobacco use, denies ETOH, denies illicit drug use. Lives with her husband of 12 years. She has four children from a previous relationship, but she and current husband have no children together. Denies unsafe living situation, denies violence in her current relationship.

Physical Exam

VS: BP 128.82, HR 68 (regular), RR 12, T 99, Ht 5'4", Wt 140 lbs

GEN: Well-appearing female in no apparent distress

HEENT: Head normocephalic without evidence of masses or trauma. PERRLA, EOMs intact. Noninjected. Fundoscopic exam unremarkable. Ear canal without redness or irritation, TMs clear, pearly, bony landmarks visible. No discharge, no pain noted. Neck supple without masses. No thyromegaly. No JVD noted. No abnormalities along hairline with some thinning noted

Skin: No redness, no warmth, no pruritus, no discharge noted. Hair distribution is noted to be thinning on scalp and sparse on trunk and extremities but in a normal distribution pattern

CV: S_1 and S_2 RRR, no murmurs, no rubs

Lungs: Clear to auscultation

Abdomen: Soft, nontender, nondistended, bowel sounds present ×4 quadrants, no organomegaly, no bruits

GU: No suprapubic, flank pain, or costovertebral tenderness on palpation. Pelvic exam with loss of lubrication and thinning of mucosa noted. No cervical motion tenderness. Rectocele palpated on examination

Rectal: Digital rectal exam negative for mucosal friability, purulent discharge, or perianal lesions. Small amount of brown stool is guaiac negative

What additional assessments/diagnostics do you need?

What is the differential diagnoses list?

What is your working diagnosis?

Additional Assessments/Diagnostics Needed[19]

Ask focused ROS questions:

▶ Assess dysfunctional uterine bleeding (DUB) to estimate blood loss. Ask Mrs. Brownlee about the number of soaked pads per day to roughly estimate flow.

▶ Vasomotor symptoms. Explore the types of vasomotor symptoms Mrs. Brownlee is experiencing, frequency of symptoms, and how these symptoms are interfering with her quality of life to determine what level of management would be recommended.

▶ Irritability. Determine if her irritability is having a negative impact on interpersonal relationships and how it may be interfering with her quality of life.

▶ Vaginal atrophy. Discuss options for lubrication, interference with sexual functioning, and impact on quality of life to determine the most appropriate management options.

▶ Changes in bowel and bladder function

Routine Labs/Diagnostics

▶ Thyroid panel
▶ CBC
▶ Cholesterol panel
▶ May consider LH and FSH
▶ Uterine ultrasound to determine if endometrial hyperplasia is present
▶ Uterine biopsy to rule out (r/o) malignancy

Differential Diagnoses List

Perimenopause

Thyroid dysfunction

Autoimmune disease

Working Diagnosis—Perimenopause

Pathophysiology

Menopause is defined as the cessation of menstruation for more than 1 year. Perimenopause is defined as the years prior to menopause where the changes from childbearing to nonchildbearing occur to the female body. Loss of estrogen and imbalance of estrogen and progesterone are largely responsible for the symptoms experienced during perimenopause. Treatment is directed at alleviation of symptoms while still paying attention to possible side effects of treatments such as hormone replacement therapy (HRT).

What Is Your Treatment Plan?[19]

Mrs. Brownlee is primarily concerned about her dysfunctional uterine bleeding as she progresses through perimenopause but not as concerned about her vasomotor symptoms at this time. While her concerns may change over the next several years until she finally reaches menopause, right now her treatment will be focused on controlling the volume and frequency of uterine blood loss.

Pharmacologic

▶ Progesterone 400 mg PO QD
▶ HRT may be considered if severe vasomotor symptoms or severe vaginal atrophy occur. Prior to initiation of HRT, careful evaluation of the risk and benefit for each patient must be considered. In females with an intact uterus, unopposed estrogen should not be recommended as HRT.
▶ Contraindications to HRT include:
  ▶ Breast cancer history or risk related to familial history
  ▶ Undiagnosed vaginal bleeding
  ▶ Endometrial hyperplasia
  ▶ History of (h/o) deep-vein thrombosis (DVT) or thromboembolism
  ▶ Myocardial infarction (MI), hypertension (HTN), liver disease
  ▶ Porphyria cutanea tarda is an absolute contraindication
▶ Vaginal cream, vaginal rings, and oral medications to address vaginal dryness and atrophy that are recalcitrant to lubricants

Bioidentical hormones are not currently recommended because of indeterminate results.

Nonpharmacologic

▶ Lubricants for sexual activity
▶ Attention to vaginal hygiene to prevent UTI

- Lifestyle modifications to help cope with vasomotor symptoms and irritability:
    - Cool environment
    - Relaxation therapy
    - Exercise
    - Avoidance of caffeine, warm areas, spicy foods, alcohol, stress
- Get enough sleep to help with memory problems and mood swings

Education/Counseling

- Nonpharmacologic treatment
- Length of time for perimenopause
- When to start and stop medications

SOAP Note

S: Mrs. Brownlee is a 50-year-old female who presents today with c/o dysfunctional uterine bleeding, night sweats, sleep disturbance, and irritability. She denies vasomotor symptoms during the day and states she is most bothered by the heavy menstrual periods that seem to be coming at "random times." Denies significant past medical history. Denies any pain, fever, cough, shortness of breath, orthopnea, or chest pain. Denies abdominal pain, nausea, vomiting, or changes in bowel habits. Denies dysuria, discharge, hesitancy, or sensation of incomplete voiding. Denies headache, dizziness, vision changes, hearing loss. Well-woman exam and mammogram 1 year ago were normal. Reports childhood immunizations up-to-date. Last tetanus booster was 4 years ago. Does not receive annual influenza vaccine. Denies tobacco use, denies ETOH, denies illicit drug use. Lives with her husband of 12 years. She has four children from a previous relationship, but she and her current husband have no children together. Denies unsafe living situation, denies violence in her current relationship.

O: *VS:* BP 128.82, HR 68 (regular), RR 12, T 99, Ht 5'4", Wt 140 lbs

GEN: Well-appearing female in no apparent distress

HEENT: Head normocephalic without evidence of masses or trauma. PERRLA, EOMs intact. Noninjected. Fundoscopic exam unremarkable. Ear canal without redness or irritation, TMs clear, pearly, bony landmarks visible. No discharge, no pain noted. Neck supple without masses. No thyromegaly. No JVD noted. No abnormalities along hairline with some thinning noted

Skin: No redness, no warmth, no pruritus, no discharge noted. Hair distribution is noted to be thinning on scalp and sparse on trunk and extremities but in a normal distribution pattern

CV: S_1 and S_2 RRR, no murmurs, no rubs

Lungs: Clear to auscultation

Abdomen: Soft, nontender, nondistended, bowel sounds present × 4 quadrants, no organomegaly, no bruits

GU: No suprapubic, flank pain, or costovertebral tenderness on palpation. Pelvic exam with loss of lubrication and thinning of mucosa noted. No cervical motion tenderness. Rectocele palpated on examination

Rectal: Digital rectal exam negative for mucosal friability, purulent discharge, or perianal lesions. Small amount of brown stool is guaiac negative

A: Perimenopause

P: Mrs. Brownlee reports vaginal dryness, atrophy, difficulty sleeping, night sweats, and dysfunctional uterine bleeding. Uterine biopsy negative for malignancy, ultrasound positive for benign hyperplasia. Begin progesterone 400 mg PO QD, over-the-counter vaginal lubricants, lifestyle modifications. Labs drawn and sent: CBC, TSH, cholesterol panel. Recheck in 2 weeks.

Health Promotion[12–14,20]

- Annual influenza vaccination
- Annual well-woman exam
- Annual mammogram
- Colonoscopy

Guidelines to Direct Care

Centers for Disease Control and Prevention. Recommended adult immunization schedule, by vaccine and age group. 2014. http://www.cdc.gov/vaccines/schedules/hcp/imz/adult.html. Accessed September 2, 2015.

Goodman NF, Cobin RH, Ginzburg SB, et al; American Association of Clinical Endocrinologists. American Association of Clinical Endocrinologists Medical Guidelines for Clinical Practice for the diagnosis and treatment of menopause: executive summary of recommendations. *Endocr Pract.* 2011;17(6):949–954.

Smith RA, Saslow D, Sawyer KA, et al; American Cancer Society. American Cancer Society guidelines for breast cancer screening: update 2003. http://onlinelibrary.wiley.com/doi/10.3322/canjclin.53.3.141/epdf

US Dept of Agriculture and US Dept of Health and Human Services. *Dietary Guidelines for Americans, 2010.* 7th ed. Washington, DC: US Government Printing Office; 2010.

US Preventive Services Task Force. Recommendations for primary care practice: published recommendations. http://www.uspreventiveservicestaskforce.org/BrowseRec/Index/browse-recommendations. Accessed September 2, 2015.

REFERENCES

1. Workowski K. In the clinic: chlamydia and gonorrhea. *Ann Intern Med.* 2013;158:ITC2-1.

2. Wong B. Gonorrhea clinical presentation. http://emedicine.medscape.com/article/218059-clinical. Accessed September 25, 2015.

3. Peterman TA, Tian LH, Metcalf CA, et al; Respect-2 Study Group. High incidence of new sexually transmitted infections in the year following a sexually transmitted infection: a case for rescreening. *Ann Intern Med.* 2006;145:564–572.

4. Mishori R, McClaskey EL, Winklerprins VJ. Chlamydia trachomatis infections: screening, diagnosis, and management. *Am Fam Phys.* 2012;86:1127–1132.

5. Centers for Disease Control and Prevention. 2015 sexually transmitted diseases treatment guidelines. http://www.cdc.gov/std/tg2015/default.htm. Accessed September 25, 2015.

6. Centers for Disease Control and Prevention. 2011 sexually transmitted diseases surveillance. http://www.cdc.gov/std/stats11/natprointro.htm. Accessed September 25, 2015.

7. LeFevre ML; US Preventive Services Task Force. Behavioral counseling interventions to prevent sexually transmitted infections: US Preventive Services Task Force recommendation statement. *Ann Intern Med.* 2014;161(12):894–901.

8. Juckett G, Hartman-Adams H. Human papillomavirus: clinical manifestations and prevention. *Am Fam Phys.* 2010;82:1209–1214.

9. Gavin L, Moskosky S, Carter M, et al. Providing quality family planning services: recommendations of CDC and the US Office of Population affairs. *MMWR.* 2014;63(RRo4):1–29.

10. Centers for Disease Control and Prevention. United States Medical Eligibility Criteria (US MEC) for contraceptive use, 2010. *MMWR.* 2010;59(RR04):1–85.

11. Lee JK, Parisi SM, Akers AY, Borrero S, Schwarz EB. The impact of contraceptive counseling in primary care on contraceptive use. *J Gen Intern Med.* 2011;26:731–736.

12. US Preventive Services Task Force. Published recommendations. http://www.uspreventiveservicestaskforce.org/BrowseRec/Index/browse-recommendations.

13. Centers for Disease Control and Prevention. Recommended adult immunization schedule by vaccine and age group. http://www.cdc.gov/vaccines/schedules/hcp/imz/adult.html.

14. US Department of Agriculture; US Department of Health and Human Services. Dietary guidelines for Americans: 2010. http://health.gov/dietaryguidelines/dga2010/dietaryguidelines2010.pdf. Published December 2010.

15. Klein DA, Poth MA. Amenorrhea: An approach to diagnosis and management. *Am Fam Physician.* 2013;87(11)781–788. http://www.aafp.org/afp/2013/0601/p781.html

16. Gordon CM. Clinical practice. Functional hypothalmic amenorrhea. *N Engl J Med.* 2010;363(4):365–371. doi: 10.1056/NEJMcp0912024

17. American Psychiatric Association. Practice guideline for the treatment of patients with eating disorders. Washington, DC: American Psychiatric Association; 2006. http://psychiatryonline.org/pb/assets/raw/sitewide/practice_guidelines/guidelines/eatingdisorders.pdf

18. American College of Obstetrician and Gynecologists (ACOG). Treatment of urinary tract infections in non-pregnant women. 2008;91. http://www.guideline.gov/content.aspx?id=12628

19. Goodman NE, Cobin RH, Ginzburg SB, Katz IA, Woode DE. American Association of Clinical Endocrinologists medical guidelines for clinical practice for the diagnosis and treatment of menopause. *Endocr Pract.* 2011;17(6). https://www.aace.com/files/menopause.pdf

20. Smith RA, Saslow D, Sawyer KA, et al; American Cancer Society. American Cancer Society guidelines for breast cancer screening: update 2003. http://onlinelibrary.wiley.com/doi/10.3322/canjclin.53.3.141/epdf

Common Men's Health Disorders in Primary Care

Joanne L. Thanavaro

Chapter Outline

Learning Objectives

Using a case-based approach, the learner will be able to:

1. Identify key history and physical examination parameters for common men's health disorders seen in primary care, including benign prostatic hypertrophy, erectile dysfunction, lower urinary tract symptoms, testicular torsion, and sexually transmitted illnesses.

2. Summarize recommended laboratory and diagnostic studies indicated for the evaluation of common men's health disorders seen in primary care.

3. State pathophysiology of common men's health disorders.

4. Document a clear, concise SOAP note for patients with common men's health disorders.

5. Identify relevant education and counseling strategies for patients with common men's health disorders.

6. Develop a treatment plan for common men's health disorders utilizing current evidence-based guidelines.

Case 1

Mr. Frank is a 65-year-old white male who presents with complaints of waking up to urinate about three times nightly. He also has urinary frequency during the day, reports problems initiating a urinary stream, and has a feeling of incomplete emptying. He noticed these symptoms about 2 years ago, but they are gradually worsening. He feels exhausted because of the nighttime awakenings, and the urinary frequency interferes with his job, which includes a fair amount of traveling. He denies pain with urination, fever, or chills. His family history is unremarkable for prostate or bladder cancer. His last prostate-specific antigen (PSA), 3 years ago, was normal. He is otherwise healthy except for some mild arthritis in his knees. He takes over-the-counter ibuprofen about three times weekly, which seems to help his joint pain. He is a nonsmoker and drinks 2–3 alcoholic beverages a week.

Physical Exam

Vital Signs (VS): Blood pressure (BP) 142/82, heart rate (HR) 70 (regular), respiratory rate (RR) 18, temperature (T) 98.6, height (Ht) 6'0", weight (Wt) 220 lbs, body mass index (BMI) 30

General (GEN): No acute distress

Heart: S_1 and S_2 regular rate and rhythm (RRR) without murmurs, rubs, or gallops

Lungs: Clear to auscultation

Abdomen: Soft, nontender with bowel sounds in all quadrants. No evidence of hernia

Genitourinary (GU): No suprapubic, flank pain, or costovertebral tenderness on palpation

Rectal: Digital rectal exam reveals no fissures or hemorrhoids. Sphincter tightens evenly. Prostate is symmetrically enlarged, smooth and firm, nontender, with a 1-cm protrusion into the rectum. Median sulcus is not appreciated. Moderate amount of brown stool is guaiac negative

What additional assessments/diagnostics do you need?

What is the differential diagnoses list?

What is your working diagnosis?

Additional Assessments/Diagnostics Needed

Review of Systems (ROS)

Assess the severity of symptoms:

- ▶ American Urology Association—Symptom Index (AUA-SI)
  - ▶ Used to assess the severity of three storage symptoms (frequency, nocturia, and urgency) and four voiding symptoms (feeling of incomplete emptying, intermittency, straining, and a weak stream)[1]
- ▶ International Prostate Symptom Score (I-PSS)
  - ▶ This index assesses the symptoms included in the AUA-SI as well as the "bother" associated with the seven symptoms with this additional question: "If you were to spend the rest of your life with your urinary condition just the way it is now, how would you feel about that?"[2]
  - ▶ The first seven questions of the I-PSS are identical to the questions appearing on the AUA-SI.
  - ▶ Each question is scored on a scale of 1 to 6, with 1 being not at all and 6 being almost always.
  - ▶ Quality of life (question 8) is scored as 1 being "delighted" and 6 being "terrible."

In the Past Month

1. How often have you had the sensation of not emptying your bladder?

2. How often have you had to urinate less than every 2 hours?

3. How often have you found you stopped and started again several times when you urinated?

4. How often have you found it difficult to postpone urination?

5. How often have you had a weak urinary stream?

6. How often have you had to strain to start urination?

7. How many times did you typically get up at night to urinate?

8. If you were to spend the rest of your urinary condition just the way it is now, how would you feel about that?

- Symptoms are categorized as follows:
  - Mild (symptom score less than or equal to 7)
  - Moderate (symptom score range 8–19)
  - Severe (symptom score range 20–35)
- Benign prostatic hyperplasia (BPH) impact index (BII)[3]
  - This questionnaire assesses the effect of symptoms on everyday life and their interference with daily activities and can be administered in conjunction with the AUA-SI.
  - Each question is scored on a scale of 0 (none, not at all) to 3 (a lot, most of the time).

Over the Past Month

1. How much physical discomfort did any urinary problems cause you?

2. How much did you worry about your health because of any urinary problems?

3. How bothersome has any trouble with urination been overall?

4. How much of the time has any urinary problem kept you from doing things you would usually do?

Routine Labs

- Urinalysis
- PSA
- Urine cultures recommended in men at risk for bladder cancer
- The routine measurement of serum creatinine levels is not recommended in the initial evaluation of men with lower urinary tract symptoms (LUTS) secondary to BPH.[4,5]

Differential Diagnoses List

Neurogenic bladder
LUTS secondary to BPH
LUTS independent of BPH
Urethral stricture
Bladder cancer
Prostate cancer
Cystitis
Pyelonephritis
Urinary calculi

Working Diagnosis—LUTS Secondary to BPH

Pathophysiology

BPH is a histologic diagnosis that refers to the proliferation of smooth muscle and epithelial cells in the transition zone of the prostate. The exact etiology is unknown, but it is theorized that BPH may result from a "reawakening" in adulthood of the embryonic induction processes. The enlarged gland is thought to contribute to lower urinary tract symptoms either by direct bladder outlet obstruction (BOO) or from increased smooth muscle tone and resistance within the enlarged gland; it is likely that both these mechanisms contribute to the symptoms. LUTS include storage and/or voiding disturbances, which are common in men as they age. In the past, a number of terms have been used to describe these symptoms, including *BPH, clinical BPH, prostate enlargement,* or *prostatism.* The AUA maintains that symptoms that occur in older males may not have an etiology in prostate enlargement; the terms *LUTS independent of BPH* and *LUTS secondary to BPH* are now recommended to clarify the broad spectrum of etiologies that may cause these symptoms. *Bladder outlet obstruction (BOO)* is the generic term for all forms of obstruction to the bladder outlet.[4]

What Is Your Treatment Plan?

Pharmacologic

- If drug therapy is considered, treatment choices should take into account coexisting overactive bladder symptoms, prostate size, and PSA levels.
- If there are coexisting BOO and overactive bladder symptoms, consider combination therapy with an alpha blocker and anticholinergic medication.
- When BOO symptoms predominate, alpha-adrenergic blocking agents are first-line drugs for LUTS due to BPH.
- Alpha blockers alone, 5-alpha-reductase inhibitors (5-ARIs) alone, or combination alpha blocker and 5-ARI therapy is most effective when the prostate is enlarged.
- All drug treatment choices should be made in conjunction with the patient's preferences.[4]
- Herbal therapies:
  - Saw palmetto is widely used, but few data support its efficacy; no differences were found in urinary symptom scores, measures of urinary flow, or prostate size with saw palmetto versus placebo.[6]
  - Beta-sitosterol improved symptoms in men with BPH, but the long-term effectiveness and safety are unknown.[7]

Nonpharmacologic

▶ Watchful waiting includes monitoring of the patient with no active intervention for BPH. The level of symptom distress that an individual patient can tolerate varies widely, so watchful waiting may be an appropriate choice even if the patient has a high AUA-SI score.

▶ Watchful waiting is acceptable for patients with mild symptoms secondary to BPH, including an AUA-SI score <8.

▶ Watchful waiting is also an acceptable strategy for men with moderate to severe symptoms who have not developed complications of LUTS.

▶ Symptom distress may be reduced with measures including avoiding decongestants and antihistamines, decreasing fluid intake at bedtime, and reducing caffeine and alcohol.

▶ Patients who are getting conservative treatment should be reassessed annually.[4]

Minimally Invasive Therapies

▶ Transurethral needle ablation (TUNA)—effective treatment alternative for bothersome moderate or severe LUTS secondary to BPH

▶ Transurethral microwave thermotherapy (TUMT)—partially relieves LUTS secondary to BPH and can be considered in men with moderate to severe symptoms[4]

Surgical Options

▶ Surgical intervention is an appropriate treatment alternative for moderate to severe LUTS and for patients who have developed acute urinary retention (AUR) or other BPH-related complications.

▶ Surgical intervention is generally reserved for patients who have failed medication therapy:

  ▸ Open prostatectomy
  ▸ Transurethral holmium laser ablation of the prostate (HoLap)
  ▸ Transurethral holmium laser enucleation of the prostate (HoLep)
  ▸ Holmium laser resection of the prostate (HoLRP)
  ▸ Photoselective vaporization of the prostate (PVP)
  ▸ Transurethral incision of the prostate (TUIP)
  ▸ Transurethral vaporization of the prostate (TUVP)
  ▸ Transurethral resection of the prostate (TURP)[8]

Education/Counseling

▶ Regulation of fluid intake especially in the evening

▶ Recommend lifestyle measures, including increasing activity and avoiding highly seasoned or irritating foods

▶ Double voiding

SOAP Note

S: Mr. Frank presents today with complaints of nocturia and urinary frequency during the day. He has problems initiating his urinary stream and feels he's unable to completely empty his bladder. These symptoms started about 2 years ago and have progressively worsened. He denies pain with urination, fever, or chills. These symptoms are now interfering with his ability to do his job, which involves frequent travel. I-PSS score is 10; BII score is 8. His family history is unremarkable for prostate or bladder cancer. His last PSA, 3 years ago, was normal. He is a nonsmoker and drinks 2–3 alcoholic beverages a week. His only medication is occasional ibuprofen for joint pain.

O: *VS:* BP 142/82, HR 70 (regular), RR 18, T 98.6, Ht 6'0", Wt 220 lbs

GEN: No acute distress

Heart: S_1 and S_2 RRR without murmurs, rubs, or gallops

Lungs: Clear to auscultation

Abdomen: Soft, nontender with bowel sounds in all quadrants. No evidence of hernia

GU: No suprapubic, flank pain, or costovertebral tenderness on palpation

Rectal: Digital rectal exam reveals no fissures or hemorrhoids. Sphincter tightens evenly. Prostate is symmetrically enlarged, smooth and firm, nontender, with a 1-cm protrusion into the rectum. Median sulcus is not appreciated. Moderate amount of brown stool is guaiac negative

Labs: Urine analysis negative, PSA 0.4

A: LUTS secondary to BPH

P: Long discussion regarding possible treatment options. Symptoms are interfering with quality of life, so he would like to try medication. Start tamsulosin 0.4 mg daily. We discussed the possibility of dizziness when medication is first started. Discussed lifestyle measures to help reduce symptoms, including limiting fluids in the evening, double voiding, and avoiding highly seasoned food, alcohol, and caffeine. Call immediately if unable to void. Follow-up here in 1 month

Health Promotion Issues

▶ Daily exercise

▶ Weight reduction diet

Guidelines to Direct Care

McVary KT, Roehrborn CG, Avins AL, et al. American Urological Association Guideline: management of benign prostatic hyperplasia. https://www.auanet.org/education/guidelines/benign-prostatic-hyperplasia.cfm. Accessed September 28, 2015.

Case 2

Mr. Little is a 56-year-old man who you are treating for coronary artery disease (CAD), diabetes mellitus (DM), and hypertension (HTN). He watches his diet carefully and exercises five times weekly by walking for 1 hour. His medications include toprol XL 50 mg daily, atorvastatin 20 mg daily, lisinopril 20 mg daily, metformin 500 mg BID, and acetylsalicylic acid (ASA) 81 mg daily. He adheres strictly to his medication regimen. His chief complaint today is that he is having difficulty achieving and maintaining an erection. This has been a problem for the last 6 months and is progressively worsening.

Physical Exam

VS: BP 130/70, HR 76 (regular), RR 14, T 98.4 Ht 5'8", Wt 170 lbs, BMI 26

Head, eyes, ears, nose, and throat (HEENT): Unremarkable

Heart: S_1 and S_2 RRR, no murmurs, gallops, or rubs

Lungs: Clear to auscultation

Abdomen: Soft, nontender, + bowel sounds, no organomegaly. No evidence of hernia

GU: No suprapubic, flank pain, or costovertebral tenderness on palpation

Rectal: Digital rectal exam reveals no fissures or hemorrhoids. Prostate is symmetrically enlarged, smooth and firm, nontender. Small amount of brown stool is guaiac negative

Neurology: Unremarkable

Extremities: Varicosities noted bilateral ankles. Dorsalis pedis and posterior tibialis pulses +2. No edema

Recent labs: Total cholesterol (TC) 196, triglycerides 155, low-density lipoproteins (LDL) 97, high-density lipoproteins (HDL) 45, aspartate aminotransferase (AST) 20, alanine aminotransferase (ALT) 30, Na 145, K 4.0, blood urea nitrogen (BUN) 20, Creatinine (Cr) 1.2, fasting blood sugar (FBS) 109, HbA1c 6.5

What additional assessments/diagnostics do you need?

What is the differential diagnoses list?

What is your working diagnosis?

Additional Assessments/Diagnostics Needed

ROS

▶ Evaluate the severity of symptoms using the Five-Item Version of the International Index of Erectile Function Questionnaire.[9]

  ▶ Each question is scored on a scale of 1 to 5, with 1 being very low (question 1) or never or almost never (questions 2–5) and 5 being very high (question 1) or almost always or always (questions 2–5).

Over the Past 6 Months

1. How do you rate your confidence that you could get and keep an erection?

2. When you had erections with sexual stimulation, how often were your erections hard enough for penetration?

3. During sexual intercourse, how often were you able to maintain your erection after you had penetrated (entered) your partner?

4. During sexual intercourse, how difficult was it to maintain your erection to completion of intercourse?

5. When you attempted sexual intercourse, how often was it satisfactory for you?

  ▶ Erectile dysfunction (ED) is classified based on these scores:

      17–21 mild

      12–16 mild to moderate

      8–11 moderate

      5–7 severe

▶ Evaluate for medications that may cause or contribute to ED.

▶ The patient's psychological state should be assessed with a focus on:[10]

  ▶ Indications of depression

  ▶ Loss of libido

  ▶ Problems and tension in the sexual relationship

  ▶ Insomnia

  ▶ Lethargy

  ▶ Moodiness

  ▶ Stress from work and other sources

Physical Exam

Physical exam should include assessment of vital signs; body habitus for central obesity; and the cardiovascular, neurologic, and genitourinary systems, including penile, testicular, and digital rectal exams.[11]

Routine Labs

▶ Limited diagnostic testing is recommended, including:

  ▶ Serum glucose level, lipid panel, thyroid-stimulating hormone (TSH), and morning testosterone level

▶ If there is no definable medical etiology for ED, consider:

  ▶ Screening for anxiety, depression, history of sexual abuse, and marital or relationship problems[11]

Differential Diagnoses List

Erectile dysfunction (ED)

Diabetes

Atherosclerosis

Stroke

Local trauma

Hyperprolactinemia

Hyperthyroidism

Cushing syndrome

Addison's disease

Multiple sclerosis

Psychogenic

Drugs

Working Diagnosis—Erectile Dysfunction Secondary to Coronary Artery Disease

Pathophysiology

Sexual activity is affected by age, health status, and gender. A number of age-associated changes in sexual function in men include delay in erection, diminished intensity and duration of orgasm, and decreased force of seminal emission. Male sexual dysfunction is a common problem for men, starting in their early 40s, and increases with advancing age. Erectile dysfunction is defined as the consistent or recurrent inability to acquire or sustain an erection to achieve sexual intercourse. Risk factors for ED include obesity, smoking, watching television, and the presence of comorbid conditions, including hypertension, obesity, dyslipidemia, cardiovascular disease, and medication use. The pathophysiologic causes are multifactorial, including neural influences, blood flow from the hypogastric arterial system into the erectile chambers, and hormones, including testosterone, gonadotropin-releasing hormone, and luteinizing hormone, and psychosocial factors.[10-12]

What Is Your Treatment Plan?

Pharmacologic

The currently available therapies that should be considered for the treatment of erectile dysfunction include the following:[13]

- ▶ Oral phosphodiesterase type 5 [PDE5] inhibitors
  - ▸ No evidence at this time to support the superiority of one agent over the others
- ▶ Intra-urethral alprostadil suppositories
  - ▸ Initial trial dose should be administered under healthcare provider (HCP) supervision due to the risk of syncope
- ▶ Intracavernous vasoactive drug injection
  - ▸ Most effective nonsurgical treatment for ED
  - ▸ Invasive and has highest potential for priapism among ED treatments

- ▸ An HCP should be present to instruct patients on the proper technique, determine initial effective dose, and monitor patients for side effects, especially prolonged erection
- ▶ Vacuum constriction devices
  - ▸ Vacuum constriction devices are often effective, low-cost treatment options for select patients with ED. These devices are available without a prescription.
  - ▸ Only vacuum constriction devices containing a vacuum limiter should be used.
- ▶ Penile prosthesis implantation
  - ▸ Prosthetic surgery should not be performed in the presence of systemic, cutaneous, or urinary tract infection.
  - ▸ Two types of penile prostheses: malleable (noninflatable) and inflatable.
  - ▸ Inflatable prostheses are recommended because of improved mechanical reliability.
  - ▸ Inflatable devices provide the patient with closer to normal flaccidity and erection.
  - ▸ Five-year mechanical rate is 6–16%.
  - ▸ Infection is a potential complication of any prosthetic surgery.
- ▶ These appropriate treatment options should be applied in a stepwise fashion with increasing invasiveness and risk balanced against the likelihood of efficacy.
- ▶ The patient and partner should be informed of the relevant treatment options and their associated risks and benefits; choice of treatment should be made jointly by the healthcare provider, patient, and partner.
- ▶ Testosterone therapy is not indicated in patients with a normal serum testosterone level.
- ▶ The use of yohimbine and trazodone is not recommended.

Guidelines for managing ED in patients with cardiovascular disease developed by the Princeton Consensus Panel recommend assigning patients to one of three risk levels based on their cardiovascular risk factors.[14]

- ▶ Treatment of ED in patients with cardiovascular disease should take into account that there is a small increase in the risk of myocardial infarction (MI) related to sexual activity independent of treatment. The absolute risk of MI during and for 2 hours following sexual activity is extremely low (20 chances per million per hour in post-MI patients; even less in men without a history of MI).
- ▶ High-risk patients are defined as those with unstable or refractory angina, uncontrolled hypertension, congestive heart failure (CHF; New York Heart Association classes III and IV), MI or a cardiovascular accident within the previous 2 weeks, high-risk arrhythmias, hypertrophic obstructive and other cardiomyopathies, or moderate to severe valvular disease.
- ▶ Patients at high risk should not receive treatment for sexual dysfunction until their cardiac condition has stabilized.

- The majority of patients treated for ED are in the low-risk category, defined as those who have asymptomatic coronary artery disease and less than three risk factors for coronary artery disease (excluding gender); controlled hypertension; mild, stable angina; a successful coronary revascularization; uncomplicated past MI; mild valvular disease; or CHF (left ventricular dysfunction and/or New York Heart Association class I).
- Patients at low risk may be considered for all first-line therapies.
- Patients whose risk is indeterminate should undergo further evaluation by a cardiologist.

In standard treatment, phosphodiesterase type 5 inhibitors are contraindicated in patients who are taking organic nitrates. PDE5 inhibitors potentiate the hypotensive effects of organic nitrates and nitrites, so their concomitant use is contraindicated. The monitoring of patients receiving continuing PDE5 inhibitor therapy should include a periodic follow-up of efficacy, side effects, and any significant change in health status, including medications.

Nonpharmacologic

- First-line therapy for ED is aimed at lifestyle changes and modifying drugs that may contribute to ED.
- Behavior therapy should be recommended in patients with no obvious medical etiology for ED.

Education/Counseling

- Maintain normal weight
- Regular exercise
- Stop smoking
- Instructions on how to take medications
- Instructions on going to emergency department for sustained erection

SOAP Note

S: Mr. Little is a 56-year-old man who presents today with difficulty achieving and maintaining an erection. He has noticed some problems in the past, but now he has been unsuccessful in maintaining an erection during sexual intercourse for the last 6 months. He has been married for 40 years and reports a good relationship with his wife. He admits to a stressful job but feels he is coping well. He had a stent placed in the right coronary artery 3 years ago when he experienced chest pain. Since that time he watches his diet carefully and exercises five times weekly by walking for 1 hour. He denies chest pain, shortness of breath (SOB), palpitations, diaphoresis, orthopnea, paroxysmal nocturnal dyspnea, and syncope. His medications include toprol XL 50 mg daily, atorvastatin 20 mg daily, lisinopril 20 mg daily, metformin 500 mg BID, and ASA 81 mg daily. He adheres strictly to his medication regimen. Erectile Function Questionnaire Score today = 10.

O: *VS:* BP 130/70, HR 76 (regular), RR 14, T 98.4, Ht 5'8", Wt 170, BMI 26

HEENT: Normal fundoscopic exam

Heart: S_1 and S_2 RRR, no murmurs, gallops, or rubs

Lungs: Clear to auscultation

Abdomen: Soft, nontender, + bowel sounds, no organomegaly. No evidence of hernia

GU: No suprapubic, flank pain, or costovertebral tenderness on palpation. Circumcised penis is without lesions. Urethral meatus is without discharge. No swelling or lumps in scrotum. Testes are smooth and rubbery; no nodules. Epididymis is nontender

Rectal: Digital rectal exam reveals no fissures or hemorrhoids. Prostate is symmetrically enlarged, smooth and firm, nontender. Small amount of brown stool is guaiac negative

Neuro: Oriented ×3. Affect appropriate. CNs II–XII grossly intact. Gait and tandem walking steady. Deep tendon reflexes (DTRs) 2+ throughout

Extremities: Varicosities noted bilateral ankles. No edema. Dorsalis pedis and posterior tibialis pulses +2. No open lesions on feet. Monofilament testing: 10/10 bilaterally

Recent labs: Total cholesterol 196, triglycerides 155, LDL 97, HDL 45, AST 20, ALT 30, Na 145, K 4.0, BUN 20, Cr 1.2, FBS 109, HA1C 6.5

Labs today: TSH = 1.34 mU/L, morning testosterone level = 400 ng/dL (normal = 280–1080)

A: ED secondary to coronary artery disease

CAD—stable

Hypertension—at JNC 8 goals

Dyslipidemia—well controlled on medication

Diabetes—well controlled on medication

P: After discussion, he agrees to try sildenafil 50 mg. Reviewed proper administration of medication, including taking ½ to 4 hours prior to intercourse. Continue all previous medications. The importance of continued strict lifestyle modifications to control cardiovascular risk factors was reinforced.

Health Promotion Issues

- Continued vigilance with heart healthy lifestyle
- Discuss PSA testing

Guidelines to Direct Care

American Urological Association Erectile Dysfunction Guideline Update Panel. *The Management of Erectile Dysfunction: An Update.* http://www.auanet.org/common/pdf/education/clinical-guidance/Erectile-Dysfunction.pdf. Accessed September 25, 2015.

Nehra A, Jackson G, Miner M, et al. The Princeton III consensus recommendations for the management of erectile dysfunction and cardiovascular disease. *Mayo Clin Proc.* 2012;87(8):766–778. http://www.ncbi.nlm.nih.gov/pmc/articles/PMC3498391/. Accessed September 25, 2015.

Case 3

Mr. Becker is a 46-year-old male who is complaining of an acute onset of dysuria, frequency, low back pain, and inhibited urinary voiding that began 2 days ago. He's concerned because he has noted blood when he voids, and he had a fever and chills last evening. He denies ever having an episode like this in the past. He is otherwise healthy and takes no medication. He is a nonsmoker and drinks 2–3 glasses of wine weekly.

▊ Physical Exam

VS: BP 126/70, HR 70 (regular), RR 12, Ht 6'0", Wt 210, BMI 28.5

HEENT: Unremarkable

Heart: S_1 and S_2 RRR, no murmurs, gallops, or rubs

Lungs: Clear to auscultation

Abdomen: Soft, nontender, + bowel sounds, no organomegaly

GU: No suprapubic, flank pain, or costovertebral tenderness on palpation

Rectal: Digital rectal exam reveals no fissures or hemorrhoids. Prostate is tender, warm, swollen, and boggy. Small amount of brown stool is guaiac negative

His urine specimen in the office today is positive for bacteria and white blood cells (WBCs).

What additional assessments/diagnostics do you need?

What is the differential diagnoses list?

What is your working diagnosis?

▊ Additional Assessments/Diagnostics Needed

▊ ROS

▶ Be sure to ask about onset and course of symptoms[15]

▶ Inquire whether patient is sexually active and whether partner is having symptoms such as dysuria

▶ Ask about previous urinary tract infections and the successes and failures of previous treatments

▶ Administer nine-question National Institutes of Health (NIH) Chronic Prostatitis Symptom Index (NIH-CPSI)[16]

Content removed due to copyright restrictions

Content removed due to copyright restrictions

Content removed due to copyright restrictions

Content removed due to copyright restrictions

Physical Exam

▶ Observe general appearance for signs of systemic illness.
▶ Be certain to perform a complete abdominal exam; bladder distention may be present.

- Assess external genitalia and scrotum.
- Carefully and gently palpate the prostate because vigorous massage can disseminate bacteria in the bloodstream, resulting in bacteremia.

Routine Labs

- For patients with acute symptoms, order both a urine analysis (u/a) and a urine culture; diagnosis of acute prostatitis is based on clinical findings and a positive u/a and culture.
- Collecting premassage urine, midstream urine, and post-prostatic-massage urine (Stamey-Meares) test is the gold standard for the diagnosis of chronic prostatitis but is infrequently used by primary care providers (not used for acute symptoms).
- If chronic bacterial prostatitis is suspected, order BUN and creatinine, and consider ordering an intravenous pyelogram and transrectal ultrasound to look for prostate calculi.
- In men older than 45 years, consider ordering a PSA, although it will probably be above normal in men with prostatic inflammation.
- Consider urodynamic testing for men with chronic nonbacterial prostatitis.
- If abscess is suspected, transrectal ultrasound can usually provide adequate imaging of the prostate.
- In older men, consider ordering urine cytologies to rule out bladder malignancy.
- Not every man needs sexually transmitted infection (STI) testing for this issue. Discuss sexual activity and test only if indicated.[15]

Differential Diagnoses List

Acute bacterial prostatitis

Chronic bacterial prostatitis

Chronic nonbacterial prostatitis

Prostatodynia

Lower urinary tract infection

Cystitis

Working Diagnosis—Acute Bacterial Prostatitis

Pathophysiology

Prostatitis is defined as an increased number of inflammatory cells in the prostate gland that may be infectious or inflammatory in origin. Acute prostatitis presents as a urinary tract infection and may be associated with risk factors, including bladder outlet obstruction secondary to BPH or an immunosuppressed state. Aerobic Gram-negative bacilli are the predominate pathogen, and *Escherichia coli* causes 50–80% of most cases. Other pathogens include Enterobacteriaceae *Enterococcus* species and nonfermenting Gram-negative bacilli (e.g., *Pseudomonas* species). Most authorities also accept *Staphylococcus* and *Streptococcus* species as pathogens. The increasing prevalence of Gram-positive pathogens may represent changing disease epidemiology (perhaps related to

fluoroquinolone therapy) or acceptance of their pathogenicity by healthcare providers.[15,17]

The National Institutes of Health (NIH) classification and definition of the categories of prostatitis are as follows:

- Category I: Acute bacterial prostatitis (i.e., acute infection of the prostate)
- Category II: Chronic bacterial prostatitis (i.e., recurrent urinary tract infection and/or chronic infection of the prostate)
- Category III: Chronic bacterial prostatitis/chronic pelvic pain syndrome (i.e., discomfort or pain in the pelvic region for at least 3 months with variable voiding and sexual symptoms and/or no demonstrable infection; by definition, the syndrome becomes chronic after 3 months)
- Category IIIA: Inflammatory chronic pelvic pain syndrome (i.e., white blood cells in semen and/or expressed prostatic secretions and/or third midstream bladder specimen)
- Category IIIB: Noninflammatory chronic pelvic pain syndrome (i.e., no white blood cells in semen and/or expressed prostatic secretions)
- Category IV: Asymptomatic inflammatory prostatitis (i.e., evidence of inflammation in biopsy samples, semen, and/or expressed prostatic secretions, but no symptoms)

What Is Your Treatment Plan?

Pharmacologic

- The mainstay of treatment is antibiotics.
- Mildly to moderately ill patients should receive:
  - Trimethoprim-sulfamethoxazole 160 mg/800 mg orally twice daily for 6 weeks OR
  - Ciprofloxacin 500 mg orally twice daily for 6 weeks
- Patients who are severely ill or have possible urosepsis:
  - Should be admitted for inpatient care
  - Ampicillin, 2 g IV every 6 hours plus gentamycin, 5 mg per kg every day or 1.5 mg per kg every 8 hours until afebrile[17–19]

Nonpharmacologic

- Hot sitz baths or a heating pad may relieve discomfort.[20]
- Rarely acute urinary retention develops and bladder drainage requires suprapubic catheterization.
- Prostatic abscess requires a urological referral.[21]

Education/Counseling

- A pillow or inflatable cushion may help if sitting is uncomfortable.
- Spicy foods and caffeinated drinks may exacerbate the symptoms.
- Avoid circumstances that may increase discomfort (bicycle riding).
- Bacterial prostatitis is not contagious.
- There is no need to discontinue normal sexual relations unless they are uncomfortable.[20]

SOAP Note

S: Mr. Becker presents with an acute onset of dysuria, frequency, low back pain, and inhibited urinary voiding that began 2 days ago. He had fever and chills last evening. He is sexually active only with his wife of many years. He denies ever having an episode like this in the past. He is otherwise healthy and takes no medication. His NIH-CPSI is 7. He is a nonsmoker and drinks 2–3 glasses of wine weekly.

O: *VS:* BP 126/70, HR 70 (regular), RR 12, T 98.1, Ht 6'0", Wt 210, BMI 28.5

Gen: Overall looks well-nourished and rested. No acute pain or distress

Heart: S_1 and S_2 RRR, no murmurs, gallops, or rubs

Lungs: Clear to auscultation

Abdomen: Soft, nontender, + bowel sounds, no organomegaly

GU: No suprapubic, flank pain, or costovertebral tenderness on palpation. No bladder distention

Rectal: Digital rectal exam reveals no fissures or hemorrhoids. Prostate is tender, warm, swollen, and boggy. Small amount of brown stool is guaiac negative

Urine analysis positive for bacteria and WBCs. Urine cultures pending.

A: Acute bacterial prostatitis

P: Trimethoprim-sulfamethoxazole 160 mg/800 mg orally twice daily for 6 weeks

Health Promotion Issues

▶ Discuss importance of healthy lifestyle, including low-fat diet and daily exercise.

▶ Discuss weight reduction.

Guidelines to Direct Care

British Association for Sexual Health and HIV (BASHH) Clinical Effectiveness Group. *United Kingdom National Guideline for the Management of Prostatitis (2008).* http://www.bashh.org/BASHH/Guidelines/Guidelines/BASHH/Guidelines/Guidelines.aspx. Accessed September 25, 2015.

National Institute for Health and Care Excellence (NICE). Lower urinary tract symptoms in men: assessment and management. 2010. http://www.nice.org.uk/guidance/cg97/chapter/1-recommendations. Accessed September 25, 2015.

Case 4

Adam, a 17-year-old male, is brought to your office by his soccer coach after he developed the acute onset of right testicular pain while at practice. The patient doesn't remember getting kicked or hit during practice and denies any fever, dysuria, or penile discharge. He doesn't have any abdominal pain. He is otherwise healthy and denies smoking, alcohol, or any medications.

Physical Exam

VS: BP 118/60, HR 90 (regular), RR 18, T 98.6, Ht 5'7", Wt 140 lbs, BMI 21.9

Gen: Mild distress due to pain

Heart: S_1 and S_2 RRR without murmurs, rubs, or gallops

Lungs: Clear to auscultation

Abdomen: Soft, nontender with bowel sounds in all quadrants. No evidence of hernia

GU: Right scrotal erythema and swelling; no penile lesions or discharge. Scrotum is diffusely tender and difficult to examine. Because his scrotum is so diffusely tender, it is difficult to examine it more closely.

Urinalysis: 3 to 5 white blood cells per high-power field

What additional assessments/diagnostics do you need?

What is the differential diagnoses list?

What is your working diagnosis?

Additional Assessments/Diagnostics Needed

ROS

▶ Inquire about nausea and vomiting.

▶ Inquire about sexual activity.

▶ Inquire about genitourinary surgeries of known urological abnormality.[22]

Physical Exam

▶ Observe patient's gait and resting position.

▶ Observe natural position of the testis in the scrotum while standing.

▶ Transillumination.

▶ Is swelling reducible?[22]

Routine Labs

▶ A urinalysis and urine culture are recommended since pyuria and/or bacteria suggest bacterial epididymitis or other infection.[23]

Imaging

▶ Color Doppler ultrasound should be done to rule out testicular torsion in equivocal cases.[23]

Differential Diagnoses List

Ischemia:

- ▶ Torsion of the testis (torsion of the spermatic cord)
- ▶ Appendiceal torsion, testis or epididymis
- ▶ Testicular infarction due to other vascular insult (cord injury, thrombosis)

Trauma:

- ▶ Testicular rupture
- ▶ Intratesticular hematoma
- ▶ Testicular contusion

Infectious conditions:

- ▶ Acute epididymitis
- ▶ Acute epididymorchitis
- ▶ Acute orchitis
- ▶ Abscess

Inflammatory conditions:

- ▶ Henoch-Schönlein purpura (vasculitis of the scrotal wall)

Hernia:

- ▶ Incarcerated or strangulated inguinal hernia; with or without associated testicular ischemia

Acute on chronic events:

- ▶ Spermatocele rupture or hemorrhage
- ▶ Hydrocele, rupture, hemorrhage, or infection
- ▶ Testicular tumor with rupture, hemorrhage, infarction, or infection
- ▶ Varicocele[24]

Working Diagnosis—Testicular Torsion

Pathophysiology

Testicular torsion is a urologic emergency usually seen in neonates and postpubertal boys, although it can occur at any age. Torsion occurs when there is inadequate fixation of the testis to the tunica vaginalis. If this fixation is insufficient, the testis can twist on the spermatic cord and can cause ischemia resulting from reduced arterial blood flow and venous outflow obstruction. Torsion may occur after a trauma or spontaneously. The testis suffers irreversible damage after 12 hours of ischemia; immediate surgical exploration with intraoperative detorsion and fixation of the testis is indicated. Delay in treatment may be associated with decreased fertility or may necessitate orchiectomy.[23,24]

What Is Your Treatment Plan?

Pharmacologic

- ▶ No pharmacologic treatments

Nonpharmacologic

- ▶ If surgery is not immediately available (within 2 hours), manually detorse the testicle.
- ▶ Because the testis usually rotates medially during torsion, it can be detorsed by rotating it outward toward the right.
- ▶ Successful detorsion is suggested by:
  - ▶ Relief of pain
  - ▶ Resolution of the transverse lie of the testis to a normal longitudinal orientation
  - ▶ Lower position of the testis in the scrotum
  - ▶ Return of normal pulsations on color Doppler study
- ▶ Manual detorsion should not delay surgery.
- ▶ Surgical exploration is needed after successful manual detorsion to secure the testicle to the scrotal wall.[24]

Education/Counseling

- ▶ Anticipatory guidance regarding need for immediate surgery

SOAP Note

S: Adam is brought to the office today by his soccer coach with complaints of sudden onset of right testicular pain while at practice. He doesn't remember getting kicked or hit during practice. He is healthy and denies any abdominal pain, nausea, vomiting, fever, dysuria. He is sexually active with one female partner but always uses condoms. He has never had genitourinary symptoms or surgery of any kind.

O: BP 118/60, HR 90 (regular), RR 18, T 98.6, Ht 5'7", Wt 140 lbs, BMI 21.9

Gen: Mild distress due to pain

Heart: S_1 and S_2 RRR without murmurs, rubs, or gallops

Lungs: Clear to auscultation

Abdomen: Soft, nontender with bowel sounds in all quadrants. No evidence of hernia

GU: Right scrotal erythema and swelling; no penile lesions or discharge. Scrotum is diffusely tender and difficult to examine. There is no testicular rise when the inner thigh is stroked and the right testicle is horizontal in position. There is no local tenderness appreciated along epididymis

Labs: Urinalysis: 3 to 5 WBCs per high-power field is likely an incidental finding

A: Acute testicular torsion associated with strenuous physical activity

P: Anticipatory guidance regarding need for immediate evaluation and likely surgery. Coach will take Adam to the nearby hospital immediately. Mother called and is on the way to the hospital; emergency room physician notified and will consult urologist and schedule operating room suite.

Health Promotion Issues

▶ Discuss monthly self-testicular exams on postoperative visit.

Guidelines to Direct Care

Royal Children's Hospital Melbourne. Clinical practice guidelines: acute scrotal pain or swelling. http://www.rch.org.au/clinicalguide/guideline_index/Acute_Scrotal_Pain_or_Swelling/. Accessed September 25, 2015.

American Urological Association. Acute scrotum. https://www.auanet.org/education/acute-scrotum.cfm. Accessed September 25, 2015.

Case 5

A 36-year-old male presents to the clinic today; the nurse has documented that he "wants a general checkup." On entering the exam room, you find a generally healthy-looking male who appears anxious. He states he's very worried because he hasn't been feeling well lately. He is vague with his complaints, including being stressed, tired, and "worried all the time." After a few more minutes of general questioning, he admits that he noticed a lesion on his penis 1 week ago. He is happily married with one child and has never had a sexually transmitted illness or a lesion on his penis before. He reports going away for the weekend with some old college friends and admits to "hooking up" with several of these men after drinking heavily. He denies abdominal, testicular, or scrotal pain; dysuria; or discharge from his penis. He has not experienced any fever or chills and admits that he is "feeling poorly" because he's worried that his wife will find out. He takes no medications and is a nonsmoker. He does admit to occasional "binge drinking" with friends.

Physical Exam

VS: BP 124/68, HR 90 (regular), RR 14, T 98.6, Ht 6'1", Wt 180 lbs, BMI 24

HEENT: Unremarkable

Heart: S_1 and S_2 RRR, no murmurs, gallops, or rubs

Lungs: Clear to auscultation

Abdomen: Soft, nontender, + bowel sounds, no organomegaly. No evidence of hernia

GU: No suprapubic, flank pain, or costovertebral tenderness on palpation. Vesicular lesions noted on his penis without exudates or erythema on the glans penis, which is mildly tender to palpitation

What additional assessments/diagnostics do you need?
What is the differential diagnoses list?
What is your working diagnosis?

Additional Assessments/Diagnostics Needed

ROS

▶ Ask about date of exposure.
▶ Ask about systemic symptoms, including fever, headache, malaise, and myalgias.
▶ Ask about prodromal symptoms, including mild tingling or shooting pains in the legs, hips, and buttocks occurring hours to days before eruption of the lesions.
▶ Ask about tender lymph nodes.[25]

Physical Exam

Examine lesions carefully.

▶ Genital herpes: Multiple shallow, tender, vesicular ulcers
▶ Syphilis: Painless, indurated, clean-based ulcer called a chancre
▶ Chancroid: Deep, undermined, purulent ulcer often associated with painful inguinal lymphadenitis[26]

Routine Labs

Confirm the diagnosis with any of the following:

▶ Viral culture
  ▶ Unroof the vesicle and send fluid for culture.
  ▶ Overall sensitivity is highest in the early stages when lesions are vesicular (about 50%).
▶ Polymerase chain reaction (PCR)
  ▶ More sensitive method of confirming herpes simplex virus (HSV) infection from genital ulcers
  ▶ Useful for detection of asymptomatic HSV sheeting
▶ Direct fluorescence antibody
  ▶ Available in many labs: Rapid type-specific direct antibody to detect HSV in clinical specimens
  ▶ Specific and reproducible

- Type-specific serologic tests
  - Type-specific antibodies to HSV develop during the first several weeks after infection and persist indefinitely.
- Cell culture and PCR-based testing are preferred in patients presenting with active lesion; PCR-based testing has the greatest overall sensitivity and specificity.

Draw labs to rule out other STIs.

- Urine for chlamydia and gonorrhea
- Rapid plasma reagin (RPR) for syphilis
- Human immunodeficiency virus (HIV)[27]

■ Differential Diagnoses List

Syphilis

Chancroid

Lymphogranuloma venereum

Genital herpes simplex virus (HSV)

Behcet's disease

■ Working Diagnosis—Genital Herpes (GH)

■ Pathophysiology

Genital herpes is a sexually transmitted illness (STI) caused by the herpes simplex virus type 1 (HSV-1) or type 2 (HSV-2). In the United States, GH-related infection is reported to be the most common ulcerative STI, followed by syphilis and chancroid. Nationwide, 15.5% of people between the ages of 14 and 49 years have HSV-2 infection.[28] This important healthcare issue is often underrecognized because infection is often subclinical. Infection is transmitted through contact with lesions, mucosal surfaces, and genital and oral secretions. The virus may also be shed from skin that looks normal. The average incubation period after exposure is anywhere from 4 to 12 days.

Primary infection refers to infection in a patient without preexisting antibodies to either HSV-1 or HSV-2. Nonprimary first episode infection is the acquisition of genital HSV-1 in a person with preexisting antibodies to HSV-1; an individual with prior orolabial herpes with a subsequent development of HSV-1 antibody response who develops genital herpes due to HSV-2 exposure. Recurrent infection is reactivation of genital HSV in which the HSV type recovered in the lesion is the same type as antibodies in the serum. All three types of infection can be either symptomatic or asymptomatic. Genital HSV infection usually begins with multiple vesicular lesions located inside the foreskin or rectum in men and may be painless. A link has been established between HSV-related genital ulcer disease and sexual transmission of HIV. [26–28]

■ What Is Your Treatment Plan?

■ Pharmacologic

- Treatment of HSV infection should be initiated before test results are available to decrease transmission and duration of ulcers.

- First clinical episode of GH:
  - All patients with newly acquired GH, even those with initially mild symptoms, can develop prolonged or severe symptoms and should receive antiviral therapy.
  - Recommended regimens include:
    - Acyclovir 400 mg orally three times daily for 7–10 days OR
    - Acyclovir 200 mg orally five times daily for 7–10 days OR
    - Famcicolvir 250 mg orally three times daily for 7–10 days OR
    - Valacyclovir 1 g orally twice daily for 7–10 days
  - Treatment can be extended if healing is incomplete after 10 days of treatment.
- Established HSV-2 infection
  - Almost all patients with a symptomatic first episode will have recurrent episodes.
  - Antiviral therapy for reoccurrences can be either as suppressive therapy with the goal of reducing the frequency of reoccurrences or episodically to shorten the duration of symptoms.
- Suppressive therapy for GH
  - Reduces the frequency of reoccurrences by 70–80% in patients with frequent recurrences; treatment is also effective for those with less frequent episodes.
  - Recommended regimens include:
    - Acyclovir 400 mg orally twice daily OR
    - Famcicolvir 250 mg orally twice daily OR
    - Valacyclovir 1 g orally daily
  - All agents appear equally effective for episodic treatment; famcicolvir is less effective for suppression of viral shedding.
  - Ease of administration and cost are important considerations for prolonged treatment.
- Episodic therapy for recurrent GH
  - Initiation of treatment should occur within 1 day of lesion onset or during the prodrome that precedes outbreaks in some patients.
  - Provide the patient with a prescription for the medication with instructions to initiate treatment immediately when symptoms begin.
  - Recommended regimens include:
    - Acyclovir 400 mg orally three times daily for 5 days OR
    - Acyclovir 800 mg orally twice daily for 5 days OR
    - Famcicolvir 125 mg orally twice daily for 5 days OR
    - Famcicolvir 1 g orally twice daily for 1 day OR
    - Famcicolvir 500 mg orally once, followed by 250 mg twice daily for 2 days OR
    - Valacyclovir 500 mg orally twice daily for 3 days OR
    - Valacyclovir 1 g orally once daily for 5 days

- Patients with GH and HIV can have prolonged or severe episodes of genital, perianal, or oral herpes; drug regimens for suppressive or episodic therapies use the same antivirals, but a higher dosage may be required.
- Aspirin, acetaminophen, or ibuprofen can ease the pain of herpes symptoms.[26]

Nonpharmacologic

- Soaking the affected area in warm water may help with pain relief.
- The area should be kept dry most of the time.
- If toweling off after bathing is uncomfortable, a hair dryer can be used.
- Wear cotton underwear to absorb moisture.[29]

Education/Counseling

- Explain the clinical designations of genital HSV infection (primary, nonprimary first episode, and recurrent infection).
- Explain there is no cure for GH, but antiviral medications can prevent or shorten outbreaks during the time that the person takes the medication.
- Daily suppressive therapy reduces the likelihood of transmission to partners.
- Nonprimary first episodes are usually associated with fewer lesions and system symptoms than primary infection.
- Reoccurrences are common but are generally less severe than primary or nonprimary infections.
- The frequency of reoccurrence depends on the severity and duration of the initial episode.
- Sexual partners:
  - The chance of a partner getting HSV-2 depends on how long the couple has been sexually intimate with each other.
  - Sex only once or twice, with the use of the condom, is less likely to cause transmission than the risk of long-term unprotected sex; you can be infected during any one encounter.
  - Symptomatic sex partners should be evaluated and treated in the same way as patients who have genital lesions.
  - Asymptomatic sex partners of patients with GH should be questioned regarding history of genital lesions and be offered type-specific serologic testing for HSV infection.
  - Correct and consistent use of latex condoms can reduce the risk of GH; outbreaks can occur in areas that are not covered by a condom.
  - Persons with GH should abstain from sexual activity with partners when sores or other symptoms of herpes are present.
- Genital HSV-2 is of great concern in pregnant women because of risk of transmission to the infant during delivery.

- Routine screening for HSV-1 or HSV-2 infection by serologic testing is not recommended by the Centers for Disease Control and Prevention (CDC).
- Although initial counseling should be provided at the first visit, many patients benefit from learning about the chronic aspects of the disease.[27,29]

SOAP Note

S: This 36-year-old male presents to the clinic today for a "general checkup." He is very worried because he hasn't been feeling well lately; he feels stressed, tired, and worries all the time. After some general discussion, he discloses that he noticed a lesion on his penis 1 week ago. He is happily married with one child and has never had a sexually transmitted illness or a lesion on his penis before. He regrets going away for the weekend with some old college friends and "hooking up" with several of these men after drinking heavily. He denies abdominal, testicular, or scrotal pain; dysuria; or discharge from his penis. He has not experienced any fever or chills, headache, malaise, or tingling or pain in his legs or hips. He believes that he is "feeling poorly" because he is worried that his wife will find out. He takes no medications and is a nonsmoker. He does admit to occasional "binge drinking" with friends.

O: *VS:* BP 124/68, HR 90 (regular), RR 14, T 98.6, Ht 6'1", Wt 180 lbs, BMI 24

GEN: Appears anxious but is otherwise healthy appearing

HEENT: Oral mucosa pink without lesions. No lymphadenopathy

Heart: S_1 and S_2 RRR, no murmurs, gallops, or rubs

Lungs: Clear to auscultation

Abdomen: Soft, nontender, + bowel sounds, no organomegaly. No evidence of hernia

GU: No suprapubic, flank pain, or costovertebral tenderness on palpation. No palpable lymph nodes. Multiple vesicular lesions noted on his penis around and under the foreskin, no exudates or erythema. The penis is mildly tender to palpation

Rectum: No redness, lumps, or lesions in the perianal area. Anal and rectal mucosa are smooth, nontender, and free of nodules and tenderness

A: Genital ulcer—genital herpes

P: Start acyclovir 400 mg orally three times daily for 10 days

Culture of genital lesion, serologic testing for syphilis and HIV

Urine culture for chlamydia and gonorrhea

Patient education regarding etiology of lesions, diagnostic workup, and need to discuss diagnoses with his wife. At this point he would like to return once the results of the diagnostic workup are complete before telling his wife. He does agree to start antiviral therapy and abstain from sex while lesions are present and to use condoms. Follow-up in 2 weeks. Continue counseling regarding genital herpes at that time and discuss binge drinking.

Health Promotion Issues

▶ Discuss reported episodes of "binge drinking" with friends.

▶ Discuss safe sex practices.

Guidelines to Direct Care

Centers for Disease Control and Prevention. 2010 STD treatment guidelines: diseases characterized by genital, anal, or perianal ulcers. http://www.cdc.gov/std/treatment/2010/genital-ulcers.htm#a2. Accessed September 25, 2015.

Centers for Disease Control and Prevention: 2015 STD treatment guidelines: diseases characterized by genital, anal or perianal ulcers. http://www.cdc.gov/std/tg2015/genital-ulcers.htm. Accessed September 25, 2015

REFERENCES

1. American Urology Association (AUA) BPH Symptom Score Index. http://cdn.dupagemedicalgroup.com/userfiles/file/patientForms/symptom-score-sheet-bph%20copy.pdf. Accessed September 25, 2015.

2. International Prostate Symptom Score (I-PSS). http://www.urospec.com/uro/Forms/ipss.pdf. Accessed September 25, 2015.

3. BPH impact index (BII). http://www.ti.ubc.ca/pages/score19.htm. Accessed September 25, 2015.

4. McVary KT, Roehrborn CG, Avins AL, et al. American Urological Association Guideline: management of benign prostatic hyperplasia. https://www.auanet.org/education/guidelines/benign-prostatic-hyperplasia.cfm. Accessed September 28, 2015.

5. Carballido J, Fourcade R, Paqliarulo A, et al. Can benign prostatic hyperplasia be identified in the primary care setting using only simple tests? Results of the Diagnosis Improvement in Primary Care Trial. *Int J Clin Pract.* 2011;65:989–996.

6. Tacklind J, Macdonald R, Rutkis I, et al. Serenoa repens for benign prostatic hyperplasia. *Cochrane Database Syst Rev.* 2012;(12): CD001043.

7. Wilt T, Ishani A, Macdonald R, Stark G, Mulrow C, Lau J. Beta-sitosterols for benign prostatic hyperplasia. *Cochrane Database Syst Rev.* 2000;(2):CDOO1042.

8. Deters LA. Benign prostatic hypertrophy. http://emedicine.medscape.com/article/437359-overview. Accessed September 25, 2015.

9. Rosen RC, Cappelleri JC, Smith MD, Lipsky J, Pena BM. Development and evaluation of an abridged, 5-item version of the International Index of Erective Function (IIEF-5) as a diagnostic tool for erectile dysfunction. *Int J Impot Res.* 1999;6:319–326.

10. Kim ED. Erectile dysfunction. http://emedicine.medscape.com/article/444220-overview. Accessed September 25, 2015.

11. Heidelbaugh JJ. Management of erectile dysfunction. *Am Fam Phys.* 2010;81:305–312.

12. Kandeel FR, Koussa VK, Swerdloff RS. Male sexual function and its disorders; physiology, pathophysiology, clinical investigation, and treatment. *Endocr Rev.* 2001;22:342–388.

13. American Urological Association Erectile Dysfunction Guideline Update Panel. *The Management of Erectile Dysfunction: An Update.* http://www.auanet.org/common/pdf/education/clinical-guidance/Erectile-Dysfunction.pdf. Accessed September 25, 2015.

14. Nehra A, Jackson G, Miner M, et al. The Princeton III consensus recommendations for the management of erectile dysfunction and cardiovascular disease. *Mayo Clin Proc.* 2012;87:766–778.

15. Sharp VJ, Takacs EB. Prostatitis: diagnosis and treatment. *Am fam Phys.* 2010;82:397–406.

16. Prostatitis Foundation. Prostatitis: the National Institutes of Health Chronic Prostatitis Symptoms Index (NIH-CPSI). http://www.prostatitis.org/nih-cpsi.html. Accessed September 25, 2015.

17. Deem SG. Acute bacterial prostatitis. http://emedicine.medscape.com/article/2002872-overview. Accessed September 25, 2015.

18. Lipsky BA, Byren I, Hoey CT. Treatment of bacterial prostatitis. *Clin Infect Dis.* 2010;50:1641–1652.

19. Urology Care Foundation. What are prostatitis and related chronic pelvic pain conditions? http://www.urologyhealth.org/urology/index.cfm?article=15. Accessed September 25, 2015.

20. Morse LP, Moller CC, Harvey E. Prostatic abscess due to *Burkholderia pseudomallei*: 81 cases from a 19-year prospective meliodosis study. *J Urol.* 2009;182:542–547.

21. Royal Children's Hospital Melbourne. Acute scrotal pain or swelling. http://www.rch.org.au/clinicalguide/guideline_index/Acute_Scrotal_Pain_or_Swelling. Accessed September 25, 2015.

22. Sharp VJ, Kieran K, Arlen AM. Testicular torsion: diagnosis, evaluation and management. *Am Fam Phys.* 2013;88:835–840.

23. American Urological Association. Acute scrotum. https://www.auanet.org/education/acute-scrotum.cfm. Accessed September 25, 2015.

24. Sessions AE, Rabinowitz R, Hulbert WC, Goldstein MM, Mevorach RA. Testicular torsion: direction, degree, duration and disinformation. *J Urol.* 2003;169:663–665.

25. Roett MA, Mayor MT, Uduhiri KA. Diagnosis and management of genital ulcers. *Am Fam Phys.* 2012;85:254–262.

26. Centers for Disease Control and Prevention. 2010 STD treatment guidelines: diseases characterized by genital, anal, or perianal ulcers. http://www.cdc.gov/std/treatment/2010/genital-ulcers.htm#a2. Accessed September 25, 2015.

27. Centers for Disease Control and Prevention. *Sexually Transmitted Disease Surveillance, 2013.* Atlanta, GA: US Dept of Health and Human Services; December 2014. http://www.cdc.gov/std/stats13/. Accessed September 25, 2015.

28. Centers for Disease Control and Prevention. Genital herpes—CDC fact sheet. http://www.cdc.gov/std/herpes/stdfact-herpes-detailed.htm. Accessed September 25, 2015.

29. WebMD. Alternative treatments for genital herpes. http://www.webmd.com/genital-herpes/guide/alternative-treatments#1. Accessed September 25, 2015.

Common Musculoskeletal Disorders in Primary Care

Karen S. Moore

Chapter Outline

E. Guidelines To Direct Care:

American College of Rheumatology 2012 recommendations for the use of nonpharmacologic and pharmacologic therapies in osteoarthritis of the hand, hip, and knee

AIM Specialty Health. Appropriate use criteria: imaging of the extremities. Chicago (IL)

AIM Specialty Health. Appropriate use criteria: imaging of the abdomen & pelvis. Chicago (IL)

American College of Radiology Appropriateness Criteria® chronic hip pain. Reston (VA) Acute hip pain suspected fracture. Reston (VA)

American College of Radiology Appropriateness Criteria® Stress (fatigue/insufficiency) fracture, including sacrum, excluding other vertebrae. Reston (VA)

US Food and Drug Administration Medication Guides. http://www.fda.gov/Drugs/DrugSafety/ucm085729.html

Case 5 - Carpal Tunnel Syndrome

A. History and Physical Exam

B. Recommended labs/diagnostics

C. Pathophysiology

D. Treatment Plan

E. Guidelines To Direct Care:

Expert Panel on Musculoskeletal Imaging. American College of Radiology Appropriateness Criteria® chronic wrist pain. Reston (VA)

Evidence-based guideline: neuromuscular ultrasound for the diagnosis of carpal tunnel syndrome

American Academy of Orthopaedic Surgeons (AAOS). Clinical practice guideline on the treatment of carpal tunnel syndrome. Rosemon (IL)

Rheumatology recommendations for the use of disease-modifying antirheumatic drugs and biologic agents in the treatment of rheumatoid arthritis.

American Diabetes Association. Standards of Medical Care for Diabetes – 2015

Learning Objectives

Using a case-based approach, the learner will be able to:

1. Identify key history and physical examination parameters for common musculoskeletal disorders seen in primary care.

2. Summarize recommended laboratory and diagnostic studies indicated for the evaluation of common musculoskeletal disorders seen in primary care.

3. State pathophysiology of common musculoskeletal disorders.

4. Document a clear, concise SOAP note for patients with common musculoskeletal disorders.

5. Identify relevant education and counseling strategies for patients with common musculoskeletal disorders.

6. Develop a treatment plan for common musculoskeletal disorders utilizing current evidence-based guidelines.

Case 1

John is a 35-year-old male with complaints of (c/o) low back pain that occurred after lifting a large box filled with heavy machine parts 4 days ago. States he was working in the construction industry at the time of the incident. States he initially felt a twinge and thought it would get better with a little rest, but it has not. States he took ibuprofen 400 mg "three or four times" without relief. States he feels unable to do his regular job, is having difficulty sleeping related to difficulty getting comfortable, and is having trouble performing activities of daily living such as bending over to put on shoes. States his pain is 2/10 at its best when he is able to find a position of comfort, 5/10 most of the time, and 7/10 if he attempts to bend over or lift anything over 5–10 pounds. Denies changes in bowel or bladder habits, denies impotence. Denies numbness, tingling, or weakness in back or lower extremities.

Denies any significant past medical history. John states he has not been seen at the office "in a while" because "if it isn't broke, don't fix it." States he was last seen approximately 2 years ago for an upper respiratory infection. No known drug allergies (NKDA), takes no medications. Childhood immunizations up-to-date, tetanus up-to-date, does not receive annual influenza vaccination. Smokes one pack per day × 20 years, alcohol (ETOH) occasional beer on the weekend but less than three per month, denies illicit drug use.

Physical Exam

Vital Signs (VS): Blood pressure (BP) 130/82, heart rate (HR) 88 regular, respiratory rate (RR) 16, temperature (T) 98.6, height (Ht) 6'2", weight (Wt) 190 lbs

General (GEN): Noted to be shifting position from side to side while sitting in examination room that he states is related to back pain. Demonstrates difficulty with position changes when moving from chair to examination table

Head, eyes, ears, nose, and throat (HEENT): Head normocephalic without evidence of masses or trauma. Pupils equal, round, react to light, accommodation (PERRLA), extraocular movements (EOMs) intact. Noninjected. Fundoscopic exam unremarkable. Ear canal without redness or irritation, tympanic membranes (TMs) clear, pearly, bony landmarks visible. No discharge, no pain noted. Neck supple without masses. No thyromegaly. No jugular vein distention (JVD) noted

Skin: No discoloration, no open areas noted. Scarring to right forearm from prior injury

Cardiovascular (CV): S_1 and S_2 regular rate and rhythm (RRR), no murmurs, no rubs

Lungs: Clear to auscultation

Abdomen: Soft, nontender, nondistended, bowel sounds present × 4 quadrants, no organomegaly, no bruits

Musculoskeletal (MS): Pain with palpation to L2–S1 region of lower back with paravertebral muscle (PVM) spasms noted bilaterally. No vertebral tenderness with palpation. Range of motion of lower back: forward flexion 40 degrees, extension 5 degrees, sidebending 5 degrees, rotation 5 degrees.

Neuro: Sensation intact to bilateral lower extremities, deep tendon reflexes (DTRs) 2+ at patellar and Achilles bilaterally. Great toe extension normal, ankle dorsiflexion normal, plantar flexion normal, heel/toe walk normal, unable to squat secondary to back pain. Bilateral lower extremity (LE) strength 5/5. Straight leg raises (SLR) 80 degrees bilaterally with pain

What additional assessments/diagnostics do you need?

What is the differential diagnoses list?

What is your working diagnosis?

Additional Assessments/Diagnostics Needed

Ask focused review of systems (ROS) questions.[1–8] It is important when a patient presents with low back pain that you elicit a detailed history and physical, paying careful attention to any red flags that may trigger the need for urgent evaluation or treatment.

Risk Factors for Low Back Pain

▶ Obesity

▶ Age

▶ Physically strenuous work or sedentary work

▶ Psychologically strenuous work

▶ Low education attainment

▶ Job dissatisfaction

▶ Psychological factors such as anxiety, depression, and somatization disorder

Potential for Underlying Systemic Diagnosis

Hints to an underlying systemic diagnosis as opposed to isolated low back pain may necessitate urgent evaluation and would include:

▶ History of cancer

▶ Unexplained weight loss

▶ Duration of pain greater than 1 month

▶ Pain that awakens the patient at night

▶ Unresponsive to previous therapies

▶ History of abdominal aortic aneurysm

▶ Infection

▶ Major trauma

▶ Neurologic changes or findings on examination

Red Flags

Reports of major trauma, infection, or troubling examination findings necessitate urgent referral. One such condition is known as cauda equina syndrome. Cauda equina syndrome is a medical emergency and must be recognized so the patient may be sent for emergent surgical decompression to prevent permanent injury. Nonspecific symptoms of cauda equina include low back pain that radiates into buttock and leg along the sciatic nerve root distribution. Specific symptoms of cauda equina syndrome include:

▶ Changes in bowel/bladder habits (incontinence, constipation)

▶ Decreased reflexes to lower extremities

▶ Decreased sensation to lower extremities

▶ Weakness in lower extremities

▶ Numbness in the groin/impotence

Exam

The physical examination for patients with low back pain (LBP) should include:

▶ Identification of red flags (fever, major trauma, cauda equina syndrome)

▶ Detailed history of the pain (has it happened before, when did it start, what is the level of pain, what makes it better or worse, how are you sleeping, positions of comfort, what have you tried to make it better—medications, ice/heat, exercise)

▶ Consider administration of Oswestry Low Back Pain Disability Questionnaire

▶ Nonsteroidal anti-inflammatory drugs (NSAIDs) as first-line medications. May include muscle relaxants in specific cases not fully helped by NSAIDs and with significant muscle spasm noted. Avoid opioids and glucocorticoids

▶ Heat

▶ Aerobic exercises and specific stretches

- Some work and activity restrictions may be needed for short term, but bed rest is not recommended
- Manipulation and mobilization may be recommended for acute LBP

Routine Labs/Diagnostics

- Imaging studies with X-ray, CT, or MRI are not recommended for acute or subacute low back injuries (4–6 weeks) unless red flags are present.

Differential Diagnoses

Lumbago

Lumbosacral sprain

Lumbar degenerative disc disease

Lumbar facet arthropathy

Lumbar spondylolysis and spondylolisthesis

Renal infection or stone

Abdominal aortic aneurysm

Osteoporosis

Working Diagnoses

Lumbosacral sprain

Lumbago

Pathophysiology

Low back pain in the United States costs an estimated $26.3 billion each year and is the second most common symptom-related reason people visit with a healthcare provider. Low back pain can be a symptom of underlying systemic illness, mechanical irritation along the lower back from a muscle sprain or strain, or arthropathies along the disc and bony elements of the vertebral column and musculoskeletal system. Uncomplicated low back pain normally resolves within 4 to 6 weeks without intervention. If low back pain does not resolve within that time frame, further evaluation and more aggressive treatment may be advised.[4–6]

What Is Your Treatment Plan?

Pharmacologic

- NSAIDs—ibuprofen 800 mg prescribed for this patient
- Proton pump inhibitors, histamine blockers for gastrointestinal (GI) protection while on NSAIDs—not done with this patient
- Muscle relaxants—cyclobenzaprine 5 mg PO HS prescribed for this patient

Nonpharmacologic

- Heat

- Home exercises
- Work/activity restrictions

Education/Counseling

- Good back hygiene—lifting technique
- Work restrictions

SOAP Note

S: John is a 35-year-old male with c/o low back pain that occurred after lifting a large box filled with heavy machine parts 4 days ago. States he was working in the construction industry at the time of the incident. States he initially felt a twinge and thought it would get better with a little rest, but it has not. States he took ibuprofen 400 mg "three or four times" without relief. States he feels unable to do his regular job, is having difficulty sleeping related to difficulty getting comfortable, and is having trouble performing activities of daily living such as bending over to put on shoes. States his pain is 2/10 at its best when he is able to find a position of comfort, 5/10 most of the time, and 7/10 if he attempts to bend over or lift anything over 5–10 pounds. Denies changes in bowel or bladder habits, denies impotence. Denies numbness, tingling, or weakness in back or lower extremities. Denies any significant past medical history. John states he was last seen approximately 2 years ago for an upper respiratory infection. NKDA, takes no medications. Immunizations up-to-date but refuses annual influenza vaccination. Twenty-pack-year history of tobacco use, ETOH less than three beers per month, denies illicit drug use.

O: *VS:* BP 130/82, HR 88 regular, RR 16, T 98.6, Ht 6'2", Wt 190 lbs

GEN: Noted to be shifting position from side to side while sitting in examination room that he states is related to back pain. Demonstrates difficulty with position changes when moving from chair to examination table

HEENT: Head normocephalic without evidence of masses or trauma. PERRLA, EOMs intact. Noninjected. Fundoscopic exam unremarkable. Ear canal without redness or irritation, TMs clear, pearly, bony landmarks visible. No discharge, no pain noted. Neck supple without masses. No thyromegaly. No JVD noted

Skin: No discoloration, no open areas noted. Scarring to right forearm from prior injury

CV: S_1 and S_2 RRR, no murmurs, no rubs

Lungs: Clear to auscultation

Abdomen: Soft, nontender, nondistended, bowel sounds present × 4 quadrants, no organomegaly, no bruits

MS: Pain with palpation to L2–S1 region of lower back with PVM spasms noted bilaterally. No vertebral tenderness with palpation. Range of motion of lower back: forward flexion

40 degrees, extension 5 degrees, sidebending 5 degrees, rotation 5 degrees.

Neuro: Sensation intact to bilateral lower extremities, DTR 2+ at patellar and Achilles bilaterally. Great toe extension normal, ankle dorsiflexion normal, plantar flexion normal, heel/toe walk normal, unable to squat secondary to back pain. Bilateral LE strength 5/5. SLR 80 degrees bilaterally with pain

A:

1. Lumbosacral sprain
2. Lumbago

P: Begin ibuprofen 800 mg PO TID with food, cyclobenzaprine 5 mg PO HS, warm compresses to lower back 15 minutes at a time at least three times daily, home exercise program provided, discussion of back hygiene with focus on lifting techniques as well as positioning at rest. Work restrictions: limit bending and twisting, limit lifting to 10 lbs, limit stooping and squatting, no ladders, no work at heights. Discussed smoking cessation and influenza vaccine. States he will "think about" vaccination and smoking cessation. Reviewed signs and symptoms (s/s) of worsening condition. Instructed to call or return if symptoms worsen. Follow-up in 1 week to reassess low back pain and work restrictions.

Health Promotion Issues

▶ Encourage influenza vaccination annually
▶ Smoking cessation recommended

Guidelines to Direct Care

AIM Specialty Health. *Appropriate Use Criteria: Imaging of the Spine.* Chicago, IL: AIM Specialty Health; 2013.

American College of Occupational and Environmental Medicine (ACOEM). *Occupational Medicine Practice Guidelines: Evaluation and Management of Health Problems and Functional Recovery in Workers.* 3rd ed. Elk Grove Village, IL: American College of Occupational and Environmental Medicine; 2011:333–796.

Centers for Disease Control and Prevention. Recommended adult immunization schedule, by vaccine and age group. 2014. http://www.cdc.gov/vaccines/schedules/hcp/imz/adult.html. Accessed September 2, 2015.

Chou R, Qaseem A, Snow V, et al; Clinical Efficacy Assessment Subcommittee of the American College of Physicians; American College of Physicians; American Pain Society Low Back Pain Guidelines Panel. Diagnosis and treatment of low back pain: a joint clinical practice guideline from the American College of Physicians and the American Pain Society. *Ann Intern Med.* 2007;147(7):479–491.

US Dept of Agriculture and US Dept of Health and Human Services. *Dietary Guidelines for Americans, 2010.* 7th ed. Washington, DC: US Government Printing Office; 2010.

US Preventive Services Task Force. Recommendations for primary care practice: published recommendations. http://www.uspreventiveservicestaskforce.org/BrowseRec/Index/browse-recommendations. Accessed September 2, 2015.

Case 2

Susan is a 25-year-old female who was involved in a motor vehicle accident (MVA) 3 days ago. States she was wearing her seat belt at the time of the accident and was struck from behind by another vehicle as she was stopped at a stoplight. States her car sustained substantial damage, and she was "thrown around a little bit," but she denies striking her head or losing consciousness. States she was seen at the emergency room (ER), X-ray studies were taken, and she was told she did not have a fracture. Complaints of (c/o) pain in posterior neck, worsened with bending or twisting her neck, and difficulty sleeping related to finding a position of comfort, and states she feels like her neck is "weak." When queried further, states she has some numbness and tingling in her right shoulder and periscapular region. Denies headache, dizziness, nausea, or vomiting. Denies striking head. Reports some bruising to her knees but denies injury to chest or abdomen. States she had a previous episode of numbness and tingling in her shoulder region in the past when she "slept wrong." Denies weakness in arms or lower extremities, denies changes in bowel/bladder habits. NKDA.

Childhood immunizations completed, unsure of last tetanus, does not receive annual influenza vaccinations. Takes no medications regularly. Regular well-woman exam completed with normal Pap 1 year ago. Employed full time as an office worker. Prescribed ibuprofen 800 mg PO TID and hydrocodone 5 mg PO Q6H PRN in the ER. Denies smoking, illicit drug use. Reports ETOH use of "a few drinks" on the weekend "occasionally."

Physical Exam

VS: BP 116/78, HR 72 regular, RR 20, T 98.8, Ht 5'5", Wt 110 lbs

GEN: No acute distress

HEENT: Head normocephalic without evidence of masses or trauma. PERRLA, EOMs intact. Noninjected. Fundoscopic exam unremarkable. Ear canal without redness or irritation, TMs clear, pearly, bony landmarks visible. No discharge, no pain noted. Neck without masses. No thyromegaly. No JVD noted

Skin: No open areas noted. Ecchymosis and slight swelling to bilateral prepatellar surfaces and right pretibial region

CV: S_1 and S_2 RRR, no murmurs, no rubs. No ecchymosis noted to thorax

Lungs: Clear to auscultation

Abdomen: Soft, nontender, nondistended, bowel sounds present × 4 quadrants, no organomegaly, no bruits. No bruising, no abrasions noted

MS: Pain with palpation to C5–7 vertebral processes with PVM spasms noted bilaterally in cervical region. Range of motion of neck: forward flexion 10 degrees, extension 0 degrees, sidebending 5 degrees, rotation 5 degrees. Spurling's negative, right shoulder abduction positive. Weakness noted on resisted sidebending of neck to the right. No pain with palpation of thoracic or lumbosacral regions

Neuro: Sensation intact to bilateral upper and lower extremities, DTR 2+ at biceps, triceps, brachioradialis, patellar, and Achilles bilaterally. Great toe extension normal, ankle dorsiflexion normal, plantar flexion normal, heel/toe walk normal. Bilateral upper extremity (UE)/lower extremity (LE) strength 5/5

What additional assessments/diagnostics do you need?

What is the differential diagnoses list?

What is your working diagnosis?

Additional Assessments/Diagnostics Needed

Ask Focused ROS Questions.[4–7]

When assessing a patient with neck pain, it is important to consider red flags such as suggestion of instability, cord compression, or systemic illness. Some issues suggestive of cord impingement to explore:

▶ Difficulty gripping or grasping

▶ Weakness in neck

▶ Weakness in upper extremities

Risk factors for neck pain with radiculopathy:

▶ Prior history of neck or back injuries or pain

▶ History of neurologic conditions that may mimic paresthesias

▶ History of sports injuries with potential for neck trauma

Potential for Underlying Systemic Diagnosis

Although the workup for Susan would be fairly straightforward given her history and physical exam, if discrepancies in history and physical occurred, systemic disease such as the following may be a consideration:

▶ Central nervous system (CNS) lesions

▶ Multiple sclerosis and other neuromuscular disorders

Exam[9]

The physical examination should focus on assessing for:

▶ Neck pain

▶ Shoulder pain

▶ Motor weakness in upper extremities

▶ Absent or diminished reflexes

▶ Sensory changes in upper extremities

▶ Scapular pain

▶ Periscapular pain

Atypical findings may include:

▶ Deltoid weakness

▶ Scapular winging

▶ Chest or deep breast pain

▶ Weakness of intrinsic muscles of the hand

▶ Headaches

Provocative tests such as shoulder abduction and Spurling's test may be done if radiculopathy is suspected.

Routine Labs/Diagnostics[9-11]

▶ NEXUS Criteria would be utilized initially to determine whether imaging is necessary for this patient with a potential C-spine injury. A "yes" response to any of the following NEXUS queries would indicate that imaging may be recommended:

   ▷ Focal neurologic deficit present

   ▷ Midline spinal tenderness present

   ▷ Altered level of consciousness

   ▷ Intoxication

   ▷ Distracting injury present

▶ MRI would be recommended in a patient such as Susan who is exhibiting signs and symptoms of radiculopathy and ligamentous weakness in the cervical region.

▶ CT without contrast could be done to diagnose or rule out C-spine fracture. A CT may be done in conjunction with an MRI if ligamentous, soft tissue, and bony injuries are suspected. If CT findings are discordant with MRI findings, a CT with myelogram may be conducted.

▶ X-ray imaging is not the preferred method of imaging in suspected C-spine injury. A lateral view may be helpful if CT reconstruction is not optimal.

Differential Diagnoses List

Brachial plexus injury

Cervical cord impingement

Cervical disc injury

Cervical discogenic pain syndrome

Cervical facet syndrome

Cervical sprain/strain with radiculopathy

Rotator cuff injury

■ *Working Diagnosis—Cervical sprain/strain with radiculopathy*

■ Pathophysiology

The cervical region of the neck is made up of ligaments, muscles, tendons, the bony vertebral column, articular cartridge such as discs and facets, as well as the spinal cord and nerve roots. A cervical acceleration/deceleration injury commonly known as "whiplash" is often seen following a motor vehicle accident. Although injury to the spinal cord and vertebral column are the primary focus of early imaging studies, injury to the surrounding tissues and structures can cause significant debilitation and pain. It is believed that injury to the muscle, tendon, and facet regions can lead to inflammation and irritation of the muscle–tendon unit, spasm, and radicular symptoms. Treatment is often aimed at reduction of inflammation and symptoms associated with the sequelae of injury such as spasm and radiculopathy.[4–7]

■ *What Is Your Treatment Plan?*

■ Pharmacologic

▶ NSAIDs

▶ Muscle relaxants

■ Nonpharmacologic

▶ CT

▶ MRI

▶ Physical therapy (PT)—PT may be initiated only after CT and MRI are completed and demonstrate no findings that would contraindicate therapy

■ Education/Counseling

▶ Sleep hygiene—to avoid neck strain and malpositioning during sleep

▶ What to anticipate in PT—may initially increase stiffness and pain

▶ Medication education

▶ Attention to work hygiene and ergonomic workstation arrangement to avoid repetitive neck flexion or sidebending and unusual postures

■ SOAP Note

S: Susan is a 25-year-old female who was involved in an MVA 3 days ago. States she was wearing her seat belt at the time of the accident and was struck from behind by another vehicle as she was stopped at a stoplight. States her car sustained substantial damage, and she was "thrown around a little bit," but she denies striking her head or losing consciousness. States she was seen at the ER, X-ray studies were taken, and she was told she did not have a fracture. C/o pain in posterior neck, worsened with bending or twisting her neck, and difficulty sleeping related to finding a position of comfort, and states she feels like her neck is "weak." When queried further, states she has some numbness and tingling in her right shoulder and periscapular region. Denies headache, dizziness, nausea, or vomiting. Denies striking head. Reports some bruising to her knees but denies injury to chest or abdomen. States she had a previous episode of numbness and tingling in her shoulder region in the past when she "slept wrong." Denies weakness in arms or lower extremities, denies changes in bowel/bladder habits. NKDA. Childhood immunizations completed, unsure of last tetanus, does not receive annual influenza vaccinations. Takes no medications regularly. Regular well-woman exam completed with normal Pap 1 year ago. Employed full time as an office worker. Prescribed ibuprofen 800 mg PO TID and hydrocodone 5 mg PO Q6H PRN in the ER. Denies smoking, illicit drug use. Reports ETOH use of "a few drinks" on the weekend "occasionally."

O: *VS:* BP 116/78, HR 72 regular, RR 20, T 98.8, Ht 5'5", Wt 110 lbs

GEN: No acute distress

HEENT: Head normocephalic without evidence of masses or trauma. PERRLA, EOMs intact. Noninjected. Fundoscopic exam unremarkable. Ear canal without redness or irritation, TMs clear, pearly, bony landmarks visible. No discharge, no pain noted. Neck without masses. No thyromegaly. No JVD noted

Skin: No open areas noted. Ecchymosis and slight swelling to bilateral prepatellar surfaces and right pretibial region

CV: S_1 and S_2 RRR, no murmurs, no rubs. No ecchymosis noted to thorax

Lungs: Clear to auscultation

Abdomen: Soft, nontender, nondistended, bowel sounds present × 4 quadrants, no organomegaly, no bruits. No bruising, no abrasions noted

MS: Pain with palpation to C5–7 vertebral processes with PVM spasms noted bilaterally. Range of motion of neck: forward flexion 10 degrees, extension 0 degrees, sidebending 5 degrees, rotation 5 degrees. Spurling's negative, shoulder abduction positive. Weakness noted on resisted sidebending of neck to the right. No pain with palpation of thoracic or lumbosacral regions

Neuro: Sensation intact to bilateral upper and lower extremities, DTR 2+ at biceps, triceps, brachioradialis, patellar, and Achilles bilaterally. Great toe extension normal, ankle dorsiflexion normal, plantar flexion normal, heel/toe walk normal. Bilateral UE/LE strength 5/5

A: Cervical sprain/strain with radiculopathy

P: Continue ibuprofen 800 mg PO TID, discontinue hydrocodone, add cyclobenzaprine 5 mg PO HS. Order CT and MRI today, with stat preliminary read. If stat read negative, will have patient follow up in 24–48 hours for discussion of final read, reassess med regimen, and order PT. Plan to update tetanus at next visit and to discuss influenza vaccination.

Health Promotion Issues

▶ Update tetanus

▶ Encourage annual flu vaccine[1-3]

Guidelines to Direct Care

AIM Specialty Health. *Appropriate Use Criteria: Imaging of the Spine.* Chicago, IL: AIM Specialty Health; 2013.

Centers for Disease Control and Prevention. Recommended adult immunization schedule, by vaccine and age group. 2014. http://www.cdc.gov/vaccines/schedules/hcp/imz/adult.html. Accessed September 2, 2015.

Expert Panels on Musculoskeletal and Neurologic Imaging. *ACR Appropriateness Criteria: Suspected Spine Trauma.* Reston, VA: American College of Radiology; 2009.

North American Spine Society. *Diagnosis and Treatment of Cervical Radiculopathy from Degenerative Disorders.* Burr Ridge, IL: North American Spine Society; 2010.

Stiell G, Clement CM, McKnight RD, et al. The Canadian C-spine rule versus the NEXUS low-risk criteria in patients with trauma. *N Engl J Med.* 2003;349(26):2510–2518.

US Preventive Services Task Force. Recommendations for primary care practice: published recommendations. http://www.uspreventiveservicestaskforce.org/BrowseRec/Index/browse-recommendations. Accessed September 2, 2015.

Case 3

Jennifer is an 18-year-old female who injured her right knee while playing soccer on her select team. States she is a midfielder and was running from the backfield to a more forward position when she planted her foot to pass the ball and felt her right knee "buckle." States she heard a loud "pop" and at the time had severe pain that persists. States she feels unable to bear full weight. States she has been using ice "around the clock" and ibuprofen every 6 hours, but states her "swelling is the worst ever." Denies any numbness or tingling. When queried, states she has played select soccer year-round since she was 7 years old. States she has had prior minor injuries "strains and sprains, but nothing serious." Denies prior surgeries. Denies history of serious illness. Vaccinations are up-to-date. Denies receiving annual influenza vaccination because she doesn't believe it works. NKDA. Denies sexual activity, denies tobacco use, denies ETOH use, denies illicit drug use. Denies relationship difficulties, being in abusive or unsafe relationships. Reports a history of a healthy diet with balanced macronutrients and micronutrients. States she pays close attention to her diet related to trying out for college scholarships soon. Denies binge/purge, restrictive dieting, or attempts at weight loss.

Physical Exam

VS: BP 104/68, HR 64 regular, RR 16, T 98.5, Ht 5'7", Wt 120 lbs

GEN: No acute distress

HEENT: Head normocephalic without evidence of masses or trauma. PERRLA, EOMs intact. Noninjected. Fundoscopic exam unremarkable. Ear canal without redness or irritation, TMs clear, pearly, bony landmarks visible. No discharge, no pain noted. Neck without masses. No thyromegaly. No JVD noted

Skin: No open areas noted. Ecchymosis and a large amount of swelling to right knee region

CV: S_1 and S_2 RRR, no murmurs, no rubs. No ecchymosis noted to thorax

Lungs: Clear to auscultation

Abdomen: Soft, nontender, nondistended, bowel sounds present × 4 quadrants, no organomegaly, no bruits. No bruising, no abrasions noted

MS: Muscular body habitus noted. Large amount of swelling and effusion noted to right knee with diffuse ecchymosis. Right knee measurement at joint line 29 cm; left knee measurement at joint line 20 cm. Pain with palpation to anterior knee and along joint line. Active range of motion with extension at −10 degrees, flexion at 60 degrees. Passive range of motion consistent with active range of motion. Anterior drawers with laxity noted, posterior drawers mild laxity, valgus and varus stressing without laxity. Unable to perform McMurray's secondary to pain and swelling. Pain noted on all provocative maneuvers and with passive and active range of motion

Neuro: Sensation intact to bilateral lower extremities, DTR 2+ at left patellar and Achilles as well as right Achilles. Right patellar reflexes deferred secondary to pain and swelling. Bilateral ankle dorsiflexion and plantar flexion normal. No pain with palpation of ankles. No ankle pain with range of motion.

Unable to bear weight on right lower extremity secondary to knee pain. Neurovascular intact.

What additional assessments/diagnostics do you need?

What is the differential diagnoses list?

What is your working diagnosis?

Additional Assessments/Diagnostics Needed

Evaluation for the patient with suspected knee injury should include:[1–4,12–14]

- A complete history and physical with special attention paid to:
  - Mechanism of injury
  - Sensations of popping, giving way, buckling, or inability to bear weight
  - Laxity on provocative maneuvers
  - Swelling, effusion, and ecchymosis
- Appropriate imaging studies based upon history and physical (H&P)

Ask focused ROS questions:

- Prior injuries
- Prior surgeries
- Associated injuries
- Sports participation

Risk Factors for Knee Injury

In the case of Jennifer, some things that put her at risk for knee injury are:

- Female
- Competitive athlete
- Stopping and starting under speed
- Planting her foot while turning/rotating

Other risk factors for an anterior cruciate ligament (ACL) injury are:

- Slowing down while running
- A tackling sport such as football
- An acceleration/deceleration sport such as soccer, football, or basketball
- Landing from a jump

Potential for Underlying Systemic Diagnosis

In this case, there is no great suspicion of underlying systemic disease or diagnosis. If imaging studies suggest, bony tumors or metabolic disturbances could be explored. These would be highly unlikely in this particular young woman.

Exam

The physical exam should focus on performing a complete knee evaluation. This should include:

- Bilateral comparison of lower extremities
- Measurement of knees bilaterally to document swelling more succinctly
- Evaluation of bony structures
- Evaluation of ligamentous structures utilizing provocative maneuvers
- Assessment of gait
- Evaluation of range of motion
- Evaluation of neurovascular status

Routine Labs/Diagnostics[12–14]

- X-ray—standard plain films are recommended to rule out bony involvement
- MRI—MRI would be strongly recommended to evaluate the ligamentous and articular surfaces

Differential Diagnoses List

ACL tear/Grade 3 sprain

ACL sprain/Grade 1 or 2

Meniscus tear

Posterior cruciate ligament (PCL) sprain/tear

Collateral ligament sprain

Working Diagnosis—ACL tear/Grade 3 sprain

Pathophysiology

The knee joint is stabilized via the collateral and cruciate ligamentous structures.[12–14] The collateral ligaments run alongside the knee on the medial and lateral positions and prevent aberrant side-to-side motion of the knee. The cruciate ligaments form an X inside the knee to stabilize the knee from the posterior and anterior positions. The anterior cruciate ligament's primary role is to prevent the tibia from sliding forward anterior to the femur. When the ACL sustains a sprain, it is classified using the following grading scale:

- Grade 1: The ACL is stretched, but the joint is not unstable.
- Grade 2: The ACL is stretched, and the joint feels some laxity. This is often referred to as a partial tear.
- Grade 3: The ACL is completely torn, and the joint is unstable. This is often referred to as a complete tear.

It is important to note that in approximately 50% of ACL tears, additional injuries to the knee are sustained.

What Is Your Treatment Plan?

Pharmacologic

- NSAIDs
- Pain medication as needed[12–14]

Nonpharmacologic

▶ Ice—recommend 15–20 minutes at a time, applying each hour initially

▶ Elevation—for comfort and to reduce swelling

▶ Imaging with X-ray and MRI—X-ray is recommended to rule out fracture, MRI to assess for ligamentous and articular injury

▶ Rest—out of sports, non-weight-bearing

▶ Bracing—bracing preferably with compression to reduce swelling and stabilize the knee until surgical correction

▶ Surgery—in a young competitive athlete with a complete tear, surgery would be recommended

Education/Counseling

▶ Rest: It is important to emphasize the need for rest and restrictions from activity with this patient.

▶ Bracing: Educate about the need and purpose of bracing. Emphasize comfort of bracing and neurovascular checks to ensure that the brace is not too tight.

▶ Return to activity: Non-weight-bearing at present time. Anticipate this will continue until after surgical correction.

▶ Return to sports: It is anticipated that this patient will require surgical correction and a course of physical therapy (PT) postoperatively. Sports participation will be restricted for an extended period of time to allow full healing of the repaired ACL.

SOAP Note

S: Jennifer is an 18-year-old female who injured her right knee while playing soccer on her select team. States she planted her foot to pass the ball and felt her right knee "buckle," heard a loud "pop," and at the time had severe pain that persists. States she feels unable to bear full weight. States she has been using ice "around the clock" and ibuprofen every 6 hours, but states her "swelling is the worst ever." Denies any numbness or tingling. States she has played select soccer year-round since she was 7 years old. States she has had prior minor injuries "strains and sprains, but nothing serious." Denies prior surgeries. Denies history of serious illness. Vaccinations are up-to-date. Denies receiving annual influenza vaccination because she doesn't believe it works. NKDA. Denies sexual activity, denies tobacco use, denies ETOH use, denies illicit drug use. Denies relationship difficulties, being in abusive or unsafe relationships. Reports a history of a healthy diet with balanced macronutrients and micronutrients. States she pays close attention to her diet related to trying out for college scholarships soon. Denies binge/purge, restrictive dieting, or attempts at weight loss.

O: *VS:* BP 104/68, HR 64 regular, T 98.5, RR 16, Ht 5'7", Wt 120 lbs

GEN: No acute distress

HEENT: Head normocephalic without evidence of masses or trauma. PERRLA, EOMs full to confrontation. Noninjected. Fundoscopic exam unremarkable. Ear canal without redness or irritation, TMs clear, pearly, bony landmarks visible. No discharge, no pain noted. Neck without masses. No thyromegaly. No JVD noted

Skin: No open areas noted. Ecchymosis and a large amount of swelling to right knee region

CV: S_1 and S_2 RRR, no murmurs, no rubs. No ecchymosis noted to thorax

Lungs: Clear to auscultation

Abdomen: Soft, nontender, nondistended, bowel sounds present × 4 quadrants, no organomegaly, no bruits. No bruising, no abrasions noted

MS: Muscular body habitus noted. Large amount of swelling and effusion noted to right knee with diffuse ecchymosis. Right knee measurement at joint line 29 cm; left knee measurement at joint line 20 cm. Pain with palpation to anterior knee and along joint line. Active range of motion with extension at –10 degrees, flexion at 60 degrees. Passive range of motion consistent with active range of motion. Anterior drawers with laxity noted, posterior drawers mild laxity, valgus and varus stressing without laxity. Unable to perform McMurray's secondary to pain and swelling. Pain noted on all provocative maneuvers and with passive and active range of motion.

Neuro: Sensation intact to bilateral lower extremities, DTR 2+ at left patellar and Achilles as well as right Achilles. Right patellar reflexes deferred secondary to pain and swelling. Bilateral ankle dorsiflexion and plantar flexion normal. No pain with palpation of ankles. No ankle pain with range of motion. Unable to bear weight on right lower extremity secondary to knee pain. Neurovascular intact.

A: ACL tear/Grade 3 sprain

P: Female competitive athlete with probable ACL tear. Ibuprofen 800 mg PO TID, compression bracing until MRI can be completed. Order X-ray and MRI. If positive, refer for surgery with PT anticipated postoperatively. Out of competitive soccer and sports for up to 6 months, dependent upon recovery. Influenza and meningitis vaccination discussed. She will consider following resolution of her current knee complaints.

Health Promotion Issues

▶ Encourage annual influenza vaccination

▶ Meningitis vaccination in anticipation of college enrollment

Guidelines to Direct Care

AIM Specialty Health. *Appropriate Use Criteria: Imaging of the Extremities.* Chicago, IL: AIM Specialty Health; 2014.

American Academy of Orthopaedic Surgeons (AAOS). *American Academy of Orthopaedic Surgeons Clinical Practice Guideline on Management of Anterior Cruciate Ligament Injuries*. Rosemont, IL: American Academy of Orthopaedic Surgeons; 2014.

Centers for Disease Control and Prevention. Recommended adult immunization schedule, by vaccine and age group. 2014. http://www.cdc.gov/vaccines/schedules/hcp/imz/adult.html. Accessed September 2, 2015.

Tuite MJ, Daffner RH, Weissman BN, et al; Expert Panel on Musculoskeletal Imaging. *ACR Appropriateness Criteria: Acute Trauma to the Knee*. Reston, VA: American College of Radiology; 2011.

US Dept of Agriculture and US Dept of Health and Human Services. *Dietary Guidelines for Americans, 2010*. 7th ed. Washington, DC: US Government Printing Office; 2010.

US Preventive Services Task Force. Recommendations for primary care practice: published recommendations. http://www.uspreventiveservicestaskforce.org/BrowseRec/Index/browse-recommendations. Accessed September 2, 2015.

■ Case 4

Mrs. Buckholz is a 66-year-old female who reports pain in her left hip that worsens with walking, bending, standing, and squatting. Denies known injury, denies stumbling, tripping, or falling. States the pain has been worsening gradually and now is almost constant if she stands or walks for a long period of time. When asked to describe where the pain occurs, she places her thumb posterior to her hip and her fingers anterior to hip, forming a C around the anterolateral hip region. Denies back pain, denies pain in posterior hip or along lateral thigh. Denies numbness, tingling, or weakness in extremities. When queried, states she walks approximately 1 mile daily since her retirement from her work as a schoolteacher 8 years ago. Past medical/surgical history significant for cholecystectomy at age 45 years and hysterectomy at age 56 years secondary to dysfunctional uterine bleeding. No hormone replacement therapy (HRT). Takes no medications. Immunizations up-to-date, including pneumonia, varicella, and annual influenza. Unsure of last mammogram. Has not yet had a colonoscopy. Denies allergies, denies illicit drug use, denies tobacco use. ETOH use of a glass of wine with dinner fewer than two times per week. Denies any changes in bowel/bladder habits. Denies fever, night sweats, cough, changes in appetite.

■ Physical Exam[15]

VS: BP 128/84, HR 80 regular, T 98.5, RR 20, Ht 5'3", Wt 130 lbs

GEN: No acute distress

HEENT: Head normocephalic without evidence of masses or trauma. PERRLA, EOMs intact. Noninjected. Fundoscopic exam unremarkable. Ear canal without redness or irritation, TMs clear, pearly, bony landmarks visible. No discharge, no pain noted. Neck without masses. No thyromegaly. No JVD noted

Skin: No open areas noted. No ecchymosis, no rashes, no swelling noted

CV: S_1 and S_2 RRR, no murmurs, no rubs

Lungs: Clear to auscultation

Abdomen: Soft, nontender, nondistended, bowel sounds present × 4 quadrants, no organomegaly, no bruits. No bruising, no abrasions noted

MS: No pain with palpation to back, spine, sacroiliac joint (SIJ), or hips. Antalgic gait noted when patient rises from seated position to standing and begins to walk. Passive and active ranges of motion of left hip noted at 75% of flexion, abduction, adduction, extension. Internal and external rotations 50% secondary to pain. FABER test (for flexion, abduction, and external rotation) positive. FADIR (for flexion, adduction, and internal rotation), Stinchfield, and Ober and Thomas tests negative

Neuro: Sensation intact to bilateral upper and lower extremities, DTR 2+ at patellar and Achilles bilaterally. Great toe extension normal, ankle dorsiflexion normal, plantar flexion normal, heel/toe walk with pain in left hip verbalized. Bilateral UE/LE strength 5/5

What additional assessments/diagnostics do you need?

What is the differential diagnoses list?

What is your working diagnosis?

■ *Additional Assessments/Diagnostics Needed*

In evaluating a patient with hip pain, it is imperative that the examiner ask specific questions to help focus the region of pain and narrow the differential diagnoses.[1–4,14–22] Hip pain can be divided into three anatomic regions: anterior, lateral, and posterior.

▶ Anterior hip pain is the most common hip complaint in primary care and predominantly originates from intra-articular surfaces, hip flexor strains, stress fractures, labral tears, and iliopsoas bursitis.

▶ Lateral hip pain has causation rooted in trochanteric bursitis, gluteus medius injury, iliotibial band syndrome, and, less commonly, meralgia paresthetica.

▶ Posterior hip pain is the least common pain pattern and is suggestive of sources outside of the hip, such as lumbosacral spinal arthropathy, disc disease, or spinal stenosis.

Ask focused ROS questions:

- When did the pain begin?
- Was it insidious or sudden in onset?
- Was it associated with injury?
- Is there any underlying history of bony pathology, congenital malformations, or degenerative conditions?
- Where is it located?
- Does it radiate from, stem from, or radiate to any other place on your body?

Risk Factors for Hip Pain

- Postmenopausal female—places patient at greater risk for osteoporosis and fracture
- Chronic or high-dose steroid use—risk of avascular necrosis
- History of sickle cell disease—risk of avascular necrosis
- Cancer history—risk of pathologic fracture or bony metastases
- History of low back pain or back issues—suggestive of radiation of symptoms to hip
- Competitive or aggressive athletic training or competition—risk of injury and musculoskeletal/tendon irritation
- Increased age—chronic conditions such as osteoarthritis
- History of chronic alcohol use—leads to bone loss and increased risk of osteoporosis

Potential for Underlying Systemic Diagnosis

In the case of this patient, she does not have a history of underlying metabolic disease, congenital anomalies, or cancer. Although it is true that she has not had routine colonoscopy screening, she denies any bleeding or changes in bowel/bladder habits. She also denies any signs or symptoms of inflammatory conditions such as fever, night sweats, rash, or joint swelling. If inflammatory conditions are suspected, a complete blood count (CBC), erythrocyte sedimentation rate (ESR), and C-reactive protein (CRP) may be considered as well as removal and evaluation of any joint fluid.

Exam

Evaluation of hip pain should include an assessment of the hips, back, abdomen, and vascular and neurologic systems. The hip evaluation itself should contain:

- Assessment of gait
- Modified Trendelenburg test—patient stands on one leg and the examiner looks for asymmetry of the iliac crest
- C sign—indicative of anterior hip pain as seen with Mrs. Buckholz
- Range of motion (ROM) testing—both active and passive
- FABER test (Patrick test) (flexion, abduction, external rotation)—a positive test of posterior hip, groin, sacroiliac joint, and lumbar spine pain is sensitive for intra-articular pathology

- FADIR test (impingement test) (flexion, adduction, internal rotation)—a positive test is pain during positioning suggestive of impingement
- Straight leg raise against resistance (Stinchfield test)—weakness is suggestive of impingement and neuronal entrapment
- Ober test—if passive adduction past midline is not possible secondary to pain or snapping of the hip, lateral etiology is suggested
- Thomas test—if click palpated during maneuver, may be indicative of a labral tear

Routine Labs/Diagnostics[14–19]

In the case of Mrs. Buckholz, routine labs are not anticipated. If inflammatory conditions are suspected a CBC, ESR, and CRP may be considered as well as removal and evaluation of any joint fluid.

Imaging studies would be recommended to determine more specific etiology of Mrs. Buckholz's pain.

- X-ray—is the appropriate first imaging study to be completed and should include the full hip series with anteroposterior (AP) and lateral views of the affected hip and perhaps pelvis films
- MRI—if X-ray imaging is not sufficient to direct care, an MRI without contrast would be the appropriate next step imaging study to be completed
- Bone scan—if fracture or osteoporosis is suggested on X-ray imaging, a bone scan may be done to further evaluate bone density and subtle bony changes

Differential Diagnoses List

Differential diagnoses for hip pain can be divided by location of pain.[14–22]

- Anterior: Osteoarthritis, inflammatory or infectious arthritis, osteomyelitis, hip flexor strains, hip flexor tendonitis, iliopsoas bursitis, hip fracture, stress fracture, labral tears, avascular necrosis, tumor
- Lateral: Greater trochanteric pain syndrome, greater trochanteric bursitis, iliotibial band syndrome, meralgia paresthetica, gluteus medius muscle dysfunction
- Posterior: Lumbosacral degenerative disc disease/arthropathy/spinal stenosis, sports injuries, hip extensor/rotator muscle strain

Because the history and physical examination of Mrs. Buckholz suggest anterior hip pain, her differential diagnoses would be:

- Osteoarthritis
- Inflammatory arthritis
- Infectious arthritis
- Hip flexor tendonitis
- Hip fracture
- Avascular necrosis

- ▶ Neoplasm
- ▶ Iliopsoas bursitis
- ▶ Labral tear

Working Diagnosis—Osteoarthritis

Pathophysiology

Osteoarthritis (OA) is a musculoskeletal disease characterized by chronic changes in the hyaline cartridge as well as inflammation and bone remodeling. OA is estimated to affect nearly 40% of adults older than the age of 75 years in the United States and is the leading cause of chronic disability.

What Is Your Treatment Plan?

Pharmacologic

- ▶ NSAIDs orally: Selection of appropriate NSAID is based on patient's comorbid conditions and medication regimen.
- ▶ Proton pump inhibitor: To be given with NSAIDs related to chronic use of NSAID and mitigation of GI side effects.
- ▶ Topical capsaicin, trolamine salicylate, or NSAIDs.
- ▶ Intra-articular glucocorticoids: Recommended if conservative treatment has not provided full relief.
- ▶ Other: Consider other pain medications such as tramadol or opioids only limitedly if other measures are not effective and joint replacement is anticipated.

Nonpharmacologic

- ▶ Heat therapy.
- ▶ Exercise program: Consider aquatic-based aerobic activities or tai chi initially and progress to other aerobic weight-bearing activities if desired.
- ▶ Mrs. Buckholz is not overweight, but weight management should be recommended for overweight patients with OA.
- ▶ Radiographs of left hip: AP and lateral views.

Education/Counseling

- ▶ Pain management
- ▶ Activity
- ▶ Medications and side effects

SOAP Note

S: Mrs. Buckholz is a 66-year-old female who reports pain in her left hip that worsens with walking, bending, standing, and squatting. Denies known injury, denies stumbling, tripping, or falling. States the pain has been worsening gradually and now is almost constant if she stands or walks for a long period of time. When asked to describe where the pain occurs, she places her thumb posterior to her hip and her fingers anterior to hip, forming a C around the anterolateral hip region. Denies back pain, denies pain in posterior hip or along lateral thigh. Denies numbness, tingling, or weakness in extremities. When queried, states she walks approximately 1 mile daily since her retirement from her work as a schoolteacher 8 years ago. Past medical/surgical history significant for cholecystectomy at age 45 years and hysterectomy at age 56 years secondary to dysfunctional uterine bleeding. No HRT. Takes no medications. Immunizations up-to-date, including pneumonia, varicella, and annual influenza. Unsure of last mammogram. Has not yet had a colonoscopy. Denies allergies, denies illicit drug use, denies tobacco use. ETOH use of a glass of wine with dinner fewer than two times per week. Denies any changes in bowel/bladder habits. Denies fever, night sweats, cough, changes in appetite.

O: *VS:* BP 128/84, HR 80 regular, T 98.5, RR 20, Ht 5'3", Wt 130 lbs

GEN: No acute distress

HEENT: Head normocephalic without evidence of masses or trauma. PERRLA, EOMs full to confrontation. Noninjected. Fundoscopic exam unremarkable. Ear canal without redness or irritation, TMs clear, pearly, bony landmarks visible. No discharge, no pain noted. Neck without masses. No thyromegaly. No JVD noted

Skin: No open areas noted. No ecchymosis, no rashes, no swelling noted

CV: S_1 and S_2 RRR, no murmurs, no rubs

Lungs: Clear to auscultation

Abdomen: Soft, nontender, nondistended, bowel sounds present × 4 quadrants, no organomegaly, no bruits. No bruising, no abrasions noted

MS: No pain with palpation to back, spine, SIJ, or hips. Antalgic gait noted when patient rises from seated position to standing and begins to walk. Passive and active ranges of motion of left hip noted at 75% of flexion, abduction, adduction, extension. Internal and external rotations 50% secondary to pain. FABER test positive. FADIR, Stinchfield, and Ober and Thomas tests negative.

Neuro: Sensation intact to bilateral upper and lower extremities, DTR 2+ at patellar and Achilles bilaterally. Great toe extension normal, ankle dorsiflexion normal, plantar flexion normal, heel/toe walk with pain in left hip verbalized. Bilateral UE/LE strength 5/5

A: Osteoarthritis

P: AP and lateral radiograph of left hip ordered and completed. Radiographic findings consistent with osteoarthritis. Begin celecoxib 200 mg PO QD, omeprazole 20 mg PO QD. Referral for aquatic aerobics. Order mammogram and colonoscopy. Return visit in 1 month to review results of colonoscopy and mammogram and to assess for response to treatment for OA.

▶ Mammogram

▶ Colonoscopy

▶ Exercise program—consider aquatic-based aerobic activities or tai chi

▶ Mrs. Buckholz is not overweight, but if she were, weight management should be recommended

Guidelines to Direct Care

AIM Specialty Health. *Appropriate Use Criteria: Imaging of the Abdomen and Pelvis.* Chicago, IL: AIM Specialty Health; 2014.

AIM Specialty Health. *Appropriate Use Criteria: Imaging of the Extremities.* Chicago, IL: AIM Specialty Health; 2014.

American College of Radiology. ACR Appropriateness Criteria: acute hip pain—suspected fracture. 2013. https://acsearch.acr.org/docs/3082587/Narrative/. Accessed September 25, 2015.

American College of Radiology. ACR Appropriateness Criteria: chronic hip pain. 2011. https://acsearch.acr.org/list. Accessed September 25, 2015.

Centers for Disease Control and Prevention. Recommended adult immunization schedule, by vaccine and age group. 2014. http://www.cdc.gov/vaccines/schedules/hcp/imz/adult.html. Accessed September 2, 2015.

Daffner RH, Weissman BN, Appel M, et al; Expert Panel on Musculoskeletal Imaging. ACR Appropriateness Criteria: stress (fatigue/insufficiency) fracture, including sacrum, excluding other vertebrae. Reston, VA: American College of Radiology; 2011.

Hochberg MC, Altman RD, April KT, et al. American College of Rheumatology 2012 recommendations for the use of nonpharmacologic and pharmacologic therapies in osteoarthritis of the hand, hip, and knee. *Arthritis Care Res* (Hoboken). 2012;64(4):465–474.

US Dept of Agriculture and US Dept of Health and Human Services. *Dietary Guidelines for Americans, 2010.* 7th ed. Washington, DC: US Government Printing Office; 2010.

US Food and Drug Administration. Medication guides. http://www.fda.gov/Drugs/DrugSafety/ucm085729.htm. Accessed September 25, 2015.

US Preventive Services Task Force. Recommendations for primary care practice: published recommendations. http://www.uspreventiveservicestaskforce.org/BrowseRec/Index/browse-recommendations. Accessed September 2, 2015.

Case 5

Ms. Moore is a 56-year-old right-hand-dominant female who reports pain, numbness, and tingling in the palmar surface of both of her hands, along the thenar eminence, thumb, and index and middle fingers. She reports that the symptoms originally started a few years ago and would wake her up at night occasionally. States she would shake her hand out, and the symptoms would subside. States that now she feels her hands are weak, and she has noticed that she has been dropping things. Past medical history is significant for diabetes, rheumatoid arthritis, hypertension, and obesity. States she has tried to lose weight multiple times but has not been able to lose more than 10 or 15 pounds. Reports that her weight restricts her ability to exercise and that makes her feel more hopeless about her ability to lose weight. States she works as an assembly-line worker at an automobile plant using a hydraulic tool to put bolts onto the vehicle chassis. States she works four 10-hour shifts per week with a half hour break for lunch and three 15-minute breaks. Reports she has worked at this same position for over 20 years. Denies changes in bowel/bladder habits. Denies dizziness, loss of consciousness, chest pain, dyspnea on exertion. Past medical/surgical history of diabetes, hypertension (HTN), rheumatoid arthritis (RA), cholecystectomy 15 years ago, appendectomy 35 years ago. Not sexually active, no pregnancies, never married. Well-woman exam and mammogram 1 year ago were normal. Has never had colonoscopy. All immunizations up-to-date. Seasonal allergies treated with over-the-counter antihistamines. Medications: metformin 1000 mg PO BID, sulfasalazine 1000 mg PO BID, lisinopril 20 mg PO QD.

Physical Exam

VS: BP 140/88, HR 84 regular, T 98.7, RR 24, Ht 5'3", Wt 210 lbs

GEN: No acute distress

HEENT: Head normocephalic without evidence of masses or trauma. PERRLA, EOMs intact. Noninjected. Fundoscopic exam unremarkable. Ear canal without redness or irritation, TMs clear, pearly, bony landmarks visible. No discharge, no pain noted. Neck without masses. No thyromegaly. No JVD noted

Skin: No open areas noted. No ecchymosis, no pruritus, no scarring, no swelling noted

CV: S_1 and S_2 RRR, no murmurs, no rubs. No ecchymosis noted to thorax

Lungs: Clear to auscultation

Abdomen: Round, obese, soft, nontender, nondistended, bowel sounds present × 4 quadrants, no organomegaly, no bruits. No bruising, no abrasions noted. Scarring right lower quadrant (RLQ) and midline consistent with surgical history reported

MS: C-spine without pain on palpation. Bilateral shoulders, elbows, and forearms without pain on palpation. Bilateral hands with nodularity noted along interphalangeal joint (IPJ) of all fingers. Pain with palpation to nodular joints. Thenar atrophy noted bilaterally. Range of motion of wrists and fingers full but painful

Neuro: Sensation diminished to bilateral third, fourth, and fifth phalanges of bilateral hands. DTR 2+ at biceps, triceps, brachioradialis. Tinel's positive, Phalen's positive, median nerve compression positive, hand elevation positive. Sensation to third, fourth, and fifth phalanges of bilateral hands diminished to 2-point discrimination, pressure and monofilament. Coolness noted to bilateral hands when compared to forearms. Grip strength 3/5 bilaterally; thumb abduction strength 2/5 bilaterally. Bilateral lower extremities with normal sensation to pressure and monofilament, pedal pulses 2+, strength 5/5

What additional assessments/diagnostics do you need?

What is the differential diagnoses list?

What is your working diagnosis?

Additional Assessments/Diagnostics Needed

Evaluation for the patient with suspected carpal tunnel syndrome (CTS) should include the following items.[1-4,23-29]

Ask focused ROS questions:

- Detailed history with exploration of:
    - Risk factors
    - Onset of symptoms
    - Time since first symptoms appeared
    - Progression of symptoms
    - Occupational history
- It is also important to explore any other potential causes for the paresthesia such as:
    - Trauma to the wrist
    - Hematoma along the carpal tunnel or volar wrist
    - History of bleeding or clotting disorder (which heightens the risk of hematoma)
    - Neck injury or causation
    - Shoulder injury or causation

Risk Factors for CTS

- Female
- Diabetes
- Rheumatoid arthritis

- Autoimmune disease
- Pregnancy
- Obesity
- Thyroid disease

Exam[25-29]

The physical examination should focus on a complete examination of bilateral upper extremities from the fingertips to the neck to assess for the causation of the paresthesia being reported. This would include:

- Comparison of bilateral upper extremities for coolness, pulses, sensation, swelling, and grip strength
- Physical examination tests to elicit paresthesia if present:
    - Tinel's
    - Phalen's
    - Median nerve compression
    - Hand elevation
- Palpation of C-spine
- Palpation of medial and lateral elbows and forearms

[Handwritten annotations: Tinel's (ext arm on table, palm up) Press on index finger down middle of palm to halfway up forearm if feels numbness, tingling (+) test; Phalen's (Press wrists together fingers down x1 minute if numbness or tingling (+)]

Routine Labs/Diagnostics[25-29]

Labs would be done to determine impact or presence of comorbid or underlying disease processes such as diabetes, thyroid disease, or autoimmune conditions. Labs for this patient would include:

- Urinalysis (UA) with glomerular filtration rate (GFR)—to evaluate renal function
- Complete metabolic panel (CMP) including blood urea nitrogen (BUN), creatinine (Cr), electrolytes, and glucose
- HbA1c
- Lipid profile
- Liver profile

Further Diagnostic Studies[25-27]

If a patient presents with complaints consistent with CTS and a physical examination that correlates, further diagnostic testing can be accomplished. These would include:

- Electrodiagnostic studies
    - Nerve conduction studies (NCS) are primary testing to determine the rate of conduction of both sensory and motor impulses along the median nerve.
    - Electromyography (EMG) is not normally performed for a suspected diagnosis of CTS but may be done if a demyelinating versus denervation process is suspected, such as multiple sclerosis (MS).
- Routine radiography is generally not performed unless trauma is suspected.
- Ultrasound of the wrist is performed only if hematoma is suspected as a possible diagnosis.

Differential Diagnoses List

Carpal tunnel syndrome

Medial epicondylitis

Lateral epicondylitis

Cervical radiculopathy

Hematoma of volar wrist

Diabetic neuropathy

Working Diagnosis—Bilateral carpal tunnel syndrome

Pathophysiology

Carpal tunnel syndrome (CTS) is a neuronal and muscular dysfunction of the hand caused by compression of the median nerve in the volar wrist.[23–29] CTS affects 3% of US adults, primarily between the ages of 40 and 60 years, with women three times more likely than men to experience it within their lifetime. Although a definitive cause for CTS is elusive, risk factors such as diabetes, pregnancy, metabolic diseases, obesity, rheumatoid arthritis, trauma, family history of the disorder, as well as repetitive forceful motions of the hand and wrist and use of vibratory tools seem to be contributory.

What Is Your Treatment Plan?

Pharmacologic[28–29]

There are no pharmacologic treatments for CTS. Ms. Moore would be maintained on her current medication regimen for her diabetes, HTN, and RA.

Nonpharmacologic

▶ Splints and braces especially at night may be utilized early in disease. At the point Ms. Moore has reached, these conservative approaches will have little impact.

▶ NCS—Ms. Moore's NCS were positive for bilateral CTS.

▶ Surgical intervention—surgery to decompress the carpal tunnel and relieve the pressure that is causing the paresthesia would be indicated for treatment of the disease. Unfortunately, at the late stage of disease exhibited in the case of Ms. Moore, full symptom resolution and neuromuscular return of function will probably not occur.

Education/Counseling

▶ Management of DM and RA to prevent further damage to nerves

▶ What to expect from NCS and surgical interventions

SOAP Note

S: Ms. Moore is a 56-year-old right-hand-dominant female who reports pain, numbness, and tingling in the palmar surface of both of her hands, along the thenar eminence, thumb, and index and middle fingers. She reports that the symptoms originally started a few years ago and would wake her up at night occasionally. States she would shake her hand out, and the symptoms would subside. States that now she feels her hands are weak, and she has noticed that she has been dropping things. Past medical history is significant for diabetes, rheumatoid arthritis, hypertension, and obesity. States she has tried to lose weight multiple times but has not been able to lose more than 10 or 15 pounds. Reports that her weight restricts her ability to exercise and that makes her feel more hopeless about her ability to lose weight. States she works as an assembly-line worker at an automobile plant using a hydraulic tool to put bolts onto the vehicle chassis. States she works four 10-hour shifts per week with a half-hour break for lunch and three 15-minute breaks. Reports she has worked at this same position for over 20 years. Denies changes in bowel/bladder habits. Denies dizziness, loss of consciousness, chest pain, dyspnea on exertion. Past medical/surgical history of diabetes, hypertension, rheumatoid arthritis, cholecystectomy 15 years ago, appendectomy 35 years ago. Not sexually active, no pregnancies, never married. Well-woman exam and mammogram 1 year ago were normal. Has never had colonoscopy. All immunizations up-to-date. Seasonal allergies treated with over-the-counter antihistamines. Medications: metformin 1000 mg PO BID, sulfasalazine 1000 mg PO BID, lisinopril 20 mg PO QD.

O: *VS:* BP 140/88, HR 84 regular, T 98.7, RR 24, Ht 5'3", Wt 210 lbs

GEN: No acute distress

HEENT: Head normocephalic without evidence of masses or trauma. PERRLA, EOMs intact. Noninjected. Fundoscopic exam unremarkable. Ear canal without redness or irritation, TMs clear, pearly, bony landmarks visible. No discharge, no pain noted. Neck without masses. No thyromegaly. No JVD noted

Skin: No open areas noted. No ecchymosis, no pruritus, no scarring, no swelling noted

CV: S_1 and S_2 RRR, no murmurs, no rubs. No ecchymosis noted to thorax

Lungs: Clear to auscultation

Abdomen: Round, obese, soft, nontender, nondistended, bowel sounds present × 4 quadrants, no organomegaly, no bruits. No bruising, no abrasions noted. Scarring RLQ and midline consistent with surgical history reported

MS: C-spine without pain on palpation. Bilateral shoulders, elbows, and forearms without pain on palpation. Bilateral hands with nodularity noted along IPJ of all fingers. Pain with palpation to nodular joints. Thenar atrophy noted bilaterally. Range of motion of wrists and fingers full but painful.

Neuro: Sensation diminished to bilateral third, fourth, and fifth phalanges of bilateral hands. DTR 2+ at biceps, triceps, brachioradialis. Tinel's positive, Phalen's positive, median nerve compression positive, hand elevation positive. Sensation to third, fourth, and fifth phalanges of bilateral hands diminished to 2-point discrimination, pressure and monofilament. Coolness noted to bilateral hands when compared to forearms. Grip strength 3/5 bilaterally; thumb abduction strength 2/5 bilaterally. Bilateral lower extremities with normal sensation to pressure and monofilament, pedal pulses 2+, strength 5/5

A:

1. Carpal tunnel syndrome
2. HTN
3. DM
4. RA

▮ Health Promotion Issues

▶ Comprehensive diabetic examination to include:[29]

  ▶ Comprehensive physical examination with height, weight, body mass index (BMI), thyroid palpation, fundoscopic eye exam, skin exam, comprehensive foot exam

  ▶ Referral for dilated diabetic eye exam

  ▶ Diabetic lab assessment

    ➤ UA with GFR

    ➤ CMP includes BUN, Cr, electrolytes, and glucose

    ➤ HbA1c

    ➤ Lipid profile

    ➤ Liver profile

  ▶ Referral to dietitian

  ▶ Referral to dentist for complete dental examination

  ▶ Discussion of medications and s/s of hypoglycemic episodes

▶ Labs for medication monitoring (in addition to CMP)

  ▶ CBC

▶ Colonoscopy[1–4,23–29]

▮ Guidelines to Direct Care

US Preventive Services Task Force. Recommendations for primary care practice: published recommendations. http://www.uspreventiveservicestaskforce.org/BrowseRec/Index/browse-recommendations. Accessed September 2, 2015.

Centers for Disease Control and Prevention. Recommended adult immunization schedule, by vaccine and age group. 2014. http://www.cdc.gov/vaccines/schedules/hcp/imz/adult.html. Accessed September 2, 2015.

US Dept of Agriculture and US Dept of Health and Human Services. *Dietary Guidelines for Americans, 2010.* 7th ed. Washington, DC: US Government Printing Office; 2010.

American College of Radiology. ACR Appropriateness Criteria: chronic wrist pain. http://www.acr.org/~/media/ACR/Documents/AppCriteria/Diagnostic/ChronicWristPain.pdf. Accessed September 25, 2015.

Cartwright MS, Hobson-Webb LD, Boon AJ, et al; American Association of Neuromuscular and Electrodiagnostic Medicine. Evidence-based guideline: neuromuscular ultrasound for the diagnosis of carpal tunnel syndrome. *Muscle Nerve.* 2012;46(2):287–293.

American Academy of Orthopaedic Surgeons (AAOS). *Clinical Practice Guideline on the Treatment of Carpal Tunnel Syndrome.* Rosemont, IL: American Academy of Orthopaedic Surgeons; 2008.

Singh JA, Furst DE, Bharat A, et al. 2012 update of the 2008 American College of Rheumatology recommendations for the use of disease-modifying antirheumatic drugs and biologic agents in the treatment of rheumatoid arthritis. *Arthritis Care Res* (Hoboken). 2012;64(5):625–639.

American Diabetes Association. Standards of medical care for diabetes—2015. *Diabetes Care.* 2015;38(Suppl 1).

REFERENCES

1. US Preventive Services Task Force. Recommendations for primary care practice: published recommendations. http://www.uspreventiveservicestaskforce.org/BrowseRec/Index/browse-recommendations. Accessed September 2, 2015.

2. Centers for Disease Control and Prevention. Recommended adult immunization schedule, by vaccine and age group. 2014. http://www.cdc.gov/vaccines/schedules/hcp/imz/adult.html. Accessed September 2, 2015.

3. US Dept of Agriculture and US Dept of Health and Human Services. *Dietary Guidelines for Americans, 2010.* 7th ed. Washington, DC: US Government Printing Office; 2010.

4. AIM Specialty Health. *Appropriate Use Criteria: Imaging of the Spine.* Chicago, IL: AIM Specialty Health; 2013.

5. Chou R, Qaseem A, Snow V, et al; Clinical Efficacy Assessment Subcommittee of the American College of Physicians; American College of Physicians; American Pain Society Low Back Pain Guidelines

Panel. Diagnosis and treatment of low back pain: a joint clinical practice guideline from the American College of Physicians and the American Pain Society. *Ann Intern Med.* 2007;147(7):479–491.

6. American College of Occupational and Environmental Medicine. *Occupational Medicine Practice Guidelines. Evaluation and Management of Health Problems and Functional Recovery in Workers.* 3rd ed. Elk Grove Village, IL: American College of Occupational and Environmental Medicine; 2011:333–796.

7. Fairbank JCT, Pynsent PB. The Oswestry Disability Index. *Spine.* 2000;25(22):2940–2953.

8. Davidson M, Keating J. A comparison of five low back disability questionnaires: reliability and responsiveness. *Phys Ther.* 2002;82:8–24.

9. North American Spine Society. *Diagnosis and Treatment of Cervical Radiculopathy from Degenerative Disorders.* Burr Ridge, IL: North American Spine Society; 2010.

10. Expert Panels on Musculoskeletal and Neurologic Imaging. *ACR Appropriateness Criteria: Suspected Spine Trauma.* Reston, VA: American College of Radiology; 2009.

11. Stiell G, Clement CM, McKnight RD, et al. The Canadian C-spine rule versus the NEXUS low-risk criteria in patients with trauma. *N Engl J Med.* 2003;349(26):2510–2518.

12. American Academy of Orthopaedic Surgeons. American Academy of Orthopaedic Surgeons Clinical Practice Guideline on Management of Anterior Cruciate Ligament Injuries. Rosemont, IL: American Academy of Orthopaedic Surgeons; 2014.

13. Tuite MJ, Daffner RH, Weissman BN, et al; Expert Panel on Musculoskeletal Imaging. *ACR Appropriateness Criteria: Acute Trauma to the Knee.* Reston, VA: American College of Radiology; 2011.

14. AIM Specialty Health. *Appropriate Use Criteria: Imaging of the Extremities.* Chicago, IL: AIM Specialty Health; 2014.

15. Wilson JJ, Furukawa M. Evaluation of the patient with hip pain. *Am Fam Phys.* 2014;89(1).

16. AIM Specialty Health. *Appropriate Use Criteria: Imaging of the Abdomen and Pelvis.* Chicago, IL: AIM Specialty Health; 2014.

17. Taljanovic MS, Daffner RH, Weissman BN, et al; Expert Panel on Musculoskeletal Imaging. *ACR Appropriateness Criteria: Chronic Hip Pain.* Reston, VA: American College of Radiology; 2011.

18. Ward RJ, Weissman BN, Kransdorf MJ, et al; Expert Panel on Musculoskeletal Imaging. *ACR Appropriateness Criteria: Acute Hip Pain—Suspected Fracture.* Reston, VA: American College of Radiology; 2013.

19. Daffner RH, Weissman BN, Appel M, et al; Expert Panel on Musculoskeletal Imaging. *ACR Appropriateness Criteria: Stress (Fatigue/Insufficiency) Fracture, Including Sacrum, Excluding Other Vertebrae.* Reston, VA: American College of Radiology; 2011.

20. Hochberg MC, Altman RD, April KT, et al. American College of Rheumatology 2012 recommendations for the use of nonpharmacologic and pharmacologic therapies in osteoarthritis of the hand, hip, and knee. *Arthritis Care Res* (Hoboken). 2012;64(4):465–474.

21. Jeffries MA, Donica M, Baker LW, Stevenson ME, Annan AC, Humphrey MB, James JA, Sawalha AH. Genome-wide DNA methylation study identifies significant epigenomic changes in osteoarthritic cartilage. *Arthritis Rheumatol.* 2014;66(10):2804–2815. doi:10.1002/art.38762.

22. US Food and Drug Administration. Medication guides. http://www.fda.gov/Drugs/DrugSafety/ucm085729.htm. Accessed September 25, 2015.

23. Carpal tunnel syndrome. In: Hegmann KT, ed. *Occupational Medicine Practice Guidelines: Evaluation and Management of Common Health Problems and Functional Recovery in Workers.* 3rd ed. Elk Grove Village, IL: American College of Occupational and Environmental Medicine; 2011:1–73.

24. Rubin DA, Weissman BN, Appel M, et al; Expert Panel on Musculoskeletal Imaging. *ACR Appropriateness Criteria: Chronic Wrist Pain.* Reston, VA: American College of Radiology; 2012.

25. Cartwright MS, Hobson-Webb LD, Boon AJ, et al. Evidence-based guideline: neuromuscular ultrasound for the diagnosis of carpal tunnel syndrome. *Muscle Nerve.* 2012;46(2):287–293.

26. American Academy of Orthopaedic Surgeons. Clinical Practice Guideline on the Treatment of Carpal Tunnel Syndrome. Rosemont, IL: American Academy of Orthopaedic Surgeons; 2008.

27. Wang L. Electrodiagnosis of carpal tunnel syndrome. *Phys Med Rehabil Clin N Am.* 2013;24(1):67–77.

28. Singh JA, Furst DE, Bharat A, et al. 2012 update of the 2008 American College of Rheumatology recommendations for the use of disease-modifying antirheumatic drugs and biologic agents in the treatment of rheumatoid arthritis. *Arthritis Care Res* (Hoboken). 2012;64(5):625–639.

29. American Diabetes Association. Standards of Medical Care for Diabetes—2015. *Diabetes Care.* 2015;38(Suppl 1).

Common Neurologic Disorders in Primary Care

Joanne L. Thanavaro

Chapter Outline

Case 1 - Headaches

A. History and Physical Exam

B. Recommended Labs/Diagnostics

C. Pathophysiology

D. Guidelines to direct care: International Headache Society (HIS) ICHD Guidelines

E. Treatment Plan

Case 2 - Dizziness

A. History and Physical Exam

B. Recommended Labs/Diagnostics

C. Pathophysiology

D. Guidelines to direct care: American Academy of Otolaryngology-Head and Neck Surgery Foundation. Clinical practice guideline: benign paroxysmal positional vertigo.

E. Treatment Plan

Case 3 - Seizure

A. History and Physical Exam

B. Risk Stratification

C. Recommended Labs/Diagnostics

D. Pathophysiology

E. Guidelines to direct care: Practice parameter: evaluating apparent unprovoked first seizure in adults (an evidence-based review). Report of the Quality Standards Subcommittee of the American Academy of Neurology and the American Epilepsy Society.

F. Treatment Plan

Case 4 - Parkinson's disease

A. History and Physical Exam

B. Recommended Labs/Diagnostics

C. Pathophysiology

D. Guidelines to direct care: Quality Standards Subcommittee of the American Academy of Neurology. Practice parameter: diagnosis and prognosis of new onset Parkinson disease (an evidence-based review). Report of the Quality Standards Subcommittee of the American Academy of Neurology.

E. Treatment Plan

Case 5 - Transient Ischemic Attacks (TIAs)

A. History and Physical Exam

B. Recommended Labs/Diagnostics

C. Pathophysiology

D. Guidelines to direct care: Guidelines for the prevention of stroke in women: a statement for healthcare professionals from the American Heart Association/American Stroke Association.

Definition and evaluation of transient ischemic attack: a scientific statement for healthcare professionals from the American Heart Association/American Stroke Association Stroke Council; Council on Cardiovascular Surgery and Anesthesia; Council on Cardiovascular Radiology and Intervention; Council on Cardiovascular Nursing; and the Interdisciplinary Council on Peripheral Vascular Disease.

Guidelines for the prevention of stroke in patients with stroke and transient ischemic attack: a guideline for healthcare professionals from the American Heart Association/American Stroke Association.

E. Treatment Plan

Learning Objectives

Using a case-based approach, the learner will be able to:

1. Identify key history and physical examination parameters for common neurologic disorders seen in primary care, including headache, dizziness, seizure, Parkinson's disease, and TIAs.

2. Summarize recommended laboratory and diagnostic studies indicated for the evaluation of common neurologic disorders seen in primary care.

3. State pathophysiology of common neurologic disorders.

4. Document a clear, concise SOAP note for patients with common neurologic disorders.

5. Identify relevant education and counseling strategies for patients with common neurologic disorders.

6. Develop a treatment plan for common neurologic disorders utilizing current evidence-based guidelines.

Case 1

Kathy is a 26-year-old female who is concerned about headaches. She has had headaches since she was a teenager, but they have been increasing in frequency and intensity for the past 4 months. The headache is usually unilateral, throbbing over her right eye and temple, and is accompanied by light sensitivity and nausea. She has noted they are always worse during her menstrual cycles. She now has headaches about two to three times weekly, and they are affecting her ability to function at her job. The pain usually occurs in the morning or afternoon. She has tried aspirin 325 mg, two tablets, at the onset of the headache as well as cold compresses to her head and lying down. These measures don't provide much relief. She takes no medications and uses a diaphragm for birth control. Her family history is remarkable for a mother who had "painful headaches that required bed rest."

Physical Exam

Vital Signs (VS): Blood pressure (BP) 118/72, heart rate (HR) 72 (regular), respiratory rate (RR) 12, afebrile, height (Ht) 5'5", weight (Wt) 120 lbs

Head, eyes, ears, nose, and throat (HEENT): Pupils equal, round, react to light, accommodation (PERRLA), extraocular movements (EOMs) full with no gaze abnormality. Fundoscopic exam shows sharp disc margins. No arteriovenous (AV) nicking or exudates. Conjunctiva clear, sclera white, corneas clear. No thyromegaly or carotid bruits

Cardiovascular (CV): S_1 and S_2 regular rate and rhythm (RRR). No murmurs, gallops, or rubs. Point of maximal impact (PMI) 5th intercostal space (ICS), midclavicular line (MCL)

Respiratory (RESP): Lungs clear to auscultation (CTA)

Gastrointestinal (GI): Abdomen soft, nontender, nondistended

Extremities (Ext): Normal muscle tone, full range of motion (ROM) in all extremities, no edema or joint deformities. Peripheral pulses +2 bilaterally

Neurologic (Neuro): Oriented ×3. Affect appropriate

What additional assessments/diagnostics do you need?

What is the differential diagnoses list?

What is your working diagnosis?

Additional Assessments/Diagnostics Needed

Review of Systems (ROS)

▶ Evaluate symptoms to determine primary headache subtypes
  ▶ Migraine
    ➤ Migraine without aura
      ■ At least 5 attacks
      ■ Episodes lasting 4–72 hours (untreated or unsuccessfully treated)
      ■ Unilateral, pulsating, moderate to severe intensity
      ■ Aggravated by routine physical activity
      ■ Associated with at least one of the following: nausea, photophobia, or phonophobia
      ■ Not better accounted for by another headache diagnosis
    ➤ Migraine with aura
      ■ At least 2 attacks
      ■ One or more of the reversible aura symptoms: visual, sensory, speech or language, motor, brain stem, retinal
      ■ At least two of the following four characteristics:
        ♦ At least one aura symptom that spreads over >5 minutes and/or two or more symptoms that occur in succession
        ♦ Each individual aura symptom lasting 5–60 minutes
        ♦ Aura is accompanied or followed by headache within 60 minutes

- Not better accounted for by another headache diagnosis, and transient ischemic attack has been excluded
  - The mnemonic POUND may be helpful in diagnosing migraine:[1]
    - P = Pulsatile
    - O = One-day duration
    - U = Unilateral
    - N = Nausea or vomiting
    - D = Disabling
- Tension-type headache
  - Episodic
    - At least 10 episodes of headache occurring on <1 day per month on average
    - Lasting from 30 minutes to 7 days
    - At least two of the following are present:
      - Bilateral location
      - Pressing or tightening quality, not pulsating
      - Mild or moderate intensity
      - Not aggravated by routine physical activity
    - Both of the following are present:
      - No nausea or vomiting
      - No more than one of photophobia or phonophobia
    - Not better accounted for by another headache diagnosis
  - Chronic
    - Headache occurring on 15 or more days/month for >3 months
    - Lasting hours to days, or unremitting
    - At least two of the following are present:
      - Bilateral location
      - Pressing or tightening (not pulsating) quality
      - Mild or moderate intensity
      - Not aggravated by routine physical activity
    - Both of the following are present:
      - No more than one of photophobia, phonophobia, or mild nausea
      - Neither moderate nor severe nausea or vomiting
    - Not accounted for by another headache diagnosis
- Trigeminal autonomic cephalagias
  - Multiple subtypes, but cluster is most common and categorized as episodic or chronic
  - Episodic cluster
    - At least 5 attacks
    - Severe or very severe unilateral orbital, supraorbital, and/or temporal pain lasting 15–180 minutes (when untreated)

- Either or both of the following:
  - At least one of the following symptoms or signs ipsilateral to the headache:
    - Conjunctival injection and/or lacrimation
    - Nasal congestion and/or rhinorrhea
    - Eyelid edema
    - Forehead and facial sweating
    - Forehead and facial flushing
    - Sensation of fullness in the ear
    - Miosis and/or ptosis
  - A sense of restlessness or agitation
  - Attacks occur one every other day—eight per day for more than half of the time when the disorder is active
  - Not better accounted for by another headache diagnosis
  - Chronic cluster
    - Attacks fulfilling criteria for cluster headache AND
    - Occurring without a remission period, or with remissions lasting for <1 month, for at least 1 year
- Other primary headache disorders include the following (see Internal Headache Society guidelines for characteristics associated with other primary headache disorders):[2]
  - Primary cough headache
  - Primary exercise headache
  - Primary headache associated with sexual activity
  - Primary thunderclap headache
  - Cold-stimulus headache
  - External-pressure headache
  - Primary stabbing headache
  - Nummular headache
  - Hypnic headache
  - New daily persistent headache (NDPH)
- Evaluate for red flags associated with secondary headaches using the mnemonic SNOOP[3]
  - S = Systemic signs or symptoms, including fever, meningismus, persistent vomiting, weight loss, malignancy, and immunosuppressed or anticoagulated patient
  - N = Neurologic symptoms associated with changes in cognition or mental functioning, including seizures, syncope, weakness, numbness, or gait disturbances
  - O = Onset that is abrupt or severe, known as "thunderclap headaches"
  - O = Older age of initial onset: age 40 years or older
  - P = Previous headache history or progression of headache, including severity, frequency, or change in location

Labs

▶ Depending on the history and physical exam, consider the following for acute onset headache:[4]

  ▸ Comprehensive metabolic panel (CMP) (hypo- or hyperglycemia)

  ▸ Complete blood count (CBC) (infection, inflammation, anemia)

  ▸ Thyroid-stimulating hormone (TSH) (hypothyroidism)

  ▸ Erythrocyte sedimentation rate (ESR) and C-reactive protein (CRP) (giant cell arteritis)

  ▸ Prothrombin time (PT)/partial thromboplastin time (PTT) (coagulopathy)

  ▸ Drug screen (opiates, cocaine, benzodiazepines)

▶ Initial labs are not routinely indicated in chronic or migraine headaches[1]

Imaging

▶ No benefit in performing imaging for primary headache disorders

▶ Central nervous system (CNS) imaging is appropriate for patients with red-flag symptoms

▶ CNS imaging may be appropriate for patients who have an increased likelihood of structural disease such as arteriovenous malformation, aneurysm, tumor, or subarachnoid hemorrhage[1]

Differential Diagnoses List

Subarachnoid hemorrhage

Frontal sinusitis

Meningitis

Trigeminal neuralgia

Tension headache

Cluster headache

Migraine

Working Diagnosis—Migraine

Pathophysiology

Migraine is one of the most common forms of primary headache and is primarily a genetically transmitted neurovascular condition. Stimulation of the trigeminovascular system, including the blood vessels and neural connections, is thought to initiate the cascade of events that cause a migraine. Neurotransmitters are secreted, including substance P and calcitonin gene-related peptide, and cause inflammation and dilatation of affected cranial blood vessels. Triggers include menstrual cycles, stress, changes in weather or barometric pressure, changes in sleep patterns, and certain foods and drinks.[5]

What Is Your Treatment Plan?

Pharmacologic

▶ Acute treatment of mild to moderate migraines[2]

  ▸ Nonsteroidal anti-inflammatory drugs (NSAIDs) used alone or with acetaminophen and caffeine

  ▸ Isometheptene/dichloralphenazone/acetaminophen (Midrin)

▶ Medications for moderate to severe migraines

  ▸ 5-HT receptor agonists (triptans)

  ▸ Ergotamines

  ▸ Antiemetics

  ▸ Opioids and butalbital-containing medications

▶ Prophylactic pharmacotherapy

  ▸ Indicated when headaches occur 15 or more times per month

  ▸ Tricyclic antidepressants (TCAs)

  ▸ Selective serotonin reuptake inhibitors (SSRIs)

  ▸ Beta-adrenergic blockers (BBs)

  ▸ Calcium channel blockers (CCBs)

  ▸ Antiepileptics (topiramate, valproate)

  ▸ Botox injections[6]

  ▸ Selection should be based on patient's age, comorbid conditions, and side effect profile

Nonpharmacologic

▶ Maintain a healthy diet

▶ Maintain a regular sleep schedule

▶ Cognitive behavioral therapy strategies to manage stress

Education/Counseling

▶ Discuss migraine triggers. Avoid common food triggers, including alcohol, chocolate, aged cheeses, monosodium glutamate (MSG), aspartame (NutraSweet), caffeine, and nuts.

▶ Discuss keeping a headache diary for 1 month to help determine other triggers and what makes the headaches better.

▶ Discuss trying a short-term preventive therapy during the perimenstrual period called a "mini prophylaxis." NSAIDs or long-acting triptans (frovatriptan, sumatriptan, or naratriptan) can be started 1 to 2 days prior to the expected onset of menstrual migraine and continued for 5 days.

▶ Take acute treatment drug at the first sign of a headache or aura. You may repeat this medication in 2 hours with a maximum of 2 tablets in 24 hours. NSAIDs may be used along with acute treatment drugs.

▶ Avoid overuse of any antimigraine medication. Overuse (more often than prescribed) can lead to medication-overuse headaches (rebound headaches).

▶ The American Headache Society (http://www.achenet.org/resources/information_for_patients/) is a reliable source for more information on headaches.

SOAP Note

S: Kathy presents today with headaches that initially began during her teenage years. Headaches are increasing in frequency and intensity over the last 4 months. The headache is a unilateral pounding sensation on the right eye and temple. Pain is rated 8/10 and does not respond to acetylsalicylic acid (ASA), cold compression, or lying down. Her headaches are associated with photophobia and phonophobia. She is frequently nauseated but has never vomited. She now has headaches about two to three times weekly, and they last 1–2 days and are affecting her ability to function at her job; she called in sick to work six times last month. She reports no aura prior to the onset of pain. She denies fever, seizures, syncope, neck pain, or thunderclap sensation. Her weight has been stable over the last few years. She takes no medications and uses a diaphragm for birth control. Her family history is remarkable for a mother who had "painful headaches that required bed rest."

O: *VS:* BP 118/72, HR 72 (regular), RR 12, afebrile, Ht 5'5", Wt 120 lbs

HEENT: PERRLA, EOMs full with no gaze abnormality. Fundoscopic exam shows sharp disc margins. No AV nicking or exudates. Conjunctiva clear, sclera white, corneas clear. No thyromegaly or carotid bruits

CV: S_1 and S_2 RRR. No murmurs, gallops, or rubs. PMI 5th ICS, MCL

RESP: LCTA

GI: Abdomen soft, nontender, nondistended

Ext: Normal muscle tone, full ROM in all extremities. No edema or joint deformities. Peripheral pulses +2 bilaterally

Neuro: Oriented ×3. Affect appropriate. Cranial nerves (CN) II–XII grossly intact. Gait and tandem walking steady. Rapid hand/foot movement intact. Deep tendon reflexes (DTRs) 2+ throughout

A: Migraine headaches without aura

P: Discussed the nature of migraine headaches. Discussed possible triggers and recommended keeping a headache diary for the next month. Will try trial "mini prophylaxis" with NSAIDs 2 days prior and continuing through the next menstrual cycle. Script for sumatriptan 100 mg to be taken at onset of migraine. May repeat dose once in 2 hours if symptoms don't resolve; do not exceed more than 2 tablets in 24 hours. Discussed avoidance of rebound headaches and discussed stress management techniques. Follow-up in 1 month to evaluate effectiveness of medication. Consider long-acting triptan if NSAIDs are not effective to prevent menstrual migraines.

Health Promotion Issues

Discuss healthy lifestyle, including diet, exercise, and consistent sleep patterns.

Guidelines to Direct Care

International Headache Society. ICHD/guidelines. http://www.ihs-headache.org/ichd-guidelines/ihs-guidelines. Accessed October 26, 2015.

Case 2

Shirley Brown is a 68-year-old slender female who presents to the office today with complaints of severe dizziness, nausea, and vomiting. She states that she has had bouts of dizziness over a 3-day period, and the nausea increased to the point that she had two vomiting episodes since awakening early this a.m. She feels like the room is spinning for a few seconds; then it stops, and she feels off-balance. She is currently being treated for hypertension with atenolol 50 mg daily and hydrochlorothiazide 25 mg daily. She occasionally uses extra-strength Tylenol (acetaminophen) for mild joint stiffness. She has never smoked and has an occasional cocktail when out to dinner with friends (one to two/month).

Physical Exam

VS: BP supine 136/68 RA (right arm), 138/88 LA (left arm), HR 76; standing 134/86 RA, 136/86 LA, HR 78; RR 20, temperature (T) 97.4

Skin: Pale, dry, turgor fair. Mucous membranes and nailbeds pink. No jaundice or bruising noted

HEENT: Eyes: No AV nicking. No exudates or hemorrhage noted. Disk well marginated. EOMs intact, peripheral vision intact, visual acuity oculus dexter (OD, right) 20/40, oculus sinister (OS, left) 20/30 corrected with glasses. Ears: Tympanic membranes (TMs) gray, light reflex present. Rinne/Weber within normal limits (WNL). Hearing Handicap Inventory for the Elderly score of 6. Neck: Thyroid nonpalpable. No venous hum over neck vessels, no carotid bruits heard

CV: S and S_2 RRR. No murmurs, gallops, or rubs

Lungs: CTA

Abdomen: Soft, nontender, bowel sounds in all four quadrants. No hepatosplenomegaly

Ext: Full range of motion (FROM) upper and lower extremities. Peripheral pulses +2, no peripheral edema

Neuro: Alert and oriented ×3, CNs I–VII, IX–XII intact. VIII diminished bilaterally to whisper test. No spontaneous nystagmus. Motor function/muscle strength/gait normal

What additional assessments/diagnostics do you need?

What is the differential diagnoses list?

What is your working diagnosis?

Additional Assessments/Diagnostics Needed

ROS

▶ Initial description may be difficult for patient to explain; focus on what type of sensation the patient is feeling

▶ Main categories of dizziness include:[7]

  ▶ Vertigo: False sense of motion, spinning sensation

  ▶ Disequilibrium: Off-balance or wobbly

  ▶ Presyncope: Feeling of "blacking out" or losing consciousness

  ▶ Lightheadedness: Vague, "feeling disconnected to the surroundings"

Physical Exam

▶ Main goal is to reproduce the patient's dizziness in the office

▶ Always obtain blood pressure and heart rate in the supine and standing positions

▶ Dix-Hallpike maneuver[8]

  ▶ Patient should be seated on exam table

  ▶ Turn patient's head 45 degrees to the side

  ▶ Patient quickly lies flat while holding the head turned to the side

  ▶ Assess for nystagmus of benign paroxysmal positional vertigo (BPPV): Initial delay of a few seconds followed by briskly torsional and upbeat nystagmus that lessens in 10–30 seconds

  ▶ If no nystagmus is noted, return patient to a sitting position and repeat on the opposite side

  ▶ The presence of this characteristic nystagmus is highly predictive of BPPV

▶ Romberg test

▶ Observation of gait

▶ Thorough cardiovascular exam: ECG, Holter, carotid duplex only if underlying cardiac cause is suspected based on physical exam findings or history of known cardiac disease

Routine Labs

In general, lab testing and imaging are not helpful in patients with no other neurologic abnormalities.[9]

Imaging

Reserved for cases of atypical nystagmus or persistent positional vertigo not responding to positioning maneuvers.[9]

Differential Diagnoses List

Vertigo

Nonspecific dizziness

Disequilibrium

Presyncope

Meniere's disease

Orthostatic hypotension

Medication related

Working Diagnosis

Vertigo—suspect BPPV

Hypertension (HTN)

Pathophysiology

BPPV is the most common type of recurrent vertigo, and the prevalence of BPPV is seven times higher in patients older than 60 years of age. BPPV is commonly attributed to calcium debris (canalithiasis) in the posterior semicircular canal of the ear, which causes the erroneous sensation of spinning when the head moves with gravity changes. Calcium debris can also occur in the anterior of horizontal ear canal or can be "torsional BPPV"; this occurs when canalithiasis involves both the anterior and posterior canals.[9]

What Is Your Treatment Plan?

Pharmacologic

▶ Medication (benzodiazepine, antihistamines) are of limited benefit in treating dizziness

▶ Antihistamines appear to relieve nausea and vomiting[8]

Nonpharmacologic

▶ Canalith repositioning maneuver is highly effective for treating posterior semicircular canal BPPV:

  ▶ Initiate maneuver when nystagmus is seen during Dix-Hallpike test.

  ▶ Without returning to sit, the patient rolls onto the unaffected side until the nose is pointed to the floor.

  ▶ Slowly return to sitting position and chin tucked with head still turned to the unaffected shoulder.

  ▶ May repeat the maneuver, starting with the Dix-Hallpike position on the affected side.

▶ Fall prevention strategies

▶ Prevention of dehydration

- Refer patients for vestibular rehabilitation for persistent symptoms of BPPV despite positioning maneuvers, atypical nystagmus, and vertigo not explained by BPPV[8]

Education/Counseling

- Discuss and demonstrate proper repositioning techniques
- Anticipatory guidance that repositioning maneuvers may cause nausea and vomiting
- Avoid neck strain during positioning maneuvers
- Anticipatory guidance on reoccurrence in 7–23% of patients after treatment, but long-term occurrence may be as high as 50%[8]

SOAP Note

S: A 68-year-old female presents today with complaints of severe dizziness that began 3 days ago. Increased nausea resulted in two vomiting episodes early this morning but has improved. She feels like the room is spinning for a few seconds; then it stops, and she feels off-balance. She denies diplopia, headache, paralysis, paresthesia, confusion, and falls; she did have an upper respiratory infection 2 weeks ago, which resolved with over-the-counter cold remedies. She has not experienced dizziness in the past and takes atenolol 50 mg and hydrochlorothiazide 25 mg daily.

O: *VS:* BP supine 136/68 RA, 138/88 LA, HR 76; standing 134/86 RA, 136/86 LA, HR 78; RR 20, T 97.4

Skin: Pale, dry, turgor fair. Mucous membranes and nailbeds pink. No jaundice or bruising noted

HEENT: Eyes: No AV nicking. No exudates or hemorrhage noted. Disk well marginated. EOMs intact, peripheral vision intact. Visual acuity OD 20/40, OS 20/30 corrected with glasses. Ears: TMs gray, light reflex present. Weber test no lateralization. Rinne air conduction greater than bone conduction. Hearing Handicap Inventory for the Elderly score of 6. Neck: Thyroid nonpalpable. No venous hum over neck vessels, no carotid bruits heard

CV: S_1 and S_2 RRR. No murmurs, gallops, or rubs

Lungs: CTA

Abdomen: Soft, nontender, bowel sounds in all four quadrants. No hepatosplenomegaly

Ext: FROM upper and lower extremities. Peripheral pulses +2, no peripheral edema

Neuro: Alert and oriented ×3, CNs I–VII, IX–XII intact. No spontaneous nystagmus. Dix-Hallpike maneuver produces rotational nystagmus consistent with BPPV. Motor function upper and lower extremities 5/5, normal sensory and vibratory sensation. Romberg negative. Normal gait

A: BPPV

Good motivation and cognitive ability to perform positioning maneuvers

HTN: At Eighth Joint National Committee (JNC 8) goals

P: Discussed probable etiology of BPPV. Demonstrated positioning maneuvers. Patient able to return demonstration of positioning with minimal difficulty. Meclizine 25 mg— use sparingly for nausea. Discussed fall prevention. Avoid driving until dizziness subsides. No driving while taking meclizine. Call back if symptoms don't resolve and will refer for vestibular rehabilitation. Continue hypertensive medications

Health Promotion Issues

- Screening for hearing loss (diseases associated with vertigo frequently have an associated hearing loss)[10]

Guidelines to Direct Care

Bhattacharyya N, Baugh RF, Orvidas L, et al; American Academy of Otolaryngology—Head and Neck Surgery Foundation. Clinical practice guideline: benign paroxysmal positional vertigo. *Otolaryngol Head Neck Surg.* 2008;139:S47–S81. (Note: Reaffirmed 2014.)

Fife TD, Iverson DJ, Lempert T, et al. Practice parameter: therapies for benign paroxysmal positional vertigo (an evidence-based review). *Neurology.* 2008;70:2067–2074.

Case 3

Ryan is a 26-year-old white male who comes to the office after his friends tell him that he passed out while he was shopping for CDs at the music store. He reports no symptoms prior to the time his friends observed him fall to the floor. His friends told him that his body began to shake and make jerking motions. He thinks it probably lasted for about 2 minutes, and his friends told him that he did not respond for another 2–3 minutes. The paramedics were called, but Ryan refused to go to the hospital. He went home and admits that he felt a little confused after the episode. Ryan's past medical history (PMH) includes a motor vehicle accident 6 years ago; he sustained a fracture of his left femur and a closed head injury with a 30-minute loss of consciousness. A CT scan of the head and cervical spine films were normal at that time. He denies any residual problems from the accident. He takes no medications, smokes one and one-half packs of cigarettes daily, and drinks two to three drinks nightly and a few more on weekends. He has a negative review of systems.

Physical Exam

VS: BP 136/78, HR 86 (regular), RR 12, afebrile

HEENT: PERRLA, EOMs full with no gaze abnormality. Hearing intact bilaterally. Mouth, good dentition. Small ulceration on tongue. Neck supple. No bruits

CV: S_1 and S_2 RRR. No murmurs, gallops, or rubs. PMI 5th ICS, MCL

RESP: LCTA

GI: Abdomen soft, nontender, nondistended. No hernias or organomegaly

Ext: Normal muscle tone, full ROM in all extremities; no cyanosis, edema, or joint deformities. Peripheral pulses +2 bilaterally

Neuro: Oriented ×3. Affect appropriate. Remote and recent memory intact. CNs II–XII grossly intact

What additional assessments/diagnostics do you need?

What is the differential diagnoses list?

What is your working diagnosis?

Additional Assessments/Diagnostics Needed

ROS

- ▶ Seizures are categorized based on presentation and etiology
- ▶ Always interview anybody who observed the seizure, if possible, to help determine the type of seizure
- ▶ The International League Against Epilepsy (ILAE) Commission on Classification and Terminology revised concepts, terminology, and approaches for classifying seizures and forms of epilepsy in 2010.[11]
- ▶ Generalized and focal are redefined:
  - ▶ Generalized—occurring in and rapidly engaging bilaterally distributed networks
  - ▶ Focal—within networks limited to one hemisphere and either discretely localized or more widely distributed
- ▶ The classification of generalized seizures is simplified, and focal seizures are described according to their manifestations.
  - ▶ Generalized seizures
    - ➤ Tonic-clonic (in any combination)
    - ➤ Absence
      - ■ Typical
      - ■ Atypical
      - ■ Absence with special features
      - ■ Myoclonic absence
      - ■ Eyelid myoclonia
      - ■ Myoclonic
    - ➤ Myoclonic atonic

- ➤ Myoclonic tonic
  - ■ Clonic
  - ■ Tonic
  - ■ Atonic
- ▶ Focal seizures
  - ➤ Descriptors of focal seizures according to degree of impairment
    - ■ No impairment of consciousness or awareness
    - ■ Observable motor or autonomic components
    - ■ Involving subjective sensory or psychic phenomena (i.e., aura)
    - ■ With impairment of consciousness or awareness
    - ■ Evolving to a bilateral convulsive seizure (involving tonic, clonic, or tonic and clonic components)
- ▶ Unknown
  - ➤ Epileptic spasms

Physical Exam

There is no standard algorithm for the evaluation of every patient with a first seizure.

A careful history and physical examination should determine imaging and laboratory testing decisions.

Routine Labs

- ▶ Glucose abnormalities and hyponatremia are the most common laboratory findings associated with seizures.
- ▶ Pregnancy testing should be performed in all premenopausal women.
- ▶ Toxicology testing should be performed when substance abuse is suspected. Drugs particularly likely to cause seizure include tricyclic antidepressants, cocaine, and other stimulants.[12]

Imaging

- ▶ Recommendations for imaging after a first seizure depend on age, seizure type, and associated risk factors.
- ▶ Immediate neuroimaging is indicated when a serious structural brain lesion is suspected and should be considered for patients with focal seizures and for those older than age 40 years.
- ▶ Neuroimaging at a later date is acceptable for patients who have completely recovered from the seizure when there is no clear etiology.
- ▶ MRI is the preferred imaging method because of its greater sensitivity to detect abnormalities.
- ▶ CT scans are usually performed first in acute seizure patients because they more accurately detect acute bleeding and are reasonably sensitive in detecting other abnormalities.[13]

Lumbar Puncture

▶ Not recommended in the routine evaluation of an adult with an apparent unprovoked first seizure unless fever is present.[12]

Differential Diagnoses List

Seizure

Syncope

Cardiac arrhythmia

Alcohol withdrawal

Drug withdrawal (cocaine, amphetamines, benzodiazepine, heroin)

Trauma

Panic attack

Migraine

Narcolepsy

Working Diagnosis—Seizure

Pathophysiology

New-onset epilepsy is the most common cause of unprovoked seizures. A seizure is the clinical manifestation of abnormal and excessive discharge of a population of neurons. There are many causes of seizure, including alcohol and illicit drug use and withdrawal, brain injury or abnormalities, central nervous system infections, epilepsy, fever, metabolic disorders, and medications. Epilepsy is a central nervous system disorder characterized by recurrent seizures.[14]

What Is Your Treatment Plan?

Pharmacologic

▶ Management of patients with seizures focuses on three main goals.

▶ Optimal treatment plans are developed based on an accurate assessment of seizure type, an evaluation of intensity and frequency of seizure, an awareness of side effect profiles of available medications, and the evaluation of potential disease-related psychosocial problems.

▶ Immediate antiepileptic drug (AED) therapy is not necessary after a single seizure, especially if the seizure was provoked by factors that resolve.

▶ AED therapy is generally started after two or more unprovoked seizures; recurrence implies that the patient has increased risk for repeated seizures, above 50%.

▶ Fifty percent of patients with newly diagnosed epilepsy will become seizure free with the first medication prescribed.

▶ No single AED is optimal for every patient and AED therapy should be individualized according to drug effectiveness for seizure type, potential side effects and interactions with other medications, age and gender, lifestyle and patient preferences, and cost.[15–17]

Nonpharmacologic

▶ Vagus nerve stimulation may reduce the frequency of generalized seizures.

▶ Callosotomy may be considered as a palliative treatment for patients with severe refractory generalized seizures.

▶ Focal cortical resection is a consideration in patients with drug-resistant focal epilepsy if the seizures arise from a region that can be resected without cognitive dysfunction of neurologic disability.[18–19]

Education/Counseling

▶ Reduce the chance of having more seizures by taking medicines exactly as directed.

▶ Avoid alcohol, which can increase the risk of seizures and the effectiveness of seizure medications.

▶ Women who are planning to get pregnant need to discuss medication options for seizure control before getting pregnant; some medications are contraindicated in pregnancy.

▶ Call your primary care physician (PCP) whenever you have a seizure; if the seizure lasts longer than 5 minutes or you don't wake up after a seizure, family members need to call 911.

▶ Don't drive until seizures are under control. The laws governing when a person can drive vary from state to state.[20]

▶ Give information for Epilepsy Foundation of America.

SOAP Note

S: Ryan is a 26-year-old white male who comes to the office today. He reports "passing out" yesterday while he was shopping for CDs with his friends. He denies any symptoms prior to the episode and was a bit confused when he woke up on the ground. A telephone conversation with a friend who witnessed this event reveals that suddenly Ryan fell to the floor and his arms and legs began to shake and make jerking motions. He did not hit his head, and the episode lasted about 2–3 minutes. He "stopped shaking" after a few minutes but seemed a little confused when he first got up. He was not incontinent during the episode. The paramedics were called, but Ryan refused to go to the hospital. Ryan denies any further episodes and reports no headache, confusion, speech difficulties, or problems with gait. He suffered a motor vehicle accident 6 years ago and sustained a fracture of his left femur and a closed head injury with a 30-minute loss of consciousness. A CT scan of the head and cervical spine films were normal at that time. He denies any residual problems from the accident. He takes no medications, smokes one and one-half packs of cigarettes daily, and drinks two to three drinks nightly and a few more on weekends. He hasn't had an alcoholic drink for the last 2 days.

O: *VS:* BP 136/78, HR 86 (regular), RR 12, afebrile

HEENT: Head atraumatic. PERRLA, no papilledema. EOMs full with no gaze abnormality. Hearing intact bilaterally. Mouth, good dentition. Small ulceration on tongue. Neck supple. No bruits

CV: S_1 and S_2 RRR. No murmurs, gallops, or rubs. PMI 5th ICS, MCL

RESP: No dullness to palpation or pain over anterior/posterior thorax. LCTA

Abdomen soft, nontender, nondistended. No organomegaly

Ext: Normal muscle tone, full ROM in all extremities; no cyanosis, edema, or joint deformities. Peripheral pulses +2 bilaterally

Neuro: Oriented ×3. Affect appropriate. Remote and recent memory intact. CNs II–XII grossly intact. DTRs +2 bilaterally upper and lower extremities. Motor strength and sensation equal in the upper extremities. Gait normal

Labs: CBC, CMP within normal limits. Toxicology screen negative

Diagnostics: Electroencephalogram (EEG) normal

Imaging: CT of the head normal with no structural abnormalities

A: Probable idiopathic first seizure

P: Discussed the etiology of seizures and explained that at this point we are uncertain of cause. Reviewed recommendation for "watchful waiting" for a first-time seizure. Encouraged no driving for the next few days. If another "passing out" episode occurs, go to the emergency department (ED) immediately.

Encouraged healthy diet and exercise; avoid sleep deprivation, alcohol, and excessive caffeine for now. Will need referral to a neurologist if second seizure occurs. Follow-up 1 month

Health Promotion Issues

▶ Discuss smoking cessation strategies. Advise to stop smoking completely.

▶ Discuss American Heart Association guidelines for alcohol intake.

Guidelines to Direct Care

French JA, Kanner AM, Bautista J, et al. Efficacy and tolerability of the new antiepileptic drugs I: treatment of new onset epilepsy. *Neurology.* 2004;62:1252–1260.

Harden CL, Huff JS, Schwartz TH, et al. Reassessment: neuro imaging in the emergency patient presenting with seizure (an evidence-based review). Report of the Therapeutics and Technology Assessment Subcommittee of the American Academy of Neurology. *Neurology.* 2007;69:1772–1780.

Krumholz A, Wiebe S, Gronseth G, et al. Practice parameter: evaluating apparent unprovoked first seizure in adults (an evidence-based review). Report of the Quality Standards Subcommittee of the American Academy of Neurology and the American Epilepsy Society. *Neurology.* 2007;69:1996–2007.

Morris GL, Gloss D, Buchhalter J, Mack KJ, Nickels K, Harden C. Evidence-based guideline update: vagus nerve stimulation for the treatment of epilepsy. Report of the Guideline Development Subcommittee of the American Academy of Neurology. *Neurology.* 2013;81:1453–1459.

Case 4

Gerald is a 65-year-old male who visits a healthcare provider only when there is a problem. He's concerned about a slight hand tremor. The tremor started about 1 year ago and initially began in his left leg and then moved to his left hand. The tremor is worse when he is sitting and remains constant unless he gets up and moves to do something. He has also noticed some soreness and stiffness in his legs, which he believes is due to "getting older." Gerald is concerned because the tremor is slowly worsening, and it's affecting both his tennis and golf games. He denies headaches, visual disturbances, changes in speech, or swallowing problems. His past medical history is significant for benign prostatic hypertrophy. He denies any history of coronary artery disease (CAD), diabetes mellitus (DM), HTN, or thyroid disease. His family history is unremarkable. He has no known allergies. Gerald denies any history of smoking and drinks four to five glasses of red wine per week. He is looking forward to retirement within the next several years.

Physical Exam

VS: BP 130/70, HR 64 (regular), RR 12, afebrile, Ht 5'8", Wt 159 lbs

HEENT: Male pattern baldness. PERRLA, EOMs full with no gaze abnormality. Hearing intact bilaterally. Mouth: Good dentition. No thyromegaly or carotid bruits

CV: S_1 and S_2 RRR. No murmurs, gallops, or rubs. PMI 5th ICS, MCL

RESP: LCTA

GI: Abdomen soft, nontender, nondistended. No hernias or organomegaly

Ext: Normal muscle tone, full ROM in all extremities; no cyanosis, edema, or joint deformities. Peripheral pulses +2 bilaterally

Skin: No rashes or pigment changes

Neuro: Oriented ×3. Affect appropriate. CNs II–XII grossly intact. At rest there is a noticeable tremor in his left leg and left hand. The hand tremor resolved when reaching for a magazine. No difficulty with the up and go test. Gait steady with decreased arm swing in left arm. Romberg negative. DTRs 2+ throughout. No Babinski or clonus

What additional assessments/diagnostics do you need?

What is the differential diagnoses list?

What is your working diagnosis?

Additional Assessments/Diagnostics Needed

ROS

- Ask about exclusion criteria for Parkinson's disease (PD), including:[21]
  - Repeated strokes with stepwise progression
  - Repeated head injury
  - Antipsychotic or dopamine-depleting drugs
  - More than one affected relative
  - Sustained remission
  - Strictly unilateral features after 3 years
  - Exposure to known neurotoxin
  - Other neurologic features: early severe dementia with disturbances of language, memory, or praxis

Physical Exam

- Assess tremor characteristics[22]
  - Rest tremor
    - Occurs in a body part that is relaxed and supported
    - Rate of tremor is usually between 3 and 6 Hz/cycle/second
    - If mild, it can be intensified by having the patient concentrate on a different task (e.g., counting backward from 100 by 7s)
    - Commonly seen in Parkinson's
  - Action tremor: Produced by voluntary muscle contraction (four types)
    - *Postural:* Produced when the affected body part maintains its position against gravity (for example, extending leg in front of the body)
    - *Kinetic:* Produced during a voluntary movement and can be either simple kinetic or intention:
      - *Simple:* Occurs with movement of the extremities
      - *Intention:* Occurs with movements that are directed toward a specific target with significant amplitude changes when approaching the target (for example, picking up a cup of coffee)
    - *Isometric:* Occurs with voluntary muscle contractions without movement

- *Task-specific tremor:* Occurs when performing a specific task such as writing or speaking
- Evaluate for diagnostic criteria for PD[21]
  - Diagnosis of parkinsonism
    - Bradykinesia and at least one of the following:
      - Muscular rigidity (cog wheeling)
      - Resting tremor 4–6 Hz
      - Postural instability not caused by a visual, vestibular, cerebellar, or proprioceptive dysfunction
  - Features that support a PD diagnosis
    - Unilateral onset
    - Rest tremor present
    - Progressive nature
    - Persistent asymmetry affecting the side of onset
    - Clinical course of ≥10 years
- Evaluate for other signs of PD, including:
  - Soft voice
  - Decreased facial expression
  - Subtle decrease in dexterity
  - Slowness in thinking
  - Depression or anhedonia

Routine Labs

There are no specific blood tests for tremor or PD, but consider serum vitamin B_{12} and vitamin D levels and thyroid function tests to identify potential underlying secondary causes of parkinsonism.[23]

Imaging

- DaTscan can be used as an aid in the diagnosis of PD.
- There is no evidence that CT or MRI can assist in the diagnosis of PD. These studies may reveal other causes of parkinsonism such as vascular insults, mass lesions, and cortical atrophy patterns suggestive of dementing illnesses.[23]

Differential Diagnoses List

Anxiety

Essential (familial) tremor

Parkinson's disease

Hyperthyroidism

Hepatic encephalopathy

Adult-onset idiopathic dystonia

Wilson's disease

Dementia

Progressive supranuclear palsy (PSP)

Multiple system atrophy (MSA)

Drugs

Working Diagnosis—Movement disorder (likely Parkinson's disease)

Pathophysiology

PD is one of the most common neurologic disorders and affects about 1% of individuals older than age 60 years. PD causes progressive disability, which can be slowed, but not cured, by treatment. Neuropathic changes in PD include loss of pigment dopaminergic neurons of the substantia nigra and the presence of Lewy bodies and Lewy neurites. The etiology of PD is likely a combination of environmental exposure and a genetic predisposition. A number of genetic mutations have been discovered that may cause PD.[23]

What Is Your Treatment Plan?

Pharmacologic

The goal of medication is to provide good motor function through the day by restoring dopamine to normal levels.[24] The major drugs available for treatment of motor symptoms include:

- Levodopa
  - Most effective drug
  - First drug of choice, especially for symptoms related to bradykinesia
- Dopamine agonists
  - Can be given as monotherapy or in combination with other antiparkinsonian drugs for more advanced disease
  - Ineffective in patients who don't respond to levodopa
  - May delay need to initiate levodopa
- Monoamine oxidase (MAO) inhibitors
  - May be useful in patients with early PD
  - Modest symptomatic benefit as monotherapy
- Anticholinergic drugs
  - Most useful as monotherapy in patients younger than 70 with disturbing tremor without bradykinesia or gait disturbance
- Amantadine
  - Weak drug with low toxicity
  - Useful in treating younger patients with early or mild PD
  - May be used later in therapy for dyskinesia
- Catechol-O-methyltransferase (COMT) inhibitors
  - Useful as adjuncts to levodopa and dopa-decarboxylase inhibitors (DDCIs)

Nonpharmacologic

- Acupuncture—anecdotal and case reports suggest a symptomatic benefit to both motor and nonmotor symptoms.

- Manual therapy—the Alexander technique (AT) involves developing awareness of posture in order to improve it. Small studies showed some outcome measures.
- Exercise therapy—improved functional outcomes with a variety of modalities.
- Speech therapy
- Occupational therapy
- Surgical treatment may improve motor symptoms and reduce side effects associated with medications.[25]

Education/Counseling

- Discuss importance of building a healthcare team that may include a neurologist, physical therapist, occupational therapist, social worker, and geriatric psychiatrist
- Discuss management of medication
  - Patients must know how long it takes their medication to work and how long it lasts.
- Discuss good nutrition. As dysphagia progresses, pureed foods may be needed to prevent aspiration
- Discuss coping with symptoms and side effects of medications
  - Cognitive impairment
  - Depression
  - Fatigue
  - Gastrointestinal issues
  - Impulsive behaviors
  - Orthostatic hypotension
  - Pain
  - Skin changes
  - Sleep disturbances
  - Speech problems
  - Swallowing and dental concerns
  - Vision changes
  - Falls
- Stress importance of staying independent
- Additional information should be discussed at the appropriate time:
  - Need for financial planning
  - Insurance issues
  - Disability application
  - Placement (assisted living, nursing home)
  - PD support group information[21]

SOAP Note

S: Gerald comes in today with concern about a slight hand tremor that began 1 year ago. Tremor started in his left leg and now is also in his left hand. Tremor is worse at rest and is affecting his tennis and golf games. He denies headaches, visual disturbances, changes in speech, or swallowing problems. His past medical history is significant for benign prostatic hypertrophy. He has no known allergies and takes no medications. He is looking forward to retirement within the next several years and wants to ensure that his tremor is nothing serious.

O: *VS:* BP 130/70, HR 64 (regular), RR 12, afebrile, Ht 5'8", Wt 159 lbs

HEENT: Normal facial expression. PERRLA, EOMs full with no gaze abnormality. Hearing intact bilaterally. Mouth: Good dentition. No thyromegaly or carotid bruits

CV: S_1 and S_2 RRR. No murmurs, gallops, or rubs. PMI 5th ICS, MCL

RESP: No dullness to palpation. Clear to auscultation

GI: Abdomen soft, nontender, nondistended. No hernias or organomegaly

Ext: Normal muscle tone, full ROM in all extremities; no cyanosis, edema, or joint deformities. Peripheral pulses +2 bilaterally

Skin: No rashes or pigment changes

Neuro: Oriented ×3. Affect appropriate. CNs II–XII grossly intact. At rest there is a noticeable tremor in his left leg and left hand. The hand tremor has a fine pill-rolling appearance. Tremor is slow frequency. Noticeable cog wheeling in left wrist. Resolution of tremor noted when reaching for a magazine. Rapidly alternating movements reveal slight bradykinesia on the left. No rigidity noticed in the larger joints. Strength in lower and upper extremities 4/5 left, 5/5 right. Performs finger–nose testing without difficulty. Get up and go test = 20 seconds. Gait steady with decreased arm swing in left arm. Romberg negative. DTRs 2+ throughout. No Babinski or clonus

Psych: Good eye contact. Asking appropriate questions regarding new diagnosis. Discusses lifestyle management issues easily with wife as well as considering retirement earlier than anticipated

Labs: TSH 0.45 mU/L, free T4 1.4 mg/dL, vitamin D 25-OH 40 ng/mL 38, vitamin B_{12} 450 mg/L

A: Movement disorder—likely Parkinson's disease

P: Long discussion regarding movement disorders and Parkinson's disease with patient and wife. Referral to neurology to confirm the diagnosis. Follow-up here after initial evaluation and medications are started. Will monitor ongoing progress here, including effectiveness of medications and strategies to help cope with PD

Health Promotion Issues

▶ Discuss importance of good sleep habits, exercise, and nutrition.

▶ Administer influenza, pneumonia, and zoster vaccines.

Guidelines to Direct Care

National Parkinson Foundation. Diagnostic criteria. http://www.toolkit.parkinson.org/content/diagnostic-criteria#Exclusion_Criteria_for_PD. Accessed October 26, 2015.

Parkinson's Disease Foundation. Managing your PD. http://www.pdf.org/en/managing_pd. Accessed October 26, 2015.

Suchowersky O, Reich S, Perlmutter J, Zesiewicz T, Gronseth G, Weiner WJ; Quality Standards Subcommittee of the American Academy of Neurology. Practice parameter: diagnosis and prognosis of new onset Parkinson disease (an evidence-based review). Report of the Quality Standards Subcommittee of the American Academy of Neurology. *Neurology.* 2006;66:968–975.

Case 5

Mrs. Smith is a 70-year-old woman who is a known patient in your clinic. You have been managing her HTN for several years. She reports having a headache 1 week ago and remembers falling to the ground. She was unable to move her left side for a while. Initially, she seems a bit confused about the circumstances surrounding this incident, but as you continue to talk with her she is able to validate the information she is giving you. Her PMH includes HTN for the past 10 years, which is generally well controlled on hydrochlorothiazide 25 mg daily. She has her BP checked regularly at the senior center in addition to being seen in the clinic every 6 months. She reports one episode of a high BP (160/100) at the senior center last week. She quit smoking 20 years ago and has an occasional drink on holidays. Her ROS is negative today.

Physical Exam

VS: BP 160/100 (supine), 162/98 (standing), HR 96 (regular), RR 12, afebrile, Ht 5'5", Wt 132 lbs

HEENT: PERRLA, EOMs full with no gaze abnormality. No facial drooping. Hearing intact bilaterally. Mouth: Good dentition. No thyromegaly or carotid bruits

CV: S_1 and S_2 RRR. +S_4

RESP: LCTA

GI: Abdomen soft, nontender, nondistended. No hernias or organomegaly

Ext: Normal muscle tone, full ROM in all extremities; no cyanosis, edema, or joint deformities. Peripheral pulses +2 bilaterally

Neuro: Oriented ×3. Affect appropriate. CNs II–XII grossly intact. Gait and heel to toe WNL, rapid alternating movement intact. Perceives pain and light touch bilaterally. Vibratory sense intact. No apparent neurologic deficits

What additional assessments do you need?

What is your differential diagnoses list?

What is your working diagnosis?

Additional Assessments/Diagnostics Needed

ROS

▶ Ask about symptoms consistent with a focal neurologic deficit and timing and resolution of symptoms

▶ Ask about symptoms and PMH that inform need for hospitalization

▶ The 2006 National Stroke Association recommends hospitalization be considered for patients with first transient ischemic attack (TIA) presenting with any of the following:[26]

  ▶ Crescendo TIAs

  ▶ Duration of symptoms >1 hour

  ▶ Symptomatic internal carotid artery stenosis >50%

  ▶ Known cardiac source of embolus, i.e., atrial fibrillation

  ▶ Known hypercoagulable state

Physical Exam

▶ Assess for signs that inform need for hospitalization

▶ Guidelines recommend that it is reasonable to hospitalize patients with TIA symptoms who present within 72 hours of symptoms and meet any of the following criteria[27]:

  ▶ ABCD^2 score of ≥3 (see Table 1)

  ▶ ABCD^2 score of 0 to 2 and uncertainty that the diagnostic workup can be completed within 2 days as an outpatient

  ▶ ABCD^2 score of 0 to 2 and other evidence that the event was caused by focal ischemia

Routine Labs

In patients with suspected TIA, consider the following labs:[26,27]

▶ CBC

▶ PT/PTT

▶ CMP

TABLE 1 ABCD 2 Score for Predicting Stroke After TIA	
Age	
≥60 years	1 point
<60 years	0 points
Blood Pressure Elevation When First Assessed After TIA	
Systolic ≥140 mm Hg or diastolic ≥90 mm Hg	1 point
Systolic <149 mm Hg *and* diastolic <90 mm Hg	0 points
Clinical Features	
Unilateral weakness	2 points
Isolated speech disturbance	1 point
Other	0 points
Duration of TIA Symptoms	
≥60 minutes	2 points
10 to 59 minutes	1 point
<10 minutes	0 points
Diabetes	
Present	1 point
Absent	0 points

Adapted from National Stroke Association. Transient Ischemic Attack (TIA): Prognosis and Key Management Considerations. www.stroke.org.

▶ ESR

▶ Lipid panel

Imaging

▶ Neuroimaging should occur within 24 hours of symptom onset:[27]

  ▶ Brain imaging with head CT and/or MRI. MRI is preferred because of sensitivity, but CT is used more commonly due to availability. If emergent CT is obtained, at follow-up MRI should be performed when available

  ▶ Cervicocephalic vasculature should be assessed for treatable atherosclerotic lesions with carotid ultrasonography, magnetic resonance angiography, or CT angiography within 1 week of symptom onset

  ▶ ECG during initial evaluation

  ▶ Echocardiography

Differential Diagnoses List

Seizures

Migraine auras

Syncope

Ischemic stroke

Intracerebral hemorrhage

Brain tumor

Peripheral causes of vertigo

Hypoglycemia

Working Diagnosis—TIA

Pathophysiology

Transient ischemic attacks are defined as a transient episode of neurologic dysfunction caused by focal cerebral, spinal cord, or retinal ischemia without acute infarction. Twenty to 50% of patients with complete symptom resolution have evidence of acute tissue infarction on MRI. TIAs and ischemic stroke are essentially due to the same pathophysiologic process; the difference is only in duration, degree of ischemia, and resultant permanent brain injury. Focal cerebral ischemia can be due to a variety of causes, including embolism from a thrombus on ulcerated plaque or vessel occlusion that causes perfusion failure, cardioembolism, or occlusion or stenosis of deep cerebral vessels. Determination of the underlying cause of TIA is crucial for risk assessment and prevention of future stroke.[28-29]

What Is Your Treatment Plan?

Pharmacologic

► Everyone with a history of TIA should be considered for treatment to reduce cardiovascular risk.

► Risk factors for recurrent cerebrovascular ischemic events should be treated appropriately, including lowering blood pressure and blood cholesterol with drug therapy.

► Antiplatelet therapy: Aspirin, extended-release dipyridamole/aspirin, and clopidogrel are acceptable first-line agents.[30,31]

Nonpharmacologic

Lifestyle modifications for hypertension: Dietary Approaches to Stop Hypertension (DASH) diet

► Lifestyle modifications for hyperlipidemia: Low-fat, low-cholesterol diet

► Exercise on most days for a minimum of 30 minutes

► Maintain a normal weight

► Smoking cessation

► For diabetic patients, maintain HbA1c <7%

► Carotid endarterectomy may benefit symptomatic patients with recent (within 2 to 4 weeks) hemispheric nondisabling carotid artery ischemic events and ipsilateral 70% to 99% carotid artery stenosis[30,31]

Education/Counseling

► Instruct patients to go to an ED immediately if symptoms recur.

► Develop individualized education plans to address lifestyle modification.[32]

SOAP Note

S: Mrs. Smith is a 70-year-old woman who comes to the clinic today reporting a headache last week. She fell to the ground while gardening and was unable to move her left side or speak for about 1–2 minutes. No one witnessed this episode. She has had no reoccurrence of symptoms. She denies memory loss, headache, blurred vision, diplopia, or weakness in arms or legs. She reports one episode of a high BP (160/100) at the senior center last week. She is taking her hydrochlorothiazide 25 mg daily. She quit smoking 20 years ago and has an occasional drink on holidays. She stays active at the community senior center and tries to eat a heart-healthy diet.

O: *VS:* BP 160/100 (supine), 162/98 (standing), HR 96 (regular), RR 12, afebrile, Ht 5'5", Wt 132 lbs, body mass index (BMI) = 22

HEENT: PERRLA, no papilledema, EOMs full with no gaze abnormality. No facial drooping. Hearing intact bilaterally. Mouth: Good dentition. No thyromegaly or carotid bruits

CV: S_1 and S_2 RRR. $+S_4$

RESP: No dullness to percussion. LCTA

GI: Abdomen soft, nontender, nondistended. No hernias or organomegaly

Ext: Normal muscle tone, full ROM in all extremities; no cyanosis, edema, or joint deformities. Peripheral pulses +2 bilaterally

Neuro: Alert and oriented ×3. Affect appropriate. CNs II–XII grossly intact. Normal finger-to-nose and heel-to-shin without nystagmus or past pointing. Motor testing 5/5 upper and lower extremities bilaterally without spasticity, clonus, or rigidity. Sensory and vibratory sensation intact. Gait normal without ataxia

Labs: CBC, CMP, PT/PTT normal

Lipids: Total cholesterol (TC) 250, low-density lipoprotein (LDL) 150, high-density lipoprotein (HDL) 40, triglycerides (TRI) 220 (atherosclerotic cardiovascular disease [ASCVD] 10-year risk 21.5%)

ECG: Normal sinus rhythm without ectopy. Left ventricular hypertrophy (LVH)

A: TIA

P: Discussed etiology of TIA and explained need for imaging today

Start aspirin 81 mg daily

Start high-intensity statin: Rosuvastatin 20 mg in light of high ASCVD score

Continue hydrochlorothiazide and start beta blocker (atenolol 50 mg daily)

Scheduled for CT scan today and carotid duplex this week

Discussed importance of lifestyle modifications, including walking 30 minutes daily and low-fat, low-cholesterol, low-sodium diet. Handouts provided

Instructed to go to ED immediately if symptoms reoccur

Follow-up next week. Will review results of CT and carotid duplex, check BP, and continue to discuss healthy lifestyle management at that time

▌ Health Promotion Issues

▶ Should focus on lifestyle modification

▌ *Guidelines to Direct Care*

Bushnell C, McCullough LD, Awad IA, et al. Guidelines for the prevention of stroke in women: a statement for healthcare professionals from the American Heart Association/American Stroke Association. *Stroke*. 2014;45:1–44.

Easton JD, Saver JL, Albers GW, et al. Definition and evaluation of transient ischemic attack: a scientific statement for healthcare professionals from the American Heart Association/American Stroke Association Stroke Council; Council on Cardiovascular Surgery and Anesthesia; Council on Cardiovascular Radiology and Intervention; Council on Cardiovascular Nursing; and the Interdisciplinary Council on Peripheral Vascular Disease. The American Academy of Neurology affirms the value of this statement as an educational tool for neurologists. *Stroke*. 2009;40:2276.

Johnston SC, Nguyen-Huynh MN, Schwarz ME, et al. National Stroke Association guidelines for the management of transient ischemic attacks. *Ann Neurol*. 2006;60:301.

Kernan WN, Ovbiagele B, Black HR, et al. Guidelines for the prevention of stroke in patients with stroke and transient ischemic attack: a guideline for healthcare professionals from the American Heart Association/American Stroke Association. *Stroke*. 2014;45:2160–2236.

REFERENCES

1. Post J, Moriates C. When does an adult with headaches need central nervous system imaging? *Cleveland Clin J Med*. 2014;81:719–720.
2. International Headache Society. ICHD/guidelines. http://www.ihs-headache.org/ichd-guidelines/ihs-guidelines. Accessed October 26, 2015.
3. Foley M. Headache warning signs. http://headaches.about.com/od/headaches101/a/warning_signs.htm. Accessed October 26, 2015.
4. Kriegler JS, Kelley NE. Acute headache. In Lynn DJ, Newton HB, Rae-Grant AD, eds. *The 5-Minute Neurology Consult*. 2nd ed. Philadelphia: Wolters Kluwer/Lippincott Williams & Wilkins; 2012.
5. Moloney MF, Cranwell-Bruce LA. Migraine headaches. *Nurse Practitioner*. 2010;35:16–23.
6. Jackson JL, Kuriyama A, Hayashino Y. Botulinum toxin A for prophylactic treatment of migraine and tension headaches in adults—a meta-analysis. *JAMA*. 2012;307:1736–1745.
7. Post RE, Dickerson LM. Dizziness: a diagnostic approach. *Am Fam Phys*. 2010;82:361–368.
8. Fife TD, Iverson DJ, Lempert T, et al. Practice parameter: therapies for benign paroxysmal positional vertigo (an evidence-based review). *Neurology*. 2008;70:2067–2074.
9. White JA. Benign paroxysmal positional vertigo. In Lynn DJ, Newton HB, Rae-Grant AD, eds. *The 5-Minute Neurology Consult*. 2nd ed. Philadelphia: Wolters Kluwer/Lippincott Williams & Wilkins; 2012.
10. Hearing Handicap Inventory for the Elderly—Screening Version (HHIE-S). http://familymed.uthscsa.edu/geriatrics/tools/Hearing_Assessment.pdf. Accessed October 26, 2015.
11. Berg AT, Berkovic SF, Brodie MJ, et al. Revised terminology and concepts for organization of seizures and epilepsies: report of the ILAE Commission on Classification and Terminology, 2005–2009. *Epilepsia*. 2010;51:676–685.
12. Wilden JA, Cohen-Gadol AA. Evaluation of first nonfebrile seizure. *Am Fam Phys*. 2012;86:334–340.
13. Harden CL, Huff JS, Schwartz TH, et al. Reassessment: neuroimaging in the emergency patient presenting with seizure (an evidence-based review). Report of the Therapeutics and Technology Assessment Subcommittee of the American Academy of Neurology. *Neurology*. 2007;69:1772–1780.
14. Adams SM, Knowles PD. Evaluation of a first seizure. *Am Fam Phys*. 2007;75:1342–1347.
15. Schlacter SC. Update in the treatment of epilepsy. *Compr Ther*. 1995;21:473.
16. Fountain NB, Van Ness PC, Swain-Eng R, et al. Quality improvement in neurology: AAN epilepsy quality measures: report of the Quality Measurement and Reporting Subcommittee of the American Academy of Neurology. *Neurology*. 2011;76:76–94.
17. Kwan P, Brodie MJ. Effectiveness of first antiepileptic drug. *Epilepsia*. 2001;42:1255.
18. Varma JK. Epilepsy, generalized. In Lynn DJ, Newton HB, Rae-Grant AD, eds. *The 5-Minute Neurology Consult*. 2nd ed. Philadelphia: Wolters Kluwer/Lippincott Williams & Wilkins; 2012.
19. Moore JL, Hall CW. Epilepsy, complex partial. In Lynn DJ, Newton HB, Rae-Grant AD, eds. *The 5-Minute Neurology Consult*. 2nd ed. Philadelphia: Wolters Kluwer/Lippincott Williams & Wilkins; 2012.
20. UpToDate. Seizures: the basics. www.uptodate.com. Krumholz A, Hopp J. Driving restrictions for patients with seizures and epilepsy. Topic last updated: Feb 12, 2015.

21. National Parkinson Foundation. Diagnostic criteria. http://www
.toolkit.parkinson.org/content/diagnostic-criteria#Exclusion
_Criteria_for_PD. Accessed October 26, 2015.

22. Struble LM. Tremors. *Nurse Practitioner*. 2010;35:18–24.

23. Elmer LW, Hauser RA. Parkinson's disease/PD dementia. In Lynn
DJ, Newton HB, Rae-Grant AD, eds. *The 5-Minute Neurology Consult*.
2nd ed. Philadelphia: Wolters Kluwer/Lippincott Williams &
Wilkins; 2012.

24. Connolly BS, Lang AE. Pharmacological treatment of Parkinson disease: a review. *JAMA*. 2014;311:1670–1683.

25. Suchowersky O, Gronseth G, Perlmutter J, Reich S, Zesiewicz T,
Weiner J. Practice parameter: neuroprotective strategies and alter-
native therapies for Parkinson disease (an evidence-based review).
Report of the Quality Standards Subcommittee of the American
Academy of Neurology. *Neurology*. 2006;66:976–982.

26. Johnston SC, Nguyen-Huynh MN, Schwarz ME, et al. National Stroke
Association guidelines for the management of transient ischemic
attacks. *Ann Neurol*. 2006;60:301.

27. Easton JD, Saver JL, Albers GW, et al. Definition and evaluation of
transient ischemic attack: a scientific statement for healthcare professionals from the American Heart Association/American Stroke
Association Stroke Council; Council on Cardiovascular Surgery and
Anesthesia; Council on Cardiovascular Radiology and Intervention; Council on Cardiovascular Nursing; and the Interdisciplinary
Council on Peripheral Vascular Disease. The American Academy of
Neurology affirms the value of this statement as an educational tool
for neurologist. *Stroke*. 2009;40:2276.

28. Cucchiara B, Kasner SE. In the clinic—transient ischemic attack.
Ann Intern Med. January 2011;ITC1-12.

29. Simmons BB, Gadegbeku AB, Cirignano B. Transient ischemic attack: part II. Risk factor modification and treatment. *Am Fam Phys*.
2012;86:527–532.

30. Kernan WN, Ovbiagele B, Black HR, et al. Guidelines for the prevention of stroke in patients with stroke and transient ischemic
attack: a guideline for healthcare professionals from the American
Heart Association/American Stroke Association. *Stroke*. 2014;45:
2160–2236.

31. Bushnell C, McCullough LD, Awad IA, et al. Guidelines for the prevention of stroke in women: a statement for healthcare professionals
from the American Heart Association/American Stroke Association. *Stroke*. 2014;45:1–44.

32. Holzemer E, Thanavaro J, Malmstrom TK, Cruz-Flores S. Modifying risk factors after TIA and stroke: the impact of intensive education. *J Nurse Practitioners*. 2011;7:372–377.

Common Psychiatric Disorders in Primary Care

Karen S. Moore

Chapter Outline

Learning Objectives

Using a case-based approach, the learner will be able to:

1. Identify key history and physical examination parameters for common psychiatric disorders seen in primary care.

2. Summarize recommended laboratory and diagnostic studies indicated for the evaluation of common psychiatric disorders seen in primary care.

3. State pathophysiology of common psychiatric disorders.

4. Document a clear, concise SOAP note for patients with common psychiatric disorders.

5. Identify relevant education and counseling strategies for patients with common psychiatric disorders.

6. Develop a treatment plan for common psychiatric disorders utilizing current evidence-based guidelines.

Case 1

Sam is a 23-year-old male who presents with complaints of (c/o) difficulty in social situations and "worrying too much." States he is unable to apply for a job because he is afraid he will be rejected; he is unable to go for interviews because he worries so much he will fail that he does not try. States people have always told him he "is a worrier," but he feels it is getting in the way of him leading a normal life. States he often refuses going out with friends because of worry and feels he is going to be "alone forever" if he "can't get this under control." States the past year has been very stressful since graduating from college. Reports when queried that he often has difficulty sleeping because he is thinking about "something over and over." States that although he can think about "one thing that is bugging" him, he often finds it difficult to concentrate on daily tasks or interactions. Denies suicidal or homicidal ideation, denies wanting to harm self or others. States he is "desperate" for the racing thoughts and anxiety to stop.

Denies any pain, fever, cough, night sweats, shortness of breath, orthopnea, or chest pain. Denies abdominal pain, nausea, vomiting, or changes in bowel habits. Denies dysuria, discharge, hesitancy, or sensation of incomplete voiding. Denies known personal or family history of mental health issues but reports he "comes from a long line of worriers." Reports immunizations are up-to-date, last tetanus was 5 years ago, receives annual influenza vaccination. Denies taking any medications. No known drug allergies (NKDA). Denies tobacco use, denies illicit drug use. States he sometimes will drink alcohol to help "calm" him but then worries that he is drinking too much. Unable to quantify the amount of alcohol he consumes when drinking but states he is now "drinking something every day to just try to help." Lives alone and is not sexually active.

Physical Exam

Vital Signs (VS): Blood pressure (BP) 130/80, heart rate (HR) 86, temperature (T) 98.6, respiratory rate (RR) 16, height (Ht) 5'11", weight (Wt) 185 lbs

General (GEN): Well-appearing male noted to be shifting in chair frequently and having difficulty maintaining eye contact

Head, eyes, ears, nose, and throat (HEENT): Head normocephalic without evidence of masses or trauma. Pupils equal, round, react to light, accommodation (PERRLA), extraocular movements (EOMs) intact. Noninjected. Fundoscopic exam unremarkable. Ear canal without redness or irritation, tympanic membranes (TMs) clear, pearly, bony landmarks visible. No discharge, no pain noted. Oropharynx without redness, masses, or exudate. Neck supple without masses. No thyromegaly. No jugular vein distention (JVD) noted. No abnormalities along hairline

Skin: No redness, no warmth, no pruritus, no discharge noted. Hair distribution in normal distribution and pattern

Cardiovascular (CV): S_1 and S_2 regular rate and rhythm (RRR), no murmurs, no rubs

Lungs: Clear to auscultation

Abdomen: Soft, nontender, nondistended, bowel sounds present × 4 quadrants, no organomegaly, no bruits

What additional assessments/diagnostics do you need?

What is the differential diagnoses list?

What is your working diagnosis?

Additional Assessments/Diagnostics Needed[1–5]

In evaluating a client with stated or observed mental health concerns, the first issues to be addressed are the safety of the client and the safety of those around the client. It is imperative that if a client appears to be at risk of harm to self or others, or has stated a desire to harm self or others, emergent inpatient management should be initiated. If it is determined, in your clinical judgment, that the outpatient clinical setting is appropriate for the interaction, then an assessment of the issues being raised can proceed. It is important to note that an appropriate evaluation of mental health concerns can be quite time consuming. Although this can be taxing for the provider, it can be overwhelming for the patient. It is imperative that the provider determine which items will be addressed today and which items will require another session or referral.

Ask Focused Review of System (ROS) Questions

It is important to guide the client through the history of the present illness and any pertinent past medical history. As Sam states, he sometimes has difficulty concentrating, so your ability as a clinician to ask appropriate, specific questions will help you to paint the true picture of Sam's current clinical situation. Some questions might be:

- When did Sam first notice these symptoms?
- Do they fluctuate in their severity (waxing and waning)?
- If so, what makes the symptoms better or worse?
- What behaviors or coping mechanisms has Sam used to try to alleviate his concerns?
- Does Sam have any other symptoms besides worry that are troubling to him (i.e., hallucinations, delusions, paranoia, aggressive behaviors, changes in libido, change in sleep, change in appetite)?
- Has Sam ever experienced this before, and if so, what was his treatment?
- Have Sam's close contacts noticed the same issues Sam is raising or do significant others have different concerns about Sam's behaviors?
- Whom does Sam identify as a resource or support system?
- What does Sam identify as the most important life events he has experienced thus far?
- How did Sam respond to those events or see himself interacting with those events?
- Does Sam have any childhood issues or traumas that he can recall?
- Has Sam felt able to maintain close relationships with family, friends, or a significant other?
- What are Sam's cultural, social, and religious beliefs?
- What is Sam's sexual history (partners, intimate violence, abuse/assault)?
- What is Sam's occupational history (is he employed, how long, what field)?
- Does Sam have any history of legal issues (arrest, incarceration, divorce, lawsuits)?
- What is Sam's family history (psychiatric history, abuse, neglect, abandonment, medical issues)?

Exam

Observe for signs and symptoms (s/s) of agitation, anxiety, confusion, delirium, hallucinations, paranoia, aggression, or withdrawal. In the history and physical (H&P), elicit information about physical manifestations of mental health issues such as weight loss/gain, sleep disturbance, sexual dysfunction, abdominal distress, and headaches.

Routine Labs/Diagnostics

There are no routine labs or diagnostics to be performed, but some diagnostics may be appropriate if pharmacotherapy is anticipated or if an organic brain disorder is suspected.

- Labs to determine safety for prescribing could include:
  - Complete blood count (CBC)
  - Comprehensive metabolic panel (CMP)
  - Liver function tests (LFTs)
- Diagnostic imaging to consider may include:
  - Brain imaging
    - CT
    - MRI
    - PET scanning

Screening tools can be very helpful in determining whether a particular disease or disorder may be present and the level to which it is affecting the client's life. In the case of Sam, the Generalized Anxiety Disorder 7 Item Scale (GAD-7) was utilized.[4] Another tool that could be helpful if a past trauma is suspected as having a role in the client's current concerns is the Primary Care Post Traumatic Stress Disorder Screen (PC-PTSD).[5]

Differential Diagnoses List

Generalized anxiety disorder
Post-traumatic stress disorder (PTSD)
Bipolar disorder
Alcohol (ETOH) use disorder

Working Diagnosis—Generalized anxiety disorder

Pathophysiology[1-3]

According to the Diagnostic Statistical Manual of Mental Disorders, fifth edition (DSM-5), generalized anxiety disorder (GAD) is a condition characterized by excessive worry about everyday problems that persists for more than 6 months. Although the exact etiology is unknown, GAD does have a familial tendency and is often identified between adolescence and midlife. While Sam's primary diagnosis is GAD, it is not uncommon for patients to have overlapping or comorbid diagnoses. For example, if Sam had a particularly distressing traumatic event in the past, he may be experiencing episodes of PTSD that are triggering his anxiety. Likewise, Sam states that he abuses alcohol to "help calm" him. This is not an unusual occurrence in mental health and must be addressed in the creation of a cohesive plan of care.

What Is Your Treatment Plan?[1–8]

Sam is experiencing severe symptoms of GAD as evidenced by his H&P and the GAD-7 score of 21/21. An urgent referral to a psych-mental health practitioner was initiated for appropriate therapies to begin. It would be anticipated that Sam would receive a combination of pharmacologic treatment and therapeutic modalities.

Pharmacologic

▶ Anti-anxiolitic medications are meant for short-term use and are habit forming, so these must be carefully monitored.

▶ Antidepressants can be helpful for persons with GAD but must be carefully monitored related to the risk of suicidal ideation that is a side effect of these medications.

Nonpharmacologic

Cognitive behavioral therapy will teach Sam new ways to assess and handle situations that cause him worry so that he is better able to cope and function.

Education/Counseling

▶ Referral to appropriate mental health provider
▶ Follow-up as needed for other health concerns

SOAP Note

S: Sam is a 23-year-old male who presents with c/o difficulty in social situations and "worrying too much." States he is unable to apply for a job because he is afraid he will be rejected; he is unable to go for interviews because he worries so much he will fail that he does not try. States people have always told him he "is a worrier," but he feels it is getting in the way of him leading a normal life. States he often refuses going out with friends because of worry and feels he is going to be "alone forever" if he "can't get this under control." States the past year has been very stressful since graduating from college. Reports when queried that he often has difficulty sleeping because he is thinking about "something over and over." States that although he can think about "one thing that is bugging" him, he often finds it difficult to concentrate on daily tasks or interactions. Denies suicidal or homicidal ideation, denies wanting to harm self or others. States he is "desperate" for the racing thoughts and anxiety to stop.

Denies any pain, fever, cough, night sweats, shortness of breath, orthopnea, or chest pain. Denies abdominal pain, nausea, vomiting, or changes in bowel habits. Denies dysuria, discharge, hesitancy, or sensation of incomplete voiding.

Denies known personal or family history of mental health issues but reports he "comes from a long line of worriers." Reports immunizations are up-to-date, last tetanus was 5 years ago, receives annual influenza vaccination. Denies taking any medications. NKDA. Denies tobacco use, denies illicit drug use. States he sometimes will drink alcohol to help "calm" him but then worries that he is drinking too much. Unable to quantify the amount of alcohol he consumes when drinking but states he is now "drinking something every day to just try to help." Lives alone and is not sexually active.

O: *VS:* BP 130/80, HR 86 regular, T 98.6, RR 16, Ht 5'11", Wt 185 lbs

GEN: Well-appearing male noted to be shifting in chair frequently and having difficulty maintaining eye contact

HEENT: Head normocephalic without evidence of masses or trauma. PERRLA, EOMs intact. Noninjected. Fundoscopic exam unremarkable. Ear canal without redness or irritation, TMs clear, pearly, bony landmarks visible. No discharge, no pain noted. Oropharynx without redness, masses, or exudate. Neck supple without masses. No thyromegaly. No JVD noted. No abnormalities along hairline

Skin: No redness, no warmth, no pruritus, no discharge noted. Hair distribution in normal distribution and pattern

CV: S_1 and S_2 RRR, no murmurs, no rubs

Lungs: Clear to auscultation

Abdomen: Soft, nontender, nondistended, bowel sounds present × 4 quadrants, no organomegaly, no bruits

A: Generalized anxiety disorder

P: Sam presents with agitation, difficulty concentrating, and high scores (21/21) on the GAD-7. Immediate urgent referral made to appropriate mental health professional, who states he will meet Sam at the emergency department (ED) to begin assessment and ensure his safety. Sam refuses EMS transport but consents to transport to ED by his sibling, who accompanied him to this visit and has been in the waiting room. Sam requests that his sibling may be told only that Sam needs transport to the ED and may not be given information about the nature of Sam's referral for mental health services. Privacy policies reinforced with Sam and reassurance provided. Sam's mental health concerns will be managed by a psychiatric mental health professional, with follow-up at this clinic on an as-needed basis for primary health concerns.

Health Promotion

Safety topics addressed:

▶ Personal safety
▶ Physical violence prevention
▶ Risk taking
▶ ETOH and driving

Guidelines to Direct Care

Centers for Disease Control and Prevention. Recommended adult immunization schedule, by vaccine and age group. 2014. http://www.cdc.gov/vaccines/schedules/hcp/imz/adult.html. Accessed September 2, 2015.

US Dept of Agriculture and US Dept of Health and Human Services. *Dietary Guidelines for Americans, 2010.* 7th ed. Washington, DC: US Government Printing Office; 2010.

US Preventive Services Task Force. Recommendations for primary care practice: published recommendations. http://www.uspreventiveservicestaskforce.org/BrowseRec/Index/browse-recommendations. Accessed September 2, 2015.

Diagnostic and Statistical Manual of Mental Disorders DSM-5. 5th ed. Arlington, Va.: American Psychiatric Association; 2013. http://www.psychiatryonline.org. Accessed October 28, 2015.

Case 2

Chloe is a 35-year-old female who presents for routine annual checkup. Chloe denies any concerns but is noted to avoid eye contact throughout the examination and to speak softly and slowly. When queried, states she has recently experienced the loss of her mother after a long illness. States, when queried about how she is coping, that she is having difficulty getting out of bed in the morning and in fact sleeps in "most days." States her mother passed away 3 weeks ago, and she has not yet returned to work. States she was missing some work prior to her mom's death related to "just not feeling well" but now seems to have little motivation to eat, work, or socialize with friends. States she feels she could sleep all day and all night, but sleep can be fretful at times. Denies suicidal or homicidal ideation, denies wanting to harm self or others.

Denies any pain, fever, cough, night sweats, shortness of breath, orthopnea, or chest pain. Denies abdominal pain, nausea, vomiting, or changes in bowel habits. Denies dysuria, discharge, hesitancy, or sensation of incomplete voiding. Denies known personal or family history of mental health issues. Reports immunizations are up-to-date, last tetanus was 5 years ago, receives annual influenza vaccination. Well-woman exam 1 year ago was normal. Denies taking any medications. No known drug allergies (NKDA). Denies tobacco use, denies ETOH use, denies illicit drug use. Lives with husband of 5 years in a mutually monogamous relationship and has no children. Employed as an administrative assistant at a bank.

Physical Exam

VS: BP 118/76, HR 64 regular, T 98.3, RR 12, Ht 5'6", Wt 140 lbs

GEN: Well-appearing, clean, and well-kempt female noted to speak slowly with difficulty maintaining eye contact

HEENT: Head normocephalic without evidence of masses or trauma. PERRLA, EOMs intact. Noninjected. Fundoscopic exam unremarkable. Ear canal without redness or irritation, TMs clear, pearly, bony landmarks visible. No discharge, no pain noted. Oropharynx without redness, masses, or exudate. Neck supple without masses. No thyromegaly. No JVD noted. No abnormalities along hairline

Skin: No redness, no warmth, no pruritus, no discharge noted. Hair distribution in normal distribution and pattern

CV: S_1 and S_2 RRR, no murmurs, no rubs

Lungs: Clear to auscultation

Abdomen: Soft, nontender, nondistended, bowel sounds present × 4 quadrants, no organomegaly, no bruits

What additional assessments/diagnostics do you need?

What is the differential diagnoses list?

What is your working diagnosis?

Additional Assessments/Diagnostics Needed[1,9–10]

In evaluating a client with stated or observed mental health concerns, the first issues to be addressed are the safety of the client and the safety of those around the client. It is imperative that if a client appears to be at risk of harm to self or others, or states a desire to harm self or others, emergent inpatient management should be initiated. If it is determined, in your clinical judgment, that the outpatient clinical setting is appropriate for the interaction, then an assessment of the issues being raised can proceed. It is important to note that an appropriate evaluation of mental health concerns can be quite time consuming. Although this can be taxing for the provider, it can be overwhelming for the patient. It is imperative that the provider determine which items will be addressed today and which items will require another session or referral.

Ask Focused ROS Questions

In the case of Chloe, addressing the issues she raised about her mother's illness and death may be helpful to explore if she is able and willing to discuss them. Inquiring about how long her mother was ill and the perception of support Chloe received during the illness and after her mother's passing could begin the conversation. Additionally, inquiring about family and personal history of depression will allow you to determine a plan that may be most helpful to her. Conversation about mood swings and feeling up and then down should also be explored to determine whether evaluation for bipolar disorder is appropriate.

▉ Routine Labs/Diagnostics

Administration of a brief depression scale such as the nine-question Patient Health Questionnaire (PHQ-9) can provide a framework for the level of disability that Chloe's depressive symptoms are causing.[10]

Labs to rule out potential metabolic causes for her depression symptoms would include:

- ▶ CBC to explore possible anemia and infection
- ▶ CMP to evaluate electrolyte disturbances, renal function
- ▶ LFTs to evaluate liver function
- ▶ Thyroid panel (thyroid-stimulating hormone [TSH], free T4, free T3, total T3, calcitonin, thyroglobulin, anti-thyroid antibody titers: TgAb, TPOAb, and TRAb)

▉ *Differential Diagnoses List*

Major depressive disorder

Bipolar disorder

Hypothyroidism

Anemia

▉ *Working Diagnosis—Depression*

▉ Pathophysiology[1,9]

The pathophysiology of major depressive disorder, which is often referred to as "depression" is not well understood but seems to have genetic, environmental, and psychological factors that predispose one to depression. Some persons will experience only one depressive episode in their lifetime, while others will experience multiple depressive episodes. While troubling events such as the loss of a loved one may trigger a depressive episode, other life changes or stressors may also be considered triggering events. Chloe exhibits depressive criteria level A traits of depressed mood, loss of interest in usual activities, and decreased energy for major depressive disorder as described in the Diagnostic Statistical Manual of Mental Disorders, fifth edition (DSM-V).

▉ *What Is Your Treatment Plan?*[1,6–10]

For patients with major depressive disorder, either goal-directed psychotherapy or pharmacologic therapies are appropriate starting points for treatment depending on patient and provider preference and perceived risks and benefits of each. A combination of psychotherapy and medications may also be utilized. For pregnant women, for whom many medication classes utilized for treatment of depression are contraindicated, psychotherapy alone should be utilized. For severe depression that has been resistant to medications and psychotherapy, electroconvulsive therapy (ECT) has been utilized. For Chloe, the decision was made jointly by provider and Chloe that she would be open to attending psychotherapy and starting on medication because she is aware of the impact her depression is having on her life, her relationship with her spouse, and her ability to perform activities of daily living (ADLs).

▉ Pharmacologic

First-line pharmacologic treatment for major depression includes the drug classes of selective serotonin reuptake inhibitors (SSRIs), serotonin-norepinephrine reuptake inhibitors (SNRIs), and tricyclic antidepressants (TCAs). For Chloe, the patient and provider agreed upon starting on an SSRI: fluoxetine 20 mg PO QD.

▉ Nonpharmacologic

Chloe and the provider agreed upon starting goal-directed psychotherapy, which for Chloe would include a provider who is well acquainted with therapy for depression as well as grief support.

▉ Education/Counseling

- ▶ Medication teaching for SSRIs
  - ▸ Side effects (suicidal ideation, QT prolongation)
  - ▸ Time line for efficacy (1–2 weeks for symptom improvement, 6–8 weeks for full efficacy)
  - ▸ Do not discontinue abruptly
- ▶ S/S of worsening of condition
- ▶ How to seek urgent help
- ▶ Healthy lifestyle choices
  - ▸ Diet
  - ▸ Exercise/activity
  - ▸ Sleep hygiene
  - ▸ General hygiene

▉ SOAP Note

S: Chloe is a 35-year-old female who presents for routine annual checkup. Chloe denies any concerns but is noted to avoid eye contact throughout the examination and to speak softly and slowly. When queried, states she has recently experienced the loss of her mother after a long illness. States, when queried about how she is coping, that she is having difficulty getting out of bed in the morning and in fact sleeps in "most days." States her mother passed away 3 weeks ago, and she has not yet returned to work. States she was missing some work prior to her mom's death related to "just not feeling well" but now seems to have little motivation to eat, work, or socialize with friends. States she feels she could sleep all day and all night, but sleep can be fretful at times. Denies suicidal or homicidal ideation, denies wanting to harm self or others.

Denies any pain, fever, cough, night sweats, shortness of breath, orthopnea, or chest pain. Denies abdominal pain, nausea, vomiting, or changes in bowel habits. Denies dysuria, discharge, hesitancy, or sensation of incomplete voiding. Denies known personal or family history of mental health issues. Reports immunizations are up-to-date, last tetanus was 5 years ago, receives annual influenza vaccination. Well-woman exam 1 year ago was normal. Denies taking any medications. NKDA. Denies tobacco use, denies ETOH use, denies illicit drug use. Lives with husband of 5 years in a mutually monogamous relationship and has no children. Employed as an administrative assistant at a bank.

O: *VS:* BP 118/76, HR 64 regular, T 98.3, RR 12, Ht 5'6", Wt 140 lbs

GEN: Well-appearing, clean, and well-kempt female noted to speak slowly with difficulty maintaining eye contact

HEENT: Head normocephalic without evidence of masses or trauma. PERRLA, EOMs intact. Noninjected. Fundoscopic exam unremarkable. Ear canal without redness or irritation, TMs clear, pearly, bony landmarks visible. No discharge, no pain noted. Oropharynx without redness, masses, or exudate. Neck supple without masses. No thyromegaly. No JVD noted. No abnormalities along hairline

Skin: No redness, no warmth, no pruritus, no discharge noted. Hair distribution in normal distribution and pattern

CV: S_1 and S_2 RRR, no murmurs, no rubs

Lungs: Clear to auscultation

Abdomen: Soft, nontender, nondistended, bowel sounds present × 4 quadrants, no organomegaly, no bruits

A: Depression

P: Chloe presents today with a history of prolonged sadness following the death of her mother. Her symptoms are troubling to her daily and interfering with her ability to work, sleep, eat, and interact with spouse and peers. Chloe has no significant medical history that she can recall of depressive episodes in her youth or identified depressive episodes in her family. Chloe identifies that her symptoms of depressive disorder are problematic for her and states she is open to beginning psychotherapy and pharmacologic management for her major depressive disorder. Chloe is being referred to a psychotherapist with experience in grief support and depression counseling. Prescription provided for fluoxetine 20 mg PO QD. Side effects of medication, time of efficacy, and discontinuation discussed with patient. Healthy lifestyle topics of sleep hygiene, general hygiene, exercise, and diet were also discussed to help her manage her disease. Chloe verbalized understanding of instructions and referral process.

▌ Health Promotion

- ▶ Exercise
- ▶ Sleep hygiene
- ▶ General hygiene
- ▶ Healthy diet

▌ *Guidelines to Direct Care*

Diagnostic and Statistical Manual of Mental Disorders DSM-5. 5th ed. Arlington, Va.: American Psychiatric Association; 2013. http://www.psychiatryonline.org. Accessed October 28, 2015.

American Psychiatric Association (APA): Practice guideline for the treatment of patients with major depressive disorder (2010). http://psychiatryonline.org/pb/assets/raw/sitewide/practice_guidelines/guidelines/mdd. Accessed October 28, 2015.

Centers for Disease Control and Prevention. Recommended adult immunization schedule, by vaccine and age group. 2014. http://www.cdc.gov/vaccines/schedules/hcp/imz/adult.html. Accessed September 2, 2015.

US Dept of Agriculture and US Dept of Health and Human Services. *Dietary Guidelines for Americans, 2010.* 7th ed. Washington, DC: US Government Printing Office; 2010.

US Preventive Services Task Force. Recommendations for primary care practice: published recommendations. http://www.uspreventiveservicestaskforce.org/BrowseRec/Index/browse-recommendations. Accessed September 2, 2015.

▌ Case 3

Charles is a 28-year-old male patient who is accompanied by his spouse to his examination. Charles agrees for his wife to be present during the initial interview and states "she is worried about some stuff, but I am fine." Charles's wife states that Charles has always been "high energy," but lately he is not sleeping more than 2 hours at night, seems "very impatient," has gotten in fights at work, and is at risk of losing his job. States in the 6 months since they married he went from a high-energy, exciting person to wanting to sleep all the time to this newly agitated state. Denies suicidal or homicidal ideation, denies wanting to harm self or others. Denies any pain, fever, cough, night sweats, shortness of breath, orthopnea, or chest pain. Denies abdominal pain, nausea, vomiting, or changes in bowel habits. Denies dysuria, discharge, hesitancy, or sensation of incomplete voiding. Denies known family history of mental health issues. Reports immunizations are up-to-date, last tetanus was 2 years ago, does not receive annual influenza vaccination. Denies taking any medications. States he was last on medication at the age of 15 years for attention deficit hyperactivity disorder (ADHD) but stopped because it made him feel "zoned out." NKDA. Reports 20-pack-year history of tobacco use; started using tobacco at age 13 years. States he drinks a six-pack during the workweek and then "parties on the weekends." Unable to quantify how much he drinks, but wife states he often has to be driven home and does not remember where he has been or what he has done. Has used marijuana in the past to "mellow" him. Lives with wife of 6 months in a mutually monogamous relationship and has no children. Employed as a dockworker at a factory.

Physical Exam

VS: BP 136/78, HR 84 regular, T 98.6, RR 16, Ht 5'8", Wt 160 lbs

GEN: Well-appearing male noted to be moving around examination room throughout interview, using arms and hands in broad sweeping motions, speaking loudly and laughing throughout the examination

HEENT: Head normocephalic without evidence of masses or trauma. PERRLA, EOMs intact. Noninjected. Fundoscopic exam unremarkable. Ear canal without redness or irritation, TMs clear, pearly, bony landmarks visible. No discharge, no pain noted. Oropharynx without redness, masses, or exudate. Neck supple without masses. No thyromegaly. No JVD noted. No abnormalities along hairline

Skin: No redness, no warmth, no pruritus, no discharge noted. Hair distribution in normal distribution and pattern

CV: S_1 and S_2 RRR, no murmurs, no rubs

Lungs: Clear to auscultation

Abdomen: Soft, nontender, nondistended, bowel sounds present × 4 quadrants, no organomegaly, no bruits

What additional assessments/diagnostics do you need?

What is the differential diagnoses list?

What is your working diagnosis?

Additional Assessments/Diagnostics Needed[1,5–8,11–13]

In evaluating a client with stated or observed mental health concerns, the first issues to be addressed are the safety of the client and the safety of those around the client. It is imperative that if a client appears to be at risk of harm to self or others, or states a desire to harm self or others, emergent inpatient management should be initiated. If it is determined, in your clinical judgment, that the outpatient clinical setting is appropriate for the interaction, then an assessment of the issues being raised can proceed. It is important to note that an appropriate evaluation of mental health concerns can be quite time consuming. Although this can be taxing for the provider, it can be overwhelming for the patient. It is imperative

that the provider determine which items will be addressed today and which items will require another session or referral.

Ask Focused ROS Questions

Charles is presenting with a clinical picture that could make it difficult to elicit a full and complete history. In his case, his wife stands by and is able to fill in details that Charles may be skimming over or that he denies the importance of in his current situation. Charles states he is comfortable allowing his wife to participate in the conversation, but that could change if Charles decides to disagree with her detailed accounting of his behaviors and history. The challenge for this client interaction is to determine the underlying cause of his current state in the most efficient manner possible. The amount of time Charles will be able to pay attention and maintain his level of communication appears to be limited. Some important questions would be:

▶ History of the present illness
  ▶ When did Charles first notice these symptoms?
  ▶ Do they fluctuate in their severity (waxing and waning)?
  ▶ If so, what makes them better or worse?
  ▶ What behaviors or coping mechanisms has Charles used to try to alleviate his concerns?
  ▶ Does Charles have any other symptoms besides agitation that are troubling to him (i.e., hallucinations, delusions, paranoia, aggressive behaviors, changes in libido, change in sleep, change in appetite)?
  ▶ Has Charles ever experienced this before, and if so, what was his treatment?
  ▶ Have others in Charles's life noticed the issues he is raising or do they have other concerns?
  ▶ Whom does Charles identify as a resource or support system?
▶ Family history (psychiatric history, abuse, neglect, abandonment, medical issues)
▶ Sexual history (partners, intimate violence, abuse/assault), although he may not be willing to share that information with his wife present
▶ Occupational history (is he employed, how long, what field)
▶ Any history of legal issues (arrest, incarceration, divorce, lawsuits)

Exam

Observe for s/s of agitation, anxiety, confusion, delirium, hallucinations, paranoia, aggression, or withdrawal. In the H&P, elicit information about physical manifestations of mental health issues such as weight loss/gain, sleep disturbance, sexual dysfunction, abdominal distress, and headaches. Charles is exhibiting physical manifestations such as agitation, intermittent aggression, alcohol use, and sleep disturbance that are interfering with important relationships at home and at work.

Routine Labs/Diagnostics[1,5,11–13]

There are no routine labs or diagnostics to be performed, but some diagnostics may be appropriate if pharmacotherapy is anticipated or if an organic brain disorder is suspected.

- Labs to determine safety for prescribing could include:
  - CBC
  - CMP
  - LFTs
- Diagnostic imaging to consider may include:
  - Brain imaging
    - CT
    - MRI
    - PET scanning

Screening tools can be very helpful in determining whether a particular disease or disorder may be present and the level to which it is affecting the client's life. Administration of a screening tool such as the Mood Disorders Questionnaire (MDQ) to screen for bipolar disorder will help Charles objectively answer questions that will aid in the identification of his current condition.[11] The MDQ is brief, estimated to take only about 5 minutes to complete, and is very effective at identifying bipolar I disorder (depression and mania), which Charles seems to be exhibiting. Bipolar disorder can occur along with other mental health conditions such as PTSD, anxiety disorders, ADHD, and substance use disorder.

Differential Diagnoses List

Mania
Psychosis
Bipolar disorder
Substance use disorder

Working Diagnosis

Bipolar I disorder
Acute mania

Pathophysiology[12]

Bipolar disorder, also known as manic-depressive illness, is characterized by mood swings that can be very destabilizing for patients and families. Bipolar disorder can be classified as:

- *Bipolar I Disorder:* Distinct manic or mixed episodes as well as depressive episodes. Manic symptoms may be so severe as to require hospitalization.
- *Bipolar II Disorder:* Depressive episodes with hypomanic episodes but no true manic or mixed episodes.
- *Bipolar Disorder Not Otherwise Specified (BP-NOS):* Symptoms exist but do not fit the criteria for either I or II.
- *Cyclothymic Disorder:* Mild form of bipolar disorder in which the patient has episodes of mild depression and hypomania

for at least 2 years, but they do not fit the clinical picture for true bipolar disorder.

- *Rapid-Cycling Bipolar Disorder:* A condition that occurs when patients present with four or more episodes of cycling between mania and depression within 1 year. This is more commonly seen in patients who experience their first bipolar episode at a younger age.

In bipolar disorder, patients may go from depression that is so severe that they remain in their room in bed for days to episodes of invincibility and high energy that place them at risk of harm. When in a manic episode, bipolar patients can be loud, brash, aggressive, boisterous, and overly confident. Differentiating this disorder from other mental health conditions can be challenging without input from the patient's significant others because the patient presents to you in one phase of illness and may not mention the "other side of the coin." Many patients with bipolar disorder do not consider their manic episodes to be problematic because they feel happy, enthusiastic, and even euphoric during those times. As with other mental health issues, it is not uncommon for patients to present with comorbid conditions and often report use of drugs or alcohol to "self-medicate" their symptoms.

What Is Your Treatment Plan?[1,6–8,12–13]

Although bipolar disorder can be managed, most patients report continued episodes even on optimal treatment. The goal of treatment is to allow for effective management of symptoms, avoid damage to relationships, and avoid harm to self or others. This will require ongoing psychotherapy as well as lifetime medication use.

Pharmacologic

Medications known as mood stabilizers will be used to manage Charles's Bipolar I Disorder.

An older medication that is still in use for mood stabilization is lithium.

Some anticonvulsants have also been found to have a mood-stabilizing effect in the treatment of bipolar disorder, and these include:

- Valproic acid — *Depakote*
- Lamotrigine — *Lamictal*
- Gabapentin
- Topiramate — *Topamax (anticonvulsant/nerve pain)*
- Oxcarbazepine — *Trileptal*

If warranted, atypical antipsychotics may be used in combination with other agents such as antidepressants to treat bipolar disorder. These medications would include olanzapine, aripiprazole, and risperidone.

Antidepressants such as sertraline, fluoxetine, and buproprion can be used along with a mood stabilizer to treat the depression associated with bipolar disorder but should not be used alone.

Charles's manic episode is severe enough to merit hospitalization for urgent stabilization. Once Charles is discharged, his mental health professional will be handling prescribing for his mood-stabilizing medications.

▌ Nonpharmacologic

Psychotherapy will be utilized to treat bipolar disorder and may include one of the following types of therapeutic approaches:

- ▶ Cognitive behavioral therapy to help the patient learn to change thought patterns and behaviors
- ▶ Family-focused therapy to provide support to the family as well as the patient and teach them how to co-manage the disease
- ▶ Interpersonal and social rhythm therapy to help patients learn how to regulate their daily activities to promote balance and rest
- ▶ Psychoeducation to help patients with bipolar disorder understand their disease and unique symptoms of cycling so they are better able to intervene early and avoid a full manic/depressive episode

ECT therapy may also be utilized to treat bipolar disorder that has not responded well to other therapies.

▌ Education/Counseling

- ▶ Medication
  - ▶ Side effects (suicidal ideation, risk to fetus in pregnant women)
  - ▶ Time line for efficacy
  - ▶ Do not discontinue abruptly
- ▶ S/S of worsening of condition
- ▶ How to seek urgent help
- ▶ Healthy lifestyle choices
  - ▶ Diet
  - ▶ Exercise/activity
  - ▶ Sleep hygiene
  - ▶ General hygiene
- ▶ Risk-taking behaviors
  - ▶ Avoid risk-taking behaviors and situations
  - ▶ Avoid drinking ETOH or using drugs and operating machinery or driving

▌ SOAP Note

S: Charles is a 28-year-old male patient who is accompanied by his spouse. Charles agrees for his wife to be present during the initial interview and states "she is worried about some stuff, but I am fine." Charles's wife states that Charles has always been "high energy," but lately he is not sleeping more than 2 hours at night, seems "very impatient," has gotten in fights at work, and is at risk of losing his job. States in the 6 months since they married he went from a high-energy, exciting person to wanting to sleep all the time, to this newly agitated state. Denies suicidal or homicidal ideation, denies wanting to harm self or others. Denies constitutional symptoms. Denies family history of mental health issues. Reports immunizations are up-to-date, last tetanus was 2 years ago, does not receive annual influenza vaccination. Denies taking any medications. States he was last on medication at the age of 15 years for ADHD but stopped because it made him feel "zoned out." NKDA. Reports 20-pack-year history of tobacco use; started using tobacco at age 13 years. States he drinks a six-pack during the workweek and then "parties on the weekends." Unable to quantify how much he drinks, but wife states he often has to be driven home and does not remember where he has been or what he has done. Has used marijuana in the past to "mellow" him. Lives with wife of 6 months in a mutually monogamous relationship and has no children. Employed as a dockworker at a factory.

O: *VS:* BP 136/78, HR 84 regular, T 98.6, RR 16, Ht 5'8", Wt 160 lbs

GEN: Well-appearing male noted to be moving around examination room throughout interview, using arms and hands in broad sweeping motions, speaking loudly and laughing throughout

HEENT: Head normocephalic without evidence of masses or trauma. PERRLA, EOMs intact. Noninjected. Fundoscopic exam unremarkable. Ear canal without redness or irritation, TMs clear, pearly, bony landmarks visible. No discharge, no pain noted. Oropharynx without redness, masses, or exudate. Neck supple without masses. No thyromegaly. No JVD noted. No abnormalities along hairline

Skin: No redness, no warmth, no pruritus, no discharge noted. Hair distribution in normal distribution and pattern

CV: S_1 and S_2 RRR, no murmurs, no rubs

Lungs: Clear to auscultation

Abdomen: Soft, nontender, nondistended, bowel sounds present × 4 quadrants, no organomegaly, no bruits

A:

1. Bipolar I disorder
2. Acute mania

P: Charles presents today in an acute manic episode. He exhibits invincibility in his thought process and states he feels "on top of the world." Charles's wife accompanies him to this visit and is very concerned about Charles's increasingly risky behaviors and aggressive confrontations with strangers. Charles completed the MDQ, which demonstrates a need for further evaluation of probable bipolar I disorder with his current manic episode. Charles is initially resistant but does agree to urgent inpatient hospitalization. Transportation arranged and calls placed to facilitate transfer. Charles is not able to concentrate and participate in much health promotion or education today, so focus was placed on safety topics. Charles will be followed by mental health providers for management of his bipolar I disorder but will follow up at this clinic as needed for primary healthcare issues. Charles and wife verbalized understanding of admission, safety topics, and follow-up.

Health Promotion

- Safety
  - Wear seat belts
  - Social awareness (listen to cues from significant other; avoid areas that are unsafe; avoid situations that would lead to confrontation)
  - Risk-taking behaviors (avoid risk-taking behaviors and unsafe situations)
- Healthy lifestyle
  - Diet
  - Exercise/activity
  - Sleep hygiene
  - General hygiene
- ETOH/drug use cessation
- Smoking cessation

Guidelines to Direct Care

Centers for Disease Control and Prevention. Recommended adult immunization schedule, by vaccine and age group. 2014. http://www.cdc.gov/vaccines/schedules/hcp/imz/adult.html. Accessed September 2, 2015.

Diagnostic and Statistical Manual of Mental Disorders DSM-5. 5th ed. Arlington, Va.: American Psychiatric Association; 2013. http://www.psychiatryonline.org. Accessed October 28, 2015.

Substance Abuse and Mental Health Services Administration and the Health Resources Services Administration. Standards for Bipolar Excellence (STABLE): A performance measurement and quality improvement project. National Coordinating Council. STABLE resource toolkit. http://www.integration.samhsa.gov/images/res/STABLE_toolkit.pdf. Accessed October 28, 2015.

US Dept of Agriculture and US Dept of Health and Human Services. *Dietary Guidelines for Americans, 2010.* 7th ed. Washington, DC: US Government Printing Office; 2010.

US Preventive Services Task Force. Recommendations for primary care practice: published recommendations. http://www.uspreventiveservicestaskforce.org/BrowseRec/Index/browse-recommendations. Accessed September 2, 2015.

Case 4

Zachary is a 32-year-old male who presents with c/o redness and irritation to his bilateral axillary areas. States the areas are reddened and painful without itching or discharge. Denies new soaps, foods, personal hygiene products. States when queried about bathing and showering habits that he takes four to five showers each day related to fear of body odor and wanting to "feel clean." States he has always been "particular," but lately he is having difficulty getting out of the house on time for work related to showering twice every morning, checking every light in the house to make sure it is turned off, and checking every door in the house twice. States he feels that his need to check everything "just to be sure" was not a problem before, but since he started a new job in management at a local paper company his behaviors seem to have increased. States, when asked whether he prefers to sit on the exam table or in the chair, that he prefers the exam table because it is "covered" in paper. Noted to be carefully avoiding touching the table and other items in the examination room. When queried as to why, patient states he "does not like germs."

Denies suicidal or homicidal ideation, denies wanting to harm self or others. Denies any pain, fever, cough, night sweats, shortness of breath, orthopnea, or chest pain. Denies abdominal pain, nausea, vomiting, or changes in bowel habits. Denies dysuria, discharge, hesitancy, or sensation of incomplete voiding. Denies

known personal or family history of mental health issues. Reports immunizations are up-to-date, last tetanus was 6 years ago, does not receive annual influenza vaccination. Denies taking any medications. NKDA. Denies tobacco use and illicit drugs and reports only occasional ETOH use such as at a wedding or large social event less than monthly. Lives alone, is not sexually active currently, although he has been in the past, and has no children.

Physical Exam

VS: BP 132/74, HR 76 regular, T 98.5, RR 16, Ht 5'8", Wt 170 lbs

GEN: Well-appearing male in no apparent distress. Noted to be sitting in the center of the paper covering on the exam table

HEENT: Head normocephalic without evidence of masses or trauma. PERRLA, EOMs intact. Noninjected. Fundoscopic exam unremarkable. Ear canal without redness or irritation, TMs clear, pearly, bony landmarks visible. No discharge, no pain noted. Oropharynx without redness, masses, or exudate. Neck supple without masses. No thyromegaly. No JVD noted. No abnormalities along hairline

Skin: Axillary region and groin at femoral triangle bilaterally excoriated with reddened, broken skin areas noted. No vesicles, no plaques, no papules, no macules appreciated. No warmth, no pruritus, no discharge noted. Bilateral hands dorsal and palmar surfaces appear reddened, dry, and excoriated. Hair distribution in normal distribution and pattern

CV: S_1 and S_2 RRR, no murmurs, no rubs

Lungs: Clear to auscultation

Abdomen: Soft, nontender, nondistended, bowel sounds present × 4 quadrants, no organomegaly, no bruits

What additional assessments/diagnostics do you need?

What is the differential diagnoses list?

What is your working diagnosis?

Additional Assessments/Diagnostics Needed[1,4,6–8,14,17]

Although Zachary appears on the surface to be calm and appropriate in his conversation and responses, he reports a level of distress with daily living that is problematic and in need of further evaluation and intervention. Zachary reports that his obsessive behaviors are affecting his ability to arrive on time to work, which can be a threat to his livelihood and career opportunities.

Ask focused ROS questions:

- Does Zachary feel his behaviors have interfered with:
  - His ability to maintain close relationships with family, friends, or a significant other?
  - His ability to get or keep a job or advance in his career?
  - His ability to attend or enjoy social gatherings?
- What behaviors or coping mechanisms has Zachary used to try to alleviate his concerns?
- Are there any events or experiences that seem to trigger Zachary's behaviors?
- Does Zachary have any other symptoms besides worry that are troubling to him (i.e., hallucinations, delusions, paranoia, aggressive behaviors, changes in libido, change in sleep, change in appetite)?
- What are Zachary's cultural, social, and religious beliefs?
- What is Zachary's sexual history (partners, intimate violence, abuse/assault)?
- Does Zachary have any history of legal issues (arrest, incarceration, divorce, lawsuits)?
- What is Zachary's family history (psychiatric history, abuse, neglect, abandonment, medical issues)?
- Has Zachary ever experienced these issues before, and if so, what was his treatment?
- Whom does Zachary identify as a resource or support system?

Exam

Observe for s/s of agitation, anxiety, confusion, delirium, hallucinations, paranoia, aggression, or withdrawal. In the H&P, elicit information about physical manifestations of mental health issues such as weight loss/gain, sleep disturbance, sexual dysfunction, abdominal distress, and headaches. In the case of Zachary, he readily identifies that his behaviors are getting in the way of his normal daily functioning and that he wants to be able to control his impulses so he can lead a "normal" life. Zachary voices frustration with his current level of coping and is now experiencing physical manifestations of his troubling behaviors in the excoriated skin from repetitive washing.

Routine Labs/Diagnostics

There are no routine labs or diagnostics to be performed, but some diagnostics may be appropriate if pharmacotherapy is anticipated or if an organic brain disorder is suspected.

- Labs to determine safety for prescribing could include:
  - CBC
  - CMP
  - LFTs
- Diagnostic imaging to consider may include:
  - Brain imaging
    - CT
    - MRI
    - PET scanning

Screening tools can be very helpful in determining whether a particular disease or disorder may be present and the level to which it is affecting the client's life. In the case of Zachary, his obsessive repetitive behaviors fall in the category of anxiety disorders, so the Generalized Anxiety Disorder 7 Item Scale (GAD-7) was utilized.[4]

Differential Diagnoses List

Generalized anxiety disorder

Post-traumatic stress disorder

Bipolar disorder

Obsessive-compulsive disorder

Skin abrasion or friction burn, multiple sites

Working Diagnosis

Obsessive-compulsive disorder

Skin abrasion or friction burn, multiple sites

Pathophysiology[1,14]

Obsessive-compulsive disorder (OCD) is a condition characterized by excessive worry and fear that causes patients to ritualistically engage in behaviors repetitively. For example, a fear of germs or "smelling bad" for Zachary caused him to wash his hands, groin, and axillae so frequently and abrasively that he excoriated the skin. Performing the ritualistic behaviors is not about deriving pleasure from repeating the actions but rather is an attempt to control the obsessive thoughts and images. Although the exact etiology is unknown, OCD does have a familial tendency and is often identified in childhood or adolescence. Although Zachary's primary diagnosis is OCD, it is not uncommon for patients to have overlapping or comorbid diagnoses. For example, if Zachary had a particularly distressing traumatic event in the past, his anxiety may be triggered by episodes of PTSD. This is not an unusual occurrence in mental health and must be addressed in the creation of a cohesive plan of care.

What Is Your Treatment Plan?[1,6–8,14]

Pharmacologic

▶ Anti-anxiolitic medications are meant for short-term use and are habit forming, so these must be carefully monitored.

▶ Antidepressants can be helpful for persons with OCD but must be carefully monitored related to the risk of suicidal ideation that is a side effect of these medications.

▶ Over-the-counter ointment will be recommended to provide moisture and a barrier to Zachary's frequent bathing.

Nonpharmacologic

Cognitive behavioral therapy will teach Zachary new ways to assess and handle situations that cause him fear and anxiety so that he is better able to cope and function.

Education/Counseling

▶ Referral to appropriate mental health provider for cognitive behavioral therapy

▶ Follow-up in 2 weeks to assess wound healing and medication

▶ Skin care
  ▶ Avoid hot water in the shower
  ▶ Shower only one to two times daily
  ▶ Do not rub or scrub skin
  ▶ After showering pat dry and apply moisturizer

SOAP Note

S: Zachary is a 32-year-old male who presents with c/o redness and irritation to his bilateral axillary areas. States the areas are reddened and painful without itching or discharge. Denies new soaps, foods, personal hygiene products. States when queried about bathing and showering habits that he takes four to five showers each day related to fear of body odor and wanting to "feel clean." States he has always been "particular," but lately he is having difficulty getting out of the house on time for work related to showering twice every morning, checking every light in the house to make sure it is turned off, and checking every door in the house twice. States he feels that his need to check everything "just to be sure" was not a problem before, but since he started a new job in management at a local

paper company his behaviors seem to have increased. States, when asked whether he prefers to sit on the exam table or in the chair, that he prefers the exam table because it is "covered" in paper. Noted to be carefully avoiding touching the table and other items in the examination room. When queried as to why, patient states he "does not like germs." Denies suicidal or homicidal ideation, denies wanting to harm self or others. Denies any pain, fever, cough, night sweats, shortness of breath, orthopnea, or chest pain. Denies abdominal pain, nausea, vomiting, or changes in bowel habits. Denies dysuria, discharge, hesitancy, or sensation of incomplete voiding. Denies known personal or family history of mental health issues. Reports immunizations are up-to-date, last tetanus was 6 years ago, does not receive annual influenza vaccination. Denies taking any medications. NKDA. Denies tobacco use and illicit drugs and reports only occasional ETOH use such as at a wedding or large social event less than monthly. Lives alone, is not sexually active currently, although he has been in the past, and has no children.

O: *VS:* BP 132/74, HR 76 regular, T 98.5, RR 16, Ht 5'8", Wt 170 lbs

GEN: Well-appearing male in no apparent distress. Noted to be sitting in the center of the paper covering on the exam table

HEENT: Head normocephalic without evidence of masses or trauma. PERRLA, EOMs intact. Noninjected. Fundoscopic exam unremarkable. Ear canal without redness or irritation, TMs clear, pearly, bony landmarks visible. No discharge, no pain noted. Oropharynx without redness, masses, or exudate. Neck supple without masses. No thyromegaly. No JVD noted. No abnormalities along hairline

Skin: Axillary region and groin at femoral triangle bilaterally excoriated with reddened, broken skin areas noted. No vesicles, no plaques, no papules, no macules appreciated. No warmth, no pruritus, no discharge noted. Bilateral hands dorsal and palmar surfaces appear reddened, dry, and excoriated. Hair distribution in normal distribution and pattern

CV: S_1 and S_2 RRR, no murmurs, no rubs

Lungs: Clear to auscultation

Abdomen: Soft, nontender, nondistended, bowel sounds present × 4 quadrants, no organomegaly, no bruits

A:

1. Obsessive-compulsive disorder

2. Skin abrasion or friction burn, multiple sites

P: Zachary presents today with skin excoriation to groin, axillae, and hands caused by repetitive washing. Zachary reports daily anxiety, obsessive thoughts, and repetitive behaviors consistent with obsessive-compulsive disorder. He denies any suicidal or homicidal ideation, denies any hallucinations or psychoses. Will start Zachary on a lanolin/petrolatum topical ointment to excoriated skin surfaces after each washing and paroxetine 20 mg PO QAM for OCD. Recheck in

1 week to titrate dose of paroxetine by 10 mg weekly until anticipated maintenance dose of 40 mg QAM. Referral for cognitive-behavioral therapy initiated. Zachary verbalized understanding of all.

Health Promotion

▸ Safety

▸ Skin care

▸ General hygiene

Guidelines to Direct Care

Centers for Disease Control and Prevention. Recommended adult immunization schedule, by vaccine and age group. 2014. http://www.cdc.gov/vaccines/schedules/hcp/imz/adult.html. Accessed September 2, 2015.

US Dept of Agriculture and US Dept of Health and Human Services. *Dietary Guidelines for Americans, 2010.* 7th ed. Washington, DC: US Government Printing Office; 2010.

US Preventive Services Task Force. Recommendations for primary care practice: published recommendations. http://www.uspreventiveservicestaskforce.org/BrowseRec/Index/browse-recommendations. Accessed September 2, 2015.

Diagnostic and Statistical Manual of Mental Disorders DSM-5. 5th ed. Arlington, Va.: American Psychiatric Association; 2013. http://www.psychiatryonline.org. Accessed October 28, 2015.

American Psychiatric Practice Guideline for the Treatment of Patients with Obsessive Compulsive Disorder. Original publication 2007, updated 2013. http://psychiatryonline.org/pb/assets/raw/sitewide/practice_guidelines/guidelines/ocd.pdf.

Case 5

Mr. Fritz is a 72-year-old male who presents for a new patient visit. Denies any concerns and states he is feeling fine. Denies any pain, fever, cough, night sweats, shortness of breath, orthopnea, or chest pain. Denies abdominal pain, nausea, vomiting, or changes in bowel habits. Denies dysuria, discharge, hesitancy, or sensation of incomplete voiding. Denies headaches, vision changes, hearing loss "other than just getting old." States he uses reading glasses now and notices he has "a little more trouble" listening to the television if it is "down low." States he feels able to hear conversations "just fine" and socializes often with his "buddies at the bar." Has never had a hearing test and has not been to the eye doctor "since the wife died." When queried about nutrition, states he eats "TV dinners" or "eats out" nightly. States his children sometimes come and have lunch and bring him some food, which he enjoys. Denies known personal or family history of mental health issues. Reports immunizations are up-to-date, last tetanus was 2 years ago, does not receive annual influenza vaccination, has not had pneumonia or shingles vaccine. Denies regular exercise or activity. States he had a colonoscopy 2 years ago and "everything was fine." Denies taking any medications. NKDA. Reports 75-pack-year history of tobacco use, starting at age 15 years. States he drinks a six-pack daily during the week for 50+ years and "more on the weekend." Unable to quantify how much he drinks on the weekend but states he usually takes a cab home. Denies illicit drug use. Lives alone since the death of his wife 5 years ago, has 5 children and 10 grandchildren. Retired from his job as an accountant.

Physical Exam

VS: BP 130/78, HR 70 regular, T 98.2, RR 12, Ht 5'11", Wt 160 lbs

GEN: Well-appearing male in no apparent distress

HEENT: Head normocephalic without evidence of masses or trauma. PERRLA, EOMs intact. Noninjected. Fundoscopic exam unremarkable. Snellen near vision 20/100 each eye uncorrected, 20/30 distance each eye uncorrected. Ear canal with slight redness but without irritation, TMs clear, pearly, bony landmarks visible. No discharge, no pain noted. Forced whisper test with hearing loss identified. Oropharynx with slight redness, no masses, no exudate. Neck supple without masses. No thyromegaly. No JVD noted. No abnormalities along hairline.

Skin: No redness, no warmth, no pruritus, no discharge noted. Hair distribution in normal distribution and pattern for a male of his age

CV: S_1 and S_2 RRR, no murmurs, no rubs

Lungs: Expiratory wheeze noted on auscultation bilaterally

Abdomen: Soft, nontender, nondistended, bowel sounds present × 4 quadrants, no organomegaly, no bruits. Liver noted to be firm and nodular on palpation

What additional assessments/diagnostics do you need?

What is the differential diagnoses list?

What is your working diagnosis?

Additional Assessments/Diagnostics Needed[1,8–10,15–17]

Mr. Fritz reports a history of prolonged frequent alcohol and tobacco use. The challenge in discussing the issues with Mr. Fritz is that he has entrenched patterns of behavior that are now reinforced by his need for connection and socialization residing at the bar. With further exploration and discussion, Mr. Fritz identified that he was "probably drinking and smoking too much, but who cares, I'm old and alone." Based upon his responses to initial inquiry, the CAGE-AID and PHQ-9 were administered to screen for alcohol, other drug abuse, and depression. His results on screening merit further exploration.

Routine Labs/Diagnostics

- CBC
- CMP
- LFTs (abnormal secondary to alcohol-related cirrhosis)

Differential Diagnoses List

Substance Use Disorder

Tobacco use

Major Depressive Disorder

Presbycusis — hearing loss c̄ age

Presbyopia — farsightedness

Nutritional deficit

Alcohol-related liver disease

Working Diagnosis

Substance Use Disorder

Tobacco use

Major Depressive Disorder

Presbycusis

Presbyopia

Nutritional deficit

Alcohol-related liver disease

Pathophysiology[1,16]

Alcoholism, also Substance Use Disorder, is a chronic progressive disease that is affected by genetic, environmental, and psychological components. Alcoholism can lead to nutritional deficits, liver cirrhosis, encephalopathy, esophageal varices, and a form of liver cancer. Psychosocially, alcoholism places the patient at increased risk for death from accidental causes such as motor vehicle accidents, falls, and assault. Alcoholism is often associated with depression and other mental health issues.

What Is Your Treatment Plan?[1,6–10,16–17]

Mr. Fritz's liver panel was abnormal and a follow-up liver biopsy confirmed alcohol-related liver cirrhosis. Discussed with Mr. Fritz the need to stop drinking alcohol, to modify his diet, and to quit or decrease smoking.

Pharmacologic

- Related to concerns over liver function, pharmacologic therapy was deferred today.

Nonpharmacologic

- Liver biopsy (cirrhosis secondary to alcohol abuse)
- Psychotherapy to address grief, alcohol use, tobacco cessation, and depression recommended

Education/Counseling

- ETOH and tobacco use discussed at length with patient. States he knows they are bad for him, but he is "too old to quit." Discussed ways to approach cutting down if not discontinuing ETOH and tobacco altogether. Stated he would "try it and see." Discussed liver biopsy results and the impact on his overall health. Verbalized understanding.
- Personal safety emphasized.
  - Discussed risk of falls and assault associated with regular frequent alcohol consumption
  - Seat belt use
  - Never drink and drive
  - Never smoke in bed or when intoxicated related to (r/t) risk of fire
  - Smoke detectors in home
  - No throw rugs
- Healthy diet
  - Low salt
  - Low fat
  - High fiber
  - High fruits/vegetables
  - Whole grains
  - Limit alcohol
- Increased activity
  - Encourage walking, golf, or swimming related to his stated preferences for activity

SOAP Note

S: Mr. Fritz is a 72-year-old male who presents for a new patient visit. Denies any concerns and states he is feeling fine. Denies any pain, fever, cough, night sweats, shortness of breath, orthopnea, or chest pain. Denies abdominal pain, nausea, vomiting, or changes in bowel habits. Denies dysuria, discharge, hesitancy, or sensation of incomplete voiding. Denies headaches, vision changes, hearing loss "other than just getting old." States he uses reading glasses now and notices he has "a little more trouble" listening to the television if it is "down low." States he feels able to hear conversations "just fine" and socializes often with his "buddies at the bar." Has never had a hearing test and has not been to the eye doctor "since the wife died." When queried about nutrition, states he eats "TV dinners" or "eats out" nightly. States his children sometimes come and have lunch and bring him some food, which he enjoys. Denies known personal or family history of mental health issues. Reports immunizations are up-to-date, last tetanus was

2 years ago, does not receive annual influenza vaccination, has not had pneumonia or shingles vaccine. Denies regular exercise or activity. States he had a colonoscopy 2 years ago and "everything was fine." Denies taking any medications. NKDA. Reports 75-pack-year history of tobacco use, starting at age 15 years. States he drinks a six-pack daily during the week for 50+ years and "more on the weekend." Unable to quantify how much he drinks on the weekend but states he usually takes a cab home. Denies illicit drug use. Lives alone since the death of his wife 5 years ago, has 5 children and 10 grandchildren. Retired from his job as an accountant.

O: *VS:* BP 130/78, HR 70 regular, T 98.2, RR 12, Ht 5'11", Wt 160 lbs

GEN: Well-appearing male in no apparent distress

HEENT: Head normocephalic without evidence of masses or trauma. PERRLA, EOMs intact. Noninjected. Fundoscopic exam unremarkable. Snellen near vision 20/100 each eye uncorrected, 20/30 distance each eye uncorrected. Ear canal with slight redness noted but without irritation, TMs clear, pearly, bony landmarks visible. No discharge, no pain noted. Forced whisper test with hearing loss identified. Oropharynx with slight redness, no masses, no exudate. Neck supple without masses. No thyromegaly. No JVD noted. No abnormalities along hairline

Skin: No redness, no warmth, no pruritus, no discharge noted. Hair distribution in normal distribution and pattern for a male of his age

CV: S_1 and S_2 RRR, no murmurs, no rubs

Lungs: Expiratory wheeze noted on auscultation bilaterally

Abdomen: Soft, nontender, nondistended, bowel sounds present × 4 quadrants, no organomegaly, no bruits. Liver noted to be firm and nodular on palpation

A:

1. Substance use disorder
2. Tobacco use
3. Major depressive disorder
4. Presbycusis
5. Presbyopia
6. Nutritional deficit
7. Alcohol-related liver cirrhosis

P: Mr. Fritz presented as a new patient with no complaints. Prolonged history of alcohol and tobacco use identified during examination. Liver function tests abnormal, liver biopsy demonstrated cirrhosis. Referral to psychotherapy for grief support, depression, smoking cessation, and alcohol cessation. Patient states he will "consider it." Referrals for ophthalmology and audiology provided. Healthy diet, safety, and activity discussed with patient. Referral to dietitian offered, but patient is not interested at this time. Pneumonia vaccination and shingles vaccination offered, but patient again wishes to think about it. Mr. Fritz verbalized understanding of all instructions but is in the pre-contemplation phase at this point. Follow-up in 1 month to assess readiness to change.

Health Promotion[6–8]

▶ Pneumonia vaccination
▶ Shingles vaccination
▶ Smoking cessation encouraged
▶ ETOH use discouraged
▶ Exercise/activity encouraged
▶ Audiologist referral
▶ Ophthalmologist referral
▶ Diet education

Guidelines to Direct Care

American Psychiatric Association (APA). Practice guideline for the treatment of patients with major depressive disorder (2010). http://psychiatryonline.org/pb/assets/raw/sitewide/practice_guidelines/guidelines/mdd. Accessed October 28, 2015.

Centers for Disease Control and Prevention. Recommended adult immunization schedule, by vaccine and age group. 2014. http://www.cdc.gov/vaccines/schedules/hcp/imz/adult.html. Accessed September 2, 2015.

US Dept of Agriculture and US Dept of Health and Human Services. *Dietary Guidelines for Americans, 2010.* 7th ed. Washington, DC: US Government Printing Office; 2010.

US Preventive Services Task Force. Recommendations for primary care practice: published recommendations. http://www.uspreventiveservicestaskforce.org/BrowseRec/Index/browse-recommendations. Accessed September 2, 2015.

Diagnostic and Statistical Manual of Mental Disorders DSM-5. 5th ed. Arlington, Va.: American Psychiatric Association; 2013. http://www.psychiatryonline.org. Accessed October 28, 2015.

Centers for Disease Control and Prevention. Alcohol and public health. http://www.cdc.gov/alcohol/. Accessed October 28, 2015.

REFERENCES

1. Diagnostic and Statistical Manual of Mental Disorders DSM-5. 5th ed. Arlington, Va.: American Psychiatric Association; 2013. http://www.psychiatryonline.org. Accessed October 28, 2015.

2. National Institute of Mental Health. Anxiety disorders. http://www.nimh.nih.gov/health/topics/anxiety-disorders/index.shtml. Accessed October 28, 2015.

3. National Institute of Mental Health. Transforming the understanding and treatment of mental health. Generalized anxiety disorder. http://www.nimh.nih.gov/health/topics/generalized-anxiety-disorder-gad/index.shtml. Accessed October 28, 2015.

4. Spitzer RL, Kroenke K, Williams JBW, Lowe B. A brief measure for assessing generalized anxiety disorder. *Arch Intern Med.* 2006; 166:1092–1097.

5. Prins A, Ouimette P, Kimerling R, et al. The primary care PTSD screen (PC-PTSD): development and operating characteristics. *Primary Care Psychia.* 2003;9(1);9–14.

6. US Preventive Services Task Force. Recommendations for primary care practice: published recommendations. http://www.uspreventiveservicestaskforce.org/BrowseRec/Index/browse-recommendations. Accessed September 2, 2015.

7. Centers for Disease Control and Prevention. Recommended adult immunization schedule, by vaccine and age group. 2014. http://www.cdc.gov/vaccines/schedules/hcp/imz/adult.html. Accessed September 2, 2015.

8. US Dept of Agriculture and US Dept of Health and Human Services. *Dietary Guidelines for Americans, 2010.* 7th ed. Washington, DC: US Government Printing Office; 2010.

9. American Psychiatric Association (APA). Practice guideline for the treatment of patients with major depressive disorder (2010). http://psychiatryonline.org/pb/assets/raw/sitewide/practice_guidelines/guidelines/mdd. Accessed October 28, 2015.

10. Pfizer. Patient Health Questionnaire (PHQ-9). http://www.integration.samhsa.gov/images/res/PHQ%20-%20Questions.pdf. Accessed October 28, 2015.

11. Hirschfield RMA. The Mood Disorders Questionnaire (MDQ). http://www.integration.samhsa.gov/images/res/MDQ.pdf. Accessed October 28, 2015.

12. National Institute of Mental Health. Bipolar disorder. http://www.nimh.nih.gov/health/topics/bipolar-disorder/index.shtml.

13. Substance Abuse and Mental Health Services Administration and the Health Resources Services Administration. Standards for Bipolar Excellence (STABLE): A performance measurement and quality improvement project. National Coordinating Council. STABLE resource toolkit. http://www.integration.samhsa.gov/images/res/STABLE_toolkit.pdf. Accessed October 28, 2015.

14. American Psychiatric Practice Guideline for the Treatment of Patients with Obsessive Compulsive Disorder. Original publication 2007, updated 2013. http://psychiatryonline.org/pb/assets/raw/sitewide/practice_guidelines/guidelines/ocd.pdf.

15. Brown RL, Rounds LA. Conjoint screening questionnaires for alcohol and other drug abuse: criterion validity in a primary care practice. *Wisc Med J.* 1995;94(3):135–140.

16. American Psychiatric Practice Guideline for the Treatment of Patients with Substance Use Disorders. Original publication 2006, updated 2007. http://psychiatryonline.org/pb/assets/raw/sitewide/practice_guidelines/guidelines/substanceuse-watch.pdf.

17. Centers for Disease Control and Prevention. Alcohol and public health. http://www.cdc.gov/alcohol/. Accessed October 28, 2015.

Common Dermatologic Disorders in Primary Care

Karen S. Moore

Chapter Outline

D. Treatment Plan

E. Guidelines To Direct Care:

American Academy of Dermatolgy: Guidelines of care for the Management of Primary Cutaneous Melanoma

American Academy of Dermatology. Melanoma Diagnosis, Treatment and Outcome.

Final version of 2009 AJCC melanoma staging and classification.

Learning Objectives

Using a case-based approach, the learner will be able to:

1. Identify key history and physical examination parameters for common dermatologic disorders seen in primary care.

2. Summarize recommended laboratory and diagnostic studies indicated for the evaluation of common dermatologic disorders seen in primary care.

3. State pathophysiology of common dermatologic disorders.

4. Document a clear, concise SOAP note for patients with common dermatologic disorders.

5. Identify relevant education and counseling strategies for patients with common dermatologic disorders.

6. Develop a treatment plan for common dermatologic disorders utilizing current evidence-based guidelines.

Case 1

Katie is a 24-year-old female who presents with complaints of (c/o) waking up at night "itching" and has noticed "bumps" on her skin. States the "bumps" originally were on her hands but now are spreading to other areas of her body. States when queried that one of the patients she cared for at an extended care facility had a "skin problem" about a month ago. States she has not been back to work on that unit since that time related to her schedule, so she is unsure of what the diagnosis or treatment plan was for the elderly male. Denies discharge, states the "bumps" and "rash" are "very itchy" but are not painful. Denies fever, night sweats, cough, respiratory illness, abdominal pain, nausea, vomiting, or diarrhea. States that "besides this" she is "very healthy." Denies any new soaps, new personal care items, exposure to new food or outdoor environments. No known allergies to food, personal care products, metals, or medications. Reports use of implanted contraceptive, but no daily medications. Childhood immunizations up-to-date, tetanus up-to-date, does receive annual influenza vaccination because of her role as a nurse's aide. Denies tobacco use; alcohol (ETOH) use consists of an occasional beer on the weekend but less than three per month; denies illicit drug use. Reports she has been living with her boyfriend and in a monogamous sexual relationship for over a year. Well-woman exam was normal 6 months ago.

Physical Exam

Vital Signs (VS): Blood pressure (BP) 110/74, heart rate (HR) 72 regular, temperature (T) 98.7, respiratory rate (RR) 12, height (Ht) 5'6", weight (Wt) 140 lbs

General (GEN): Well-appearing female noted to be scratching hands and wrists intermittently throughout examination

Head, eyes, ears, nose, and throat (HEENT): Head normocephalic without evidence of masses or trauma. Pupils equal, round, react to light, accommodation (PERRLA), extraocular movements (EOMs) intact. Noninjected. Fundoscopic exam unremarkable. Ear canal without redness or irritation, tympanic membranes (TMs) clear, pearly, bony landmarks visible. No discharge, no pain noted. Neck supple without masses. No thyromegaly. No jugular vein distention (JVD) noted. No abnormalities along hairline, no evidence of nits or infestation

Skin: Raised papular rash in linear distribution noted to web space of fingers and along volar wrists. Pruritus noted throughout examination. No discharge noted

Cardiovascular (CV): S_1 and S_2 regular rate and rhythm (RRR), no murmurs, no rubs

Lungs: Clear to auscultation

Abdomen: Soft, nontender, nondistended, bowel sounds present × 4 quadrants, no organomegaly, no bruits

What additional assessments/diagnostics do you need?

What is the differential diagnoses list?

What is your working diagnosis?

Additional Assessments/Diagnostics Needed

Ask focused review of systems (ROS) questions.[1,2] In assessing a patient with skin conditions, it is important to pay attention to potential exposures to infectious agents as well as systemic disease that may be manifesting in a cutaneous pattern. In this case, Katie is a 24-year-old, healthy, sexually active female who works in an extended care facility as a nurse's aide. She denies any new potential exposures to allergens, denies any medications. With this review of her history you can narrow your focus away from potentially allergic or systemic causes to possible infectious exposures. Although sexual activity cannot be fully excluded as the cause of her potential infectious issue, Katie's job as a nurse's aide and exposure to a patient with a recent skin condition merit attention.

Exam

The physical examination for patients with skin conditions should include:

- Identification of red flags (fever, recent medication changes, abnormal labs)
- Detailed history of the skin eruption (has it happened before, when did it start, what makes it better or worse, how are you sleeping, does the skin/eruption itch/burn/hurt, what have you tried to make it better [skin creams, medications, lotions, avoidance of potential irritants])
- Description of the skin eruption (macular, papular, discharge, vesicles)

Routine Labs/Diagnostics[1,2]

- Depending on the differential diagnosis, the following diagnostics may be considered:
  - Scraping of the area with microscopic evaluation of the scraping to identify any potential mites or infestations
  - Laboratory testing if systemic issues such as lupus or leukemia are suspected
  - Laboratory testing for allergy panels if allergic cause is suspected
- In the case of Katie, a skin scraping and microscopic evaluation would be completed.

Differential Diagnoses List

Scabies

Norwegian scabies

Contact dermatitis

Working Diagnosis—Scabies

Pathophysiology

The skin reaction seen in human scabies infection is caused by an allergic response to the burrowing of an adult female *Sarcoptes scabiei* mite as she lives, deposits waste, and lays her eggs in the epidermis of her human host.[1,2] The serpiginous-shaped burrows often begin in the web space of the fingers and spread to wrists, hands, and other skin surfaces. Scabies is transmitted by close skin-to-skin contact such as during sexual activity or in the sharing of bedding and personal care items in institutional settings such as prisons and healthcare facilities. Although scabies requires direct prolonged skin-to-skin contact for transmission, in the case of Norwegian crusted scabies, the crusted regions may contain up to 2 million mites, making the mites more easily transmitted with only limited contact, as occurs in extended care

facilities. Upon initial infestation with the scabies mite, the irritation and itching may not be seen for 2 to 6 weeks postinfection, but the mite infestation is still able to be transmitted to others. Once a person has experienced a prior scabies infection, the itching and rash will occur more rapidly, often within 24–48 hours of infestation.

What Is Your Treatment Plan?

Pharmacologic

Pharmacologic treatment should include treatment of the patient with the known infestation as well as close household contacts and sexual partners for the month preceding recognition of infestation.[1-5] If the infected person works in an institutional setting or if the infestation was caused by contact in an institutional setting, treatment of all potentially infected persons, laundering of linens, and reporting to the health department should be completed.

- Permethrin cream 5% is the preferred first-line treatment for scabies infection in persons older than the age of 2 months. Treatment consists of application of the cream to cover the entire body from the neck down in adults, including the hairline in children or those with suspected Norwegian scabies infestation. Patients should be instructed to follow the instructions carefully, wash the cream off fully following application, and anticipate retreatment approximately 1 week after the first application.
- Alternative pharmacologic treatments have varying levels of efficacy and are not recommended for all patients. They are as follows:
  - Crotamiton cream or lotion 10% is FDA approved for adults, but not children. Treatment failure has been reported.
  - Lindane 1% is FDA approved but is not recommended as first-line therapy related to a concerning side effect profile.
  - Ivermectin is an oral antiparasitic agent that may be used to treat scabies in children >15 kg and adults who are not pregnant or nursing. This treatment regimen should be reserved for scabies infestation that has not been effectively treated with topical agents.
- Additionally, pharmacologic treatment may be required to address the pruritus experienced by patients, which may be severe. An oral antihistamine such as diphenhydramine or hydroxyzine could be considered.

Nonpharmacologic

- Bed linens should be washed in very hot water and dried on high heat to kill the scabies mites. Mites cannot survive temperatures of 122°F for longer than 10 minutes.
- Any items that are unable to be laundered in the conventional manner may be bagged in dark trash bags, and the bags should remain unopened for 72 hours. Scabies mites do not

live for more than 72 hours when not in contact with their human host.

Education/Counseling

▶ Work restrictions. Patients should be instructed to stay off work until effective treatment for scabies has been completed if the patient has frequent skin-to-skin contact with others. This would include careers in institutional settings, laundry rooms or with linens, child care, massage therapy, and cosmetology/esthetics.

▶ Patients should be advised that the itching may continue for several weeks following effective treatment, but itching that persists past 4 weeks following treatment, the appearance of new burrows, or new areas of rash indicate that retreatment is necessary.

▶ Patients should be advised to refrain from sexual activity until effective treatment has been completed. Sexual partners should be treated at the same time to avoid reinfestation.

SOAP Note

S: Katie is a 24-year-old female who presents with c/o waking up at night "itching" and has noticed "bumps" on her skin. States the "bumps" originally were on her hands but now are spreading to other areas of her body. States when queried that one of the patients she cared for at an extended care facility had a "skin problem" about a month ago. States she has not been back to work on that unit since that time, so she is unsure of what the diagnosis or treatment plan was for the elderly male. Denies discharge, states the "bumps" and "rash" are "very itchy" but are not painful. Denies fever, night sweats, cough, respiratory illness, abdominal pain, nausea, vomiting, or diarrhea. States that "besides this" she is "very healthy." Denies any new soaps, new personal care items, exposure to new food or outdoor environments. No known allergies to food, personal care products, metals, or medications. Reports use of implanted contraceptive, but no daily medications. Childhood immunizations up-to-date, tetanus up-to-date, does receive annual influenza vaccination because of her role as a nurse's aide. Denies tobacco use; ETOH use consists of an occasional beer on the weekend but less than three per month; denies illicit drug use. Reports she has been living with her boyfriend and in a monogamous sexual relationship for over a year. Well-woman exam was normal 6 months ago.

O: *VS:* BP 110/74, HR 72 regular, T 98.7, RR 12, Ht 5'6", Wt 140 lbs

GEN: Well-appearing female noted to be scratching hands and wrists intermittently throughout examination

HEENT: Head normocephalic without evidence of masses or trauma. PERRLA, EOMs intact. Noninjected. Fundoscopic exam unremarkable. Ear canal without redness or irritation, TMs clear, pearly, bony landmarks visible. No discharge, no pain noted. Neck supple without masses. No thyromegaly. No JVD noted. No abnormalities along hairline, no evidence of nits or infestation

Skin: Raised papular rash in linear distribution noted to web space of fingers and along volar wrists. Pruritus noted throughout examination. No discharge noted

CV: S_1 and S_2 RRR, no murmurs, no rubs

Lungs: Clear to auscultation

Abdomen: Soft, nontender, nondistended, bowel sounds present × 4 quadrants, no organomegaly, no bruits

A: Scabies

P: Permethrin 5% cream at bedtime tonight. Apply to entire body from neck to toes, leave on according to package instructions, and wash off completely prior to going to bed for the night. Treat all bed linens with hot water wash and hot dryer setting. Work restrictions: Off work at extended care facility until reassessment in 2 weeks. If infestation appears cleared, may resume work at that time. Sexual partner should be treated at the same time as Katie. Contact made with employer regarding infestation, and it is confirmed that the patient Katie reported caring for was treated for scabies. Health department contacted and aware of work-related infestation. Reviewed signs and symptoms (s/s) of worsening condition, medications, and side effects with Katie. Instructed to call or return if symptoms worsen. Follow-up in 2 weeks to reassess and determine whether further work restrictions are necessary.

Health Promotion Issues

▶ Continue healthy behaviors such as well-woman exam and influenza vaccination annually.

Guidelines to Direct Care

Centers for Disease Control and Prevention. Parasites: scabies: crusted scabies cases (single or multiple). http://www.cdc.gov/parasites/scabies/health_professionals/crusted.html. Accessed October 28, 2015.

Centers for Disease Control and Prevention. Recommended adult immunization schedule, by vaccine and age group. 2014. http://www.cdc.gov/vaccines/schedules/hcp/imz/adult.html. Accessed September 2, 2015.

Centers for Disease Control and Prevention. 2015 sexually transmitted diseases treatment guidelines: ectoparasitic infections. http://www.cdc.gov/std/tg2015/ectoparasitic.htm. Accessed October 28, 2015.

US Dept of Agriculture and US Dept of Health and Human Services. *Dietary Guidelines for Americans, 2010.* 7th ed. Washington, DC: US Government Printing Office; 2010.

US Preventive Services Task Force. Recommendations for primary care practice: published recommendations. http://www.uspreventiveservicestaskforce.org/BrowseRec/Index/browse-recommendations. Accessed September 2, 2015.

Case 2

Josiah is a 28-year-old male who presents with c/o itching and a rash that presented after he was walking in the woods over the weekend. States it was pretty warm this past weekend, but he was wearing long pants and a short-sleeved shirt. States that the rash is "really bad" and keeping him awake at night. States he has tried topical lotions and oral diphenhydramine, but the itching persists. Denies any fever, cough, or upper respiratory complaints. States he has allergic rhinitis, but that does not seem to be bothering him right now. States the "rash" has "some blisters" that "keep getting bigger." Denies pain, fever, night sweats, shortness of breath, chest pain, or cough. Josiah's past medical history (PMH) is significant for asthma, eczema, and gastroesophageal reflux disease (GERD). Allergies to cats, pollens, mold, minocycline, and sulfa medications. Medications taken daily include omeptrazole, albuterol MDI, fluticasone propionate MDI. Uses no medications for his eczema regularly but treats with "creams or something as needed." Childhood immunizations up-to-date. Denies any vaccinations since high school graduation. Does not receive annual influenza immunizations. Denies tobacco use, ETOH "sometimes" but refuses to elaborate, denies illicit drug use. Lives alone, not currently sexually active, but with prior history of sexual activity with female partner, use of condoms for sexually transmitted infection (STI) prevention.

Physical Exam

VS: BP 128/82, HR 64 regular, T 98.3, RR 12, Ht 6'1", Wt 185 lbs

GEN: Well-appearing male in no acute distress

HEENT: Head normocephalic without evidence of masses or trauma. PERRLA, EOMs intact. Noninjected. Fundoscopic exam unremarkable. Ear canal without redness or irritation, TMs clear, pearly, bony landmarks visible. No discharge, no pain noted. Oropharynx without redness or discharge. Neck supple without masses or lymph nodes palpable. No thyromegaly. No JVD noted

Skin: Bilateral volar forearms with pruritic erythematous rash with multiple vesicles arranged in a linear distribution pattern. No lesions or rash noted to lower extremities, trunk, genitourinary (GU) region, or buttocks. No lymph nodes palpable

CV: S_1 and S_2 RRR, no murmurs, no rubs

Lungs: Clear to auscultation

Abdomen: Soft, nontender, nondistended, bowel sounds present × 4 quadrants, no organomegaly, no bruits

Musculoskeletal (MS): Joints of bilateral upper and lower extremities without swelling, pain, or erythema. Full active range of motion demonstrated

What additional assessments/diagnostics do you need?

What is the differential diagnoses list?

What is your working diagnosis?

Additional Assessments/Diagnostics Needed

Ask focused ROS questions.[6–8] In assessing a patient with skin conditions, it is important to pay attention to potential exposures to infectious agents as well as systemic disease that may be manifesting in a cutaneous pattern. This review of Josiah's history reveals a history of atopy, with multiple allergies, asthma, and eczema, which should make you consider allergic causes for his new skin eruption. Additionally, Josiah reports a recent foray into a wooded area wearing short sleeves, which suggests potential exposure to skin irritants such as plants, insects, and wildlife. The distribution of his skin eruption and description of the vesicles with pruritus and erythema coupled with his probable exposure to topical irritants in the woods leads to a working diagnosis of contact dermatitis.

Exam

The physical examination for patients with skin conditions should include:

▶ Identification of red flags (fever, recent medication changes, abnormal labs)

▶ Detailed history of the skin eruption (has it happened before, when did it start, what makes it better or worse, how are you sleeping, does the skin/eruption itch/burn/hurt, what have you tried to make it better [skin creams, medications, lotions, avoidance of potential irritants])

▶ Description of the skin eruption (macular, papular, discharge, vesicles)

Routine Labs/Diagnostics

▶ Depending on the differential diagnosis, the following diagnostics may be considered:

▷ Skin biopsy to determine the etiology of the skin eruption

▷ Laboratory testing for allergy panels if systemic allergic cause is suspected

▶ In the case of Josiah, no diagnostic testing would need to be completed based upon his history and physical examination.

Differential Diagnoses List

Contact dermatitis

Allergic response to medication

Sunburn

Insect bites

Working Diagnosis—Contact dermatitis (rhus dermatitis)

Pathophysiology

Rhus dermatitis, also known as *Toxicodendron* dermatitis, is a skin eruption caused by contact with plants from the genus

Toxicodendron.[6-8] Plants from this family, such as poison ivy, poison oak, and poison sumac, produce a chemical irritant known as urushiol. Contact with damaged leaves, as occurs when walking through the woods, pulling weeds in a garden, or interacting with a pet that has come in contact with the plants allows the urushiol sap to be deposited on clothing, hands, and skin. The allergic response occurs within 10 minutes and may be reinitiated by contact with contaminated clothing or transfer of urushiol to other body areas via scratching. Exposure to urushiol may also come from inhalation caused by the burning of leaves.

What Is Your Treatment Plan?

Pharmacologic[6-8]

▶ Topical antihistamines and steroid creams may be used to decrease irritation.

▶ Oral antihistamines such as diphenhydramine can be used if drowsiness is not a consideration.

▶ Oral glucocorticoids may be used if the allergic response is severe or involves the respiratory system, face, or genitals. Taper dosing should be utilized to avoid rebound.

▶ Barrier skin creams containing bentoquatam can be used if exposure to the offending leaves and sap is unavoidable. Barrier creams should be washed off and reapplied twice daily if exposure persists.

Nonpharmacologic

▶ Immediate washing of skin with warm soapy water should be initiated. Areas of suspected exposure should be carefully washed with an emphasis on avoiding contamination of non-exposed skin surfaces via sap transfer during washing.

▶ Immediate hot water washing of clothing must be done to avoid recontamination.

▶ Immediate washing of shoes and garden tools with isopropyl alcohol should be completed.

▶ Clipping of nails to avoid scratching and transfer of sap should be performed.

▶ Oatmeal baths can be utilized to soothe skin and relieve itching.

Education/Counseling

Patient education and counseling should include the following:

▶ Avoidance and identification of urushiol-containing plants

▶ Cleaning and decontamination of equipment

▶ Cleaning of clothing and person

▶ Medication teaching, including skin barrier creams

SOAP Note

S: Josiah is a 28-year-old male who presents with c/o itching and a rash that presented after he was walking in the woods over the weekend. States it was pretty warm this past weekend, but he was wearing long pants and a short-sleeved shirt. States that the rash is "really bad" and keeping him awake at night. States he has tried topical lotions and oral diphenhydramine, but the itching persists. Denies any fever, cough, or upper respiratory complaints. States he has allergic rhinitis but that does not seem to be bothering him right now. States the "rash" has "some blisters" that "keep getting bigger." Denies pain, fever, night sweats, shortness of breath, chest pain, or cough. Josiah's PMH is significant for asthma, eczema, and GERD. Allergies to cats, pollens, mold, minocycline, and sulfa medications. Medications taken daily include omeprazole, albuterol MDI, fluticasone propionate MDI. Uses no medications for his eczema regularly but treats with "creams or something as needed." Childhood immunizations up-to-date. Denies any vaccinations since high school graduation. Does not receive annual influenza immunizations. Denies tobacco use, ETOH "sometimes" but refuses to elaborate, denies illicit drug use. Lives alone, not currently sexually active, but with prior history of sexual activity with female partner, use of condoms for STI prevention.

O: *VS:* BP 128/82, T 98.3, HR 64 regular, RR 12, Ht 6'1", Wt 185 lbs

GEN: Well-appearing male in no acute distress

HEENT: Head normocephalic without evidence of masses or trauma. PERRLA, EOMs intact. Noninjected. Fundoscopic exam unremarkable. Ear canal without redness or irritation, TMs clear, pearly, bony landmarks visible. No discharge, no pain noted. Oropharynx without redness or discharge. Neck supple without masses or lymph nodes palpable. No thyromegaly. No JVD noted

Skin: Bilateral volar forearms with pruritic erythematous rash with multiple vesicles arranged in a linear distribution pattern. No lesions or rash noted to lower extremities, trunk, GU region, or buttocks. No lymph nodes palpable

CV: S_1 and S_2 RRR, no murmurs, no rubs

Lungs: Clear to auscultation

Abdomen: Soft, nontender, nondistended, bowel sounds present × 4 quadrants, no organomegaly, no bruits

MS: Joints of bilateral upper and lower extremities without swelling, pain, or erythema. Full active range of motion demonstrated

A: Contact dermatitis—rhus dermatitis

P: Continue oral diphenhydramine, begin topical hydrocortisone cream. Oatmeal baths three times daily. Cleaning of clothing and shoes discussed. Avoidance and identification of offending plants discussed. Immunizations recommended: influenza and TdaP. Education regarding medications, alcohol use, and safe sex.

Health Promotion Issues[3-5]

▶ Encourage influenza vaccination annually

▶ Encourage TdaP booster

- Administer CAGE questionnaire to allow for discussion of ETOH use
- Safe sex and STI discussion

Guidelines to Direct Care

American Academy of Allergy, Asthma and Immunology. Consultation and referral guidelines: citing the evidence: how the allergist–immunologist can help. *J Allergy Clin Immunol.* 2011;117(2 Suppl Consultation):S495–523.

Centers for Disease Control and Prevention. Recommended adult immunization schedule, by vaccine and age group. 2014. http://www.cdc.gov/vaccines/schedules/hcp/imz/adult.html. Accessed September 2, 2015.

Eichenfield LF, Tom WL, Chamlin SL, et al. Guidelines of care for the management of atopic dermatitis. *J Am Acad Dermatol.* 2014;70(2):338–351.

US Dept of Agriculture and US Dept of Health and Human Services. *Dietary Guidelines for Americans, 2010.* 7th ed. Washington, DC: US Government Printing Office; 2010.

US Preventive Services Task Force. Recommendations for primary care practice: published recommendations. http://www.uspreventiveservicestaskforce.org/BrowseRec/Index/browse-recommendations. Accessed September 2, 2015.

Case 3

Sarah is a 17-year-old female with a history of prior asthma who presents with new complaints of "rough patches" on the skin of her elbows and the back of her legs that are making her self-conscious about wearing shorts this summer. States she notices that sometimes the rough areas have "some bumps, but not all the time and not right now." PMH significant for asthma and seasonal allergies. States she uses albuterol MDI PRN but has not needed the medication for a month. States she uses her inhaler primarily in the spring and fall when her seasonal allergies exacerbate. Has taken steroid in the past with asthma exacerbation but "not for several years." States she participates in basketball at her school and will occasionally need to use albuterol prior to activity. Denies medication allergies, reports food allergies to strawberries, mangoes, and peaches as well as a severe anaphylactic allergy to latex. States when queried that she "had some kind of skin problem" when she was much younger and skin dryness in the winter, but "this is the worst it's been." Denies pain, fever, night sweats, shortness of breath, chest pain, or cough. Denies changes in personal hygiene products, foods, or medications. Immunizations up-to-date, including tetanus, human papillomavirus (HPV), meningitis, and annual influenza. Denies tobacco use, denies ETOH use, denies illicit drug use. Lives with mother and one sibling aged 19 years, and both are well. Denies being sexually active. Last menstrual period (LMP) 1 week prior to this visit.

Physical Exam

VS: BP 117/72, HR 58 regular, T 98.8, RR 12, Ht 5'11", Wt 145 lbs

GEN: Well-appearing female in no acute distress

HEENT: Head normocephalic without evidence of masses or trauma. PERRLA, EOMs intact. Noninjected. Fundoscopic exam unremarkable. Ear canal without redness or irritation, TMs clear, pearly, bony landmarks visible. No discharge, no pain noted. Oropharynx without redness or discharge. Neck supple without masses or lymph nodes palpable. No thyromegaly. No JVD noted

Skin: Bilateral preolecranon and posterior popliteal fossa regions with erythematous, papular region with lichenified scaling noted. No lesions or rash noted to trunk, GU region, or buttocks. No lymph nodes palpable

CV: S_1 and S_2 RRR, no murmurs, no rubs

Lungs: Clear to auscultation

Abdomen: Soft, nontender, nondistended, bowel sounds present × 4 quadrants, no organomegaly, no bruits

MS: Joints of bilateral upper and lower extremities without swelling, pain, or erythema. Full active range of motion demonstrated

What additional assessments/diagnostics do you need?

What is the differential diagnoses list?

What is your working diagnosis?

Additional Assessments/Diagnostics Needed

Ask focused ROS questions.[7-9] In assessing a patient with skin conditions, it is important to pay attention to potential exposures to infectious agents as well as systemic disease that may be manifesting in a cutaneous pattern. Sarah's history reveals a history of atopy, with multiple allergies, asthma, and prior skin eruptions, which should make you consider chronic allergic as well as systemic atopic causes for the skin complaints she is currently experiencing. The absence of other systemic symptoms such as fever, general malaise, or reports of self- or familial illness lessen the possibility of systemic causes other than allergies and atopy.

Exam

The physical examination for patients with skin conditions should include:

- Identification of red flags (fever, recent medication changes, abnormal labs)
- Detailed history of the skin eruption (has it happened before, when did it start, what makes it better or worse, how are you sleeping, does the skin/eruption itch/burn/hurt, what have you tried to make it better [skin creams, medications, lotions, avoidance of potential irritants])
- Description of the skin eruption (macular, papular, discharge, vesicles)

Routine Labs/Diagnostics[7–9]

- Depending on the differential diagnosis, the following diagnostics may be considered:
  - Skin biopsy to determine the etiology of the skin eruption
  - Laboratory testing for allergy panels if systemic allergic cause is suspected
- In the case of Sarah, diagnostic testing would be aimed at determining triggering factors for this seemingly chronic skin eruption.

Differential Diagnoses List

Contact dermatitis

Systemic allergic reaction

Eczema

Psoriasis

Working Diagnosis—Eczema, chronic

Pathophysiology[7–9]

Eczema is a family of skin conditions that present with varying levels of pruritus, rash, vesicles, and scaling. Eczema can be divided into acute, subacute, and chronic presentations. The acute presentation is often mistaken for simple contact dermatitis with vesicles, inflammation, erythema, and pruritus. In subacute eczema, the presentation manifests as scaling, erythematous patches of papules, and plaques with irregular borders. In the chronic phase, lichenification is present with varying degrees of inflammation and pruritus. Eczema is an inflammatory skin response to various triggers such as allergens and contact irritants that can be exacerbated by stress and hormonal fluctuation. The exact mechanism of eczema is not fully understood.

What Is Your Treatment Plan?

Pharmacologic[7–9]

Pharmacologic management of eczema is divided into daily management and exacerbation management. Daily management of moisturizers is recommended for all patients with eczema. For some patients with eczema that is not well controlled, medications used for exacerbation may need to be utilized daily. Exacerbation management should be applied as directed to only affected skin areas and discontinued when the skin inflammation resolves.

- Topical steroid creams/ointments/lotions such as clobetasol or betamethasone may be used to decrease irritation. These medications do have common side effects of skin thinning, striae, and skin discoloration. These side effects are worsened by inappropriate use of these medications.
- Topical calcineurin inhibitors such as pimecrolimus and tacrolimus do not contain steroids and are also an effective treatment for eczema. They do not cause the common side effects associated with topical steroid use.
- Systemic immunosuppressant therapy has been utilized when topical approaches to disease management have failed. They include cyclosporine, methotrexate, and mycophenolate mofetil. Because these medications are systemic, their side effect profile must be carefully weighed prior to initiation of treatment, and ongoing monitoring of lab testing may be necessary.

Nonpharmacologic[7–9]

Good daily skin hygiene should be encouraged for all patients with eczema, including:

- Take short, warm baths or showers that are no longer than 10–15 minutes.
- Avoid overly hot baths or showers that can dry skin.
- Use mild, fragrance-free and dye-free cleansers that do not dry or irritate skin.
- Use daily, gentle, nonallergenic skin moisturizers. Apply within 3 minutes of bathing to "lock in" moisture.
- Do not rub or scrub skin. Pat skin dry after bathing/showering.
- Use a humidifier when indoor air quality dictates, such as in the winter.
- Keep fingernails trimmed to avoid scratching.

In addition to skin hygiene and pharmacologic treatment, persons with eczema may benefit from:

- Trigger avoidance. By identifying and avoiding irritants that cause an exacerbation of their eczema, patients will reduce the side effect burden of exacerbation medication.
- Phototherapy has been shown to be effective in some patients with eczema. The exact mechanism is unknown, but it appears to have an anti-inflammatory and antimicrobial effect.
- Psychological techniques to reduce the itch–scratch cycle seen in eczema include biofeedback, hypnosis, relaxation, and meditation.

► Alternative therapies have also been attempted to decrease the negative impact of eczema and may include various wraps and special baths as well as acupuncture.

Education/Counseling

Patient education and counseling should include the following:

► Skin hygiene regarding daily bathing, cleansing, and moisturizing.

► Eczema triggers and avoidance techniques.

► Medication counseling for prevention and treatment. It is important that patients understand how to apply their treatment medications appropriately and when to initiate and discontinue treatment regimens. Discussion and verification of understanding of side effects of each treatment regimen initiated are important.

SOAP Note

S: Sarah is a 17-year-old female with a history of prior asthma who presents with new complaints of "rough patches" on the skin of her elbows and the back of her legs that are making her self-conscious about wearing shorts this summer. States she notices that sometimes the rough areas have "some bumps, but not all the time and not right now." PMH significant for asthma and seasonal allergies. States she uses albuterol MDI PRN but has not needed the medication for a month. States she uses her inhaler primarily in the spring and fall when her seasonal allergies exacerbate. Has taken steroid in the past with asthma exacerbation but "not for several years." States she participates in basketball at her school and will occasionally need to use albuterol prior to activity. Denies medication allergies, reports food allergies to strawberries, mangoes, and peaches as well as a severe anaphylactic allergy to latex. States when queried that she "had some kind of skin problem" when she was much younger and skin dryness in the winter, but "this is the worst it's been." Denies pain, fever, night sweats, shortness of breath, chest pain, or cough. Denies changes in personal hygiene products, foods, or medications. Immunizations up-to-date, including tetanus, HPV, meningitis, and annual influenza. Denies tobacco use, denies ETOH use, denies illicit drug use. Lives with mother and one sibling aged 19 years, and both are well. Denies being sexually active. LMP 1 week prior to this visit.

O: *VS:* BP 117/72, T 98.8, HR 58 regular, RR 12, Ht 5'11", Wt 145 lbs

GEN: Well-appearing female in no acute distress

HEENT: Head normocephalic without evidence of masses or trauma. PERRLA, EOMs intact. Noninjected. Fundoscopic exam unremarkable. Ear canal without redness or irritation, TMs clear, pearly, bony landmarks visible. No discharge, no pain noted. Oropharynx without redness or discharge. Neck supple without masses or lymph nodes palpable. No thyromegaly. No JVD noted.

Skin: Bilateral preolecranon and posterior popliteal fossa regions with erythematous, papular region with lichenified scaling noted. No lesions or rash noted to trunk, GU region, or buttocks. No lymph nodes palpable

CV: S_1 and S_2 RRR, no murmurs, no rubs

Lungs: Clear to auscultation

Abdomen: Soft, nontender, nondistended, bowel sounds present × 4 quadrants, no organomegaly, no bruits

MS: Joints of bilateral upper and lower extremities without swelling, pain, or erythema. Full active range of motion demonstrated

A: Eczema—chronic variant

P: Discussion of skin hygiene, daily cleansing, and moisturizing. Initiate treatment with clobetasol ointment 0.05%, apply to affected areas BID. Health promotion topics discussed: immunizations, safe sex, and sexual violence. Recheck in 2 weeks to assess for medication response.

Health Promotion Issues[3–5,10]

► Encourage influenza vaccination annually
► Discussion of safe sex and sexual violence

Guidelines to Direct Care

American Academy of Allergy, Asthma and Immunology. Consultation and referral guidelines: citing the evidence: how the allergist–immunologist can help. *J Allergy Clin Immunol.* 2011;117(2 Suppl Consultation):S495–523.

Centers for Disease Control and Prevention. Injury prevention and control: Division of Violence Prevention: sexual violence. http://www.cdc.gov/ViolencePrevention/sexualviolence/index.html. Accessed October 28, 2015.

Centers for Disease Control and Prevention. Recommended adult immunization schedule, by vaccine and age group. 2014. http://www.cdc.gov/vaccines/schedules/hcp/imz/adult.html. Accessed September 2, 2015.

Eichenfield LF, Tom WL, Chamlin SL, et al. Guidelines of care for the management of atopic dermatitis. *J Am Acad Dermatol.* 2014;70(2):338–351.

US Dept of Agriculture and US Dept of Health and Human Services. *Dietary Guidelines for Americans, 2010.* 7th ed. Washington, DC: US Government Printing Office; 2010.

US Preventive Services Task Force. Recommendations for primary care practice: published recommendations. http://www.uspreventiveservicestaskforce.org/BrowseRec/Index/browse-recommendations. Accessed September 2, 2015.

Case 4

Mr. Zamboni is a 42-year-old high school wrestling coach who presents to you with c/o a "spider bite" on his left lower leg. When queried further states the area began as a raised reddened "bite" that over a day or so progressed to become hard and painful. States today he noticed a "whitehead" that he "scratched off" and believes the size of the reddened area has increased. When queried about possible contact with biting or stinging insects, patient denies any known exposures, denies any work in basements or closets. States he used an antibiotic ointment on it and kept it covered, but it seems to be getting bigger and more painful, so he presents for care. States he would rate the pain at present 5/10. Denies itching, but reports warmth and redness as well as some mucopurulent discharge "from the scabbed area." Denies significant past medical history. Denies recent infections or systemic illness. No known drug allergies (NKDA), takes no medications. Childhood immunizations up-to-date, tetanus up-to-date, does not receive annual influenza vaccination. Denies tobacco use; ETOH "a few drinks once in a while"; denies illicit drug use. Last physical examination 6 months ago with complete blood count (CBC), cholesterol panels, comprehensive metabolic panel (CMP) normal. Patient is sexually active and in a monogamous relationship with a female partner.

Physical Exam

VS: BP 138/86, HR 72 regular, T 99.5, RR 20, Ht 5'10", Wt 225 lbs

GEN: Obese male in no apparent distress

HEENT: Head normocephalic without evidence of masses or trauma. PERRLA, EOMs intact. Noninjected. Fundoscopic exam unremarkable. Ear canal without redness or irritation, TMs clear, pearly, bony landmarks visible. No discharge, no pain noted. Neck supple without masses. No thyromegaly. No JVD noted

Skin: Left lateral leg approximately 12 cm above lateral malleolus of ankle with 10-cm round area of redness with central mucopurulent raised weeping area noted. Warm and painful to touch. Discharge expresses readily with minimal palpation. Pain with very light palpation noted. No lymph nodes palpable

CV: S_1 and S_2 RRR, no murmurs, no rubs

Lungs: Clear to auscultation

Abdomen: Soft, nontender, nondistended, bowel sounds present × 4 quadrants, no organomegaly, no bruits

MS: Joints of bilateral upper and lower extremities without swelling, pain, or erythema. Full active range of motion demonstrated

What additional assessments/diagnostics do you need?

What is the differential diagnoses list?

What is your working diagnosis?

Additional Assessments/Diagnostics Needed

Ask focused ROS questions.[11–13] In assessing Mr. Zamboni, it is important to pay attention to the patient's stated history and evaluate that in relationship to potential exposures to infectious agents and insect stings or bites. Mr. Zamboni does not have a history consistent with spider bite because he denies being in basements, closets, or cleaning areas where spiders and insects may go unseen. As a wrestling coach, Mr. Zamboni would have contact with mats and equipment that have been exposed to skin contact, allowing for infectious disease spread.

Exam

The physical examination for patients with skin conditions should include:

- Identification of red flags (fever, recent medication changes, abnormal labs, systemic illness)
- Detailed history of the skin eruption (has it happened before, when did it start, what makes it better or worse, how are you sleeping, does the skin/eruption itch/burn/hurt, what have you tried to make it better [skin creams, medications, lotions, avoidance of potential irritants])
- Description of the skin eruption (macular, papular, discharge, vesicles)

Mr. Zamboni's examination is concerning related to the condition of the wound as well as his low-grade temperature.

Routine Labs/Diagnostics[11–13]

- Wound discharge should be sent for:
  - Gram stain
  - Culture
  - Sensitivity
- A CBC should be drawn and sent related to febrile illness and potential for systemic spread of infection.

Differential Diagnoses List

Obesity

Hypertension

Skin condition:

- Community-associated methicillin-resistant *Staphylococcus aureus* (CA-MRSA)
- Cellulitis
- Spider bite
- Furuncle
- Carbuncle

Working Diagnosis

Obesity
Elevated blood pressure
CA-MRSA

Pathophysiology[11–13]

CA-MRSA is a form of a commonly occurring skin surface bacteria that has grown resistant to the antibiotic methicillin and is spread in the community setting. Close skin contact with contaminated persons or surfaces increases the risk of contracting the condition. Initially the skin irritation begins as a raised, painful bump that may be red, warm and full of purulent discharge. The area can progress into a deep abscess and systemic illness if left untreated.

What Is Your Treatment Plan?

An incision and drainage (I&D) is recommended to treat the skin abscess and allows for collection of a wound culture for further specification of treatment regimens.

Pharmacologic

▶ Antibiotic treatment after incision and drainage may be initiated. Trimethoprim-sulfamethoxazole DS PO BID as empiric therapy may be utilized but the antibiotic regimen may require adjustment following sensitivity results. Recommended antibiotics that may be used to treat MRSA include vancomycin, linezolid, clindamycin, daptomycin, ceftaroline, doxycycline, minocycline, and trimethoprim-sulfamethoxazole

▶ Nonsteroidal anti-inflammatory drugs (NSAIDs) for pain relief

Nonpharmacologic

▶ Exquisite hygiene measures to prevent spread
  ▶ Hand washing with soap and water after any care and frequently throughout the day should be conscientiously observed. Use of pump soap is preferred to avoid contamination of bar soap.
  ▶ Use of disposable towels with hand washing and wound care should be utilized. For bathing, towels should be used only once and laundered separately from the clothing and linens of others in the household.
  ▶ Disposable gloves should be used if anticipating wound contact.
  ▶ Change bed linens daily or more frequently if soiled. Launder separately.
▶ Sports participation
  ▶ Cleaning of all sports equipment, including mats, with a product that is registered with the EPA as effective against MRSA
  ▶ No whirlpool use

▶ No sharing of equipment
▶ Exclusion from participation in contact sports until wound is properly covered and not at risk for becoming uncovered. As a coach, Mr. Zamboni would need only coverage of his wound to avoid contact with others, but he should consider evaluation of the team to determine whether any athletes have experienced similar infections.

Education/Counseling

▶ Wound care
▶ Antibiotic therapy
▶ Appropriate disinfection of equipment
▶ Hygiene practices
▶ Signs or symptoms of worsening
▶ Weight loss
▶ Elevated blood pressure

SOAP Note

S: Mr. Zamboni is a 42-year-old high school wrestling coach who presents to you with c/o a "spider bite" on his left lower leg. When queried further states the area began as a raised reddened "bite" that over a day or so progressed to become hard and painful. States today he noticed a "whitehead" that he "scratched off" and believes the size of the reddened area has increased. When queried about possible contact with biting or stinging insects, patient denies any known exposures, denies any work in basements or closets. States he used an antibiotic ointment on it and kept it covered, but it seems to be getting bigger and more painful, so he presented for care. States he would rate the pain at present 5/10. Denies itching, but reports warmth and redness as well as some mucopurulent discharge "from the scabbed area." Denies significant past medical history. Denies recent infections or systemic illness. NKDA, takes no medications. Childhood immunizations up-to-date, tetanus up-to-date, does not receive annual influenza vaccination. Denies tobacco use; ETOH "a few drinks once in a while"; denies illicit drug use.

O: *VS:* BP 138/86, HR 72 regular, T 99.5, RR 20, Ht 5'10", Wt 225 lbs

GEN: Obese male in no apparent distress

HEENT: Head normocephalic without evidence of masses or trauma. PERRLA, EOMs intact. Noninjected. Fundoscopic exam unremarkable. Ear canal without redness or irritation, TMs clear, pearly, bony landmarks visible. No discharge, no pain noted. Neck supple without masses. No thyromegaly. No JVD noted

Skin: Left lateral leg approximately 12 cm above lateral malleolus of ankle with 10-cm round area of redness with central mucopurulent raised weeping area noted. Warm and painful to touch. Discharge expresses readily with minimal palpation. Pain with very light palpation noted. No lymph nodes palpable

CV: S_1 and S_2 RRR, no murmurs, no rubs

Lungs: Clear to auscultation

Abdomen: Soft, nontender, nondistended, bowel sounds present × 4 quadrants, no organomegaly, no bruits

MS: Joints of bilateral upper and lower extremities without swelling, pain, or erythema. Full active range of motion demonstrated

A:

1. Obesity
2. Elevated blood pressure
3. CA-MRSA

P: Risk and benefit of I&D discussed and consent received prior to procedure. I&D completed with approximately 0.5 cc of mucopurulent discharge removed. Gram stain, culture and sensitivity (C&S) of wound drainage sent. Bleeding well controlled. Wet to dry dressing packed into wound and occlusive dressing placed. Blood testing performed and sent for CBC evaluation. Begin trimethoprim-sulfamethoxazole DS PO BID × 3 days until sensitivity results are available. Will reevaluate antibiotic regimen at day 3 and make adjustments as needed based upon results. Prescription for ibuprofen 800 mg PO TID provided to patient for pain relief following procedure. Follow-up tomorrow for dressing change and wound evaluation. Immunizations recommended, and patient states he will "think about them." Vaccination declined at visit today. Medications, diet, immunizations, wound care, hygiene, symptoms of worsening, disinfection regimen for sports equipment, and home disinfection discussed. Patient verbalized understanding.

Health Promotion Issues[3–5]

▶ Encourage influenza vaccination annually
▶ Hepatitis B vaccination discussed, but declined
▶ Weight loss recommended
▶ Blood pressure monitoring to evaluate for persistent elevation

Guidelines to Direct Care

US Preventive Services Task Force. Recommendations for primary care practice: published recommendations. http://www.uspreventiveservicestaskforce.org/BrowseRec/Index/browse-recommendations. Accessed September 2, 2015.

Centers for Disease Control and Prevention. Recommended adult immunization schedule, by vaccine and age group. 2014. http://www.cdc.gov/vaccines/schedules/hcp/imz/adult.html. Accessed September 2, 2015.

US Dept of Agriculture and US Dept of Health and Human Services. *Dietary Guidelines for Americans, 2010.* 7th ed. Washington, DC: US Government Printing Office; 2010.

Stevens DL, Bisno AL, Chambers HF, et al; Infectious Diseases Society of America. Practice guidelines for the diagnosis and management of skin and soft tissue infections: 2014 update by the Infectious Diseases Society of America. *Clin Infect Dis.* 2014:59(2):e10–52.

Liu C, Bayer A, Cosgrove SE, et al; Infectious Diseases Society of America. Clinical practice guidelines by the Infectious Diseases Society of America for the treatment of methicillin-resistant *Staphylococcus aureus* infections in adults and children. *Clin Infect Dis.* 2011;52(3):e18–55.

Environmental Protection Agency. List H: EPA's registered products effective against MRSA and vancomycin resistant Enterococcus faecalis or faecium (VRE). http://www2.epa.gov/pesticide-registration/list-h-epas-registered-products-effective-against-methicillin-resistant. Accessed November 13, 2015.

Case 5

Mr. Woodard is a 78-year-old male who is at the clinic for a routine examination. States when queried that he is not really concerned about "anything in particular" and that he is just "here to get checked out." Denies any changes in bowel/bladder habits, denies respiratory issues, denies allergies. Denies pain, fever, night sweats, shortness of breath, chest pain, cough, abdominal pain, visual changes. Reports PMH of diverticulitis without any recent exacerbations and "a little arthritis here and there." States when queried that he has noticed some hearing loss, but it is being monitored by an audiologist. States he is playing golf three times weekly, as has been his practice since retirement at the age of 62 years. When asked about skin changes, patient reports he was told by his golf partner that he has a "spot" on "the back" of his neck, but he has not been able to "get a good look at it." Denies any pain, itching, or bleeding from the area. States he can "feel it," and it sometimes bothers him when his collar rubs on it, but otherwise it "isn't causing a problem." States he receives his annual influenza vaccination, had a pneumonia vaccine and shingles vaccine last year. Tetanus immunization is up-to-date. Childhood illness history of measles, mumps, rubella, and varicella without sequelae. Reports he is a widower and is not sexually active at this time. States he lives in a senior condominium complex and enjoys an active social life with frequent golf and evening card games. Denies current tobacco use, but reports he used to smoke cigars on the weekend for about

35 years until he "gave it up" 5 years ago. Reports ETOH use consists of one beer after his golf games, denies illicit drug use. States his appetite is good and he has no difficulties with chewing or swallowing food. States he feels happy in his life and enjoys frequent visits from his 4 children and 10 grandchildren.

Physical Exam

VS: BP 132/74, HR 76 regular, T 98.2, RR 12, Ht 6'0", Wt 170 lbs

GEN: Well-appearing elderly male in no apparent distress

HEENT: Head normocephalic without evidence of masses or trauma. PERRLA, EOMs intact. Noninjected. Fundoscopic exam unremarkable. Ear canal without redness or irritation, TMs clear, pearly, bony landmarks visible. No discharge, no pain noted. Neck supple without masses. No thyromegaly. No JVD noted

Skin: Posterior neck with 8-mm darkened, slightly raised area with an asymmetric border, variation in coloring noted across lesion, no ulceration, no discharge. No pain with palpation, no erythema, no pruritus noted

CV: S_1 and S_2 RRR, no murmurs, no rubs

Lungs: Clear to auscultation

Abdomen: Soft, nontender, nondistended, bowel sounds present × 4 quadrants, no organomegaly, no bruits

MS: Joints of bilateral upper and lower extremities without swelling, pain, or erythema. Full active range of motion demonstrated

Neurologic: Sensation intact to bilateral lower extremities, deep tendon reflexes (DTRs) 2+ at patellar and Achilles bilaterally. Great toe extension normal, ankle dorsiflexion normal, plantar flexion normal, heel/toe walk normal. Bilateral lower extremity (LE) strength 5/5. Patient moves throughout examination room and from chair to table without difficulty or hesitation.

What additional assessments/diagnostics do you need?
What is the differential diagnoses list?
What is your working diagnosis?

Additional Assessments/Diagnostics Needed

Routine Labs/Diagnostics[14–16]

- ▶ Surgery
  - ▶ Biopsy
    - ➤ The suspected lesion should be excised to the point of a clean margin and a depth sufficient to remove the entire lesion in one piece.
    - ➤ Depth of the tumor (commonly known as Breslow's depth) will be used as part of the American Joint Commission on Cancer's melanoma staging system to determine overall treatment plan and prognosis. In

addition to depth of the tumor, ulceration and mitotic rate will be derived from the biopsy and will assist in staging the disease. Final staging will be based upon assessment of the tumor, involvement of lymph nodes, and distant metastases identified.

- ➤ The excised lesion will be sent for pathology and staging.
- ▷ Mohs surgery is done by a specially trained surgeon and requires that the cancerous lesion is removed layer by layer with microscopic examination performed on each layer as the surgery progresses. The surgery is complete when a layer is found to be without any cancer cells.
- ▶ Sentinel lymph node biopsy (SLNB) may be necessary to fully stage the disease and determine an appropriate plan of care.
- ▶ CT scans will be performed if metastases are suspected.
- ▶ Baseline laboratory testing may be performed such as CBC, liver function tests (LFTs), and CMP to determine overall physical suitability for potential treatment regimens[14–16]

Differential Diagnoses List

Malignant melanoma

Squamous cell carcinoma

Basal cell carcinoma

Actinic keratosis

Nevus

Working Diagnosis—Probable malignant melanoma

Pathophysiology[14–15]

Malignant melanoma is a skin cancer that occurs when skin cells known as melanocytes abnormally divide as they go through their normal cell division and regeneration cycle. Although people of all races can develop melanoma, having fair skin that frequently burns with sun exposure and rarely tans, along with light hair and blue or green eyes, places an individual at a higher risk. Ultraviolet radiation exposure from the sun, tanning beds, or sunlamps increases risk in all individuals. A family history of melanoma, personal history of immune dysfunction, and having multiple nevi further increase risk. Although melanoma is seen in all age categories, it is noted to be on the rise in males older than the age of 50 years and in teens and young adults.

What Is Your Treatment Plan?[14–16]

Prior to formalization of a treatment plan, results would be required to verify the presumptive diagnosis of malignant melanoma and to determine the staging of the disease. In Mr. Woodard's case, his melanoma was in situ, which requires no treatment beyond removal of the melanoma and observation for recurrent or new lesions.

Pharmacologic

Pharmacologic agents that may be employed in the treatment of melanoma are:

- ▶ Chemotherapy agents
- ▶ Immunotherapy such as interferon and interleukin 2
- ▶ Experimental targeted therapy such as adoptive T cell therapy

Nonpharmacologic

No specific nonpharmacologic instructions are required prior to biopsy of a skin lesion. Preoperative instructions on what to anticipate for the day of biopsy, the process of staging of the lesion, and the overall diagnostic process should be thoroughly discussed with the patient. Once staging is completed, in addition to the pharmacologic agents listed above, external beam radiation therapy may be used to treat melanoma.

Education/Counseling

- ▶ Sun safety. Apply sunscreen according to package directions, reapply frequently, and be sure to apply to often missed areas of posterior neck and ears. Wear long sleeves and hats to protect neck and ears when possible.
- ▶ Skin inspection process. Teach the patient to inspect his skin regularly using a full-length mirror and handheld mirror so he is able to see the posterior surfaces of his skin.

SOAP Note

S: Mr. Woodard is a 78-year-old male who is at the clinic for a routine examination. States when queried that he is not really concerned about "anything in particular" and that he is just "here to get checked out." Denies any changes in bowel/bladder habits, denies respiratory issues, denies allergies. Denies pain, fever, night sweats, shortness of breath, chest pain, cough, abdominal pain, visual changes. Reports PMH of diverticulitis without any recent exacerbations and "a little arthritis here and there." States when queried that he has noticed some hearing loss, but it is being monitored by an audiologist. States he is playing golf three times weekly, as has been his practice since retirement at the age of 62 years. When asked about skin changes, patient reports he was told by his golf partner that he has a "spot" on "the back" of his neck, but he has not been able to "get a good look at it." Denies any pain, itching, or bleeding from the area. States he can "feel it," and it sometimes bothers him when his collar rubs on it, but otherwise it "isn't causing a problem." States he receives his annual influenza vaccination, had a Pneumovax and shingles vaccine last year. Tetanus immunization is up-to-date. Childhood illness history of measles, mumps, rubella, and varicella without sequelae. Reports he is a widower and is not sexually active at this time. States he lives in a senior condominium complex and enjoys an active social life with frequent golf and evening card games. Denies current tobacco use, but reports he used to smoke cigars on the weekend for about 35 years until he "gave it up" 5 years ago. Reports ETOH use consists of one beer after his golf games, denies illicit drug use. States his appetite is good and he has no difficulties with chewing or swallowing food. States he feels happy in his life and enjoys frequent visits from his 4 children and 10 grandchildren.

O: *VS:* BP 132/74, HR 76 regular, T 98.2, RR 12, Ht 6'0", Wt 170 lbs

GEN: Well-appearing elderly male in no apparent distress

HEENT: Head normocephalic without evidence of masses or trauma. PERRLA, EOMs intact. Noninjected. Fundoscopic exam unremarkable. Ear canal without redness or irritation, TMs clear, pearly, bony landmarks visible. No discharge, no pain noted. Neck supple without masses. No thyromegaly. No JVD noted

Skin: Posterior neck with 8-mm darkened, slightly raised area with an asymmetric border, variation in coloring noted across lesion, no ulceration, no discharge. No pain with palpation, no erythema, no pruritus noted

CV: S_1 and S_2 RRR, no murmurs, no rubs

Lungs: Clear to auscultation

Abdomen: Soft, nontender, nondistended, bowel sounds present × 4 quadrants, no organomegaly, no bruits

MS: Joints of bilateral upper and lower extremities without swelling, pain, or erythema. Full active range of motion demonstrated

Neuro: Sensation intact to bilateral lower extremities, DTRs 2+ at patellar and Achilles bilaterally. Great toe extension normal, ankle dorsiflexion normal, plantar flexion normal, heel/toe walk normal. Bilateral LE strength 5/5. Patient moves throughout examination room and from chair to table without difficulty or hesitation.

A: Probable malignant melanoma

P: Mr. Woodard is referred to Dr. Sam for surgical removal of the skin lesion. Treatment recommendations will await staging determination. Discussion of the surgical referral process discussed with patient. Surgery will be scheduled prior to discharge today. Sun safety and risk reduction discussed with patient and will be reinforced at future visits to ensure full understanding. Patient reports concern over potential for skin cancer but states he is confident "it will all be all right." Follow-up to be determined by staging and treatment recommendations from surgeon.

Health Promotion Issues[3–5,14–15]

- ▶ Encourage sun safety, including sunscreen use
- ▶ Continue annual influenza vaccination

Guidelines to Direct Care

Balch CM, Gershenwald JE, Soong S-J, et al. Final version of 2009 AJCC melanoma staging and classification. *J Clin Oncol*. 2009;27(36):6199–6206.

Bichakjian CK, Halpern AC, Johnson TM, et al; American Academy of Dermatology. Guidelines of care for the management of primary cutaneous melanoma. American Academy of Dermatology. *J Am Acad Dermatol*. 2011;65(5):1032–1047.

Centers for Disease Control and Prevention. Recommended adult immunization schedule, by vaccine and age group. 2014. http://www.cdc.gov/vaccines/schedules/hcp/imz/adult .html. Accessed September 2, 2015.

US Dept of Agriculture and US Dept of Health and Human Services. *Dietary Guidelines for Americans, 2010*. 7th ed. Washington, DC: US Government Printing Office; 2010.

US Preventive Services Task Force. Recommendations for primary care practice: published recommendations. http://www.uspreventiveservicestaskforce.org/BrowseRec/Index/browse-recommendations. Accessed September 2, 2015.

REFERENCES

1. Centers for Disease Control and Prevention. 2015 sexually transmitted diseases treatment guidelines: ectoparasitic infections. http://www.cdc.gov/std/tg2015/ectoparasitic.htm. Accessed October 28, 2015.

2. Centers for Disease Control and Prevention. Parasites: scabies: crusted scabies cases (single or multiple). http://www.cdc.gov/parasites/scabies/health_professionals/crusted.html. Accessed October 28, 2015.

3. US Preventive Services Task Force. Recommendations for primary care practice: published recommendations. http://www.uspreventiveservicestaskforce.org/BrowseRec/Index/browse-recommendations. Accessed September 2, 2015.

4. Centers for Disease Control and Prevention. Recommended adult immunization schedule, by vaccine and age group. 2014. http://www.cdc.gov/vaccines/schedules/hcp/imz/adult.html. Accessed September 2, 2015.

5. US Dept of Agriculture and US Dept of Health and Human Services. *Dietary Guidelines for Americans, 2010*. 7th ed. Washington, DC: US Government Printing Office; 2010.

6. Centers for Disease Control and Prevention. The National Institute for Occupational Safety and Health (NIOSH): poisonous plants. http://www.cdc.gov/niosh/topics/plants/. Accessed October 28, 2015.

7. Eichenfield LF, Tom WL, Chamlin SL, et al. Guidelines of care for the management of atopic dermatitis. *J Am Acad Dermatol*. 2014;70(2):338–351.

8. American Academy of Allergy, Asthma and Immunology. Consultation and referral guidelines: citing the evidence: how the allergist–immunologist can help. *J Allergy Clin Immunol*. 2011;117(2 Suppl Consultation):S495–523.

9. National Eczema Association. Eczema. http://nationaleczema.org/eczema/. Accessed October 28, 2015.

10. Centers for Disease Control and Prevention. Injury prevention and control: Division of Violence Prevention: sexual violence. http://www.cdc.gov/ViolencePrevention/sexualviolence/index.html. Accessed October 28, 2015.

11. Stevens DL, Bisno DL, Chambers HF, et al; Infectious Diseases Society of America. Practice guidelines for the diagnosis and management of skin and soft tissue infections: 2014 update by the Infectious Diseases Society of America. *Clin Infect Dis*. 2014;59(2):e10–52.

12. Liu C, Bayer A, Cosgrove SE, et al; Infectious Diseases Society of America. Clinical practice guidelines by the Infectious Diseases Society of America for the treatment of methicillin-resistant *Staphylococcus aureus* infections in adults and children. *Clin Infect Dis*. 2011;52(3):e18–55.

13. Environmental Protection Agency. List H: EPA's registered products effective against MRSA and vancomycin resistant Enterococcus faecalis or faecium (VRE). http://www2.epa.gov/pesticide-registration/list-h-epas-registered-products-effective-against-methicillin-resistant. Accessed November 13, 2015.

14. Bichakjian CK, Halpern AC, Johnson TM, et al; American Academy of Dermatology. Guidelines of care for the management of primary cutaneous melanoma. American Academy of Dermatology. *J Am Acad Dermatol*. 2011;65(5):1032–1047.

15. American Academy of Dermatology. Melanoma: signs and symptoms. https://www.aad.org/dermatology-a-to-z/diseases-and-treatments/m---p/melanoma/signs-symptoms. Accessed October 28, 2015.

16. Balch CM, Gershenwald JE, Soong S-J, et al. Final version of 2009 AJCC melanoma staging and classification. *J Clin Oncol*. 2009;27(36):6199–6206.

Common Geriatric Issues in Primary Care

Joanne L. Thanavaro

Chapter Outline

Case 1 - Cognitive Impairment and Dementia

A. History and Physical Exam

B. Recommended labs/diagnostics

C. Pathophysiology

D. Guidelines to direct care: Criteria for major neurocognitive disorder (DSM-5). American Psychiatric Association.

Screening for cognitive impairment in older adults: An Evidence update for the U.S. Preventative Services Task Force Synthesis No. 107.

Current Pharmacologic Treatment of dementia: A clinical practice guideline from the American College of Physicians and the American Academy of Family Physicians.

E. Treatment Plan

Case 2 - Frality

A. History and Physical Exam

B. Recommended labs/diagnostics

C. Pathophysiology

D. Treatment Plan

Case 3 - Driving Issues

A. History and Physical Exam

B. Recommended labs/diagnostics

C. Overview

D. Guidelines to direct care:

American Medical Association, US Dept of Transportation National Highway Traffic Safety Administration. Physician's guide to assessing and counseling older drivers.

Practice parameter update: evaluation and management of driving risk in dementia. Report of the Quality Standards Subcommittee of the American Academy of Neurology.

National Highway Traffic Safety Administration, American Association of Motor Vehicle Administration. Driver fitness medical guidelines

E. Treatment Plan

Case 4 - Elder Abuse and Neglect

A. History and Physical Exam

B. Recommended labs/diagnostics

C. Overview

D. Guidelines to direct care: *Elder Abuse Prevention*. Iowa City: University of Iowa College of Nursing, John A. Hartford Foundation Center of Geriatric Nursing Excellence

E. Treatment Plan

Case 5 - End-of Life Issues

A. History and Physical Exam

B. Recommended labs/diagnostics

C. Overview

D. Guidelines to direct care:

National Hospice Organization; Medical Guidelines Task Force. *Medical Guidelines for Determining Prognosis in Selected Non-Cancer Diseases.*

Evidence-based interventions to improve the palliative care of pain, dyspnea, and depression at the end of life: a clinical practice guideline from the American College of Physicians

E. Treatment Plan

Learning Objectives

Using a case-based approach, the learner will be able to:

1. Identify key history and physical examination parameters for geriatric issues seen in primary care, including delirium and dementia, frailty, driving, elder abuse and neglect, and end-of-life issues.

2. Summarize recommended laboratory and diagnostic studies indicated for the evaluation of common geriatric issues seen in primary care.

3. State pathophysiology of common geriatric issues.

4. Document a clear, concise SOAP note for patients with common geriatric issues.

5. Identify relevant education and counseling strategies for patients with common geriatric issues.

6. Develop a treatment plan for common geriatric issues utilizing current evidence-based guidelines.

Case 1

Mr. Johnson is a 70-year-old male who is well known to your practice. He comes in with his wife today, who is very concerned about his "confusion" lately. She reports he is having difficulty "remembering things" and seems disinterested in going out with friends and planning their annual trip to the lake. She wanted him to be "checked out" when she realized he was unable to balance their checkbook. She reports that he seems to be repeating stories about his former job as a chief executive officer of a large healthcare system. Mr. Johnson is adamant that there is not a problem, but his wife reports she has noticed a gradual increase in these symptoms for the last 4 to 5 months. Mr. Johnson's past medical history is significant for coronary artery disease and chronic obstructive pulmonary disease. He quit smoking 10 years ago when he suffered a heart attack. He has one glass of wine nightly with dinner and tries to walk daily for about 30 minutes. His current medications include one aspirin daily, metoprolol 50 mg daily, fluticasone propionate/salmeterol inhaled 250/50, 1 puff inhaled every 12 hours, and albuterol, 1–2 puffs q 4–6 hours as needed for shortness of breath.

Physical Exam

Vital Signs (VS): Blood pressure (BP) 130/82, heart rate (HR) 68 (regular), respiratory rate (RR) 18, temperature (T) 98.6, height (Ht) 6'0", weight (Wt) 152 lbs, body mass index (BMI) 21

General (GEN): No acute distress

Heart: S_1 and S_2 regular rate and rhythm (RRR); grade 2/6 systolic murmur unchanged

Lungs: Clear to auscultation with decreased breath sounds in all lung fields

Abdomen: Soft, nontender with bowel sounds in all quadrants

Extremities (Ext): Normal muscle tone, full range of motion (ROM) in all extremities, no edema or joint deformities. Peripheral pulses +2 bilaterally

Neurologic (Neuro): Oriented × 3. Affect appropriate

What additional assessments/diagnostics do you need?

What is the differential diagnoses list?

What is your working diagnosis?

Additional Assessments/Diagnostics Needed

Review of Systems (ROS)

▶ The history should be obtained from the patient and a reliable family member or close friend. Ask about the following:

  ▶ The nature of symptom onset (insidious or sudden) and duration

  ▶ Areas of impairment

   ➤ Memory (recent and remote) and learning

   ➤ Geographic and temporal disorientation

   ➤ Remembering appointments and medications

   ➤ Language impairment (word finding, difficulty expressing self)

   ➤ Behavior or personality changes

  ▶ The presence of psychiatric symptoms (apathy, hallucinations, suspicions, delusions, paranoia)

  ▶ Extent of impairment in activities of daily living (ADLs)

   ➤ Managing finances

   ➤ Driving

   ➤ Use of telephone

   ➤ Hygiene, including bathing, dressing, and continence

  ▶ Information on living situation

  ▶ Family history

  ▶ Medications that could impair cognition

  ▶ Screening for depression and alcohol or drug abuse

▶ *Diagnostic and Statistical Manual of Mental Disorders,* 5th edition (*DSM-5*), criteria for major neurocognitive disorder (previously dementia) (see Table 1)[1,2]

▶ Screen for depression.

TABLE 1 Criteria for Major Neurocognitive Disorder

Content removed due to copyright restrictions

Physical Exam

▶ Complete physical and neurologic exam
▶ Neurologic exam should focus on focal neurologic deficits that may represent prior strokes, signs of Parkinson disease (PD), gait abnormalities or slowing, and eye movements. Alzheimer's disease (AD) patients generally have no motor deficits.
▶ Cognitive screening tools. A variety of screening tools are available to guide assessment:
  ▸ Cognitive assessment instruments (see Table 2)[3]
  ▸ Domains assessed by six cognitive screening instruments (see Table 3)[4]

Routine Labs

▶ Recommend labs include complete blood count (CBC), comprehensive metabolic panel (CMP), thyroid panel, vitamin B_{12}, and syphilis serology[5,6]
▶ The use of genetic testing for AD in patients with dementia is controversial because of the potential for both false positives and false negatives. Many genes, including epsilon 4 allele of the gene encoding apolipoprotein E (APOE), have

TABLE 2 Cognitive Assessment Instruments

Instrument	Items	Maximum Score	Time to Administer	Sensitivity	Specificity
MMSE	19	30	10 min	69–91%	87–99%
3MS	15	100	15 min	83–94%	85–90%
CDT	1	4–10	3 min	88%	71%
Mini-Cog	2	5	3–5 min	76–99%	89–93%
MoCA	12	30	10 min	100%	87%
SLUMS	11	30	7 min	92–95%	76–81%

CDT, Clock Drawing Test; MMSE, Mini-Mental State Exam; MoCA, Montreal Cognitive Assessment; SLUMS, Saint Louis University Mental Status; 3MS, Modified Mini-Mental State.
Adapted from Segal-Gidan FI. Cognitive screening tools. Clin Rev. 2013;23:12–18.

TABLE 3 Domains Assessed by Cognitive Screening Instruments

	Executive Function	Abstract Reasoning	Attention and Working Memory	New Verbal Learning/Recall	Expressive Language	Visuospatial Construction
MMSE			X	X	X	X
3MS	X	X	X	X	X	X
CDT	X		X			X
Mini-Cog	X			X		X
MoCA	X	X	X	X	X	X
SLUMS	X		X	X	X	X

CDT, Clock Drawing Test; MMSE, Mini-Mental State Exam; MoCA, Montreal Cognitive Assessment; SLUMS, Saint Louis University Mental Status; 3MS, Modified Mini-Mental State.

been associated with Alzheimer's disease, but their value for diagnosis remains uncertain. A formal genetics consultation is recommended if genetic testing is being considered[7]

▮ Imaging

- ▶ MRI of the head to rule out normal pressure hydrocephalus, subdural hematoma, and cerebrovascular disease. MRI is of limited use in distinguishing between types of dementia[8]

▮ *Differential Diagnoses List*

Neurologic diseases:

- ▶ Alzheimer's disease
- ▶ Lewy body dementia
- ▶ Vascular dementia
- ▶ Frontal lobe dementia
- ▶ Parkinson's disease
- ▶ Huntington's chorea
- ▶ Brain tumor
- ▶ Subdural hematoma
- ▶ Normal pressure hydrocephalus
- ▶ Encephalitis

Systemic processes:

- ▶ Metabolic disease (renal, hepatic)
- ▶ Vitamin B_{12} deficiency
- ▶ Neurosyphilis
- ▶ Thyroid disease
- ▶ Hypercalcemia
- ▶ Depression
- ▶ Delirium
- ▶ HIV
- ▶ Cerebral vasculitis[9]

▮ *Working Diagnosis—Cognitive impairment—early dementia*

▮ Pathophysiology

Dementia is a progressive deterioration of cognitive function in memory and at least one of the following cognitive domains: orientation, learning, language, comprehension, and judgment. Dementia increases with age, and there is a 30% incidence in people older than 85 years of age. About 5 million people in the United States have dementia; nearly twice as many people have mild cognitive impairment that does not meet the criteria for dementia. Seventy percent of persons diagnosed with dementia have Alzheimer's disease (AD).[9]

Four distinct types of dementia have been identified. In AD, the pathologic hallmarks are senile plaques and neurofibrillary tangles that result in an imbalance between neuronal injury and repair as well as loss of synaptic connections, neurons, and

neurotransmitters. The brain areas involved are the entorhinal cortex, the hippocampus, the limbic lobes, and the neurocortex. Dementia with Lewy bodies is the second most common type of dementia. There is some overlap of this dementia with both AD and PD. Lewy bodies are eosinophilic cytoplasmic inclusions that contain deposits of protein called alpha-synuclein.[10] The diagnosis of vascular dementia (VaD) is based on the presence of clinical or radiographic evidence of cerebrovascular disease in a patient with dementia. Frontotemporal dementia (FTD) (formerly known as Pick disease) is one of the most common forms of dementia; onset of symptoms usually occurs in the fifth decade. The etiology is unknown, but pathologic changes include atrophy and neuronal loss in the frontal and temporal lobes of the brain and subsequent gradual and progressive decline in behavior or language.[11]

▮ *What Is Your Treatment Plan?*

▮ Pharmacologic

- ▶ Cholinesterase inhibitors (CIs)
  - ▸ Patients with AD have reduced cerebral content of choline acetyl transferase that impairs cortical cholinergic function. CIs increase transmission by inhibiting cholinesterase at the synaptic cleft
  - ▸ Recommended for patients with Mini-Mental State Exam (MMSE) scores of 10 to 26
- ▶ N-methyl-D aspartate (NMDA) receptor antagonist (memantine)
  - ▸ Proposed to be neuroprotective
  - ▸ The NMDA receptor is involved in learning and memory
  - ▸ Blocking these receptors may protect against further damage in patients with VaD
- ▶ Combination therapy memantine plus CIs
  - ▸ Recommended for patients with MMSE scores <17[12]
- ▶ Pain management
  - ▸ PAINAD: Pain Assessment in Advanced Dementia Scale can be used to assess pain in demented patients.
  - ▸ Observe patients for 5 minutes before performing this assessment.
  - ▸ Total scores range from 0 to 10: 0 = no pain; 10 = severe pain.
  - ▸ General principles:
    - ➤ Prescribe a trial of scheduled analgesics.
    - ➤ Use a stepped-care approach to analgesic prescribing.
    - ➤ Start low, go slow, but use enough.
    - ➤ Monitor the patient to balance risks and benefits of pain treatment.
    - ➤ Typical doses of analgesics may be less effective in cognitively impaired patients.[12]
- ▶ Recognition and treatment of delusions, hallucinations, depression, agitation, and aggression[14,15]

Nonpharmacologic

- Participation in structured group cognitive stimulation programs[6]
- Advanced care planning
  - Critical for managing patients with advanced dementia
- Hospice care[15]
  - According to medical eligibility guidelines, patients with a primary diagnosis of dementia must meet both of the following requirements:
    - Stage 7c or beyond on the Functional Assessment Staging (FAST) scale: At this level patients are dependent in all ADLs, are at least occasionally incontinent of urine and stool, are unable to ambulate without assistance, and have no meaningful verbal communication during an average day.
    - The occurrence of at least one of the following six specified medical complications in the prior year:
      - Aspiration pneumonia
      - Pyelonephritis or other upper urinary tract infection
      - Septicemia
      - Multiple decubitus ulcers ≥stage 3
      - Recurrent fever after antibiotics
      - Inability to maintain sufficient fluid and calorie intake with 10% weight loss during the previous 6 months or have a serum albumin <2.5 g/dL
  - Patients are considered to have a life expectancy of ≤6 months by Medicare if they meet specific criteria for a decline in clinical status that is not reversible.

Education/Counseling

Future visits should include education for patient and wife about common issues surrounding dementia including:

- Advance directives
- Driving
- Home safety
- Wandering
- Caregiver assistance

SOAP Note

S: Mr. Johnson is a 70-year-old male and comes in today with his wife, who is concerned about cognitive changes. She reports being "suspicious" of problems over the last 4–5 months, and she is now certain the symptoms are worsening. She reports he is having trouble remembering things, is apathetic about going out and planning their annual vacation, and is unable to balance their checkbook. He is constantly repeating old stories from work.

Mr. Johnson reports "feeling fine" and thinks his wife doesn't "understand the normal changes associated with aging." He denies chest pain, palpations, lightheadedness, or headaches. He reports his dyspnea on exertion (DOE) is about the same and is because of his lung problems. He denies any changes in his ability to function at home or drive. He's in good spirits and sleeps well but just isn't interested in going out or planning vacation. His past medical history is significant for coronary artery disease and chronic obstructive pulmonary disease (COPD). He no longer smokes, has a glass of wine nightly with dinner, and tries to walk 30 minutes daily.

O: *VS:* BP 130/82, HR 68 (regular), RR 18, T 98.6, Ht 6'0", Wt 152 lbs, BMI 21

GEN: No acute distress

Heart: S_1 and S_2 RRR; grade 2/6 systolic murmur unchanged from prior visits

Lungs: Clear to auscultation with decreased breath sounds in all lung fields

Abdomen: Soft, nontender with bowel sounds in all quadrants

Ext: Normal muscle tone, full ROM in all extremities, no edema or joint deformities. Peripheral pulses are +2 bilaterally

Neuro: Oriented × 3. Affect appropriate. Cranial nerves (CNs) II–XII grossly intact. No tremor at rest or with activity. Strength in lower and upper extremities 5/5 left, 5/5 right. Performs finger-to-nose testing without difficulty. Get up and go test = 5.6 seconds. Gait steady with normal arm swing. Romberg negative. Deep tendon reflexes (DTRs) 2+ throughout. No Babinski or clonus. MMSE = 20

Labs: CBC, CMP, thyroid panel, vitamin B_{12}, and syphilis serology are negative

A: Cognitive impairment—likely early dementia

Coronary artery disease (CAD)—stable

Hypertension (HTN)—at Eighth Joint National Committee (JNC 8) goals

COPD—stable

P: MRI of the head. Long discussion regarding the possibility that these symptoms represent early changes associated with dementia. Discussed medications, and patient is willing to try donepezil 5 mg at bedtime. Explained that this dosage will likely need to be increased at the next visit and that the purpose of this medication is to slow down the progression of symptoms. Offered selective serotonin reuptake inhibitor (SSRI) agent, but patient declines "for now." Encouraged continued healthy eating and daily exercises. Assured patient and wife that he will be monitored carefully and will have future visits to discuss long-term care issues. Continue taking all other prescribed medications for CAD and COPD. Follow-up 1 month.

Health Promotion Issues

- There are no proven strategies to prevent mild cognitive impairment (MCI) or dementia.
- Control of vascular factors, including HTN, dyslipidemia, and diabetes, may reduce the risk of both AD and VaD.

- Regular physical activity may be an important strategy for reducing risk.
- Cognitive activities such as mental exercises may reduce risk.
- Moderate alcohol intake and nutrition strategies may reduce risk.
- Smoking and depression are linked to increased risk: screening and intervention for both are recommended.
- Gingko biloba, nonsteroidal anti-inflammatory drugs (NSAIDs), statins, estrogens, and vitamin E have failed to delay or prevent dementia in large clinical trials.[14]

Guidelines to Direct Care

Lin JS, O'Connor E, Rossom RC, et al. *Screening for Cognitive Impairment in Older Adults: An Evidence Update for the U.S. Preventive Services Task Force Evidence Synthesis No. 107.* Rockville, MD: Agency for Healthcare Research and Quality; 2013. AHRQ Publication No. 14-05198-EF-1. http://www.ncbi.nlm.nih.gov/books/NBK174643/. Accessed October 28, 2015.

National Institute for Health and Care Excellence. Dementia: supporting people with dementia and their carers in health and social care: guidance. https://www.nice.org.uk/guidance/cg42. Accessed October 29, 2015.

Petersen RC, Stevens JC, Ganguli M, Tangalos EG, Cummings JL, DeKosky ST. Practice parameter: early detection of dementia: mild cognitive impairment (an evidence-based review). *Neurology.* 2001;56:1133–1142.

Case 2

Mrs. McArthur is a 92-year-old widow who is well known to your practice. She is a retired college professor. She currently lives with her daughter, who works full-time but who has arranged for her next-door neighbor to "check in" on her mom every day around lunchtime to make sure she is doing okay. Mrs. McArthur's past medical history (PMH) includes cardiovascular disease, dyslipidemia, hypertension, and arthritis.

Mrs. McArthur has had several falls at home, which she attributes to worsening eyesight and difficulty walking as a result of chronic low back pain. Her daughter reports she has a poor appetite and that she has lost 5 lbs in the last 2 months. Mrs. McArthur admits to minimal physical activity now because she always feels exhausted.

Physical Exam

VS: BP 110/70, HR 65 regular, RR 14, T 98.2, Ht 5'2", Wt 102, BMI 18.7

CV: S_1 and S_2 RRR without murmurs, gallops, or rubs

Pulmonary: Lungs clear to auscultation

Gastrointestinal (GI): Abdomen soft, nontender with good bowel sounds. No bruits

Musculoskeletal (MS): Upper and lower extremities with full ROM (FROM). Strength in upper extremities 3/5 bilaterally, lower extremities 4/5. Gait slightly unstable, slow. Unable to rise from chair without using arms. Alert and oriented × 3

What additional assessments/diagnostics do you need?

What is the differential diagnoses list?

What is your working diagnosis?

Additional Assessments/Diagnostics Needed

ROS

- Multiple tools are available to assess frailty. There is no consensus on which measure to use.
  - Rockwood Frailty Index[12]
    - Uses 70 variables that focus on medical conditions to functional decline
    - The higher the score, the more frail the individual
    - Uses historical measurements rather than physical measurements
  - Groningen Frailty Indicator (GFI)[18]
    - Validated, 15-item questionnaire
    - Assesses physical, cognitive, social, and psychological domains
    - Score range is from 0 to 15; a score of 4 or greater is considered the cutoff point for frailty
  - Frailty Index (FI)[19]
    - This index is constructed as the proportion of deficits present in an individual out of the total number of age-related health variables considered
    - Deficits can be any diseases, signs, symptoms, laboratory abnormalities, or functional or cognitive impairments
  - Clinical Frailty Scale[20]
    - A 9-point clinical assessment tool that classifies persons as very fit to terminally ill (see Table 4)

TABLE   4 Clinical Frailty Scale

Content removed due to copyright restrictions

- ▶ Frail Scale (Morley)[21]
  - ➤ F = Fatigue
  - ➤ R = Resistance (climbing 1 flight of stairs)
  - ➤ A = Aerobic (walks 1 block)
  - ➤ I = Illness (5 or more)
  - ➤ L = Loss of weight (>5% in the last year)
    - ▪ 1 or 2 positive = prefrail
    - ▪ 3 or more = frail
  - ➤ Benefit is it can be quickly administered; probably the clinical instrument of choice

Physical Exam

Assessment should include not only all components of a medical history but also a physical exam specific to older persons, including functional capacity, quality of life, cognition and mental health, nutrition, vision, hearing, and fecal and urinary incontinence. Balance and fall prevention, osteoporosis, and polypharmacy should be included in the evaluation.[22]

- ▶ A rolling evaluation can be helpful in the busy clinical practice setting; rolling assessment over several visits is a viable option.
- ▶ A multidisciplinary approach, including the healthcare provider, nutritionist, social worker, and physical and occupational therapists, is ideal.
- ▶ Patient-driven assessment instruments are helpful, including:
  - ▶ Katz Index of Independence in Activities of Daily Living
  - ▶ Nutritional Health Checklist
  - ▶ Screening Version of the Hearing Handicap Inventory for the Elderly
  - ▶ Tinetti Balance and Gait Evaluation
  - ▶ Geriatric Depression Scale

Routine Labs

- ▶ CBC
- ▶ CMP
- ▶ Urinalysis
- ▶ Calcium and phosphate
- ▶ Thyroid-stimulating hormone (TSH)
- ▶ Vitamin B_{12}
- ▶ Folate levels
- ▶ Albumin
- ▶ Total cholesterol
- ▶ Vitamin D[22]

Imaging

- ▶ Dual-energy X-ray absorptiometry (DEXA) of the total hip, femoral neck, and lumbar spine to diagnose osteoporosis[22]

Differential Diagnoses List

Failure to thrive
Anemia
Autoimmune disorder
Malignancy
Depression

Working Diagnosis—Frailty

Etiology/Epidemiology

Frailty definitions are not precise, but frailty may be understood as a state of increased vulnerability to adverse outcomes.[23–26] The most widely used definition in clinical practice is the presence of three or more of the following: weight loss, exhaustion, weakened grip strength, slow walking, and low physical activity. Frailty is not the same as old age or disease, but the incidence of frailty increases with age. At some point, frailty is likely for most individuals. Frailty is a state of increased vulnerability to stressors resulting from age-related declines in reserves in the neuromuscular, metabolic, and immune systems and represents a loss of reserves and redundancy of complex systems that result in difficulty maintaining homeostasis.

The frailty syndrome affects about 7% of patients older than age 65 years and 25–40% of those 80 years and older. Frailty is a challenge for most healthcare providers because there is almost never one chief complaint from the patient. Frailty leads to recurrent hospitalization, institutionalization, acute events, and death. This syndrome is potentially reversible, and screening and intervention should be a priority when caring for elderly patients.

What Is Your Treatment Plan?

Pharmacologic

- ▶ Reduce polypharmacy
- ▶ Drug therapy for depression
- ▶ Treat anemia
- ▶ Testosterone in males with low testosterone levels
- ▶ Vitamin D 1,000 IU daily

Nonpharmacologic

- ▶ Correcting orthostasis[21]
- ▶ Aggressive referral to physical therapy, including for limitations in dual tasking
- ▶ Exercise therapy
  - ▶ Aerobic
  - ▶ Resistance
  - ▶ Balance
- ▶ Diet
  - ▶ High protein (1.2–1.5 g/kg)
  - ▶ Leucine-enriched amino acid supplements between meals
- ▶ Referral for Complex Geriatric Assessment (CGA)[27]
  - ▶ Identification for referral for CGA includes:
    - ➢ Age
    - ➢ Medical comorbidities, including heart failure or cancer
    - ➢ Psychosocial disorders, including depression or isolation
    - ➢ Specific geriatric conditions, including dementia, falls, or functional disability
    - ➢ Previous or predicted high healthcare utilization
    - ➢ Consideration of living conditions (independent living to assisted living, nursing home, or in-home caregivers)

- ▶ General goals of CGA
  - ➢ Improve physical and psychological function
  - ➢ Optimize medical prescription use
  - ➢ Decrease placement in nursing homes, hospitalization, and mortality
  - ➢ Improve patient satisfaction
- ▶ Outpatient Programs of All-Inclusive Care for the Elderly (PACE)[28]
  - ▶ Outpatient management model where primary care is delivered to community-dwelling older adults by an interdisciplinary team in a day care setting
  - ▶ General goals
    - ➢ Improve function
    - ➢ Overcome environmental challenges
    - ➢ Keep older adults living in the community by preventing institutionalization

Education/Counseling

- ▶ Exercise
- ▶ Nutritional counseling
- ▶ Support services

SOAP Note

S: Mrs. McArthur, a 92-year-old widow, presents today with her daughter. Her daughter is concerned that mom is losing weight and doesn't do much physical activity. Mrs. McArthur has had several falls in the last few months. She admits to minimal physical activity, and she attributes this to difficulty walking because of chronic low back pain and fatigue; it's now hard to climb a flight of stairs. She is having difficulty with her eyesight and always feels exhausted. She has lost about 10 lbs over the last year; her appetite is "just not what it used to be." She reports today that she knows her daughter is worried about her because she has a neighbor check on her every day at lunchtime while the daughter is at work. She doesn't think this is really necessary. She is having no difficulty taking her daily medications. She denies chest pain, shortness of breath, palpitations, and syncope. Admits to occasional "loss of urine" with sneezing but is otherwise not incontinent.

O: *VS:* BP 110/70, HR 65 regular, RR 14, T 98.2, Ht 5'2", Wt 102, BMI 18.7

Skin: No rashes or pigment changes

Head, eyes, ears, nose, and throat (HEENT): Pupils equal, round, react to light, accommodation (PERRLA), extraocular movements (EOMs) full with no gaze abnormality. Vision 20/80 with glasses on. Fundoscopic exam consistent with beginning cataracts, both eyes. Hearing bilaterally intact. Normal whisper test. Rinne test—air conduction better than bone conduction. Weber test—no lateralization. Mouth: Good dentition. No thyromegaly or carotid bruits

Cardiovascular (CV): S_1 and S_2 RRR. No murmurs, gallops, or rubs. Point of maximal impact (PMI) 5th intercostal space (ICS), midclavicular line (MCL)

Respiratory (RESP): Lungs clear to auscultation (LCTA)

GI: Abdomen soft, nontender, nondistended. No hernias or organomegaly

BACK: No spinous process or costovertebral angle (CVA) tenderness on palpation. Negative straight level raises

Ext: Decreased muscle tone, full ROM in all extremities, no venous status changes or edema. + Heberden nodes bilateral hands. Peripheral pulses +2 bilaterally. Monofilament testing 10/10 bilaterally

Neuro: Oriented × 3. MMSE = 22. CNs II–XII grossly intact. Upper and lower extremities with FROM. Strength in upper extremities 3/5 bilaterally, lower extremities 4/5. Gait slightly unstable, slow. Unable to rise from chair without using arms. Get up and go test = 12 seconds. No tremor at rest or with activity. Romberg negative. DTRs 2+ throughout. No Babinski or clonus.

Psych: Slightly anxious but answers questions without hesitancy. Affect appropriate. Good eye contact

A:

Dyslipidemia—lipid panel 3 months ago; good control with statin therapy

HTN—at JNC 8 goal

Arthritis—pain daily; not taking anything for discomfort

Frailty

P:

Dyslipidemia: Continue atorvastatin 20 mg daily

HTN: Continue lisinopril 20 mg daily

Arthritis: Try Tylenol (acetaminophen) 2 tablets three times daily

Frailty

▶ Take home following patient assessment tools: Katz Index, Nutritional Health Checklist, Hearing Handicap Inventory. Daughter agrees to help her complete these questionnaires

▶ Schedule eye exam

▶ Referral to physical therapy for gait and balance evaluation

  ▶ Encourage physical activity at least 30 minutes daily

▶ Weight loss

  ▶ Encouraged foods of choice and small, frequent feedings

  ▶ Recommended nutritional supplement (Ensure)

▶ Fatigue

  ▶ Discussed strategies for energy conservation

  ▶ Recommended modifying daily procedures (for example, sitting rather than standing in shower)

▶ Mood

  ▶ Will evaluate frequently for depression and prescribed SSRIs if indicated

▶ Fall prevention

  ▶ Referral to home health for environmental assessment, including home safety

▶ Labs: CBC, CMP, calcium and phosphate, TSH, vitamin B12, folate, vitamin D, urine analysis

▶ Imaging: DEXA

Health Promotion Issues

▶ Confirm that vaccinations are up-to-date, including annual influenza, pneumococcal (PPSV23) and pneumococcal conjugate (PCV12), and Zoster vaccine

▶ Discuss importance of daily exercise as tolerated. Follow recommendations from physical therapy

▶ Diet: High-protein, low-fat diet

▶ Fall prevention strategies

Guidelines to Direct Care

There are currently no evidence-based guidelines that focus specifically on frailty. Recommended guidelines that may be helpful in directing care include the following:

Academy of Nutrition and Dietetics. Unintended weight loss (UWL) in older adults guideline (2009). http://www.andeal.org/topic.cfm?menu=5294&cat=3651. Accessed October 29, 2015.

American Geriatrics Society. AGS/BGS clinical practice guideline: prevention of falls in older persons. http://www.americangeriatrics.org/health_care_professionals/clinical_practice/clinical_guidelines_recommendations/prevention_of_falls_summary_of_recommendations. Accessed October 29, 2015.

Brosseau L, Wells GA, Finestone HM, et al. Clinical practice guidelines for gait training. *Top Stroke Rehabil.* Spring 2006; 13(2):34–41. http://www.guideline.gov/popups/printView.aspx?id=9913. Accessed October 29, 2015.

Watts NB, Bilezikian JP, Camacho PM, et al. American Association of Clinical Endocrinologists medical guidelines for clinical practice for the diagnosis and treatment of postmenopausal osteoporosis. https://www.aace.com/files/osteo-guidelines-2010.pdf. Accessed October 29, 2015.

Case 3

Mr. Hill is an 80-year-old male well known to your practice. He comes in today for his annual preventive exam. His daughter is accompanying him and asks to speak with you before her father is evaluated. She tells you she is concerned about her father's driving; he almost hit an oncoming car on the way to this visit. He has had several "fender benders" in the last year with no injuries to himself or others. She thinks he should stop driving and would like you to address this problem today. Mr. Hill has been in relatively good health with well-controlled hypertension and diabetes. His arthritis causes daily mild pain. He denies chest pain, shortness of breath (SOB), palpitations, lightheadedness, or syncope. He is a widower and lives alone but stays active by attending many senior citizens' activities, including bingo and exercise classes. He drives himself to these activities and feels he is a safe driver because he only drives during the day, stays within the speed limit, and avoids the highways. His recent "fender benders" involved hitting a car from behind and making a mistake estimating his turn.

Physical Exam

VS: BP 132/80, HR 76 regular, RR 14, T 98.2, Ht 5'8", Wt 156 lbs, BMI 25

CV: S_1 and S_2 RRR without murmurs, gallops, or rubs.

Pulmonary: Lungs clear to auscultation

GI: Abdomen soft, nontender with good bowel sounds. No bruits

MS: Upper and lower extremities with FROM. Strength in upper extremities 4/5 bilaterally, lower extremities 5/5. Gait stable. Alert and oriented × 3

What additional assessments/diagnostics do you need?

What is the differential diagnoses list?

What is your working diagnosis?

Additional Assessments/Diagnostics Needed

ROS

▶ Assess for conditions with an increased relative crash risk[29,30]
  ▶ Slight to moderate odds ratio:
    ➤ Cardiovascular disease
    ➤ Cerebrovascular disease
    ➤ Traumatic brain injury
    ➤ Depression
    ➤ Diabetes mellitus
    ➤ Musculoskeletal disorders
    ➤ Vision disorders

  ▶ Moderately high odds ratio:
    ➤ Alcohol abuse and dependence
    ➤ Dementia
    ➤ Epilepsy
    ➤ Schizophrenia
    ➤ Obstructive sleep apnea

▶ Assess for characteristics that increase risk of unsafe driving:[31]
  ▶ Clinical Dementia Rating Scale
  ▶ Caregiver's rating of a person's driving ability as marginal or unsafe
  ▶ History of traffic citations
  ▶ History of crashes
  ▶ Reduced driving mileage
  ▶ Self-reported situational avoidance
  ▶ MMSE scores of <24
  ▶ Aggressive or impulsive personality characteristics

Physical Exam

▶ Complete physical exam with particular attention to the Assessment of Driving Related Skills (ADReS)[32]
  ▶ Visual field by confrontation testing
  ▶ Visual acuity—Snellen E chart
  ▶ Rapid Pace Walk
    ➤ This is a measure of lower limb strength, endurance, range of motion, and balance
    ➤ Have patient walk distance of 20 feet
    ➤ >9 seconds is abnormal and referral for driving evaluation and/or evaluation of gait disorder is recommended
  ▶ Range of motion
    ➤ Neck rotation
    ➤ Shoulder and elbow flexion
    ➤ Finger curl
    ➤ Ankle plantar flexion
    ➤ Ankle dorsiflexion
  ▶ Motor strength
    ➤ Shoulder adduction, abduction, and flexion
    ➤ Wrist flexion and extension
    ➤ Hand-grip strength
    ➤ Hip flexion and extension
    ➤ Ankle dorsiflexion and plantar flexion
  ▶ Trail-Making Test, Part B
    ➤ Tests general cognitive function, including working memory, visual processing, visuospatial skills, selective and divided attention, and psychomotor coordination

- Clock Drawing Test
  - May assess a patient's long-term memory, visual perception, visuospatial skills, selective attention, abstract thinking, and executive skills

Routine Labs

- Labs should be ordered to rule out any underlying medical condition that may affect driving

Working Diagnosis—Possible impaired driving ability

Overview

Life expectancy continues to rise, and by the year 2030, the population of adults older than age 65 will more than double to approximately 70 million people.[33] There will be an increase in the number of older drivers not only as a result of the aging population but also because the United States is a highly mobile society and older adults use their automobiles for necessary chores, employment, and social and recreational needs. A driver's license is a symbol of independence, and studies of driving cessation have demonstrated an increase in depressive symptoms and increased social isolation with decreased out-of-home activities.[34,35] Older drivers often realize that they may have limitations related to slower reaction time, chronic healthcare problems, and medication effects; many successfully self-regulate their driving behavior by eliminating long highway trips, driving less often, driving only during the day, or driving slower. Slow driving and limiting driving miles actually may increase the risk of motor vehicle crashes.[36]

As the number of older drivers with medical conditions increases, patients and families will turn to healthcare providers (HCPs) for guidance on safe driving and driving cessation. HCPs can assist their older patients to maintain safe mobility by providing effective treatment and preventive health care and by determining the ability of older adults to drive safely.

What Is Your Treatment Plan?

Pharmacologic

- Evaluate for medications that are associated with an elevated risk of crash

Nonpharmacologic

- Vision—recommendations are subject to each state's licensing requirements.[32]
  - For visual acuity more impaired than 20/40
    - Ensure underlying cause of vision loss is adequately treated
    - Referral to ophthalmologist
    - Recommend that the patient uses the appropriate glasses or contact lenses
    - Recommend restricting travel to less-risk areas and conditions (familiar surrounds, non-rush-hour traffic, low-speed areas, daytime, and good weather conditions)
    - Consider more frequent assessment of visual acuity to detect further visual decline
  - For visual acuity more impaired than 20/70
    - Follow recommendations above
    - Recommend an on-road assessment performed by a driver rehabilitation specialist (DRS) to evaluate the patient's performance while driving
  - For visual acuity more impaired than 20/100
    - Recommend that the patient not drive unless safe driving ability is demonstrated in an on-road assessment
- Visual fields—recommendations are subject to each state's licensing requirements.
  - Visual field loss can significantly affect driving safety
  - Recommendations for visual field defects noted on clinical exam
    - Ensure that underlying cause of visual field loss is adequately treated if possible
    - Referral to ophthalmologist: automated visual field testing may help define the extent of the defect
    - For binocular visual field of questionable adequacy, refer to DRS for on-road assessment
    - Retest visual fields more frequently to determine changes due to chronic, progressive diseases
- Rapid Pace Walk
  - Longer than 9 seconds requires intervention, including evaluation for cause of gait speed and/or referral to a DRS
- Range of motion
  - If ROM is not within normal limits (includes excessive pain and hesitation with movement), intervention is needed.
  - Assess whether movements cause muscle or joint pain.
  - Assess whether movements cause a loss of balance.
  - Encourage the patient to drive a vehicle with power steering and an automatic transmission.
  - Recommend a consistent regimen of physical activity, including cardiovascular exercise, strengthening exercise, and stretching.
  - Refer the patient to physical therapy or occupational therapy for exercises to improve strength and/or range of motion.
  - Provide effective pain control if indicated.
  - Many medications have the potential of impairing driving ability; assess whether pain management is worth impairing driving ability.

- Refer to specialist for management of any joint disease, podiatry issues, or neuromuscular problems.
- Recommend an on-road assessment by a DRS.
- Post-stroke patients with deficits that interfere with driving should be referred. DRS may prescribe adaptive devices to compensate for deficits and will also train the patient in their use.

▶ Motor strength
- Less than grade 4/5 strength in either upper extremity or the right lower extremity requires an intervention such as vehicle modification.

▶ Trail Making
- A time for completion of longer than 3 minutes requires an intervention, including causes for the abnormal result (dementia, sedating medication) and/or a referral to DRS.

▶ Clock Drawing Test
- Any incorrect or missing element on the Clock Scoring Criteria requires evaluation for dementia and/or referral to DRS.
  ➤ Criteria for clock drawing
    ▪ Only the numbers 1–12 are included (no duplicates or omissions).
    ▪ The numbers are drawn inside the clock circle.
    ▪ The numbers are equally or nearly equally spaced from each other.
    ▪ The numbers are equally or nearly equally spaced from the edge of the circle.
    ▪ One clock hand correctly points to 2 (instruct the patient to draw the clock showing 2 o'clock).
    ▪ There are only two clock hands.
    ▪ There are no intrusive marks, writing, or hand indicating incorrect time.

Education/Counseling

▶ Patients who perform well on all sections of the ADReS should be advised that there are no medical contraindications to driving and that no further workup or treatment is needed.

▶ Patients who score poorly on any section of the ADReS, but the causes of poor performance are medically correctable, should be counseled regarding which medical treatments are recommended. Instruct the patient to limit driving until treatment strategies result in improvement in performance on repeat administration of the ADReS.

▶ If poor performance can't be medically corrected, refer to DRS. Counsel that driving may need to be discontinued.

▶ Recommendations for counseling patients who are no longer safe to drive:
- Explain why it's important to stop driving.
- Give the patient a prescription stating "Do Not Drive, For Your Safety and the Safety of Others."
- Discuss transportation options.

- Encourage family or caregiver assistance.
- Discuss and acknowledge the patient's feelings of loss associated with driving cessation. Explore how the patient may feel if he or she were to get in an accident and injure self or others.
- Discuss state reporting requirements. If mandatory reporting is required, inform your patient that you are required by law to inform your local Department of Motor Vehicles (DMV) of medical conditions that could affect safe operation of a vehicle.
- In states with voluntary laws, a referral to DMV may be appropriate because patients may need to hear that they will be reported if they drive against medical advice.
- Send your patient a follow-up letter reviewing the need for driving cessation and place a copy into the electronic medical record.
- Reinforce driving cessation at each visit.

SOAP Note

S: Mr. Hill is here today for his annual preventive exam accompanied by his daughter, who is concerned about her father's driving abilities. He almost hit an oncoming car on the way to this visit and has had two "fender benders in the last year"; these accidents did not cause injury to her father or the other drivers. Mr. Hill reports he is doing well. He is taking his medications as directed, but his arthritis causes some mild-moderate daily pain. He denies chest pain, SOB, palpitations, lightheadedness, or syncope. All other questions in the review of systems are unremarkable. He lives alone and has no difficulty caring for himself. He stays active by attending bingo twice weekly and exercise class three times a week at the nearby senior citizen center. He drives himself to these activities and feels he is a safe driver because he only drives during the day, stays within the speed limit, and avoids the highways. His recent "fender benders" involved hitting a car from behind and making a mistake estimating his turn.

O: *VS:* BP 132/80, HR 76 regular, RR 14, T 98.2, Ht 5'8", Wt 156 lbs, BMI 25

HEENT: Head atraumatic. PERRLA, EOMs intact. Funduscopic exam c/w grade 1 hypertensive retinopathy changes. Vision 20/70, both eyes with glasses. Visual fields by confrontation c/w decreased peripheral vision. TMs normal. Pharynx: No redness or exudates. Neck: Supple, no thyroid enlargement, no carotid bruits

CV: S_1 and S_2 RRR without murmurs, gallops, or rubs

Pulmonary: Lungs clear to auscultation

GI: Abdomen soft, nontender with good bowel sounds. No bruits

MS: FROM with neck rotation, elbow flexion, ankle plantar flexion, and ankle dorsiflexion. Decreased range of motion of shoulders bilaterally. Motor strength 4/5 for shoulder adduction, abduction, and flexion. 5/5 wrist flexion and extension.

Hand grip 4/5 bilaterally. Motor strength for hip flexion and extension, ankle dorsiflexion, and plantar flexion 5/5. Rapid Pace Walk accomplished in 8 seconds with stable gait.

Ext: No edema. Varicosities on ankles bilaterally. No venous status changes

Neuro: Alert and oriented × 3. Cranial nerves II–IX intact. MMSE 23 (unable to subtract by sevens). Trail-Making Test completed correctly in 160 seconds. Clock Drawing Test normal for all 7 elements

Labs: CMP, CBC, TSH, HbA1c, lipids, and urine analysis today

A:

▶ Annual preventive exam normal with the exception of concerns about visual acuity and decreased upper motor strength; both may affect driving abilities. No significant cognitive decline appreciated.

▶ HTN at JNC-8 goals.

▶ Diabetes mellitus (DM) well controlled with current medications.

P:

Referral to ophthalmology for complete visual exam.

Referral to physical therapy for evaluation and exercise plan for decreased upper body motor strength. After a discussion with Mr. Hill and his daughter, it is decided that it may be helpful for him to have a referral with the driver rehabilitation specialist for an evaluation of driving ability. Mr. Hill acknowledges that he has had some minor accidents recently and will take the driving

evaluation test so his daughter doesn't worry. He understands that the evaluation is important for his safety and the safety of others. He is instructed to continue to take medications as prescribed, eat a heart-healthy diet, and exercise daily.

▍ Health Promotion Issues

▶ Counsel on health maintenance by providing the Successful Aging Tips and Tips for Safe Driving handouts (*Physician's Guide*).

▍ *Guidelines to Direct Care*

American Medical Association, US Dept of Transportation National Highway Traffic Safety Administration. Physician's guide to assessing and counseling older drivers. http://www.nhtsa.gov/people/injury/olddrive/olderdriversbook/pages/Contents.html. Accessed October 29, 2015.

Iverson DJ, Gronseth GS, Reger MA, Classen S, Dubinsky RM, Rizzo M. Practice parameter update: evaluation and management of driving risk in dementia. Report of the Quality Standards Subcommittee of the American Academy of Neurology. *Neurology*. 2010;74:1316–1324.

National Highway Traffic Safety Administration, American Association of Motor Vehicle Administration. Driver fitness medical guidelines. September 2009. DOT HS 811 210. http://main.diabetes.org/dorg/PDFs/Advocacy/Discrimination/driver-fitness-medical-guidelines.pdf. Accessed October 28, 2015.

▍ Case 4

Mrs. Jacobs, a 75-year-old woman, comes in today accompanied by her son. She is seeing you today for a follow-up visit after cataract surgery. She was doing quite well until she fell down the steps last week. She is complaining of "rib pain" that is affecting her ability to take a deep breath. When asked about the fall, she responds, "I tripped at the top of the steps." Mrs. Jacobs is a widow and now lives with her 50-year-old son and daughter-in-law, who have one son. She moved into their home after the death of her husband because of financial issues. On prior visits she has always talked fondly of her current living arrangement. Her past medical history is significant for hypertension and chronic kidney disease. She sees the renal specialist quarterly and anticipates needing dialysis in the near future. She seems very quiet today and a bit nervous when you inquire about how she fell down the stairs. The medical assistant mentioned to you that the son insisted on staying in the exam room, even when Mrs. Jacobs changed into her gown.

▍ Physical Exam

VS: BP 136/80, HR 70 regular, RR 14, T 98.2, Ht 5'5", Wt 142 lbs (down 10 lbs since last visit), BMI 23.6

Skin: Bilateral bruising encircling both arms

HEENT: PERRLA, EOMs full with no gaze abnormality. Normal fundoscopic exam

CV: S_1 and S_2 RRR. No murmurs, gallops, or rubs. PMI 5th ICS, MCL

Resp: LCTA. Point tenderness right lateral thoracic area, T4–T6 with ecchymosis

GI: Abdomen soft, nontender, nondistended. No hernias or organomegaly

Back: No spinous process or CVA tenderness on palpation. Negative straight level raises

Ext: Full ROM in all extremities, no edema. Bilateral peripheral pulses +2 throughout

Neuro: Oriented × 3. Anxious, poor eye contact. Is hesitant when answering questions regarding fall and bruising of arms

What additional assessments/diagnostics do you need?
What is the differential diagnoses list?
What is your working diagnosis?

■ *Additional Assessments/Diagnostics Needed*

■ ROS

▶ Inquire about types of elder abuse[37]

  ▶ Physical

    ➤ Physical contact that may result in any type of pain or injury

    ➤ May include unwarranted administration of drugs, physical restraints, force feeding, or physical punishment

  ▶ Sexual

    ➤ Sexual contact or behavior of any kind that is against their will or with an older adult who is incapable of providing consent

  ▶ Psychological/emotional

    ➤ Words or actions that cause emotional stress

  ▶ Financial

    ➤ The misuse of finances or possessions for another's gain

  ▶ Neglect

    ➤ Failure to provide any care or responsibilities that must be provided for the patient

    ➤ Can be active or passive or intentional or nonintentional

▶ Evaluate risk for elder abuse

  ▶ Risk for suffering from abuse

    ➤ Living in the same household

    ➤ Socially isolated

    ➤ Conditions that increase dependence (advanced age, lack of financial sophistication, disability, recent personal loss [partner])

  ▶ Risk for committing abuse

    ➤ History of physical abuse in the past

    ➤ History of mental illness

    ➤ Substance abuse

    ➤ Elder dependence (financial or emotional)

➤ Single caregiver

➤ Stress related to caregiving

▶ Administer Elder Abuse Suspicion Index (EASI) (see Table 5)[38]

  ➤ All questions are answered Yes, No, or Did Not Answer

  ➤ Questions 1–5 are answered by the patient

  ➤ Question 6 is answered by the HCP

  ➤ A response of yes on one or more of questions 2–6 may establish concern

Exam

▶ Assess for signs/symptoms of elder abuse[37]

  ▶ Physical

    ➤ Pattern of bruising, including bruises that encircle the arms, legs, or torso

    ➤ Pattern of burns; burns in the shape of an object

    ➤ Broken bones, sprains, dislocations

    ➤ Open wounds and cuts

    ➤ Untreated injuries

  ▶ Sexual

    ➤ Bruising or bleeding around the genitals or chest

    ➤ Unexplained sexually transmitted illnesses

    ➤ Stained, torn, or bloody underwear

    ➤ Unusual or inappropriate relationship between the patient and potential abuser

  ▶ Psychological or emotional

    ➤ Functional decline

    ➤ Significant weight loss or gain

    ➤ Behavior changes

    ➤ Worsening of current medical conditions

    ➤ New medical conditions

  ▶ Financial

    ➤ Patient living well below their financial means

    ➤ Discomfort, evasiveness, or ambiguity when discussing finances

---

TABLE 5 Elder Abuse Suspicion Index (EASI)

Content removed due to copyright restrictions

- ➤ Unexplained ability to buy food or medication or pay bills
- ➤ Unexplained changes in legal documents
- ▶ Neglect
  - ➤ Malnutrition
  - ➤ Dehydration
  - ➤ Poor hygiene
  - ➤ Inadequate or inappropriate clothing
  - ➤ Decubitus ulcers
  - ➤ Absence of needed assistive devices (glasses, wheelchairs, dentures)
- ▶ Assess for depression

■ Routine Labs

- ▶ Labs should be drawn to evaluate any underlying medical problems.

■ Imaging

- ▶ Chest X-ray (CXR) with rib detail

■ *Differential Diagnoses List*

Osteoporosis

Frequent falls

Metabolic disorders

Psychiatric disorder

Cognitive impairment

Dementia

Neurologic disorders

Malignancy

Malabsorption syndrome

■ *Working Diagnosis—Suspected elder abuse (EA)*

■ Overview

Elder abuse can have a detrimental impact on the health and well-being of older adults, and its incidence is increasing. Data suggest that in the United States, more than 2 million older adults suffer from at least one form of elder mistreatment (EM) each year.[37] There are now two large-scale, population-based studies that estimate the prevalence of elder abuse in the United States. Laumann, Leitsch, and White[40] surveyed 3,005 community-dwelling persons, ages 57 to 85 years, and found that 9% experienced verbal, financial, or physical abuse. According to the National Elder Mistreatment Study,[41] 5,777 community-dwelling adults ages 60 years and older experienced the following types of abuse: emotional mistreatment (4.6%), physical mistreatment (1.6%), sexual mistreatment (0.6%), current potential neglect (5.1%), and lifetime

financial exploitation (6.5%). Even though 44 states and the District of Columbia have legally required mandated reporting, EM is severely underreported. Barriers to reporting elder abuse may include fear, embarrassment, or concerns about repercussions; some patients may be unable to report because of cognitive impairment or social isolation. There is a lack in uniformity across the United States on how cases of EM are handled. The most recent major studies on incidence reported that 7.6–10% of study participants experienced abuse in the prior year.[42]

■ *What Is Your Treatment Plan?*

■ Pharmacologic

- ▶ Drug therapy may be appropriate for treating medical conditions related to elder abuse.

■ Nonpharmacologic

- ▶ Documentation
  - ▸ Documentation of abuse or neglect should be completed regardless of the healthcare setting.
  - ▸ Documentation should include a complete medical and social history.
  - ▸ Record the chief complaint in the patient's own words.
  - ▸ If appointments are repeatedly canceled, document the name of the caller.
  - ▸ If injuries are present, document:
    - ➤ Type, size, location, and color
    - ➤ Patient's overall state of health
    - ➤ Resolution of problems
    - ➤ An opinion on whether injuries are adequately explained by the history
    - ➤ All labs and imaging studies
  - ▸ Diagnosis of elder mistreatment should be included on the patient's problem list
- ▶ Reporting
  - ▸ Legal requirements on reporting vary from state to state.
  - ▸ Knowing your state's reporting system is crucial.
  - ▸ Most states mandate HCPs report elder abuse; some have voluntary reporting systems.
  - ▸ In some states, HCPs can be found negligent if they fail to report suspected mistreatment.
  - ▸ See the National Center of Elder Abuse website for a state directory of help lines, hotlines, and elder abuse prevention resources.
- ▶ Ongoing care planning
  - ▸ Ensure that medical and safety needs have been met.
  - ▸ If hospitalization is not required, the home environment must be assessed.

- Ensure that there is home assistance for functionally or cognitively impaired patients.
- Schedule a social work consultation or visit from an Adult Protective Services (APS) specialist.
▶ Assessment of decision-making capacity
▶ Social service intervention
  ▶ APS or similar entities provide social interventions in almost every jurisdiction in the United States.
  ▶ Functions of the APS specialists include:[43]
    ➤ Investigate abuse and neglect for clients by responding to referrals, interviewing client and collateral contacts, analyzing collected information to determine whether criminal actions have occurred, and preparing investigation reports and submitting recommendations.
    ➤ Develop plans to address mistreatment issues by working closely with victims, families, and other involved parties to ensure that services provided reflect the patient's preferences and maximize the older adult's independence.
    ➤ APS specialists are bound by statutory limitation and may not impose services, such as medical care, if the patient is capable of making decisions.
▶ Legal interventions
  ▶ Law enforcement is generally involved in cases in which crimes are committed against older adults.
  ▶ Members of law enforcement and legal professionals help connect older persons with agencies and other resources available for victims of crime.

Education/Counseling

▶ Abuse protection support
▶ Caregiver support
▶ Coping enhancement strategies
▶ Decision-making support
▶ Emotional support
▶ Support groups
▶ Surveillance and safety[44]

SOAP Note

S: Mrs. Jacobs, a 75-year-old female, is here today for a follow-up visit after cataract surgery. She is recovering well after her surgery except for a fall down the steps last week; "she tripped on the carpet and fell down about 5 or 6 steps." She is complaining of "rib pain" that is affecting her ability to take a deep breath. She denies chest pain, palpitations, lightheadedness, or syncope. She attributes her recent weight loss to a poor appetite. She denies dysuria. Her past medical history is significant for hypertension and chronic kidney disease. She sees the renal specialist quarterly and is aware that she will require dialysis in the near future. She has been taking her medications daily, including lisinopril 40 mg, hydrochlorothiazide 25 mg, and 81 mg aspirin.

Mrs. Jacobs is a widow and now lives with her 50-year-old son and daughter-in-law, who have one son. She moved into their home after the death of her husband because of financial issues. She seems very quiet today and a nervous when describing her recent fall. Her son reluctantly agreed to leave the examination room when asked to do so for the physical examination. Mrs. Jacobs seems a bit more relaxed and tells you she thinks she will need to find another place to live. She admits that her 22-year-old grandson has been charged with taking care of her during the day and "he often screams at me when I watch TV or try to talk with him … He gets mad if I ask for help with getting lunch; and he's grabbed me by my arms several times when I walk too slow.… He calls me a stupid old hag and wishes I would just die so he could have the house by himself during the day." States he has threatened to take her in the car and leave her someplace where she can't get back home. "He's a bad egg; he barely graduated from high school and is often in trouble with the police; he has no job and doesn't plan to get one." When asked about how she really fell, she reports her grandson pushed her down the steps. She hasn't told her son about the problem with her grandson because she doesn't think he will believe her. Her EASI score today is 4 (positive for questions 1, 3, 5, and 6). Patient Health Questionnaire 9 (PHQ-9) depression questionnaire score 10, consistent with moderate depression

O: *VS:* BP 136/80, HR 70 regular, RR 14, T 98.2, Ht 5'5", Wt 142 lbs (down 10 lbs since last visit), BMI 23.6

Skin: Bilateral bruising encircling both arms

HEENT: Head nontraumatic. PERRLA, EOMs full with no gaze abnormality. Normal fundoscopic exam

CV: S_1 and S_2 RRR. No murmurs, gallops, or rubs. PMI 5th ICS, MCL

Resp: LCTA. Point tenderness right lateral thoracic area, T4–T6 with ecchymosis

GI: Abdomen soft, nontender, nondistended. No hernias or organomegaly

Back: No spinous process or CVA tenderness on palpation. Negative straight level raises

Ext: Full ROM in all extremities, no edema. Bilateral peripheral pulses +2 throughout

Neuro: Oriented × 3. MMSE = 23, CNs II–XII intact. Anxious, poor eye contact. Is hesitant when answering questions regarding fall and bruising of arms

Labs: CBC, CMP, lipids unremarkable with exception of unchanged elevated blood urea nitrogen (BUN) and creatinine

Imaging: Head CT negative; CXR with rib detail c/w 3 fractured ribs 9–12 on the right, no pneumothorax

A:

▶ Hypertension—at JNC-8 goals
▶ Chronic kidney disease—stable

- Fractured ribs—sustained from fall down the steps
- Weight loss—likely related to home situation
- Depression
- Elder abuse—physical and emotional by grandson

P:

- Hypertension: Continue current medications. Encouraged no-sodium diet
- Chronic kidney disease: Keep follow-up appointments with renal specialist
- Fractured ribs: Pain control: Ibuprofen 400 mg TID; hydrocodone 5 mg (reduced dosage due to CKD) BID for severe pain; incentive spirometry to avoid atelectasis
- Weight loss: Referral to dietitian
- Depression: Citalopram 10 mg daily

- Elder abuse: Long discussion with patient and son regarding elder abuse. Son appears genuinely concerned about mother's well-being. Explained legal obligation to report elder mistreatment. They should expect call from the APS specialist shortly. Son agrees to take mother to his sister's home (lives 15 miles away) for now and will get counseling for son.

Follow-up here 2 weeks

Health Promotion Issues

- Develop and discuss a safety plan for patient.[45]

Guidelines to Direct Care

Daly JM. *Elder Abuse Prevention*. Iowa City: University of Iowa College of Nursing, John A. Hartford Foundation Center of Geriatric Nursing Excellence; 2010.

Case 5

Mrs. Bell, a 70-year-old female, comes in today to discuss end-of-life issues. She had been relatively healthy with the exception of hypothyroidism and osteoarthritis until 2 years ago when she presented with a pulsating abdominal mass of 2-week duration and accompanying nausea. A CT scan of the abdomen and pelvis revealed a mass that was highly suspicious for mesenteric lymphoma. She was subsequently diagnosed with unresectable undifferentiated pleomorphic sarcoma and underwent chemotherapy with adriamycin and several courses of radiation. Since her diagnosis she has been hospitalized three times: once for gastric ulcer, once for gastric obstruction, and once for a right total hip arthroplasty for progressively worsening hip pain that was unresponsive to steroid injections.

She is having more trouble eating now, and nausea is a problem despite medications that include the following: aspirin 81 mg daily, Ativan (lorazepam) 0.5 mg at HS prn, calcium/vitamin D two tablets once daily, esomeprazole 40 mg BID, fish oil capsule 1 daily, levothyroid 125 mcg daily, ondansetron 8 mg every 8 hours prn for nausea, and prochloraperazine 5 mg, 2 tablets every 8 hours for nausea. She has oncology visits every 3 months for serial chest, abdomen, and pelvis CTs; she has been told that her mesenteric mass is consistent with stable disease and there is no PET or CT evidence of distal metastasis. She comes in with her husband today and has questions about long-term care planning.

Physical Exam

VS: BP 148/77, HR 72, RR 16, T 98.1, Wt 98 lbs

HEENT: PERRLA. EOMs intact. Oropharynx is clear. Neck is supple without lymphadenopathy

Resp: Lungs clear to auscultation

CV: Heart RRR without gallops, rubs, or murmurs

Abdomen: Soft, nontender, nondistended. Bowel sounds are positive

Ext: Extremities demonstrate no clubbing, cyanosis, or edema

Labs: White blood cells (WBCs) 4.3, hemoglobin and hematocrit (H&H) 12.1/37, platelets 217, Na 139, K 4.1, glucose 147, BUN/Cr 14/0.82, calcium 9.1, plasma protein 7, albumin 4.2, alkaline phosphatase 92, aspartate transaminase (AST) 34, alanine transaminase (ALT) 35

What additional assessments/diagnostics do you need?

What is the differential diagnosis list?

What is your working diagnosis?

Additional Assessments/Diagnostics Needed

ROS

- Determine Eastern Cooperative Oncology Group (ECOG) Performance Status (see Table 6)[46]
  - Used to assess how a patient's disease is progressing and how the disease affects daily living abilities and to determine appropriate treatment and prognosis

Physical Exam

- Appropriate for the underlying disease process to evaluate progression of disease

Labs/Imaging

- Appropriate for the underlying disease process to evaluate progression of disease

TABLE   6 Eastern Cooperative Oncology Group Performance Status

Content removed due to copyright restrictions

▌ *Working Diagnosis*

Unresectable undifferentiated pleomorphic sarcoma
End-of-life care

▌ Overview

When patients are diagnosed with cancer, or other life-threatening diseases, HCPs often are responsible for delivering the bad news, discussing the prognosis, and making appropriate referrals. Assessment of the patient's emotional state, readiness to discuss long-term care planning, and understanding of the condition are essential. It is important to be sensitive to how much information the patient wants to know; information should be accurate and should not give false hope. Coordination of all healthcare providers involved with care is the responsibility of the primary care provider and is vital so that mixed messages are not given to the patient and family. Reassessment of treatment effectiveness and the patient's values, goals, and preferences should be ongoing, and cultural factors that may affect end-of-life discussions should be explored. Discussions regarding palliative care should occur early in the course of the disease when the patient is still feeling well. Primary care providers are uniquely positioned to discuss these difficult issues by virtue of their long-term trusting relationships with their patients.[47]

▌ *What Is Your Treatment Plan?*

▌ Pharmacologic

- ▶ Management of pain[48]
  - ▶ NSAIDs (first line)
  - ▶ Opioids
  - ▶ Bisphosphonates (bone pain)
  - ▶ Radiotherapy for patients with cancer
- ▶ Management of common symptoms[49]
  - ▶ Depression
    - ➤ Tricyclic antidepressants
    - ➤ Selective serotonin reuptake inhibitors
- ▶ Fatigue[50]
  - ➤ Corticosteroids
  - ➤ Psychostimulants
  - ➤ Antidepressants
  - ➤ Erythropoietin
- ▶ Anorexia and cachexia
  - ➤ Dexamethasone
  - ➤ Megestrol
  - ➤ Dronabinol
  - ➤ Androgens
  - ➤ Aggressive alimentation in patients with wasting syndromes related to cancer may increase discomfort
- ▶ Nausea and vomiting
  - ➤ Corticosteroids
  - ➤ Dopamine antagonists
  - ➤ Histamine antagonists
  - ➤ Acetylcholine antagonists
  - ➤ Anxiolytics
  - ➤ Prokinetic agents
  - ➤ Antacids
- ▶ Constipation[51]
  - ➤ Psyllium
  - ➤ Hyperosmolar nonabsorbable agents
  - ➤ Magnesium and phosphorous salts
  - ➤ Glycerin suppositories
  - ➤ Sorbitol
  - ➤ Lactulose
  - ➤ Senna
  - ➤ Bisacodyl
- ▶ Delirium
  - ➤ Haloperidol
- ▶ Dyspnea
  - ➤ Duramorph
  - ➤ Oral opioids

- ➢ Beta agonists (for patients with COPD)
- ➢ Diuretics
- ➢ Oxygen

▋ Nonpharmacologic[52]

- ▶ Depression
  - ▶ Education
  - ▶ Behavioral therapy
  - ▶ Informational interventions
  - ▶ Individual and group support
- ▶ Discussing prognosis
  - ▶ Recommendations for patient-centered communication:
    - ➢ Prioritize what you want to accomplish during the discussion
    - ➢ Practice and prepare for giving bad news; ensure a quiet environment
    - ➢ Assess patient understanding by starting with open questions
    - ➢ Determine patient preferences by asking what and how much information the patient wants to know
    - ➢ Present information using language that is easy to understand and that is free from medical jargon
    - ➢ Provide emotional support by allowing time for the patient to express emotions; respond with empathy
- ▶ Advance directives[53]
  - ▶ Advance care planning involves meeting with patients and their family members to facilitate a shared understanding of diagnosis, prognosis, treatment options, and relevant values and goals.
  - ▶ Discussions should be accurately documented.
  - ▶ A written advance directive or Physician Orders for Life-Sustaining Treatment (POLST) form should be used to document aspects of advance care planning discussions.
  - ▶ There are two general categories of directives:
    - ➢ Substantive: These communicate patient's values and treatment preferences should the patient become incapacitated (living wills)
    - ➢ Process: These directives are used by patients to state who should make their decisions should they become incapacitated (healthcare power of attorney, durable power of attorney)
  - ▶ Determining whether expressed wishes conflict with best interest of the patient
    - ➢ Five-point framework recommended[54]
    - ➢ Does the urgency of the clinical situation require a time-sensitive decision, are the patient's previously expressed wishes clear, and are the advance planning documents completed and available?
    - ➢ Considering the patient's preferences and goals of care, determine whether the burdens of intervention are likely to overshadow the benefits
    - ➢ Is the advance directive appropriate in the current situation?
    - ➢ How much leeway does the surrogate have to interpret the patient's advance directive?
    - ➢ Is the surrogate acting in the patient's best interests?
- ▶ Referral and management of hospice patients[55]
  - ▶ Available for any terminally ill patient who chooses a palliative care approach.
  - ▶ Hospice care is built on the concept that the dying patient experiences physical, social, and spiritual aspects of suffering.
  - ▶ Hospice is a philosophy, not a place. It can be provided in the patient's home, nursing home, or hospital setting.
  - ▶ Primary care providers should recognize the need and recommend hospice care.
    - ➢ Discussions with patients and families about hospice should be approached in the context of the larger goals of care.
  - ▶ Patients should be referred when their prognosis is still longer than 2–3 months.
  - ▶ Hospice should be considered when the patient has:
    - ➢ New York Heart Association Class IV heart failure
    - ➢ Severe dementia
    - ➢ Activity-limiting lung disease
    - ➢ Metastatic cancer
  - ▶ Hospice benefits cover all expenses related to the terminal illness, including medication, nursing care, and equipment.
  - ▶ Even after hospice is initiated, the PCP is expected to remain in charge of the patient's care, including writing orders, seeing the patient for office visits, and completing and signing the death certificate.
- ▶ Tools for determining prognosis in terminally ill patients:
  - ▶ National Hospice Organization Medical Guidelines for Determining Prognosis in Non-Cancer Diseases[55,56]
  - ▶ Palliative Prognosis Score (PaP)[57]

▋ Education/Counseling[58]

- ▶ A wide variety of patient and family caregiver palliative care tools have been developed or adapted by Promoting Excellence in End-of-Life Care demonstration projects and national workgroups and can be accessed at http://www.promotingexcellence.org/tools/patient-family_education.html.

▋ SOAP Note

S: Mrs. Bell, a 70-year-old female, comes in today to discuss end-of-life issues. She made this appointment today because she wants to get her "ducks in a row." She is seeing her oncologist routinely and is happy to report that her recent scans show her cancer is stable and there is no indication of metastasis. She is feeling well and her pain is well controlled with ibuprofen twice daily. She is concerned about losing a little weight, but she thinks it's because she is having nausea on most days. She has not taken her medication for nausea because she's been trying to "tough it out." She would like to take as little medication as possible. She is fatigued but takes a daily nap and that helps. She denies vomiting, diarrhea, constipation, or headaches. She is trying to stay very active by walking daily and visiting friends and family. She enjoys reading and is choosing books that have a spiritual message. She's looking forward to a planned trip to see distant relatives with her husband. She admits to "feeling anxious" sometimes, especially at night before she goes to sleep. She is worrying about preparing for care when she gets "really sick." She is using her Ativan most nights before bedtime.

O: *VS:* BP 148/77, HR 72, RR 16, T 98.1, Wt 98 lbs (down 1 lb from last visit)

Skin: Good turgor, no open lesions

HEENT: PERRLA. EOMs intact. Oropharynx is clear. Neck is supple without lymphadenopathy.

Resp: Lungs clear to auscultation

CV: Heart RRR without gallops, rubs, or murmurs

GI: Abdomen is soft, nontender, nondistended. Bowel sounds are positive

Back: No spinous process or CVA tenderness on palpation

Ext: Full ROM in all extremities, no edema. Bilateral peripheral pulses +2 throughout

Neuro: Oriented × 3

Psych: Good eye contact. No hesitation while describing current healthcare issues. Reaches out to hold husband's hand on occasion

Recent Labs: WBCs 4.3, H&H 12.1/37, platelets 217, Na 139, K 4.1, glucose 147, BUN/Cr 14/0.82, calcium 9.1, plasma protein 7, albumin 4.2, alkaline phosphatase 92, AST 34, ALT 35

ECOG = 0

A:

Undifferentiated pleomorphic sarcoma—stable

Nausea

Pain

End-of-life planning

P:

Undifferentiated pleomorphic sarcoma: Follow-ups with oncology

Nausea: Encouraged to eat small frequent meals and take nausea medication routinely

Pain: Well controlled with current medications

End-of-life planning: Mrs. Bell is willing to discuss end-of-life issues today. After an explanation of the purpose and services available from hospice, she believes that in-home hospice would be her preference. She requests a referral to hospice for an initial discussion, although she feels she doesn't need services at this time. She has prepared a will but doesn't have written advance directives. She has thought about this for some time now, and her wishes are (1) no life-sustaining treatments (including cardiopulmonary resuscitation); if life-sustaining treatments are started, they should be discontinued; (2) no artificial nutrition and hydration started if they would be the main treatments sustaining life; (3) to be kept as comfortable and free of pain as possible, even if such care prolongs dying or shortens her life. She has no additional wishes or directions about her medical care today but is assured that discussions will continue and changes will be made as needed. She would like to appoint her husband as durable power of attorney for health care. The preferences of Mrs. Bell are agreeable to her husband, and I am in agreement that these wishes are in her best interest. She is given a sample advance directive form to complete after she reviews her wishes with her children.[56]

Guidelines to Direct Care

National Hospice Organization; Medical Guidelines Task Force. *Medical Guidelines for Determining Prognosis in Selected Non-Cancer Diseases.* 2nd ed. Arlington, VA: National Hospice Organization; 1996.

Qasseem A, Snow V, Shekelle P, Casey DE, Cross JT, Owens DK. Evidence-based interventions to improve the palliative care of pain, dyspnea, and depression at the end of life: a clinical practice guideline from the American College of Physicians. *Ann Intern Med.* 2008;148:141–146.

REFERENCES

1. Sink KM, Yaffe K. Cognitive impairment and dementia. In Williams BA, Chang A, Ahalt C, Chen H, Conant R, Landefeld S, Ritchie C, Yukawa M, eds. *Current Diagnosis and Treatment: Geriatrics.* 2nd ed. New York, NY: McGraw-Hill Education; 2014.
2. American Psychiatric Association. *Diagnostic and Statistical Manual of Mental Disorders.* 5th ed. Arlington, VA: American Psychiatric Association; 2013.
3. Segal-Gidan FI. Cognitive screening tools. *Clin Rev.* 2013;23:12–18.
4. Segal-Gidan FI. More on cognitive screening tools: response to an interested reader. *Clin Rev.* 2013;27:28–29.
5. Anderson HS. Alzheimer disease workup. http://emedicine.medscape.com/article/1134817-workup#aw2aab6b5b2. Accessed October 29, 2015.

6. National Institute for Health and Care Excellence. Dementia: supporting people with dementia and their carers in health and social care: guidance. https://www.nice.org.uk/guidance/cg42. Accessed October 29, 2015.

7. Mayeux AU, Saunders R, Shea S, et al. Utility of the apolipoprotein E genotype in the diagnosis of Alzheimer's disease. Alzheimer's Disease Centers Consortium on Apolipoprotein E and Alzheimer's Disease. *N Engl J Med.* 1998;338:506–511.

8. American College of Radiology. ACR Appropriateness Criteria for dementia and movement disorders. http://www.acr.org/Quality-Safety/Appropriateness-Criteria. Accessed October 29, 2015.

9. Moylan KC, Lin TL. *The Washington Manual—Geriatrics Subspecialty Consult.* Philadelphia, PA: Lippincott Williams & Wilkins; 2004.

10. Neef D, Walling AD. Dementia with Lewy bodies: an emerging disease. *Am Fam Phys.* 2006;73:1223–1229.

11. Cardarelli R, Kertesz A, Knebl JA. Frontotemporal dementia: a review for primary care physicians. *Am Fam Phys.* 2010;82:1372–1377.

12. Qaseem A, Snow V, Cross T, Forciea MA, Hopkins R, Shelkelle P et al. Current pharmacologic treatment of dementia: a clinical practice guideline from the American College of Physicians and the American Academy of Family Physicians. *Ann In Med.* 2008;148:370–379.

13. Warden V, Hurley AC, Volicer V. Development and psychometric evaluation of the Pain Assessment in Advanced Dementia (PAINAD) scale. *J Am Med Dir Association.* 2003;4:9–15.

14. McLachlan AJ, Bath S, Naganathan V, et al. Clinical pharmacology of analgesic medicines in older people: impact of frailty and cognitive impairment. *Br J Clin Pharmacol.* 2011;3:351–364.

15. McLachlan AJ, Bath S, Naganathan V, et al; National Council of Certified Dementia Practitioners, Centers for Medicare & Medicaid Services. Local coverage determination (LCD) for hospice determining terminal status (L32015). legacyhospice.net/home/download/phys_portal/CGS%20Guidelines.pdf. Accessed October 29, 2015.

16. Daviglus ML, Bell CC, Berrettini W, et al. National Institutes of Health State-of-the-Science Conference Statement: preventing Alzheimer's disease and cognitive decline. *NIH Consens State Sci Statements.* April 26–28, 2010;27(4):1–27.

17. Rockwood K, Andrew M, Mitniski A. A comparison of two approaches to measuring frailty in elderly people. *J Gerontol A Biol Sci Med Sci.* 2007;62:738–743.

18. Drubbel I, Bleijenbe N, Kranenburg G, et al. Identifying frailty. Do the Frailty Index and Groningen Frailty Indicator cover different clinical perspectives? A cross-sectional study. *BMC Fam Prac.* 2013;14:64.

19. Pena FG, Theou O, Wallace L, et al. Comparison of alternate scoring of variables on the performance of the Frailty Index. *BMC Geriatrics.* 2014;14:25.

20. Rockwood K, Stadynyk K, MacKnight C, McDowell I, Hébert R, Hogan DB. A brief clinical instrument to classify frailty in elderly people. *Lancet.* 1999;353:205–206.

21. Morley JE. Frailty: diagnosis and management. *J Nutr Health Aging.* 2011;15:667–670.

22. Elsawy B, Higgins KE. The geriatric assessment. *Am Fam Phys.* 2011;83:48–56.

23. Walston J, Hadley EF, Ferrucci L, et al. Research agenda for frailty in older adults: toward a better understanding of physiology and etiology: summary from the American Geriatrics Society/National Institute on Aging Research Conference on Frailty in Older Adults. *J Am Geriatr Soc.* 2006;54:991–1001.

24. Fried LO, Tangen CM, Walston, et al. Frailty in older adults: evidence for a phenotype. *J Gerontol A Biol Sci Med Sci.* 2001;56:M146–M156.

25. DeLepelaire J, Illife S, Mann E, Degryse JM. Frailty: an emerging concept for general practice. *Br J Gen Pract.* 2009;59:177–181.

26. Lacas A, Rockwood K. Frailty in primary care: a review of its conceptualization and implications for practice. *BMC Med.* 2012;10:4.

27. Stuck AE, Siu AL, Wieland GD, Adams J, Rubenstein Z. Comprehensive geriatric assessment: a meta-analysis of controlled trials. *Lancet.* 1993;342:1032–1036.

28. National PACE Association. What is PACE? http://www.npaonline.org/website/article.asp?id=12&title=Who,_What_and_Where_Is_PACE? Accessed October 29, 2015.

29. Marshal SC. The role of reduced fitness to drive due to medical impairments in explaining crashes involving older drivers. *Traffic Injury Prev.* 2008;9:291–298.

30. US Dept of Transportation. Reports: how medical conditions impact driving. http://www.fmcsa.dot.gov/regulations/medical/reports-how-medical-conditions-impact-driving. Accessed October 29, 2015.

31. Hoover L. AAN updates guidelines on evaluating driving risk in patients with dementia. *Am Fam Phys.* 2010;82:1145–1147.

32. American Medical Association, US Dept of Transportation National Highway Traffic Safety Administration. Physician's guide to assessing and counseling older drivers. http://www.nhtsa.gov/people/injury/olddrive/olderdriversbook/pages/Contents.html. Accessed October 29, 2015.

33. West LA, Cole S, Goodkind D, He W. 65+ in the United States: 2010—current population reports. 2014. https://www.census.gov/content/dam/Census/library/publications/2014/demo/p23-212.pdf

34. Marottoli RA, de Leon CFM, Glass TA, Williams CS, Cooney LM Jr, Berkman LF. Consequences of driving cessation: decreased out-of-home activity levels. *J Gerontol Series B Psychol Sci Soc Sci.* 2000;55:S334–340.

35. Ragland DR, Satarian WA, MacLeod KE. Driving cessation and increased depressive symptoms. *J Gerontol Series A Bio Sci Med Sci.* 2005;60:399–403.

36. Kostyniuk LP, Molnar LJ. Self-regulatory driving practices among older adults: health, age and sex effect. *Accid Anal Prev.* 2008;40:1576–1580.

37. Del Carmen T, Lachs MS. Detecting, assessing and responding to elder mistreatment. In Williams BA, Chang A, Ahalt C, Chen H, Conant R, Landefeld S, Ritchie C, Yukawa M, eds. *Current Diagnosis and Treatment: Geriatrics.* 2nd ed. New York, NY: McGraw-Hill Education, 2014.

38. Yaffe MJ, Wolfson C, Lithwick M, Weiss D. Development and validation of a tool to improve physician identification of elder abuse: The Elder Abuse Suspicion Index (EASI). *J Elder Abuse Neglect.* 2008;20(3):276–300.

39. Bonnie RJ, Wallace RB, eds.; Panel to Review Risk and Prevalence of Elder Abuse and Neglect, National Research Council. *Elder Mistreatment: Abuse, Neglect, and Exploitation in an Aging America.* Washington, DC: National Academics Press; 2003.

40. Laumann EO, Leitsch SA, Waite LJ. Elder mistreatment in the United States: prevalence estimates from a nationally representative study. *J Gerontol Series B Soc Sci.* 2008;63:S248–254.

41. Acierno R, Hernandez-Tejacda M, Muzzy W, Steve, K. *National Elder Mistreatment Study. Report to the National Institute of Justice.* Rockville, MD: National Institute of Justice; 2009. Project no. 2007-WG-BX-0009.

42. Lifespan of Greater Rochester, Inc., Weill Cornell Medical Center of Cornell University. Under the radar: New York state elder abuse prevalence study. 2011. http://ocfs.ny.gov/main/reports/Under%20 the%20Radar%2005%2012%2011%20final%20report.pdf

43. San Diego County Human Resources. Job descriptions: senior adult protective services specialist. 2009. http://agency.governmentjobs .com/sdcounty/default.cfm?action=viewclassspec&classSpecID= 80840&viewOnly=yes

44. Daly JM. *Elder Abuse Prevention*. Iowa City: University of Iowa College of Nursing, John A. Hartford Foundation Center of Geriatric Nursing Excellence; 2010.

45. Hoover RM. Detecting elder abuse and neglect: assessment and intervention. *Am Fam Phys*. 2014;88:453–460.

46. Oken MM, Creech RH, Tormey DC, et al. Toxicity and response criteria of the Eastern Cooperative Oncology Group. *Am J Clin Oncol*. 1982;5:649–655.

47. Weckman MT. The role of the family physician in the referral and management of hospice patients. *Am Fam Phys*. 2008;77:807–812.

48. Groninger H, Vijayan J. Pharmacologic management of pain at the end of life. *Am Fam Phys*. 2014;90:26–32.

49. Widera EW, Block SD. Managing grief and depression at the end of life. *Am Fam Phys*. 2012;86:259–264.

50. Ross DD, Alexander CS. Management of common symptoms in terminally ill patients: part I. Fatigue, anorexia, cachexia, nausea and vomiting. *Am Fam Phys*. 2001;64:807–815.

51. Ross DD, Alexander CS. Management of common symptoms in terminally ill patients: part II. Constipation, delirium and dyspnea. *Am Fam Phys*. 2001;64:1019–1027.

52. Ngo-Metzger Q, August KJ. End-of-life care: guidelines for patient-centered communication. *Am Fam Phys*. 2008;77:167–174.

53. Talebreza S, Widera E. Advanced directives: navigating conflicts between expressed wishes and best interests. *Am Fam Phys*. 2015; 91:480–484.

54. Smith AL, Lo B, Sudore R. When previously expressed wishes conflict with best interests. *JAMA Intern Med*. 2013;173:1241–1245.

55. Stuart B. The NHO medical guidelines for non-cancer disease and local medical review policy: hospice access for patients with diseases other than cancer. *Hosp J*. 1999;14(3–4):139–154.

56. National Hospice Organization; Medical Guidelines Task Force. *Medical Guidelines for Determining Prognosis in Selected Non-Cancer Diseases*. 2nd ed. Arlington, VA: National Hospice Organization; 1996.

57. Maltoni M, Nanni O, Pirovano M, et al. Successful validation of the palliative prognostic score in terminally ill cancer patients. Italian Multicenter Study Group on Palliative Care. *J Pain Symptom Manage*. 1999;17(4):240–247.

58. Sample advance directive form. *Am Fam Phys*. 1999;59:617–620. http://www.aafp.org/afp/1999/0201/p617.html. Accessed October 29, 2015.

Appendix

Chapter 1: Common EENT Disorders in Primary Care

1. A 17-year-old lifeguard presents to your office with c/o fullness and pressure in his left ear. You would:
   a. Advise against swimming until symptoms resolve
   b. Promote ear hygiene
   c. Prescribe otic antibiotic drops
   d. All of the above

2. A 42-year-old reports he has noticed itching and irritation in his ear for the past week or so. Upon examination, you note that the external auditory canal is reddened and slightly erythematous, TM normal, bony landmarks visible. The preferred treatment regimen would include:
   a. Fluoroquinolone drops (Cipro)
   b. Oral penicillinase
   c. Mupirocin ointment
   d. Oral macrolide

3. The preferred antibiotic for acute moderate to severe otitis media in an adult client is:
   a. Cipro HC otic
   b. Amoxicillin PO
   c. Mupirocin ointment otic
   d. Erythromycin PO

4. A 52-year-old female patient presents with c/o tinnitus, vertigo, and nausea. Denies hearing loss, denies ear pain, denies significant PMH. Reports recent URI with "cough and stuffy nose." On exam, the ear canal is clear, TM pearly without exudate, bony landmarks present. Neuro examination is normal except for dizziness. Your recommended treatment would include:
   a. Meclizine
   b. Cipro otic
   c. Vancomycin IV
   d. Amoxicillin PO

5. A 38-year-old patient reports he is having ear pain that recently occurred. He has no significant past medical history. Given that brief information, what would you consider in your differential diagnoses?
   a. Otitis externa, otitis media, periodontal disease
   b. Otitis media, otitis externa, mumps
   c. Tumor, otitis interna, varicella
   d. Otitis interna, measles, pharyngitis

6. A 68-year-old male patient with a PMH of DM presents with c/o severe ear pain and facial numbness. Examination is significant for T 104, with necrotic tissue noted in left ear canal and marked facial palsy. Your diagnosis and treatment plan would include:
   a. Malignant otitis externa with emergent transfer to hospital
   b. Otitis media with oral antibiotics
   c. Malignant otitis media with IV antibiotics
   d. Otitis interna with antiviral medication

7. Differential diagnoses for red eye should include:
   a. Allergic conjunctivitis
   b. Bacterial conjunctivitis
   c. Viral conjunctivitis
   d. Corneal abrasion
   e. All of the above

8. Treatment for allergic conjunctivitis may include:
   a. Antihistamines PO
   b. Allergen avoidance
   c. Antihistamines OU
   d. All of the above

9. Treatment for bacterial conjunctivitis should include:
   a. Antibiotic eye gtts
   b. Good hand and eye hygiene
   c. No work or school for 24 hours after initiation of treatment
   d. All of the above

10. Treatment for uncomplicated viral conjunctivitis should include:
    a. Antibiotic eye gtts
    b. Good hand and eye hygiene
    c. Oral antiviral medications
    d. Steroid eye gtts

11. Red flags for red eye are:
    a. Vision loss
    b. Severe pain
    c. Corneal ulcer
    d. All of the above

12. Ocular emergencies that require immediate referral to an eye specialist include:
    a. Vision loss, blepharitis, corneal ulcer
    b. Corneal ulcer, severe pain, conjunctival redness
    c. Globe penetration, vision loss, severe pain
    d. Light sensitivity, conjunctival redness, blepharitis

13. Treatment for corneal abrasion should include:
    a. Complete eye exam with fluorescein staining
    b. Antibiotic eye gtts
    c. Assessment for vision loss and/or extension of abrasion into visual field
    d. Both A and C
    e. All of the above

14. The most common cause or causes of vision loss in the United States are:
    a. Cataract and glaucoma
    b. Macular degeneration
    c. Diabetic retinopathy
    d. All of the above

15. Differential diagnoses for stuffy nose should include:
    a. Allergic rhinitis, vasomotor rhinitis
    b. Viral influenza, acute sinusitis
    c. Mechanical obstruction of nares, chronic sinusitis
    d. All of the above

16. Clinical picture of allergic rhinitis includes:
    a. Sneezing, dry cough, runny nose, watery eyes
    b. Sneezing, productive cough, red eyes
    c. Productive cough, runny nose, sore throat
    d. Sore throat, sneezing, productive cough

17. Treatment for allergic rhinitis should include:
    a. Oral antihistamines
    b. Intranasal steroid sprays
    c. Allergen avoidance
    d. All of the above

18. Red flags for a nasal congestion should include:
    a. Severe painful headache
    b. Visual changes
    c. Difficulty swallowing
    d. All of the above

19. Signs and symptoms of sinus infection usually include:
    a. Purulent nasal discharge
    b. Fever higher than T 39°C (102.2°F)
    c. Headache with facial pain
    d. All of the above

20. First-line treatment for acute bacterial rhinosinusitis in a non-PCN-allergic adult includes:
    a. Amoxicillin/clavulanate
    b. Azithromycin
    c. Levaquin
    d. Doxycycline

21. Treatment for chronic sinusitis may include:
    a. CT (if suppurative symptoms)
    b. Antibiotic therapy
    c. Saline nasal sprays, humidification, and increased PO fluids
    d. All of the above

22. Risk factors for chronic sinusitis in adults include:
    a. Allergy to shellfish
    b. Recent respiratory tract infection
    c. Nasal polyps or obstruction
    d. Varicella infection

23. John is a 19-year-old soccer player who is in to see you following an injury he sustained in a recent game. He was seen at an emergency room and diagnosed with a nasal fracture. You know that John is at risk for:
    a. Upper respiratory infection
    b. Sinusitis
    c. Pneumonia
    d. Ear pain

24. When you provide patient teaching for a client with chronic sinusitis, it is important to include information about which of the following topics? *allergies predispose to sinusitis*
    a. Allergen avoidance
    b. Surgical options
    c. Prophylactic antibiotics
    d. All of the above

25. A patient with chronic sinusitis is considering RAST testing. She asks what allergy testing entails. Which of the following is the best response? *RAST is not skin sensitivity*
    a. RAST testing requires a series of pinpricks to her back or arm.
    b. RAST testing requires a small tube of blood be sent for laboratory analysis.
    c. Allergy testing doesn't hurt, so no worries.
    d. Allergy testing is 25% effective in diagnosing the cause of her allergies.

26. What health-promoting behaviors would you recommend for an adult patient with allergies and sinusitis?
    a. Influenza vaccination, smoking cessation
    b. Allergen avoidance, meningitis vaccination
    c. Tetanus booster, polio booster
    d. All of the above

27. Allergen immunotherapy should be considered in patients whose allergies have been resistant to control using avoidance and other immune-modifying medications.
    a. True
    b. False

28. Susie is an 18-year-old female soccer player with c/o sudden-onset sore throat and high fever. She states that several members of her team have also recently been ill with similar symptoms. Which is your next action in the treatment of Susie?
    a. Prescribe penicillin for a 10-day course
    b. Perform a rapid antigen detection test
    c. Perform a throat culture
    d. All of the above

29. To which of the following do the Centor criteria award one point each?
    a. Absence of cough, swollen tender anterior cervical nodes
    b. Temperature >100.4°F (38°C), tonsillar exudates or swelling
    c. Age between 12 and 24 years, excessive salivation
    d. Both A and B

30. Sammy is 14 years old and comes to you with c/o severe sore throat pain and difficulty swallowing. On examination, you note enlarged painful LN, sour-smelling breath, and 3+ tonsils with exudate. RADT negative, culture negative. You diagnose Sammy with:
    a. Tonsillitis
    b. Uveitis
    c. GAS pharyngitis
    d. None of the above

31. Steven is a 15-year-old who presents with c/o severe sore throat and fever. He is accompanied by his mother, and you note he is speaking very little and in a muffled "hot potato" voice, and wiping his mouth frequently. On exam, he exhibits trismus and ear pain. You consider the following in his differential diagnoses:
    a. Peritonsillar abscess
    b. Epiglottitis
    c. Infectious mononucleosis
    d. All of the above

32. Steven is a 15-year-old who presents with c/o severe sore throat and fever. He is accompanied by his mother, and you note he is speaking very little and in a muffled "hot potato" voice, and wiping his mouth frequently. On exam, he exhibits trismus and ear pain. What is your final diagnosis for Steven?
    a. Peritonsillar abscess
    b. Epiglottitis
    c. Infectious mononucleosis
    d. All of the above

33. Treatment for peritonsillar abscess should include:
    a. Referral to ENT for drainage
    b. Antibiotic therapy
    c. Analgesia
    d. All of the above

34. John is a 21-year-old male with c/o sudden-onset sore throat and high fever. He has a positive RADT in your office. What is your next action in John's treatment?
    a. Prescribe penicillin for a 10-day course
    b. Perform a rapid antigen detection test
    c. Perform a throat culture
    d. All of the above

35. In addition to antibiotic therapy, what treatment might you recommend for John's GAS pharyngitis?
    a. Analgesia
    b. Rest, fluids
    c. Do not share utensils or food
    d. All of the above

36. Suppurative complication of GAS pharyngitis include:
    a. Mastoiditis
    b. Peritonsillar abscess
    c. Cervical lymphadenitis
    d. All of the above

37. In an adult with nonanaphylactic PCN allergy, what would you prescribe to treat GAS pharyngitis?
    a. Clindamycin 5 days
    b. Clarithromycin 7 days
    c. First-generation cephalosporin 10 days
    d. None of the above

    or a 10 D course of clind or 5D course of azithno

38. Differential diagnoses for sore throat include:
    a. GAS pharyngitis
    b. Viral pharyngitis
    c. Peritonsillar abscess
    d. All of the above

39. What does the abbreviation GAS in "GAS pharyngitis" stand for?
    a. Group A streptococcal
    b. Group A staphylococcal
    c. Genu varum Arboretum synovial
    d. None of the above

40. If untreated or not fully treated, GAS infection can lead to:
    a. Cardiac complications
    b. Renal complications
    c. Scarlet fever
    d. All of the above

Chapter 1: Answers and Rationales

1. D. According to the American Academy of Otolaryngology, the preferred treatment for swimmer's ear includes advising against swimming until symptoms resolve, promoting ear hygiene, and prescribing otic antibiotic drops.

   Rosenfeld RM, Schwartz SR, Cannon CR, et al. Clinical practice guideline: acute otitis externa. *Otolaryngol Head Neck Surg.* 2014;150(1 suppl):S1–S24. Originally issued in 2006, revised in 2013. http://www.guideline.gov/content .aspx?id=47795&search=otitis. Accessed September 2, 2015.

2. A. According to the American Academy of Family Practice and based upon the American Academy of Otolaryngology Clinical Practice Guidelines, the preferred treatment for otitis externa is topical antibiotics such as ciprofloxacin otic.

   Schaefer P, Baugh RF. Acute otitis externa: an update. *Am Fam Physician.* 2012;86(11):1055–1061. http://www.aafp.org/ afp/2012/1201/p1055.html. Accessed December 15, 2015.

   Rosenfeld RM, Schwartz SR, Cannon CR, et al. Clinical practice guideline: acute otitis externa. *Otolaryngol Head Neck Surg.* 2014;150(1 suppl):S1–S24. Originally issued in 2006, revised in 2013. http://www.guideline.gov/content .aspx?id=47795&search=otitis. Accessed September 2, 2015.

3. A. According to the 2015 edition of the *Sanford Guide to Antimicrobial Therapy*, the preferred antibiotic for a moderate to severe case of otitis media in an adult client is an otic drop such as Cipro HC.

4. A. Otitis interna/labyrinthitis is commonly caused by a viral infection. As such, routine treatment is focused on symptom management and includes medications such as meclizine to assist with the patient's vertigo.

Shupert CL, Kulick B. Labyrinthitis and vestibular neuritis: infections of the inner ear. Vestibular Disorders Association. 2015. https://vestibular.org/labyrinthitis-and-vestibular-neuritis.

5. B. Considerations for differentials for ear pain should include infectious agents with propensity for swelling and inflammation near the ear and ear canal.

Schaefer P, Baugh RF. Acute otitis externa: an update. *Am Fam Physician.* 2012;86(11):1055–1061. http://www.aafp.org/afp/2012/1201/p1055.html. Accessed December 15, 2015.

Rosenfeld RM, Schwartz SR, Cannon CR, et al. Clinical practice guideline: acute otitis externa. *Otolaryngol Head Neck Surg.* 2014;150(1 suppl):S1–S24. Originally issued in 2006, revised in 2013. http://www.guideline.gov/content.aspx?id=47795&search=otitis. Accessed September 2, 2015.

Centers for Disease Control and Prevention. Mumps: signs and symptoms of mumps. 2015. http://www.cdc.gov/mumps/about/signs-symptoms.html.

6. A. Malignant otitis externa is a medical emergency with a high degree of morbidity and potential for mortality.

Schaefer P, Baugh RF. Acute otitis externa: an update. *Am Fam Physician.* 2012;86(11):1055–1061. http://www.aafp.org/afp/2012/1201/p1055.html. Accessed December 15, 2015.

7. E. When evaluating a red eye, determine whether injury, infection, or emergent eye conditions exist.

Centers for Disease Control and Prevention. Conjunctivitis (pink eye): treatment. 2014. http://www.cdc.gov/conjunctivitis/about/treatment.html. Accessed December 16, 2015.

American Academy of Ophthalmology. Policy statement: referral of persons with possible eye diseases or injury. 2014. http://www.aao.org/clinical-statement/guidelines-appropriate-referral-of-persons-with-po. Accessed September 2, 2015.

Cronau H, Kankanala R, Mauger T. Diagnosis and management of red eye in primary care. *Am Fam Physician.* 2010;81(2):137–144. http://www.aafp.org/afp/2010/0115/p137.html. Accessed December 15, 2015.

8. D. Avoidance of allergens and control of histamine release are important factors in the treatment of allergic conjunctivitis.

Centers for Disease Control and Prevention. Conjunctivitis (pink eye): treatment. 2014. http://www.cdc.gov/conjunctivitis/about/treatment.html. Accessed December 16, 2015.

9. D. Bacterial conjunctivitis is treated with a combination of antibiotic eye drops and avoidance of infection of other eye or other persons.

Centers for Disease Control and Prevention. Conjunctivitis (pink eye): treatment. 2014. http://www.cdc.gov/conjunctivitis/about/treatment.html. Accessed December 16, 2015.

10. B. Uncomplicated viral conjunctivitis is treated with symptom management and infection control only.

Centers for Disease Control and Prevention. Conjunctivitis (pink eye): treatment. 2014. http://www.cdc.gov/conjunctivitis/about/treatment.html. Accessed December 16, 2015.

11. D. Eye conditions with vision loss or threatened vision loss should be immediately referred for emergent care by an appropriate ophthalmic specialist.

Centers for Disease Control and Prevention. Conjunctivitis (pink eye): treatment. 2014. http://www.cdc.gov/conjunctivitis/about/treatment.html. Accessed December 16, 2015.

American Academy of Ophthalmology. Policy statement: referral of persons with possible eye diseases or injury. 2014. http://www.aao.org/clinical-statement/guidelines-appropriate-referral-of-persons-with-po. Accessed September 2, 2015.

12. C. Eye conditions with vision loss or threatened vision loss should be immediately referred for emergent care by an appropriate ophthalmic specialist.

Centers for Disease Control and Prevention. Conjunctivitis (pinkeye): treatment. 2014. http://www.cdc.gov/conjunctivitis/about/treatment.html. Accessed December 16, 2015.

American Academy of Ophthalmology. Policy statement: referral of persons with possible eye diseases or injury. 2014. http://www.aao.org/clinical-statement/guidelines-appropriate-referral-of-persons-with-po. Accessed September 2, 2015.

13. D. According to the AAOP, care of the patient with corneal abrasions should include determination of severity of the abrasion and encroachment on the visual field.

Cronau H, Kankanala R, Mauger T. Diagnosis and management of red eye in primary care. *Am Fam Physician.* 2010;81(2):137–144. http://www.aafp.org/afp/2010/0115/p137.html. Accessed December 15, 2015.

American Academy of Ophthalmology. Policy statement: referral of persons with possible eye diseases or injury. 2014. http://www.aao.org/clinical-statement/guidelines-appropriate-referral-of-persons-with-po. Accessed September 2, 2015.

14. D. The Centers for Disease Control and Prevention lists the leading causes of blindness as the degenerative conditions of cataract, glaucoma, macular degeneration, and diabetic retinopathy.

Centers for Disease Control and Prevention. Vision Health Initiative: common eye disorders. 2013. http://www.cdc.gov/visionhealth/basic_information/eye_disorders.htm. Accessed December 15, 2015.

15. D. According to the Infectious Disease Society of America (IDSA) Clinical Practice Guideline for acute bacterial rhinosinusitis in children and adults, all of the diagnoses should be considered when a patient presents with a stuffy nose.

Chow AW, Benninger MS, Brook I, et al. IDSA clinical practice guideline for acute bacterial rhinosinusitis in children and adults. *Clin Infect Dis.* 2012;54(8):e72–e112. http://www.guideline.gov/content.aspx?id=36681. Accessed September 2, 2015.

16. A. According to the Infectious Disease Society of America (IDSA) Clinical Practice Guideline for acute bacterial rhinosinusitis in children and adults, the clinical presentation of allergic rhinitis includes dry cough, sneezing, runny nose, and watery eyes.

Chow AW, Benninger MS, Brook I, et al. IDSA clinical practice guideline for acute bacterial rhinosinusitis in children and adults. *Clin Infect Dis.* 2012;54(8):e72–e112. http://www.guideline.gov/content.aspx?id=36681. Accessed September 2, 2015.

17. D. According to the Infectious Disease Society of America (IDSA) Clinical Practice Guideline for acute bacterial rhinosinusitis in children and adults, treatment of allergic rhinitis should include multiple-line therapies to control and manage symptoms.

Chow AW, Benninger MS, Brook I, et al. IDSA clinical practice guideline for acute bacterial rhinosinusitis in children and adults. *Clin Infect Dis.* 2012;54(8):e72–e112. http://www.guideline.gov/content.aspx?id=36681. Accessed September 2, 2015.

18. D. According to the Infectious Disease Society of America (IDSA) Clinical Practice Guideline for acute bacterial rhinosinusitis in children and adults, severe painful headache, visual changes, and difficulty swallowing should be considered red flags for nasal congestion.

Chow AW, Benninger MS, Brook I, et al. IDSA clinical practice guideline for acute bacterial rhinosinusitis in children and adults. *Clin Infect Dis.* 2012;54(8):e72–e112. http://www.guideline.gov/content.aspx?id=36681. Accessed September 2, 2015.

19. D. According to the Infectious Disease Society of America (IDSA) Clinical Practice Guideline for acute bacterial rhinosinusitis in children and adults, the clinical presentation of sinus infection includes fever, headache, facial pain, and purulent nasal drainage.

Chow AW, Benninger MS, Brook I, et al. IDSA clinical practice guideline for acute bacterial rhinosinusitis in children and adults. *Clin Infect Dis.* 2012;54(8):e72–e112. http://www.guideline.gov/content.aspx?id=36681. Accessed September 2, 2015.

20. A. The Infectious Disease Society of America (IDSA) Clinical Practice Guideline for acute bacterial rhinosinusitis in children and adults recommends amoxicillin/clavulanate as the first-line therapy for acute bacterial rhinosinusitis.

Chow AW, Benninger MS, Brook I, et al. IDSA clinical practice guideline for acute bacterial rhinosinusitis in children and adults. *Clin Infect Dis.* 2012;54(8):e72–e112.

http://www.guideline.gov/content.aspx?id=36681. Accessed September 2, 2015.

21. D. According to the American Academy of Otolaryngology practice guideline, chronic sinusitis treatment may include humidification, nasal sprays, and fluids as well as additional imaging with CT and antibiotic therapy.

Rosenfeld RM, Piccirillo JF, Chandrasekhar SS, et al. Clinical practice guideline (update): adult sinusitis. *Otolaryngol Head Neck Surg.* 2015 Apr;152(2 Suppl).

22. C. According to the CDC, risk factors for sinusitis include structural issues within the sinus and nasal polyps.

Centers for Disease Control and Prevention. Get smart: know when antibiotics work: sinus infection (sinusitis). 2015. http://www.cdc.gov/getsmart/community/for-patients/common-illnesses/sinus-infection.html. Accessed December 15, 2015.

23. B. One risk factor for sinusitis is nasal obstruction. A nasal fracture places John at risk of a deviated septum and nasal obstruction.

Centers for Disease Control and Prevention. Get smart: know when antibiotics work: sinus infection (sinusitis). 2015. http://www.cdc.gov/getsmart/community/for-patients/common-illnesses/sinus-infection.html. Accessed December 15, 2015.

24. A. The Centers for Disease Control and Prevention notes that allergies predispose a person to sinusitis. Allergen avoidance is one tool to reduce chronic sinusitis.

Centers for Disease Control and Prevention. Get smart: know when antibiotics work: sinus infection (sinusitis). 2015. http://www.cdc.gov/getsmart/community/for-patients/common-illnesses/sinus-infection.html. Accessed December 15, 2015.

25. B. According to the Joint Task Force on Practice Parameters (which represents the American Academy of Allergy, Asthma and Immunology; the American College of Allergy, Asthma and Immunology; and the Joint Council of Allergy, Asthma and Immunology), immunoassays such as RAST are utilized to determine allergen sensitivity. RAST testing is a blood test and not a skin sensitivity test.

Wallace D, Dykewicz M, Bernstein D, et al. The diagnosis and management of rhinitis: an updated practice parameter. *J Clin Immunol.* 2008;122(2):S1–84. http://www.aaaai.org/Aaaai/media/MediaLibrary/PDF%20Documents/Practice%20and%20Parameters/rhinitis2008-diagnosis-management.pdf. Accessed December 15, 2015.

26. A. The Centers for Disease Control and Prevention recommends influenza vaccination for all adults, with special emphasis on those with asthma. Smoking cessation decreases upper respiratory irritation and chronic inflammation of the nares and airway.

Centers for Disease Control and Prevention. Recommended adult immunization schedule, by vaccine and age group. 2014.

http://www.cdc.gov/vaccines/schedules/hcp/imz/adult.html. Accessed September 2, 2015.

27. A. According to the Joint Task Force on Practice Parameters (which represents the American Academy of Allergy, Asthma and Immunology; the American College of Allergy, Asthma and Immunology; and the Joint Council of Allergy, Asthma and Immunology), allergen immunotherapy should be considered in patients who have failed to be fully managed with more conservative treatment methodologies.

Wallace D, Dykewicz M, Bernstein D, et al. The diagnosis and management of rhinitis: an updated practice parameter. *J Clin Immunol.* 2008;122(2):S1–84. http://www.aaaai.org/Aaaai/media/MediaLibrary/PDF%20Documents/Practice%20and%20Parameters/rhinitis2008-diagnosis-management.pdf. Accessed December 15, 2015.

28. B. The Infectious Diseases Society of America Clinical Practice Guideline for the diagnosis and management of group A streptococcal (GAS) pharyngitis recommends a rapid antigen detection test (RADT) prior to initiation of antibiotic therapy to differentiate between viral pharyngitis and GAS pharyngitis. If the RADT is negative, a throat culture may then be performed. If the RADT is positive, a confirmative culture is not necessary.

Shulman ST, Bisno AL, Clegg HW, et al. Clinical practice guideline for the diagnosis and management of group A streptococcal pharyngitis: 2012 update by the Infectious Diseases Society of America. *Clin Infect Dis.* September 9, 2012. doi:10.1093/cid/cis629.

29. D. The Centor criteria awards one point for each of the following: absence of cough, swollen and tender anterior cervical nodes, temperature >100.4°F (38°C), tonsillar exudates or swelling, age between 3 and 14 years. The Centor criteria awards zero points for age between 15 and 44 years and deducts one point for age 45 years and older.

Shulman ST, Bisno AL, Clegg HW, et al. Clinical practice guideline for the diagnosis and management of group A streptococcal pharyngitis: 2012 update by the Infectious Diseases Society of America. *Clin Infect Dis.* September 9, 2012. doi:10.1093/cid/cis629.

Choby BA. Diagnosis and treatment of streptococcal pharyngitis. American Academy of Family Physicians; 2009. http://www.aafp.org/afp/2009/0301/p383.pdf. Accessed September 2, 2015.

Centers for Disease Control. Acute pharyngitis in adults: physician information sheet. http://www.cdc.gov/getsmart/community/materials-references/print-materials/hcp/adult-acute-pharyngitis.html. Accessed September 2, 2015.

30. A. Tonsillitis can be caused by a viral or bacterial agent. In the absence of a rapid antigen detection test (RADT) and/or culture positive for strep, group A streptococcal (GAS)

pharyngitis is not an appropriate diagnosis. The Infectious Diseases Society of America Clinical Practice Guideline for the diagnosis and management of group A streptococcal pharyngitis recommends a rapid antigen test prior to initiation of antibiotic therapy to differentiate between viral pharyngitis and GAS pharyngitis. If the RADT is negative, a throat culture may then be performed. If the RADT is positive, a confirmative culture is not necessary.

Shulman ST, Bisno AL, Clegg HW, et al. Clinical practice guideline for the diagnosis and management of group A streptococcal pharyngitis: 2012 update by the Infectious Diseases Society of America. *Clin Infect Dis.* September 9, 2012. doi:10.1093/cid/cis629.

31. D. Infectious Diseases Society of America guidelines describe the differentials listed for consideration in Steven's case.

Shulman ST, Bisno AL, Clegg HW, et al. Clinical practice guideline for the diagnosis and management of group A streptococcal pharyngitis: 2012 update by the Infectious Diseases Society of America. *Clin Infect Dis.* September 9, 2012. doi:10.1093/cid/cis629.

Galioto NJ. Peritonsillar abscess. *Am Fam Physician.* 2008; 77(2):199–202. http://www.aafp.org/afp/2008/0115/p199.html. Accessed December 15, 2015.

32. A. Signs and symptoms of peritonsillar abscess are important to recognize. It is important with this diagnosis to be aware of the potential for airway obstruction.

Shulman ST, Bisno AL, Clegg HW, et al. Clinical practice guideline for the diagnosis and management of group A streptococcal pharyngitis: 2012 update by the Infectious Diseases Society of America. *Clin Infect Dis.* September 9, 2012. doi:10.1093/cid/cis629.

Galioto NJ. Peritonsillar abscess. *Am Fam Physician.* 2008; 77(2):199–202. http://www.aafp.org/afp/2008/0115/p199.html. Accessed December 15, 2015.

33. D. Appropriate referral to an ears, nose, and throat (ENT) clinician for urgent drainage of the abscess is the appropriate first step to prevent complications such as airway obstruction and to allow for management of the underlying infection.

Shulman ST, Bisno AL, Clegg HW, et al. Clinical practice guideline for the diagnosis and management of group A streptococcal pharyngitis: 2012 update by the Infectious Diseases Society of America. *Clin Infect Dis.* September 9, 2012. doi:10.1093/cid/cis629.

Galioto NJ. Peritonsillar abscess. *Am Fam Physician.* 2008; 77(2):199–202. http://www.aafp.org/afp/2008/0115/p199.html. Accessed December 15, 2015.

34. A. The Infectious Diseases Society of America Clinical Practice Guideline for the diagnosis and management of group A streptococcal pharyngitis recommends a rapid antigen detection test prior to initiation of antibiotic therapy to differentiate between viral pharyngitis and group A streptococcal (GAS) pharyngitis. If the RADT is negative, a throat culture may then be performed. In John's case, the RADT is positive, so a confirmative culture is not necessary. First-line treatment for GAS pharyngitis is Penicillin V (Pen V).

Shulman ST, Bisno AL, Clegg HW, et al. Clinical practice guideline for the diagnosis and management of group A streptococcal pharyngitis: 2012 update by the Infectious Diseases Society of America. *Clin Infect Dis*. September 9, 2012. doi:10.1093/cid/cis629.

35. D. Treatment for group A streptococcal (GAS) pharyngitis includes rest, pain relief, and avoiding exposure of others via salivary transfer.

Shulman ST, Bisno AL, Clegg HW, et al. Clinical practice guideline for the diagnosis and management of group A streptococcal pharyngitis: 2012 update by the Infectious Diseases Society of America. *Clin Infect Dis*. September 9, 2012. doi:10.1093/cid/cis629.

36. D. Avoidance of suppurative complications of group A streptococcal (GAS) pharyngitis is recommended.

Shulman ST, Bisno AL, Clegg HW, et al. Clinical practice guideline for the diagnosis and management of group A streptococcal pharyngitis: 2012 update by the Infectious Diseases Society of America. *Clin Infect Dis*. September 9, 2012. doi:10.1093/cid/cis629.

37. C. Recommended treatment for penicillin (PCN)-allergic patients with nonanaphylactic response is a first-generation cephalosporin for 10 days (preferred), or a 10-day course of clindamycin or clarithromycin, or a 5-day course of azithromycin.

Shulman ST, Bisno AL, Clegg HW, et al. Clinical practice guideline for the diagnosis and management of group A streptococcal pharyngitis: 2012 update by the Infectious Diseases Society of America. *Clin Infect Dis*. September 9, 2012. doi:10.1093/cid/cis629.

38. D. It is important to consider multiple causative agents when treating patients with a sore throat.

Shulman ST, Bisno AL, Clegg HW, et al. Clinical practice guideline for the diagnosis and management of group A streptococcal pharyngitis: 2012 update by the Infectious Diseases Society of America. *Clin Infect Dis*. September 9, 2012. doi:10.1093/cid/cis629.

39. A. GAS stands for group A streptococcal or group A Streptococcus. The Centers for Disease Control and Prevention describes GAS pharyngitis here: http://www.cdc.gov/Features/StrepThroat/.

Centers for Disease Control and Prevention. Is it strep throat? 2015. http://www.cdc.gov/Features/StrepThroat/. Accessed December 15, 2015.

40. D. The Infectious Diseases Society of America guidelines and the Centers for Disease Control and Prevention list

complications of untreated and undertreated strep infection, some of which are cardiac or renal complications and scarlet fever.

Shulman ST, Bisno AL, Clegg HW, et al. Clinical practice guideline for the diagnosis and management of group A streptococcal pharyngitis: 2012 update by the Infectious Diseases Society of America. *Clin Infect Dis*. September 9, 2012. doi:10.1093/cid/cis629.

Chapter 2: Common Cardiovascular Disorders in Primary Care

1. Primary care providers need to feel confident in the assessment and treatment of atrial fibrillation to prevent hospitalizations for this common arrhythmia. In the past 20 years, what has been the increase in hospitalizations caused by atrial fibrillation?
   a. 25%
   b. 33%
   c. 66%
   d. 75%

2. A 76-year-old woman presents to your clinic today following a recent hospitalization for new-onset atrial fibrillation. Her medical history is notable for hypertension and diabetes. She has no history of stroke or TIA. Her current meds include ASA 81 mg, glyburide, lisinopril, and verapamil. Her AF is under good rate control. What is this patient's calculated CHA_2DS_2-VASc score?
   a. 2
   b. 3
   c. 4
   d. 5

3. Definitions of AF are important because they guide treatment regimens. Regarding AF, which of the following statements is true?
   a. Paroxysmal AF occurs briefly once and then never reoccurs.
   b. Persistent AF lasts more than 24 hours.
   c. Long-standing persistent AF lasts more than 6 months.
   d. Permanent AF implies that persistent AF is present and the patient and provider have decided not to restore or maintain sinus rhythm.

4. A basic workup for atrial fibrillation includes all of the following *except*:
   a. ECG
   b. Transthoracic echocardiogram
   c. A thallium stress test
   d. Labs of thyroid, renal, and hepatic function

5. You see a new patient in the office today who has a history of atrial fibrillation. He stopped all his medications 3 months ago when he moved from Indianapolis. Today in the office his ECG shows no P waves and an irregularly regular ventricular rate of 70. His past medical history is significant for

a mechanical aortic valve replacement 3 years ago. Which agent is the best choice for anticoagulation for this patient?
a. Dabigatran (Pradaxa)
b. Rivaroxaban (Xarelto)
c. No anticoagulation is needed
d. Warfarin (Coumadin)

6. Which of the following is an appropriate reason for not anticoagulating a patient with AF?
a. Inability to comply with INR monitoring
b. Predisposition to falling or head trauma
c. Severe alcohol abuse within 2 years
d. All of the above

7. Which of the following does not increase risk for bleeding in patients receiving anticoagulation according to the HAS-BLED Bleeding Risk Score?
a. Uncontrolled hypertension
b. Bleeding history
c. Abnormal electrolytes
d. Abnormal renal/liver function

8. A 68-year-old female presents to the office today reporting a racing heart since last evening. She reports shortness of breath (SOB), lightheadedness, and some chest pressure at the onset of the episode last evening. She currently has no chest pain. Her past medical history is remarkable for hypertension and dyslipidemia; her current medications include hydrochlorothiazide and simvastatin. Her BP today is 98/76 mm Hg. Her ECG is consistent with AF with a ventricular rate of 180 beats per minute. What is the appropriate management for this patient?
a. Calculate a CHA_2DS_2-VASc score to help you determine whether anticoagulation is needed.
b. Start a beta blocker to help lower the heart rate.
c. Start an antiarrhythmic agent to try to restore normal sinus rhythm.
d. Hospitalize the patient.

9. Which statement is untrue regarding treatment options for AF?
a. Drug therapy and ablation are effective treatment options for rate and rhythm control.
b. Drugs and/or cardioversion are usually first-line choices for rhythm control in AF.
c. In young patients with AF, long-term drug therapy is preferred over ablation because of the risk of damaging electrical pathways permanently.
d. The need for anticoagulation in patients with AF is based on stroke risk.

10. A 63-year-old female presents to your office with a mild ankle sprain and is found to have a blood pressure of 150/102 mm Hg, possibly elevated as a result of pain. On follow-up, her BP on two occasions is 142/88 mm Hg despite good dietary habits and reasonable exercise. Her history and physical are essentially normal except that she had a hysterectomy. Basic lab evaluation reveals no significant abnormalities. Based on recent recommendations from JNC-8, which of the following is accurate information to give her?
a. At age > 50 years, high diastolic BP becomes a more important cardiovascular risk factor than high systolic pressure.
b. A thiazide diuretic or beta blocker should be started to achieve a BP goal of 130/80 mm Hg.
c. Continue therapeutic lifestyle changes and monitor BP measurements.
d. Initiating therapy with two antihypertensive agents would be preferred based on her current BP.

11. You are treating a 49-year-old male for hypertension. He is an engineer and consistently brings in his blood pressure logs to all visits. They are neatly documented on graph paper and indicate that his BP values at home are running at 120–130/ 70–80 mm Hg. BPs taken in your office are consistently above 140/90 mm Hg. According to JNC-8 guidelines, how should you manage this patient?
a. Have the patient continue documenting his home BPs and don't change his medication regimen.
b. Order an echocardiogram.
c. Do nothing. Home BP measurements are more reliable than office measurements.
d. Order ambulatory BP monitoring.

12. Which statement is not consistent with the 2014 guidelines for the management of high blood pressure?
a. When initiating therapy, African American patients without known chronic kidney disease should be prescribed calcium channel blockers and thiazide-type diuretics instead of ACE inhibitors.
b. ACE inhibitors and angiotensin receptor blockers should not be used in the same patient simultaneously.
c. Patients older than 75 years of age with impaired kidney function can be safely prescribed ACE inhibitors and angiotensin receptor blockers.
d. Use of ACE inhibitors and angiotensin receptor blockers is recommended in all patients with chronic kidney disease regardless of ethnic background.

13. Which one of the following tests is not recommended prior to initiating drug therapy for high blood pressure?
a. Urine albumin/creatinine ratio
b. Urine analysis
c. Serum potassium
d. Fasting lipid profile

14. Which of the following should be included in the initial physical exam for a patient recently diagnosed with hypertension?
a. Examination of the optic fundus
b. Auscultation for carotid, abdominal, and femoral bruits
c. Palpation of the lower extremities for edema and pulses
d. All of the above

15. Which one of the following drug categories is recommended as later-line (not first-line) medication based on the results of randomized control trials?

a. Beta blockers *(circled)*
b. Thiazide-type diuretics
c. Calcium channel blockers
d. ACE inhibitors

[handwritten: this study was compared to an ARB]

16. Which one of the following is most likely to be found on the ECG of a patient with uncontrolled hypertension?

a. ST depression
b. ST elevation
c. Left ventricular hypertrophy *(circled)*
d. Ectopy

[handwritten: evidence target organ damage 2° to pressure/volume overload]

17. What counseling information is it important to review with a patient being treated for hypertension?

a. Limit alcohol consumption to no more than three drinks daily.
b. Weight reduction will not significantly decrease blood pressure.
c. Following a low-sodium diet can help with blood pressure control. *(circled)*
d. Smoking cessation reduces the risk of cardiovascular disease.

18. A 60-year-old white male just moved to town and needs to establish care. His past medical history is significant for coronary artery disease. Preferring a "natural approach," he has been very conscientious about low-fat, low-cholesterol eating habits and a daily exercise program. Over time, he has gradually eliminated a number of prescription medications (he doesn't recall their names) that he was on at the time of hospital discharge. His past history is negative for hypertension, diabetes, and smoking. The lipid panel you obtain shows the following:

Total cholesterol 198 mg/dL; triglycerides 160 mg/dL; HDL 42; LDL (calculated) 124

Which of the following recommendations would most optimally treat his lipid status?

a. Continue current dietary efforts and exercise.
b. Calculate his ASCVD risk and start an HMG-CoA reductase inhibitor. *(circled)*
c. Add a fibric acid derivative such as gemfibrozil (Lopid).
d. Review previous medications and resume an angiotensin-converting enzyme inhibitor.

19. A 58-year-old male has a history of hypertension and asks about reducing his risk for myocardial infarction. His lipid profile shows HDL cholesterol of 32 mg/dL. According to the newest lipid guidelines, what would you recommend to this patient?

a. Aspirin, one tablet daily
b. Vitamin E, 400 IU daily
c. Folic acid plus pyridoxine (vitamin B_6)
d. Therapy based on his ASCVD risk calculation *(circled)*

20. Your 65-year-old male patient comes in to discuss his recent lipid profile. His results are as follows:

Total cholesterol 198; LDL 130; HDL 45; triglycerides 650. Which one of the following medications should be recommended?

a. Niacin
b. Fenofibrate *(circled)*
c. Atorvastatin
d. Omega-3 fatty acids

[handwritten: Fenofibrate to tx triglycerides 7500 omega 3's won't work that high]

21. Your patient has a prior history of AMI. You have him on the combination agent Vytorin (Zetia and Zocor [ezetimibe and simvastatin]), and his lipid profiles are at goal. He has tried monotherapy in the past but was unable to achieve a goal lipid profile. He now comes to you complaining of muscle cramps that are interfering with his quality of life. What might you suggest?

a. If CK levels are normal, retry another statin agent at a low dose. *(circled)*
b. Take him off Vytorin and give him monotherapy with Zetia.
c. IF CK levels are normal, start nicotinic acid.
d. Stop all hypolipidemic drugs and suggest diet and exercise alone.

22. Your 40-year-old female patient is overweight, smokes, has elevated BP readings, and has dyslipidemia. Because she is asymptomatic and has no family history of heart disease, she is reluctant to start any medication. She is particularly resistant to taking a statin because she is fearful of potential side effects. As the nurse practitioner, which strategy may be helpful in convincing the patient to start appropriate treatment for dyslipidemia?

a. Tell her you can treat her now or treat her later after she has her first MI.
b. Tell her that no one ever really gets side effects from these medications.
c. Don't bother trying to convince her because she's already made up her mind.
d. Calculate her ASCVD risk so she is aware of her actual risk for developing CAD. *(circled)*

23. Which one of the following groups of patients would not benefit from a statin?

a. Patients with clinical atherosclerotic cardiovascular disease
b. Patients without ASCVD or diabetes who are between the ages of 40 and 75 years with a 10-year ASCVD risk of 5% *(circled)*
c. Patients with primary elevations of LDL-C > 190 mg/dL
d. Diabetics aged 40–75 years with LDL-C between 70 and 189 mg/dL without clinical ASCVD

24. Which statement is correct regarding statin therapy?

a. High-intensity statin therapy will lower LDL-C by approximately 50%. *(circled)*
b. Low-intensity statin therapy will lower LDL-C by approximately 10%.
c. Low-intensity statin therapy should not be used for patients who cannot tolerate a high- or moderate-dose statin.
d. There is good evidence to support adding a nonstatin to a statin medication regimen to help reduce cardiovascular risk.

25. Which statement is accurate regarding recommended changes associated with the new dyslipidemia guidelines?
    a. There are no new recommendations for weight and lifestyle measures.
    b. Rather than monitoring lipid profile numbers, the new guidelines focus on understanding risk of ASCVD and trying to lower cholesterol numbers by a certain percentage based on that risk.
    c. Patients diagnosed with heart disease and diabetes may not need statin therapy.
    d. If providers follow the new guidelines, fewer patients will be placed on statin therapy.

26. Which statement is not accurate regarding hospitalization of patients with heart failure?
    a. Heart failure is the primary diagnosis in more than 1 million hospitalizations annually.
    b. Patients hospitalized for heart failure have a 1-month readmission rate of 25%.
    c. In 2013, office visits for heart failure cost $1.8 billion.
    d. The total cost of heart failure in the United States exceeds $30 billion annually; over 80% of this cost is spent on hospitalization.

27. Which one of the following is not a risk factor for heart failure?
    a. Hypertension
    b. Depression
    c. Chest pain
    d. Dyslipidemia

28. Which group of diagnostics is not indicated for the initial evaluation of heart failure?
    a. Lipid profile and urinalysis
    b. CBC, CMP, TSH
    c. ECG and 2D echo with color flow
    d. Radionuclide ventriculography or magnetic resonance imaging

29. Which statement is consistent with treatment recommendations for patients with heart failure?
    a. All patients with stage A heart failure should receive an ACE inhibitor.
    b. All patients with stage A heart failure should have hypertension and lipid disorders controlled in accordance with contemporary guidelines.
    c. Beta blockers should be avoided for patients with stage B heart failure.
    d. Combined use of an ACE inhibitor, an ARB, and an aldosterone inhibitor may be beneficial in patients with heart failure and a reduced ejection fraction.

30. Which of the following findings is useful in identifying patients with advanced heart failure?
    a. Progressive deterioration of renal function
    b. Frequent systolic BP less than 90 mm Hg
    c. The need to escalate diuretic treatment to maintain volume status
    d. All of the above

31. A 50-year-old man with alcohol-induced cardiomyopathy states that he becomes dyspneic even with walking to the bathroom but has no difficulty with shortness of breath when he is resting. Which of the following best describes his NYHA functional classification?
    a. I
    b. II
    c. III
    d. IV

32. You accept a new patient into your practice with NYHA class II heart failure. He has mild dyspnea and leg edema. You are working on titrating his medications up to target doses. How often will you schedule follow-up visits?
    a. Every 6 months
    b. Every 3 months
    c. Every 2–4 weeks
    d. Weekly

33. Which one of the following cardiac patients should not be evaluated in an outpatient setting?
    a. A 56-year-old patient with a history of HTN, COPD, and DM who complains of chest pain that occurred last evening
    b. A 76-year-old patient with chronic angina that hasn't changed in frequency or duration over the last year
    c. A 53-year-old patient who reports chest pain associated with syncope that occurred this morning
    d. A 42-year-old patient with mitral valve replacement requiring anticoagulation therapy

34. A 22-year-old otherwise healthy white female presents to the office with chest pressure, dizziness, numbness in both hands, and a feeling of impending doom, which began while walking in the mall. She takes no medication and her physical exam is normal. The most appropriate direction to take in the management plan would be which of the following?
    a. Exercise stress testing and echocardiography
    b. Empiric proton pump therapy
    c. Chest CT scan
    d. Reassurance plus a discussion of current life stressors

35. A 34-year-old male presents with substernal discomfort. The symptoms are worse after meals, particularly a heavy evening meal, and are sometimes associated with hot/sour fluid in the back of his throat along with nocturnal awakening. The patient denies difficulty swallowing, pain on swallowing, and weight loss. These symptoms have been present for 6 weeks. The patient also reports gaining 20 pounds in the past 2 years. Which of the following is the most appropriate initial approach?
    a. A therapeutic trial of an H_2 antagonist
    b. Exercise testing with thallium imaging
    c. CT scan of the chest
    d. Esophagogastroduodenoscopy

36. What ECG change would you expect to see in a patient with unstable angina?
    a. New onset of a right bundle branch block pattern
    b. Marked ST-T wave changes
    c. Significant Q waves
    d. Irregularly irregular heart rate

    See pg 515

37. Which statement is inconsistent with guideline recommendations for patients with stable ischemic heart disease?
    a. All patients should be counseled about the need for lifestyle modification, including weight control, increased physical activity, alcohol moderation, and sodium reduction.
    b. All patients should be treated for hypertension with a goal BP measurement of 120/90 mm Hg.
    c. It is reasonable to consider screening for depression and to refer and/or treat when indicated.
    d. Treatment with aspirin and clopidogrel may be reasonable in certain high-risk patients.

38. Which one of the following categories of medication should be prescribed as initial therapy for relief of ischemic symptoms in patients with stable ischemic heart disease?
    a. Calcium channel blockers
    b. Beta blockers
    c. Long-acting nitrates
    d. All of the above

    Beta blocker #1

39. Which of the following statements is consistent with current guidelines for the clinical evaluation of patients with chest pain?
    a. A thorough history and physical examination to assess for the probability of ischemic heart disease should be done prior to additional testing.
    b. A resting ECG is recommended in patients who do not have an obvious, noncardiac cause of chest pain.
    c. Standard exercise ECG testing is recommended for patients with a low pretest probability of ischemic heart disease, an interpretable ECG, and no disabling comorbidity.
    d. All of the above

40. What is the recommended follow-up for patients with ischemic heart disease?
    a. Periodic follow-ups should be at least annually.
    b. Surveillance should include monitoring for cardiac risk factors and complications, including heart failure and arrhythmias.
    c. Follow-up visits should assess for adequacy and adherence to recommended lifestyle changes and medical therapy.
    d. All of the above

Chapter 2: Answers and Rationales

1. C. Hospitalizations for atrial fibrillation have increased dramatically in recent years. The public health burden is expected to increase over the next decades.

Wattigney WA, Mensah GA, Croft JB. Increasing trends in hospitalization for atrial fibrillation in the United States, 1985 through 1999: implications for primary prevention. *Circulation.* 2003;108:711–716.

2. D. This patient's CHA_2DS_2-VASc score is 5 and is calculated as follows: hypertension $= 1$, diabetes $= 1$, age $> 75 = 2$, gender $= 1$. Based on the 2012 ESC Guidelines, this patient should be considered for oral anticoagulation for antithrombotic therapy for her atrial fibrillation.

January CT, Wann LS, Alpert JS, et al. 2014 AHA/ACC/HRS guideline for the management of patients with atrial fibrillation: executive summary. *J Am Coll Cardiol.* 2014; 64(21):2246–2280. http://content.onlinejacc.org/article.aspx?articleid=1854231. Accessed September 4, 2015.

ClinCalc. CHA_2DS_2-VASc calculator for atrial fibrillation. http://clincalc.com/Cardiology/Stroke/CHADSVASC.aspx. Accessed December 15, 2015.

3. D. Acceptance of atrial fibrillation (AF) represents a therapeutic attitude on the part of the patient and clinician rather than an inherent pathophysiologic attribute of this arrhythmia. According to the most recent guidelines, acceptance of AF may change as symptoms, efficacy of therapeutic interventions, and patient and clinician preferences evolve.

January CT, Wann LS, Alpert JS, et al. 2014 AHA/ACC/HRS guideline for the management of patients with atrial fibrillation: executive summary. *J Am Coll Cardiol.* 2014; 64(21):2246–2280. http://content.onlinejacc.org/article.aspx?articleid=1854231. Accessed September 4, 2015.

4. C. Exercise testing can be useful to evaluate the adequacy of rate control but is not considered part of the initial workup for atrial fibrillation.

January CT, Wann LS, Alpert JS, et al. 2014 AHA/ACC/HRS guideline for the management of patients with atrial fibrillation: executive summary. *J Am Coll Cardiol.* 2014; 64(21):2246–2280. http://content.onlinejacc.org/article.aspx?articleid=1854231. Accessed September 4, 2015.

5. D. Current guidelines do not recommend new novel agents for patients with mechanical valves. Warfarin is the treatment of choice for anticoagulation for patients with atrial fibrillation and mechanical valves because no data support using novel agents.

January CT, Wann LS, Alpert JS, et al. 2014 AHA/ACC/HRS guideline for the management of patients with atrial fibrillation: executive summary. *J Am Coll Cardiol.* 2014; 64(21):2246–2280. http://content.onlinejacc.org/article.aspx?articleid=1854231. Accessed September 4, 2015.

6. D. Situations which increase the risk of bleeding from anticoagulation should be evaluated carefully and may be an indication to withhold anticoagulation therapy.

January CT, Wann LS, Alpert JS, et al. 2014 AHA/ACC/HRS guideline for the management of patients with atrial fibrillation: executive summary. *J Am Coll Cardiol.* 2014; 64(21):2246–2280. http://content.onlinejacc.org/article.aspx ?articleid=1854231. Accessed September 4, 2015.

7. C. According to the HAS-BLED Bleeding Risk Score, abnormal electrolytes does not increase the risk for bleeding.

MDCalc. HAS-BLED score for major bleeding risk. http:// www.mdcalc.com/has-bled-score-for-major-bleeding-risk . Accessed December 15, 2015.

8. D. Patients who present with a rapid rate heart rate and who are hypotensive, as in this case, should be hospitalized for evaluation and treatment.

January CT, Wann LS, Alpert JS, et al. 2014 AHA/ACC/ HRS guideline for the management of patients with atrial fibrillation: executive summary. *J Am Coll Cardiol.* 2014; 64(21):2246–2280. http://content.onlinejacc.org/article.aspx ?articleid=1854231. Accessed September 4, 2015.

9. C. Young patients with atrial fibrillation (AF) may benefit from ablation because it is likely to remove the necessity for long-term medication therapy.

January CT, Wann LS, Alpert JS, et al. 2014 AHA/ACC/ HRS guideline for the management of patients with atrial fibrillation: executive summary. *J Am Coll Cardiol.* 2014; 64(21):2246–2280. http://content.onlinejacc.org/article.aspx? articleid=1854231. Accessed September 4, 2015.

10. C. Current guidelines recommend that in the general population older than 60 years, pharmacologic treatment should be initiated to treat a systolic blood pressure ≥ 150 mm Hg or a diastolic blood pressure ≥ 90 mm Hg as long as the patient doesn't have diabetes or chronic kidney disease.

James PA, Oparil S, Carter BL, et al. 2014 evidence-based guideline for the management of high blood pressure in adults: report from the panel members appointed to the Eighth Joint National Committee (JNC 8). *JAMA.* 2014; 311(5):507–520. http://jama.jamanetwork.com/article.aspx ?articleid=1791497. Accessed December 15, 2015.

11. D. The use of ambulatory blood pressure monitoring is not included in the 2014 guidelines for the management of high blood pressure in adults. In JNC-7 guidelines, ambulatory blood pressure monitoring is recommended for the evaluation of "white coat" hypertension in the absence of target organ injury. Ambulatory blood pressure monitoring provides information about BP during daily activities and during sleep.

Chobanian AV, Bakris GL, Black HR; Joint National Committee on Prevention, Detection, Evaluation, and Treatment of High Blood Pressure. National Heart, Lung, and Blood Institute; National High Blood Pressure Education Program Coordinating Committee. Seventh report of the Joint National Committee on Prevention, Detection, Evaluation, and Treatment of High Blood Pressure. *Hypertension.* 2003;42(6):1206–1252.

12. C. Calcium channel blockers and thiazide-type diuretics should be used instead of angiotensin-converting enzyme (ACE) inhibitors and angiotensin receptor blockers (ARBs) in patients older than the age of 75 years with impaired kidney function because of the risk of hyperkalemia, increased creatinine, and further renal impairment.

James PA, Oparil S, Carter BL, et al. 2014 evidence-based guideline for the management of high blood pressure in adults: report from the panel members appointed to the Eighth Joint National Committee (JNC 8). *JAMA.* 2014; 311(5):507–520. http://jama.jamanetwork.com/article.aspx ?articleid=1791497. Accessed December 15, 2015.

13. A. The urine albumin/creatinine ratio is used to screen patients with high blood pressure to identify early stages of kidney disease; it is not essential to have this result prior to initiating drug therapy for hypertension and is considered optional.

Chobanian AV, Bakris GL, Black HR; Joint National Committee on Prevention, Detection, Evaluation, and Treatment of High Blood Pressure. National Heart, Lung, and Blood Institute; National High Blood Pressure Education Program Coordinating Committee. Seventh report of the Joint National Committee on Prevention, Detection, Evaluation, and Treatment of High Blood Pressure. *Hypertension.* 2003;42(6):1206–1252. http://www.nhlbi.nih.gov/files/docs/ guidelines/express.pdf. Accessed December 15, 2015.

14. D. Evaluation of patients with documented hypertension should include all of the above to identify disorders that may affect prognosis and to guide treatment.

Chobanian AV, Bakris GL, Black HR; Joint National Committee on Prevention, Detection, Evaluation, and Treatment of High Blood Pressure. National Heart, Lung, and Blood Institute; National High Blood Pressure Education Program Coordinating Committee. Seventh report of the Joint National Committee on Prevention, Detection, Evaluation, and Treatment of High Blood Pressure. *Hypertension.* 2003;42(6):1206–1252. http://www.nhlbi.nih.gov/files/docs/ guidelines/express.pdf. Accessed December 15, 2015.

15. A. Beta blockers (BBs) are not recommended for initial treatment because in one study BB use resulted in a higher composite rate of cardiovascular death, myocardial infarction (MI), or stroke compared to use of angiotensin receptor blockers (ARBs). Other studies that compared BBs to the other four recommended drug classes showed that BBs performed similarly to the other drugs, or the evidence was insufficient to make a determination.

Dahlöf B, Devereux RB, Kjeldsen SE, et al; Life Study Group. Cardiovascular morbidity and mortality in the Losartan Intervention For Endpoint reduction in hypertension study (LIFE): a randomised trial against atenolol. *Lancet.* 2002: 359(9311):995–1003.

James PA, Oparil S, Carter BL, et al. 2014 evidence-based guideline for the management of high blood pressure in adults: report from the panel members appointed to the Eighth Joint National Committee (JNC 8). *JAMA*. 2014; 311(5):507–520. http://jama.jamanetwork.com/article.aspx ?articleid=1791497. Accessed December 15, 2015.

16. C. Left ventricular hypertrophy is evidence of target organ damage and may occur in patients with hypertension secondary to pressure or volume overload.

Chobanian AV, Bakris GL, Black HR; Joint National Committee on Prevention, Detection, Evaluation, and Treatment of High Blood Pressure. National Heart, Lung, and Blood Institute; National High Blood Pressure Education Program Coordinating Committee. Seventh report of the Joint National Committee on Prevention, Detection, Evaluation, and Treatment of High Blood Pressure. *Hypertension*. 2003;42(6):1206–1252. http://www.nhlbi.nih.gov/files/docs/ guidelines/express.pdf. Accessed December 15, 2015.

17. C. Adoption of a healthy lifestyle is paramount to the management of hypertension. It is recommended that dietary sodium intake be not more than 2.4 g of sodium daily. Dietary sodium reduction may reduce systolic blood pressure (BP) by 2 to 8 mm Hg.

Chobanian AV, Bakris GL, Black HR; Joint National Committee on Prevention, Detection, Evaluation, and Treatment of High Blood Pressure. National Heart, Lung, and Blood Institute; National High Blood Pressure Education Program Coordinating Committee. Seventh report of the Joint National Committee on Prevention, Detection, Evaluation, and Treatment of High Blood Pressure. *Hypertension*. 2003;42(6):1206–1252. http://www.nhlbi.nih.gov/files/docs/ guidelines/express.pdf. Accessed December 15, 2015.

18. B. Guidelines now recommend that atherosclerotic cardiovascular disease (ASCVD) risk be calculated on all patients prior to initiating treatment. However, this patient is in a high-risk category because of his history of coronary artery disease and should be on a statin medication. He should be encouraged to continue his healthy lifestyle.

Stone NJ, Robinson JG, Lichtenstein AH, et al; American College of Cardiology/American Heart Association Task Force on Practice Guidelines. 2013 ACC/AHA guideline on the treatment of blood cholesterol to reduce atherosclerotic cardiovascular risk in adults: a report of the American College of Cardiology/American Heart Association Task Force on Practice Guidelines. *J Am Coll Cardiol*. 2014;63(25 Pt B): 2889–2934. doi:10.1016/j.jacc.2013.11.002.

19. D. Guidelines now recommend that atherosclerotic cardiovascular disease (ASCVD) risk be calculated on all patients prior to initiating treatment.

Stone NJ, Robinson JG, Lichtenstein AH, et al; American College of Cardiology/American Heart Association Task

Force on Practice Guidelines. 2013 ACC/AHA guideline on the treatment of blood cholesterol to reduce atherosclerotic cardiovascular risk in adults: a report of the American College of Cardiology/American Heart Association Task Force on Practice Guidelines. *J Am Coll Cardiol*. 2014;63(25 Pt B): 2889–2934. doi:10.1016/j.jacc.2013.11.002.

20. B. When triglyceride levels exceed 500 mg/dL, a fenofibrate is a reasonable treatment choice to reduce triglyceride levels. Omega-3 fatty acids are unlikely to achieve a meaningful drop in levels this high.

Stone NJ, Robinson JG, Lichtenstein AH, et al; American College of Cardiology/American Heart Association Task Force on Practice Guidelines. 2013 ACC/AHA guideline on the treatment of blood cholesterol to reduce atherosclerotic cardiovascular risk in adults: a report of the American College of Cardiology/American Heart Association Task Force on Practice Guidelines. *J Am Coll Cardiol*. 2014;63(25 Pt B): 2889–2934. doi:10.1016/j.jacc.2013.11.002.

21. A. This patient is in one of the four groups that have compelling indications for statin therapy because he has clinical atherosclerotic cardiovascular disease (ASCVD). He may be able to tolerate a different statin agent at a lower dose.

Stone NJ, Robinson JG, Lichtenstein AH, et al; American College of Cardiology/American Heart Association Task Force on Practice Guidelines. 2013 ACC/AHA guideline on the treatment of blood cholesterol to reduce atherosclerotic cardiovascular risk in adults: a report of the American College of Cardiology/American Heart Association Task Force on Practice Guidelines. *J Am Coll Cardiol*. 2014;63(25 Pt B): 2889–2934. doi:10.1016/j.jacc.2013.11.002.

22. D. Guidelines now recommend that atherosclerotic cardiovascular disease (ASCVD) risk be calculated on all patients prior to initiating treatment. Calculating and discussing her ASCVD risk score will enable this patient to make an informed decision about whether she is willing to start medication to reduce her risk.

Stone NJ, Robinson JG, Lichtenstein AH, et al; American College of Cardiology/American Heart Association Task Force on Practice Guidelines. 2013 ACC/AHA guideline on the treatment of blood cholesterol to reduce atherosclerotic cardiovascular risk in adults: a report of the American College of Cardiology/American Heart Association Task Force on Practice Guidelines. *J Am Coll Cardiol*. 2014;63(25 Pt B): 2889–2934. doi:10.1016/j.jacc.2013.11.002.

23. B. According to the newest guidelines, statins should be initiated when the atherosclerotic cardiovascular disease (ASCVD) risk score is 7.5% or higher in patients with no comorbid conditions. Therapeutic lifestyle instructions should be recommended to this patient.

Stone NJ, Robinson JG, Lichtenstein AH, et al; American College of Cardiology/American Heart Association Task

Force on Practice Guidelines. 2013 ACC/AHA guideline on the treatment of blood cholesterol to reduce atherosclerotic cardiovascular risk in adults: a report of the American College of Cardiology/American Heart Association Task Force on Practice Guidelines. *J Am Coll Cardiol.* 2014;63(25 Pt B): 2889–2934. doi:10.1016/j.jacc.2013.11.002.

24. A. Daily doses of high-intensity statin therapy are estimated to lower LDL-C on average by ≥ 50%. High-intensity statins include atorvastatin 40–80 mg and rosuvastatin 20–40 mg.

    Stone NJ, Robinson JG, Lichtenstein AH, et al; American College of Cardiology/American Heart Association Task Force on Practice Guidelines. 2013 ACC/AHA guideline on the treatment of blood cholesterol to reduce atherosclerotic cardiovascular risk in adults: a report of the American College of Cardiology/American Heart Association Task Force on Practice Guidelines. *J Am Coll Cardiol.* 2014;63(25 Pt B): 2889–2934. doi:10.1016/j.jacc.2013.11.002.

25. B. Guidelines now recommend that atherosclerotic cardiovascular disease (ASCVD) risk be calculated on all patients prior to initiating treatment. The expert panel defined the intensity of statin therapy based on the average expected LDL-C response to a specific statin and dose.

    Stone NJ, Robinson JG, Lichtenstein AH, et al; American College of Cardiology/American Heart Association Task Force on Practice Guidelines. 2013 ACC/AHA guideline on the treatment of blood cholesterol to reduce atherosclerotic cardiovascular risk in adults: a report of the American College of Cardiology/American Heart Association Task Force on Practice Guidelines. *J Am Coll Cardiol.* 2014;63(25 Pt B): 2889–2934. doi:10.1016/j.jacc.2013.11.002.

26. D. Heart failure is the primary diagnosis in > 1 million hospitalizations annually. The total cost of heart failure exceeds $30 billion annually in the United States, but about half of these costs are spent on hospitalization.

    Yancy CW, Jessup M, Bozkurt B, et al; American College of Cardiology Foundation; American Heart Association Task Force on Practice Guidelines. 2013 ACCF/AHA guideline for the management of heart failure: a report of the American College of Cardiology Foundation/American Heart Association Task Force on Practice Guidelines. *J Am Coll Cardiol.* 2013;62(16):e147–239. doi:10.1016/j.jacc.2013.05.019.

27. C. Many conditions or comorbidities are associated with an increased risk for structural heart disease. Identification of these conditions may help to forestall the onset of heart failure. Chest pain, in and of itself, is not a risk factor because it may be secondary to many causes. Patients with known atherosclerotic disease are likely to develop heart failure.

    Yancy CW, Jessup M, Bozkurt B, et al; American College of Cardiology Foundation; American Heart Association Task Force on Practice Guidelines. 2013 ACCF/AHA guideline for the management of heart failure: a report of the American College of Cardiology Foundation/

American Heart Association Task Force on Practice Guidelines. *J Am Coll Cardiol.* 2013;62(16):e147–239. doi:10.1016/j.jacc.2013.05.019.

28. D. Radionuclide ventriculography or magnetic resonance imaging can be useful to assess left ventricular ejection fraction (LVEF) and volume when echocardiography is inadequate. It is not indicated for the initial evaluation of heart failure. (Level of Evidence: C.)

    Yancy CW, Jessup M, Bozkurt B, et al; American College of Cardiology Foundation; American Heart Association Task Force on Practice Guidelines. 2013 ACCF/AHA guideline for the management of heart failure: a report of the American College of Cardiology Foundation/American Heart Association Task Force on Practice Guidelines. *J Am Coll Cardiol.* 2013;62(16):e147–239. doi:10.1016/j.jacc.2013.05.019.

29. B. Patients with stage A heart failure do not have structural heart disease and are asymptomatic. Hypertension and lipid disorders should be controlled according to the most recent guidelines to lower the risk of developing heart failure.

    Yancy CW, Jessup M, Bozkurt B, et al; American College of Cardiology Foundation; American Heart Association Task Force on Practice Guidelines. 2013 ACCF/AHA guideline for the management of heart failure: a report of the American College of Cardiology Foundation/American Heart Association Task Force on Practice Guidelines. *J Am Coll Cardiol.* 2013;62(16):e147–239. doi:10.1016/j.jacc.2013.05.019.

30. D. Progressive decline in labs or vital signs and the need to increase medications to control symptoms are indicators of advancing heart failure.

    Yancy CW, Jessup M, Bozkurt B, et al; American College of Cardiology Foundation; American Heart Association Task Force on Practice Guidelines. 2013 ACCF/AHA guideline for the management of heart failure: a report of the American College of Cardiology Foundation/American Heart Association Task Force on Practice Guidelines. *J Am Coll Cardiol.* 2013;62(16):e147–239. doi:10.1016/j.jacc.2013.05.019.

31. C. This patient's symptoms are consistent with the defining characteristics of Stage III New York Heart Association (NYHA) Functional Classification, including marked limitation of physical activity, comfortable at rest, but less than ordinary activity causes symptoms of heart failure.

    Yancy CW, Jessup M, Bozkurt B, et al; American College of Cardiology Foundation; American Heart Association Task Force on Practice Guidelines. 2013 ACCF/AHA guideline for the management of heart failure: a report of the American College of Cardiology Foundation/American Heart Association Task Force on Practice Guidelines. *J Am Coll Cardiol.* 2013;62(16):e147–239. doi:10.1016/j.jacc.2013.05.019.

32. C. Titrating of medications requires careful monitoring, and patients should be evaluated frequently so that efficacy of treatment and changes in medications can be measured and initiated in a timely fashion. Although follow-up visits must

be assessed on an individual basis, every 2–4 weeks is reasonable for many patients.

Yancy CW, Jessup M, Bozkurt B, et al; American College of Cardiology Foundation; American Heart Association Task Force on Practice Guidelines. 2013 ACCF/AHA guideline for the management of heart failure: a report of the American College of Cardiology Foundation/American Heart Association Task Force on Practice Guidelines. *J Am Coll Cardiol.* 2013;62(16):e147–239. doi:10.1016/j.jacc.2013.05.019.

33. C. Patients with chest pain and syncope are likely to have a cardiac reason for their symptoms, including structural heart disease, pulmonary embolus, or acute myocardial infarction. These patients should be hospitalized for evaluation because they are high risk for poor outcomes.

Gauer RL. Evaluation of syncope. *Am Fam Physician.* 2011; 84:640–650.

34. D. This patient's clinical presentation is likely caused by a panic attack, not a cardiac problem. Generalized anxiety disorder and panic disorder are among the most common mental disorders in the United States. Evaluation of stressors and management to reduce anxiety is recommended.

Locke AB, Kirst N, Shultz CG. Diagnosis and management of generalized anxiety disorder and panic disorder in adults. *Am Fam Physician.* 2015;91:617–624.

35. A. This patient's clinical presentation is likely caused by a gastric esophageal reflux, not a cardiac problem. A therapeutic trial of an H_2 antagonist is first-line treatment.

Katz PO, Gerson LB, Vela MF. Diagnosis and management of gastroesophageal reflux disease. *Am J Gastroenterol.* 2013;108:308–328. http://gi.org/guideline/diagnosis-and-managemen-of-gastroesophageal-reflux-disease/. Accessed December 15, 2015.

36. B. Patients with unstable angina may present with transient ST-segment elevation, ST-segment depression more than 1 mm, or deep symmetrical T wave inversion.

Wadud A. What is unstable angina? 2014. http://nstemi.org/unstable-angina/. Accessed December 15, 2015.

37. B. In patients with stable ischemic heart disease (SIHD) with a blood pressure (BP) of 140/90 mm Hg or higher, antihypertensive drug therapy should be initiated in addition to, or after, a trial of lifestyle modification. Specific treatment goals for patients with chronic IHD remain controversial.

Fihn SD, Gardin JM, Abrams J; American College of Cardiology Foundation/American Heart Association Task Force. 2012 ACCF/AHA/ACP/AATS/PCNA/SCAI/STS guideline for the diagnosis and management of patients with stable ischemic heart disease. *Circulation.* April 22, 2014;129(16):e463. http://content.onlinejacc.org/article.aspx?articleid=1391404. Accessed December 15, 2015.

38. B. Beta blockers are recommended as the initial agents to relieve symptoms in most patients with stable ischemic heart disease (SIHD). Long-term beta-blocker treatment is well

tolerated and has proven beneficial in SIHD by reducing ischemic burden and threshold and improving survival in patients with left ventricular (LV) dysfunction or a history of myocardial infarction.

Fihn SD, Gardin JM, Abrams J; American College of Cardiology Foundation/American Heart Association Task Force. 2012 ACCF/AHA/ACP/AATS/PCNA/SCAI/STS guideline for the diagnosis and management of patients with stable ischemic heart disease. *Circulation.* April 22, 2014;129(16):e463. http://content.onlinejacc.org/article.aspx?articleid=1391404. Accessed December 15, 2015.

39. D. History, physical exam, electrocardiogram (ECG), and stress testing are all important components of the diagnostic workup of chest pain. Patients who are unable to exercise should receive chemical stress testing.

Fihn SD, Gardin JM, Abrams J; American College of Cardiology Foundation/American Heart Association Task Force. 2012 ACCF/AHA/ACP/AATS/PCNA/SCAI/STS guideline for the diagnosis and management of patients with stable ischemic heart disease. *Circulation.* April 22, 2014;129(16):e463. http://content.onlinejacc.org/article.aspx?articleid=1391404. Accessed December 15, 2015.

40. D. Patients with ischemic heart disease should receive regular follow-up to monitor symptoms and progression of disease. Follow-up should occur at least annually and should focus on assessment for new risk factors, monitoring and counseling regarding therapeutic lifestyle measures, and ensuring that medical management is optimal.

Fihn SD, Gardin JM, Abrams J; American College of Cardiology Foundation/American Heart Association Task Force. 2012 ACCF/AHA/ACP/AATS/PCNA/SCAI/STS guideline for the diagnosis and management of patients with stable ischemic heart disease. *Circulation.* April 22, 2014;129(16):e463. http://content.onlinejacc.org/article.aspx?articleid=1391404. Accessed December 15, 2015.

Chapter 3: Common Respiratory Disorders in Primary Care

1. A 44-year-old man has a long-standing history of moderate persistent asthma that is normally well controlled by fluticasone with salmeterol (Advair) via metered-dose inhaler, one puff twice daily, and the use of albuterol 1 to 2 times a week as needed for wheezing. Three days ago he developed a sore throat, clear nasal discharge, body aches, and a dry cough. In the past 24 hours, he has had intermittent wheezing that necessitated the use of albuterol, 2 puffs every 3 hours, which produced partial relief. Your next most appropriate action is to obtain a:

a. Chest X-ray
b. Measurement of oxygen saturation (SaO_2)
c. Peak expiratory flow (PEF) measurement
d. Sputum smear for white blood cells (WBCs)

helps to determine severity of exacerbations

2. You examine a 24-year-old woman who presents with an acute asthma flare. She is using budesonide (Pulmicort) and albuterol as directed and continues to have difficulty with coughing and wheezing. Today she reports her dyspnea is interfering with her usual activity, and her PEF is 55% of predicted level. Her medication regimen should be adjusted to include:
   a. Theophylline
   b. Salmeterol (Serevent)
   c. Prednisone
   d. Montelukast (Singulair)

3. Which of the following is most likely to appear on chest radiography of a person during an acute asthma attack?
   a. Hyperinflation
   b. Atelectasis
   c. Consolidation
   d. Kerley B signs

   Narrowing of airway causes hyperinflation

4. Which of the following is not consistent with the diagnosis of asthma?
   a. A troublesome nocturnal cough
   b. Cough or wheeze after exercise
   c. Morning sputum production
   d. Colds that "go to the chest" or take more than 10 days to clear

   Sputum not likely c̄ asthma as its chronic.
   Likely Viral

5. The cornerstone of moderate persistent asthma drug therapy is the use of:
   a. Oral theophylline
   b. Mast cell stabilizers
   c. Short-acting beta agonists
   d. Inhaled corticosteroids → *used for long term control of asthma*

6. Sharon is a 29-year-old woman with moderate persistent asthma. She is not using prescribed inhaled corticosteroids but is using albuterol PRN to relieve her cough and wheeze. Currently, she uses about two albuterol metered-dose inhalers per month and is requesting a prescription refill. You respond that:
   a. Albuterol use may be continued.
   b. Excessive albuterol use is associated with an increased risk of an acute exacerbation that requires an ED visit or hospitalization.
   c. She should also use salmeterol (Serevent) to reduce her albuterol use.
   d. Theophylline should be added to her treatment plan.

7. An 18-year-old high school senior presents asking for a letter stating that he should not participate in gym class because he has asthma. The most appropriate response is to:
   a. Write the note because gym class participation may trigger an asthma flare
   b. Excuse him from outdoor activities only in order to avoid pollen exposure
   c. Remind him that with appropriate asthma care he should be capable of participating in gym class
   d. Excuse him from indoor activities only in order to avoid dust mite exposure

8. What is the most accurate method of classifying the severity of chronic obstructive pulmonary disease (COPD)?
   a. Assessment of airflow limitation using spirometry
   b. Dyspnea on exhalation
   c. Elevated diaphragms noted on X-ray
   d. Polycythemia noted on complete blood cell count

9. Which of the following symptoms should prompt the NP to consider a diagnosis of COPD?
   a. Dyspnea which is intermittent and doesn't worsen over time
   b. Chronic cough which may be intermittent and may be unproductive or productive
   c. History of exposure to animals
   d. Family history of celiac disease

10. According to the GOLD COPD guidelines, which of the following medications are indicated for all patients with Stages II to IV COPD?
    a. Inhaled bronchodilators
    b. Inhaled corticosteroids
    c. Mucolytic agents
    d. Theophylline

11. Inhaled corticosteroids may be used in COPD patients. Which statement regarding these medications is not consistent with GOLD guidelines?
    a. COPD patients with FEV_1 < 80 predicted may benefit from regular treatment with inhaled corticosteroids.
    b. Inhaled corticosteroids may improve quality of life in patients with COPD.
    c. Inhaled corticosteroids are associated with an increased risk of pneumonia.
    d. Withdrawal from treatment with inhaled corticosteroids may lead to exacerbations in some patients.

    see pg.

12. Which of the following symptoms signals that antibiotics should be prescribed for an exacerbation of COPD?
    a. Increased dyspnea
    b. Increased sputum volume
    c. Increased sputum purulence
    d. All of the above

13. It's early October and many of your patients are requesting a seasonal flu vaccine. Which one of the following patients should not be given the vaccine requested?
    a. A 36-year-old female with a fish allergy
    b. A 28-year-old female and her 2-year-old daughter
    c. An 18-year-old male with minor cold symptoms and a low-grade fever 2 days ago
    d. A 72-year-old man who wants nasal spray flu vaccine because he "hates shots"

    nasal spray approved 2-49

14. The severity of influenza in a given year is related to:
    a. How well the vaccine is matched to the influenza viruses causing illness
    b. The availability of the vaccine, including time and amount
    c. The number of people who get vaccinated
    d. All of the above

15. Common signs and symptoms of influenza include all of the following *except*:
a. Fever, cough, and chills
b. Runny nose and sore throat
c. Vomiting and diarrhea
d. Muscle aches and headache

16. Complications of influenza include all of the following *except*:
a. Bacterial pneumonia and death
b. Ear and sinus infections
c. Worsening of CHF and asthma
d. All of the above

17. Which of the following statements is accurate regarding influenza vaccination?
a. Patients ideally should be vaccinated yearly in early October.
b. All trivalent and quadrivalent vaccines are appropriate for all age groups.
c. The trivalent vaccine protects against two influenza A and influenza B viruses.
d. Patients who are allergic to eggs cannot be vaccinated for influenza.

18. Which one of the following statements is inaccurate regarding acute uncomplicated bronchitis?
a. Cough is the most common symptom for which adult patients visit their primary care provider.
b. Evaluation of patients with suspected acute uncomplicated bronchitis should focus on ruling out pneumonia.
c. Colored sputum always indicates a bacterial infection.
d. In most cases, a chest X-ray is not indicated for the diagnosis of acute uncomplicated bronchitis.

19. Which one of the following treatment options for acute uncomplicated bronchitis is not consistent with CDC guidelines?
a. Cough suppressants
b. First-generation antihistamines
c. Decongestants
d. Antibiotics

20. The absence of which finding strongly suggests a pulmonary cause of dyspnea with coexisting COPD and heart failure?
a. Feeling of suffocation
b. Pursed-lip breathing
c. Orthopnea
d. Tripod positioning

21. Under the most recent CDC guidelines, which of the following patients with latent TB infection (LTBI) is considered ineligible for the 12-week DOT of INH-RPT therapy?
a. A 32-year-old patient with HIV and a CD4 count of 600 who is currently receiving antiretroviral therapy
b. A 13-year-old healthy patient with conversion of tuberculin skin test from negative to positive and exposure to contagious TB

c. A 45-year-old HIV-positive prisoner not taking antiretroviral treatment who was exposed to contagious TB
d. A 28-year-old homeless patient with healed pulmonary TB on X-ray and conversion to positive tuberculin skin test

22. A 50-year-old man with LTBI is started on 12 weeks of DOT with (isoniazid and rifapentine) NIH-RPT. Which of the following is not considered a requirement for monitoring therapy?
a. Routine liver function monitoring at baseline and 4, 8, and 12 weeks
b. Discontinuation of therapy if AST level is 5 times or higher than normal without symptoms
c. Vigilance for hypersensitivity reactions
d. Monthly patient interview and physical exam

23. According to the National Comprehensive Cancer Network guidelines, which one of the following patients should have low-dose CT screening for lung cancer?
a. All patients with a 10-pack-year smoking history
b. A 73-year-old male with a 20-pack-year smoking history and smoking cessation for 8 years
c. A 45-year-old male with a 15-pack-year smoking history and COPD
d. None of the above

24. In the United States, the majority of lung cancers are directly related to:
a. Environmental exposure
b. Tobacco smoking
c. Alpha-1 antitrypsin deficiency
d. Asbestosis

25. Which one of the following severity-of-illness scores can be used to identify patients with community-acquired pneumonia (CAP) who may be candidates for outpatient treatment?
a. Disease Risk Index
b. ASCVD risk score
c. CURB-65 criteria
d. CHADS$_2$ score

Confusion, RR, uremia, BP, age 65 or older Scoring System to determine if outpatient tx of CAP

26. Which one of the following statements is inaccurate regarding pneumococcal disease?
a. Pneumococcal meningitis can cause hearing loss, seizures, blindness, and paralysis.
b. Symptoms are usually gradual in nature.
c. In the elderly, symptoms may be atypical.
d. Eighty-five percent of invasive pneumococcal disease occurs in adults.

27. The CDC recommends only the 23-valent pneumococcal polysaccharide vaccine (PPSV23) for which one of the following types of patients?
a. All cigarette smokers
b. All patients 65 years and older
c. Residents of long-term or chronic care facilities
d. All of the above

28. The CDC recommends both the 23-valent pneumococcal polysaccharide vaccine (PPSV23) and the 13-valent pneumococcal conjugate vaccine (PCV13) for all of the following patients *except*:
    a. Patients 19 years and older with immunocompromising conditions
    b. Patients 19 years and older with functional or anatomic asplenia
    c. Patients 19 years and older who are Alaska Native and/or American Indian
    d. Patients 19 years and older with cochlear implants or cerebrospinal fluid leaks

29. According to the Infectious Diseases Society of America and the American Thoracic Society consensus guideline, which statement regarding diagnostic testing for etiology of community-acquired pneumonia is unsupported?
    a. Routine diagnostic tests to identify an etiology are optional for outpatients with CAP.
    b. Pretreatment Gram stain and culture of expectorated sputum should always be collected prior to initiation of antibiotic treatment.
    c. Patients with CAP should be investigated for specific pathogens that would significantly alter standard empirical management decisions.
    d. Hospitalized patients who are critically ill with CAP are candidates for extensive diagnostic testing.

30. Which outpatient treatment option for CAP is not consistent with the Infectious Diseases Society of America and the American Thoracic Society consensus guideline?
    a. A macrolide is an appropriate antibiotic for the outpatient treatment of CAP in a previously healthy patient who has not used antimicrobials within the last 3 months.
    b. In patients with comorbidities such as diabetes or immunosuppressive conditions, a respiratory fluoroquinolone is appropriate outpatient therapy for the treatment of CAP.
    c. In patients who have used antimicrobials within the previous 3 months, a beta-lactam plus a macrolide is appropriate therapy for the outpatient treatment of CAP.
    d. Vancomycin is an appropriate antibiotic for the outpatient treatment of CAP for patients allergic to penicillin.

31. Criteria indicating clinical instability in a patient with CAP include all of the following *except*:
    a. Temperature $\leq 36°C$
    b. Heart rate ≥ 110 beats/minute
    c. Normal mental status
    d. Systolic blood pressure 90 mm Hg

32. Which pathogens are most likely responsible for CAP in patients with COPD and/or smokers?
    a. *Haemophilus influenzae, Streptococcus pneumoniae, Moraxella catarrhalis,* and *Chlamydia pneumoniae*
    b. Oral anaerobes

    c. *Bordetella pertussis* and *Pseudomonas aeruginosa*
    d. CA-MRSA, oral anaerobes, and fungal pneumonia

33. According to the updated 2015 GOLD guidelines, which of the following should be assessed for a new patient known or thought to have COPD?
    a. Pattern of symptom development
    b. Social and family support available to the patient
    c. Impact of the disease on quality of life
    d. All of the above

34. Which one of the following is not consistent with the yellow zone on the Asthma Action Plan?
    a. Symptoms such as cough, wheeze, chest tightness, or shortness of breath
    b. Waking at night because of symptoms
    c. Peak flow 50–79% of the patient's best peak flow measurement
    d. Quick-relief medications have not helped *(Red zone)*

35. What is the purpose of the COPD Assessment Test (CAT)?
    a. To determine health status impairment in patients with COPD
    b. To measure clinical control in patients with COPD
    c. To determine exacerbation risk in patients with COPD
    d. To measure severity of airflow limitation

36. Chest X-ray findings associated with COPD include all of the following *except*:
    a. Elevated diaphragm on the lateral chest film
    b. Increased volume of the retrosternal air space
    c. Hyperlucency of the lung
    d. Rapid tapering of the vascular markings

37. Which one of the following interventions has the greatest capacity to influence the natural history of COPD?
    a. Oxygen therapy
    b. Smoking cessation
    c. Influenza and pneumococcal vaccinations
    d. Long-term steroids

38. Your 76-year-old patient comes to the office today complaining of increasing SOB, chest pain, tachycardia, and blood-tinged sputum. She is currently treated with dabigatran for atrial fibrillation. She admits to not taking this medication for the last month. Which diagnostic test should be ordered?
    a. MRA of the pulmonary arteries with and without contrast
    b. Ultrasound of the lower extremities with Doppler
    c. CT pulmonary angiogram with contrast
    d. Transesophageal echocardiogram

39. The pulmonary embolism rule-out criteria (PERC) is a clinical prediction rule that can help exclude the presence of pulmonary embolism. Which variable is not consistent with the PERC tool?
    a. Pulse rate > 99 beats per minute
    b. Patient age > 65 years
    c. Patient taking exogenous estrogen
    d. History of surgery or trauma requiring hospitalization in the past 4 weeks

40. Which statement regarding obstructive sleep apnea <u>is not</u> <u>consistent</u> with the 2013 American College of Physicians clinical guidelines for sleep apnea?

    a. OSA is caused by obstruction of the upper airway during sleep that causes reduced or transient complete airflow cessation.

    b. Common symptoms include daytime sleepiness, unrefreshing sleep, insomnia, and snoring.

    c. Adverse clinical outcomes of OSA include cardiovascular disease, hypertension, cognitive impairment, and metabolic abnormalities.

    d. All smokers should get screening polysomnography to rule out OSA.

Chapter 3: Answers and Rationales

1. C. Peak flow monitoring during exacerbations helps determine the severity of the exacerbation and guide therapeutic decisions.

National Heart, Lung, and Blood Institute. *Expert Panel Report 3: guidelines for the diagnosis and management of asthma.* https://www.nhlbi.nih.gov/files/docs/guidelines/04_sec3_comp.pdf. Accessed September 16, 2015.

2. C. Oral systemic corticosteroids should be initiated with careful monitoring of symptoms; some symptoms may last for 1–2 days. Instruct the patient to go to the emergency department (ED) if symptoms worsen or don't improve significantly. Follow-up visit in 1 month.

National Heart, Lung, and Blood Institute. *Expert Panel Report 3: guidelines for the diagnosis and management of asthma.* https://www.nhlbi.nih.gov/files/docs/guidelines/04_sec3_comp.pdf. Accessed September 16, 2015.

3. A. The narrowing of airways causes lung hyperinflation.

Langer D, Ciavaglia CE, Neder JA, Webb KA, O'Donnell DE. Lung hyperinflation in chronic obstructive pulmonary disease: mechanisms, clinical implications and treatment. *Expert Rev Resp Med.* 2014;8:731–749.

4. C. Sputum production is not expected in asthma patients because the pathophysiology of this disease is a chronic inflammatory disorder. Consider a viral respiratory infection if sputum production occurs.

National Heart, Lung, and Blood Institute. *Expert Panel Report 3: guidelines for the diagnosis and management of asthma.* https://www.nhlbi.nih.gov/files/docs/guidelines/03_sec2_def.pdf. Accessed December 21, 2015.

5. D. Inhaled corticosteroids are used in the long-term control of asthma because they block late reactions to allergens, reduce airway hyperresponsiveness, and inhibit inflammatory cell migration and activation.

National Heart, Lung, and Blood Institute. *Expert Panel Report 3: guidelines for the diagnosis and management of asthma.*

https://www.nhlbi.nih.gov/files/docs/guidelines/07_sec3_comp4.pdf. Accessed December 21, 2015.

6. B. Use of two albuterol metered-dose inhalers per month is an excessive amount of rescue medication and is an indication that asthma control has not been achieved. It's important that the patient understand that excessive use of rescue medications can have serious side effects, including death.

National Heart, Lung, and Blood Institute. *Expert Panel Report 3: guidelines for the diagnosis and management of asthma.* http://www.nhlbi.nih.gov/files/docs/guidelines/07_sec3_comp4.pdf. Accessed December 21, 2015.

7. C. When asthma is well controlled, it is expected that patients can routinely participate in normal daily activities, including exercise. Education is an important component of quality asthma care.

National Heart, Lung, and Blood Institute. Expert Panel Report 3: guidelines for the diagnosis and management of asthma. http://www.nhlbi.nih.gov/health-pro/guidelines/current/asthma-guidelines. Accessed December 21, 2015.

8. A. The classification of severity of COPD is based on the degree of airflow limitation and is defined as mild, moderate, severe, and very severe on the basis of postbronchodilator FEV_1 on spirometry.

Global Initiative for Chronic Obstructive Lung Disease. *Pocket Guide to COPD Diagnosis, Management, and Prevention.* http://www.goldcopd.org/uploads/users/files/GOLD_Pocket_2015_Feb18.pdf. Accessed December 21, 2015.

9. B. In patients with chronic cough, COPD should be considered in the differential diagnosis. Any pattern of chronic sputum production may indicate COPD, but some patients may have an unproductive cough.

Global Initiative for Chronic Obstructive Lung Disease. *Pocket Guide to COPD Diagnosis, Management, and Prevention.* http://www.goldcopd.org/uploads/users/files/GOLD_Pocket_2015_Feb18.pdf. Accessed December 21, 2015.

10. A. Pharmacologic therapy is used to reduce symptoms, reduce frequency and severity of exacerbations, and improve health and exercise tolerance. Bronchodilators are central to symptom management in COPD.

Global Initiative for Chronic Obstructive Lung Disease. *Pocket Guide to COPD Diagnosis, Management, and Prevention.* http://www.goldcopd.org/uploads/users/files/GOLD_Pocket_2015_Feb18.pdf. Accessed December 21, 2015.

11. A. COPD patients with $FEV_1 < 60$ predicted may benefit from regular treatment with inhaled corticosteroids.

Global Initiative for Chronic Obstructive Lung Disease. *Pocket Guide to COPD Diagnosis, Management, and Prevention.* http://www.goldcopd.org/uploads/users/files/GOLD_Pocket_2015_Feb18.pdf. Accessed December 21, 2015.

12. D. The three cardinal symptoms that require antibiotic therapy are increased dyspnea, sputum volume, and sputum purulence. The GOLD guidelines recommend treatment when all three cardinal symptoms are present, when there is increased sputum purulence and one other cardinal symptom, and in patients who require mechanical ventilation.

Global Initiative for Chronic Obstructive Lung Disease. *Pocket Guide to COPD Diagnosis, Management, and Prevention.* http://www.goldcopd. org/uploads/users/files/GOLD_ Pocket_2015_Feb18.pdf. Accessed December 21, 2015.

13. D. The nasal spray vaccine is approved for use only in people ages 2 through 49 years.

Centers for Disease Control and Prevention. Influenza (flu): key facts about influenza (flu) and flu vaccine. http://www .cdc.gov/flu/keyfacts.htm. Accessed December 21, 2015.

14. D. How well the flu vaccine works varies from season to season. All the factors listed in the question affect the severity of influenza in a given community. During years when the flu vaccine is not well matched to circulating viruses, it is possible that no benefit from flu vaccination may be observed. During years when there is a good match between the flu vaccine and circulating viruses, there are substantial benefits from vaccination in terms of preventing flu illness.

Centers for Disease Control and Prevention. Influenza (flu): key facts about influenza (flu) and flu vaccine. http://www .cdc.gov/flu/keyfacts.htm. Accessed December 21, 2015.

15. C. Vomiting and diarrhea may sometimes occur but more commonly in children than in adults.

Centers for Disease Control and Prevention. Influenza (flu): key facts about influenza (flu) and flu vaccine. http://www .cdc.gov/flu/keyfacts.htm. Accessed December 21, 2015.

16. D. Influenza can cause all of the complications listed in the question. Certain people are at a greater risk for serious complications if they get the flu including older people, young children, pregnant women, and people with asthma, diabetes, or heart disease.

Centers for Disease Control and Prevention. Influenza (flu): key facts about influenza (flu) and flu vaccine. http://www .cdc.gov/flu/keyfacts.htm. Accessed December 21, 2015.

17. A. The ideal time to get vaccinated is early October. Getting vaccinated later can be protective as long as flu viruses are in circulation. Influenza activity peaks in January or later, and it is recommended that people get vaccinated early before influenza begins spreading to the community.

Centers for Disease Control and Prevention. Influenza (flu): key facts about influenza (flu) and flu vaccine. http://www .cdc.gov/flu/keyfacts.htm. Accessed December 21, 2015.

18. C. The presence or absence of colored sputum does not reliably differentiate between bacterial and viral respiratory tract infections.

Albert RH. Diagnosis and treatment of acute bronchitis. *Am Fam Physician.* 2010;82:1345–1350.

19. D. Antibiotics are generally not indicated for bronchitis and should only be used if pertussis is suspected to reduce transmission or if the patient is at an increased risk of developing pneumonia.

Albert RH. Diagnosis and treatment of acute bronchitis. *Am Fam Physician.* 2010;82:1345–1350.

Centers for Disease Control and Prevention. Acute cough illness (acute bronchitis) physician information sheet (adults). http:// www.cdc.gov/getsmart/community/materials-references/ print-materials/hcp/adult-acute-cough-illness.html. Accessed September 16, 2015.

20. C. Orthopnea is an early symptom of heart failure and occurs rapidly with recumbency.

Dumitru I. Heart failure clinical presentation. http://emedicine .medscape.com/article/163062-clinical#b7. Accessed December 21, 2015.

21. A. The 12-dose regimen is a treatment option for latent tuberculosis (TB) primarily for otherwise healthy people. The 12-dose regimen is not recommended for young children, pregnant women or women who expect to become pregnant during treatment, and HIV-infected people taking antiretroviral therapy. These people should be treated with other existing latent TB infection treatment regimens.

Centers for Disease Control and Prevention. New, simpler way to treat latent TB infection. http://www.cdc.gov/Features/ TuberculosisTreatment/. Accessed December 21, 2015.

22. A. Because of the short duration of treatment, baseline hepatic chemistry blood tests (at least aspartate aminotransferase [AST]) is indicated for those with HIV, those with liver disorders, those with regular alcohol usage, and those taking medications for chronic medical conditions. Subsequent blood tests should be considered only for patients with abnormal baseline testing and for others at risk for liver disease.

Recommendations for use of isoniazid-rifapentine regimen with direct observation to treat latent *Myocbacterium tuberculosis* infection. *MMWR.* 2011;60:1650–1653. http://www.cdc .gov/mmwr/preview/mmwrhtml/mm6048a3.htm. Accessed December 21, 2015.

23. B. Lung cancer screening should be considered in high-risk patients who are candidates for definitive treatment. A 73-year-old male with a 20-pack-year history of smoking and smoking cessation for 8 years is considered high risk.

National Comprehensive Cancer Network. NNCN Clinical Practice Guidelines in Oncology (NNCN Guidelines). *Lung Cancer Screening.* http://www.nccn.org/professionals/ physician_gls/pdf/lung_screening.pdf.

24. B. Tobacco smoking is a major modifiable risk factor in the development of lung cancer and accounts for 85% of all lung-cancer-related deaths.

NNCN Clinical Practice Guidelines in Oncology (NNCN Guidelines). *Lung Cancer Screening.* http://www.nccn.org/professionals/physician_gls/pdf/lung_screening.pdf.

25. C. The CURB-65 criteria (confusion, uremia, respiratory rate, low blood pressure, and age 65 or older) is one scoring system that can help identify patients who may be candidates for outpatient treatment of CAP.

    Mandell LA, Wunderink RG, Anzueto A, et al. Infectious Diseases Society of America/American Thoracic Society Consensus guidelines on the management of community-acquired pneumonia in adults. *Clin Infect Dis.* 2007;44:S27–72.

26. B. Symptoms of pneumococcal disease usually develop suddenly and vary by clinical presentation.

    National Foundation for Infectious Diseases. *Pneumococcal Disease.* http://www.adultvaccination.org/professional-resources/public-health-toolkit/pneumo-fact-sheet-hcp.pdf. Accessed December 21, 2015.

27. D. The Centers for Disease Control and Prevention (CDC) recommends PPSV23 for all patients listed in the question and for persons ages 19 to 64 years with asthma; diabetes; lung, heart, or liver disease; or alcoholism.

    National Foundation for Infectious Diseases. *Pneumococcal Disease.* http://www.adultvaccination.org/professional-resources/public-health-toolkit/pneumo-fact-sheet-hcp.pdf. Accessed December 21, 2015.

28. C. The Centers for Disease Control and Prevention (CDC) recommends only the 23-valent pneumococcal polysaccharide vaccine (PPSV23) for patients 19 years and older who are Alaska Native and/or American Indian.

    National Foundation for Infectious Diseases. *Pneumococcal Disease.* http://www.adultvaccination.org/professional-resources/public-health-toolkit/pneumo-fact-sheet-hcp.pdf. Accessed December 21, 2015.

29. B. Pretreatment Gram stain and culture of expectorated sputum are not required prior to initiation of antibiotic treatment, and pretreatment Gram stain should be performed only if a good-quality specimen can be obtained and quality performance measures for collection, transport, and processing of samples can be met.

    Mandell LA, Wunderink RG, Anzueto A, et al. Infectious Diseases Society of America/American Thoracic Society Consensus guidelines on the management of community-acquired pneumonia in adults. *Clin Infect Dis.* 2007;44:S27–72.

30. D. Vancomycin is reserved for inpatient therapy and should be given intravenously based on body weight.

    Mandell LA, Wunderink RG, Anzueto A, et al. Infectious Diseases Society of America/American Thoracic Society Consensus guidelines on the management of community-acquired pneumonia in adults. *Clin Infect Dis.* 2007;44:S27–72.

31. C. Patients who are clinically unstable are likely to have changes in mentation.

Mandell LA, Wunderink RG, Anzueto A, et al. Infectious Diseases Society of America/American Thoracic Society Consensus guidelines on the management of community-acquired pneumonia in adults. *Clin Infect Dis.* 2007;44:S27–72.

32. A. The predominate pathogens are *Haemophilus influenzae, Streptococcus pneumoniae, Moraxella catarrhalis,* and *Chlamydia pneumoniae.* Antibiotic treatment is typically initiated on an empiric basis but should be directed by which pathogens are most likely.

    Mandell LA, Wunderink RG, Anzueto A, et al. Infectious Diseases Society of America/American Thoracic Society Consensus guidelines on the management of community-acquired pneumonia in adults. *Clin Infect Dis.* 2007;44:S27–72.

33. D. According to the GOLD guidelines, COPD has multiple symptomatic effects, and a comprehensive assessment should include more than just a measure of breathlessness. Symptom development, social and family support, and the impact of the disease on quality of life are recommended as important key variables for a comprehensive assessment.

    Global Initiative for Chronic Obstructive Lung Disease. *Global Strategy for the Diagnosis, Management, and Prevention of Chronic Obstructive Pulmonary Disease.* http://www.goldcopd.com/uploads/users/files/GOLD_Report_2014_Oct30.pdf. Accessed December 21, 2015.

34. D. Ineffective quick-relief medications is a red zone component of the Asthma Action Plan.

    National Heart, Lung, and Blood Institute. *Asthma Action Plan.* https://www.nhlbi.nih.gov/files/docs/public/lung/asthma_actplan.pdf. Accessed December 21, 2015.

35. A. The COPD Assessment Test (CAT) is a validated, short (eight-item) patient-completed questionnaire that is designed to be used in clinical practice to measure the health status of patients with chronic obstructive pulmonary disease (COPD).

    Jones PW, Harding G, Berry P, et al. Development and first validation of the COPD Assessment Test. *Eur Respir J.* 2009;34:648–654. http://www.catestonline.org/images/pdfs/CATest.pdf. Accessed December 21, 2015.

36. A. Chest X-ray (CXR) findings are usually abnormal in patients with severe chronic obstructive pulmonary disease (COPD) but may not show changes in up to one-half of patients with moderate disease. CXR findings associated with COPD include flattening (not elevation) of the diaphragm.

    Dewar M, Curry RW. Chronic obstructive pulmonary disease: diagnostic considerations. *Am Fam Physician.* 2006;73:669–676.

37. B. Smoking cessation has the biggest impact on slowing the progression of chronic obstructive pulmonary disease (COPD), and all healthcare providers should provide clear, consistent, repeated nonsmoking messages and assist with smoking cessation strategies.

Global Initiative for Chronic Obstructive Lung Disease. *Pocket Guide to COPD Diagnosis, Management, and Prevention.* http://www.goldcopd.org/uploads/users/files/GOLD_Pocket_2015_Feb18.pdf. Accessed December 21, 2015.

38. C. With this clinical presentation, pulmonary embolus must be ruled out. CT angiogram with contrast is recommended as the best imaging method for pulmonary embolism.

American College of Radiology. ACR Appropriateness Criteria. http://www.acr.org/Quality-Safety/Approrpiateness-Criteria. Accessed December 21, 2015.

39. B. The variable of age is a patient older than 49 years.

Dachs R, Endres J, Graber MA. Pulmonary embolism rule-out criteria: a clinical decision rule that works. *Am Fam Physician.* 2013;15:98–100.

40. D. There is no recommendation from the American College of Physicians that suggests that all smokers should be screened for obstructive sleep apnea (OSA).

Qassee A, Holty JE, Owens DK, et al. Management of obstructive sleep apnea in adults: clinical practice guideline from the American College of Physicians. *Ann Intern Med.* 2013;159:471–483. http://annals.org/article.aspx?articleid=1742606. Accessed December 21, 2015.

Chapter 4: Common Gastrointestinal Disorders in Primary Care

1. A 75-year-old patient comes to the office with a complaint of nonspecific abdominal pain for the last 12 hours. His white blood cell count (WBC) is normal. Vital signs are stable, and he is afebrile. Which one of the following diagnoses can be ruled out?
   a. All abdominal infections because of a normal temperature and white blood cell count
   b. Appendicitis because the pain didn't start in the umbilicus and radiate to the right lower quadrant
   c. Biliary disease because his WBC is not elevated
   d. None of the above

2. Which one of the following is the recommended imaging modality for diagnosing appendicitis in an elderly patient?
   a. Computed tomography of the abdomen and pelvis with contrast
   b. Ultrasound
   c. Abdominal X-ray
   d. None of the above

3. Which one of the following is the most common cause of a small bowel obstruction?
   a. Mass
   b. Surgical adhesions
   c. Hernia
   d. Inflammatory bowel disease

[handwritten: first line regimen]

[handwritten: → CVD + DM are risk factors]

4. Which statement is not consistent with the American College of Gastroenterology clinical guideline on colon ischemia (CI)?
   a. Symptoms of CI include sudden, mild abdominal cramping, urgent desire to defecate, and passage of bloody diarrhea.
   b. Risk factors include Crohn's disease and celiac disease.
   c. CT with intravenous and oral contrast should be the first imaging modality.
   d. Early colonoscopy should be performed within 48 hours to confirm the diagnosis.

5. Which one of the following is the most common underlying cause of abnormal liver function tests?
   a. Hepatitis C virus (HCV)
   b. Hepatitis B virus (HBV)
   c. Cholelithiasis
   d. Nonalcoholic fatty liver disease *[handwritten: → d/t ↑ obesity rates]*

6. The rate of HCV infection in the United States is highest in which group of patients?
   a. Elderly adults
   b. Young children *[handwritten: → 1970's + 80's these pt's had ↑ rates]*
   c. Patients born from 1945 to 1965
   d. Adolescents and young adults

7. What percentage of people who develop acute HCV infection clear the virus spontaneously?
   a. 5%
   b. 10% *[handwritten: for unknown reasons]*
   c. 20%
   d. 33%

8. Although not required for the average patient with gastroesophageal reflux disease (GERD), endoscopy may be appropriate if:
   a. Reflux develops in a patient older than 50 years of age.
   b. GERD has been untreated for more than 5 years.
   c. Bleeding is present.
   d. All of the above

9. What percentages of patients with proven GERD are able to eventually discontinue proton pump inhibitor (PPI) therapy?
   a. 10–15%
   b. 20–25% *[handwritten: about 1/4]*
   c. 25–33%
   d. 40–50%

10. A 36-year-old man presents for a well-patient exam. He gives a history that, over the past 20 years, he has had three episodes of abdominal pain and hematemesis, the most recent of which occurred several years ago. He was told that he had an ulcer. You obtain a serum assay for *Helicobacter pylori* IgG, which is positive. What is the most effective regimen to eradicate this organism?
   a. Omeprazole (Prilosec) 20 mg PO daily for 6 weeks
   b. Ranitidine (Zantac) 300 mg PO at bedtime for 6 weeks
   c. Omeprazole 20 mg BID, amoxicillin 1000 mg BID, clarithromycin (Biaxin) 500 mg BID for 14 days
   d. Pepto-Bismol and metronidazole (Flagyl) BID for 7 days

11. A 25-year-old medical student is stuck with a hollow needle during a procedure on a patient known to have hepatitis B viral infection but who is HIV negative. The student's baseline laboratory studies include serology: hepatitis B surface antigen (HBsAG) negative, total antibody hepatitis B core antigen (Anti-HBc) negative, immunoglobulin M antibody hepatitis B core antigen (IgM Anti-HBc) negative, and antibody to hepatitis B surface antigen (Anti-HBs) positive. Which of the following is true regarding this medical student's hepatitis status?
    a. Prior vaccination with hepatitis B vaccine
    b. Acute infection with hepatitis B virus
    c. Prior infection with hepatitis B virus
    d. The student was vaccinated for hepatitis B but is not immune

12. What postexposure prophylaxis should the student described in question 11 receive?
    a. Hepatitis B immune globulin (HBIg)
    b. Oral lamivudine
    c. Intravenous immune globulin (IVIg)
    d. Draw a titer to determine the serum antibody level for HBV

13. A 34-year-old male presents with substernal discomfort. The symptoms are worse after meals, particularly a heavy evening meal, and are sometimes associated with hot/sour fluid in the back of the throat and nocturnal awakening. The patient denies difficulty swallowing, pain on swallowing, or weight loss. The symptoms have been present for 6 weeks. The patient has gained 20 pounds in the past 2 years. Which of the following is the most appropriate initial approach?
    a. An 8-week course of a proton pump inhibitor
    b. Exercise test with thallium imaging
    c. CT scan of the chest
    d. Esophagogastroduodenoscopy

14. A 32-year-old white female complains of abdominal pain off and on since the age of 17 years. She notices abdominal bloating relieved by defecation as well as alternating diarrhea and constipation. She has no weight loss, GI bleeding, or nocturnal diarrhea. On examination, she has slight LLQ tenderness and gaseous abdominal distention. Lab studies, including CBC, are normal. Which of the following is the most appropriate initial approach?
    a. Recommend increased dietary fiber, antispasmodics as needed, and follow-up exam in 2 months.
    b. Refer to gastroenterologist for colonoscopy.
    c. Obtain antiendomysial antibodies.
    d. Order UGI series with small bowel follow-through.

15. Mr. Hauptman is a 72-year-old man who presents with occasional dyspepsia. Which one of the following is an expected gastrointestinal change associated with aging?
    a. Decreased risk of diverticular disease
    b. Increased appetite
    c. Alteration of drug effectiveness
    d. Improved absorption of calcium

16. A 40-year-old cigarette smoker complains of epigastric pain, well localized, nonradiating, and described as burning. The pain is partially relieved by eating. There is no weight loss. He has not used nonsteroidal anti-inflammatory agents. The pain has gradually worsened over several months, and he now is experiencing dysphagia. Which of the following is the most sensitive way to make a specific diagnosis?
    a. Barium X-ray
    b. Endoscopy
    c. Serologic test for *Helicobacter pylori*
    d. Serum gastrin

17. A 24-year-old man presents with a 3-month history of upper abdominal pain. He describes it as an intermittent, centrally located "burning" feeling in his upper abdomen, most often occurring 2 to 3 hours after meals. Recently, the pain has been awakening him at night. His presentation is most consistent with the diagnosis of:
    a. Acute gastritis
    b. Pancreatitis
    c. Peptic ulcer disease
    d. Cholecystitis

18. A 43-year-old female has a 12-hour history of sudden onset of right upper quadrant abdominal pain with radiation to the shoulder, fever and chills, and nausea and vomiting. She has had similar, milder episodes in the past, especially after eating fast foods. Examination reveals marked tenderness to right upper quadrant on abdominal palpation. Her most likely diagnosis is:
    a. Hepatoma
    b. Acute cholecystitis
    c. Acute hepatitis
    d. Cholelithiasis

19. Which one of the following statements is accurate regarding diverticular disease?
    a. The etiology of diverticular disease includes a low-fiber diet and reduced fecal volume related to colonic muscle shortening and thickening.
    b. Colonoscopy is considered the test of choice for the diagnosis of diverticulitis.
    c. In most cases, diverticulitis occurs in the transverse colon.
    d. Surgery is the only definitive treatment for diverticulosis.

20. The best method for determining the progression and severity of liver disease in patients with chronic hepatitis C is:
    a. Viral load
    b. ALT and AST levels
    c. CT of the liver
    d. Liver biopsy

21. Which one of the following is not an indication for diagnostic evaluation of diarrhea?
    a. Profuse watery diarrhea with signs of hypovolemia
    b. Passage of many small-volume stools containing blood and mucus
    c. Bloody diarrhea
    d. Temperature < 100°F

22. Obtaining stool cultures on initial presentation is appropriate for which group of patients?
- a. Patients with underlying inflammatory bowel disease in which distinction between a flare and superimposed infection is critical
- b. All patients over the age of 50 years
- c. All patients with diarrhea lasting more than 48 hours
- d. None of the above

23. Which statement is inaccurate regarding obtaining stool for ova and parasites?
- a. Sending stool samples for ova and parasites is not cost effective for the majority of patients with acute diarrhea.
- b. Stool for ova and parasites in a patient with persistent diarrhea with exposure to infants in day care centers is reasonable to rule out *Giardia* and *Cryptosporidium*.
- c. Patients with bloody diarrhea with few or no fecal leukocytes should be cultured to rule out intestinal amebiasis.
- d. The benefit of sending multiple samples is important to increase the diagnostic yield.

24. Which pharmacologic treatment is appropriate for patients with *Clostridium difficile* infection (CDI)?
- a. Drugs are never indicated.
- b. Clindamycin.
- c. Metronidazole. → 500 mg TID X 10D
- d. Trimethoprim-sulfamethoxazole.

25. When is it appropriate to treat patients with acute diarrhea symptomatically with loperamide (Imodium)?
- a. When patients are afebrile
- b. When patients have a low-grade fever
- c. When patients' stools are not bloody
- d. All of the above

The combo of Loperamide + Simethicone is better together then Loperamide alone

26. Adequate nutrition and oral hydration during an episode of acute diarrhea are important. Which one of the following statements is inaccurate regarding dietary recommendations for the patient with acute diarrhea?
- a. If patients are anorectic, a short period of consuming only liquids will not be harmful.
- b. Boiled starches and cereals are recommended for patients with watery diarrhea.
- c. Avoidance of lactose-containing foods is unnecessary. → no supporting data
- d. Foods with high fat content should be avoided until diarrhea subsides.

27. Which statement is inaccurate regarding irritable bowel syndrome (IBS)?
- a. IBS is defined as abdominal discomfort or pain associated with altered bowel habits that has occurred for at least 3 months.
- b. IBS affects more men than women.
- c. IBS is more common in populations with lower socioeconomic status.
- d. Patients with IBS have lower productivity and higher absenteeism.

28. Which statement is inaccurate regarding the clinical presentation of IBS?
- a. Crampy abdominal pain is the most common symptom.
- b. Emotional stress and eating may worsen the pain.
- c. Pain is often progressive and awakens patients from sleep.
- d. Altered bowel habits associated with IBS include diarrhea, constipation, or both.

29. Which statement is true regarding the initial evaluation of IBS?
- a. The HCP should consider routine testing for celiac disease in patients with diarrhea-predominant or mixed presentation IBS. 4% + c̄ bx for Celiac's
- b. CBC, serum chemistries, and thyroid function tests should be obtained in all patients.
- c. Stool testing for ova and parasites has a high yield and should be ordered.
- d. Colonoscopy is necessary for diagnosis for most patients.

30. Which of the following choices is an alarm symptom for IBS that warrants investigation for other diseases?
- a. Anemia, rectal bleeding, and weight loss
- b. A family history of colorectal cancer and/or inflammatory bowel disease
- c. Onset of symptoms after age 50 years
- d. All of the above

31. Which one of the following is not recommended for the treatment of IBS?
- a. Antispasmodics
- b. Limited exercise
- c. Probiotics
- d. Antidepressants

32. Which medication may be helpful for women with severe diarrhea-predominant IBS whose symptoms are refractory to conventional therapy?
- a. Alosetron (Lotronex)
- b. Tegaserod (Zelnorm)
- c. Hyoscyamine (Levsin)
- d. Metoclopramide (Reglan)

33. Testing for celiac disease should be considered in which of the following patients?
- a. Patients with symptoms of malabsorption and weight loss
- b. Patients without other explanations for signs and symptoms of iron-deficiency anemia, folate deficiency, or vitamin B_{12} deficiency
- c. Patients with type 1 DM and first-degree relatives of individuals with celiac disease
- d. None of the above

34. Which laboratory study should be ordered for the evaluation of celiac disease?
- a. Anti-Smith antibody
- b. Immunoglobulin A (IgA anti-tissue transglutaminase)
- c. Immunoglobulin M (IgM monoclonal antibody)
- d. Anti-Rhodamine antibody

35. What is the best treatment for celiac disease?
  a. Mediterranean diet
  b. Low-sodium diet
  c. Gluten-free diet
  d. Egg allergy diet

36. Your patient has recently been diagnosed with celiac disease and is trying to follow her diet carefully. Which of the following are acceptable to eat?
  a. Rice and corn
  b. Bread and pasta
  c. Beers and malt vinegars
  d. All spreads and condiments

37. The diagnosis of drug-induced liver injury (DILI) requires:
  a. A serum alanine aminotransferase (ALT) > 2 times the upper limit   ↑ALT or AP > 2 times limit
  b. An alkaline phosphatase (AP) > 4 times the upper limit
  c. A causality assessment score of > 10
  d. Clinical symptoms, including abdominal pain, nausea, and jaundice

38. The major factors in the development of DILI are:
  a. Length of medication use and drug dosage
  b. The weight and height of the patient
  c. The baseline creatinine level
  d. The concomitant use of herbal medicines

39. The primary treatment for drug-induced liver injury is:
  a. Liver transplantation
  b. Chelation therapy
  c. Intravenous fluids
  d. Early drug discontinuation

40. Establishing the diagnosis of subclinical celiac disease is important because of:
  a. The presence of associated nutritional excesses
  b. The danger of malignancy and associated autoimmune disease
  c. The association of infants with autism in affected mothers
  d. All of the above

Chapter 4: Answers and Rationales

1. D. Acute abdominal pain is common in older patients and presentations may differ from that of a young patient because of coexistent disease, delays in presentation, and physical and social barriers.

Lyon C, Clark DC. Diagnosis of acute abdominal pain in older patients. *Am Fam Physician.* 2006;74:1537–1544. http://www.aafp.org/afp/2006/1101/p1537.html. Accessed December 21, 2015.

2. A. According to the American College of Radiology (ACR), computed tomography (CT) is the most accurate imaging for evaluating patients without a clear clinical diagnosis of appendicitis.

American College of Radiology. ACR Appropriateness Criteria. https://acsearch.acr.org/docs/69357/Narrative/. Accessed December 21, 2015.

3. B. The most common causes of intestinal obstruction include adhesions, neoplasms, and herniation. Adhesions resulting from past abdominal surgery are the predominant cause of small bowel obstruction, accounting for about 60% of cases.

Jackson PG, Raiji M. Evaluation and management of intestinal obstruction. *Am Fam Physician.* 2011;83:159–165. http://www.aafp.org/afp/2011/0115/p159.html. Accessed December 21, 2015.

4. B. Cardiovascular disease and diabetes mellitus are risk factors for colon ischemia (CI). Chronic kidney disease is associated with increased mortality from CI.

Brandt LJ, Feuerstadt P, Longstreth GF, Boley SJ. ACG clinical guideline: epidemiology, risk factors, patterns of presentation, diagnosis, and management of colon ischemia (CI). *Am J Gastroenterol.* 2015;110:18–44. http://gi.org/wp-content/uploads/2015/01/ACG_Guideline_Colon-Ischemia_January_2015.pdf. Accessed December 21, 2015.

5. D. Nonalcoholic fatty liver disease is the leading cause of mild transaminase elevations and will likely become more prevalent as the obesity rate in the United States increases.

Oh RC, Hustead TR. Causes and evaluations of mildly elevated liver transaminase levels. *Am Fam Physician.* 2011; 84:1003–1008. http://www.aafp.org/afp/2011/1101/p1003.html. Accessed December 21, 2015.

6. C. Infection is most prevalent among persons born from 1945 to 1965, the majority of whom were likely infected during the 1970s and 1980s when the rates were highest. This is the reason for the recommendation that all persons born between these dates should be tested once for HCV.

Centers for Disease Control and Prevention. Viral hepatitis: hepatitis C information. http://www.cdc.gov/hepatitis/hcv/hcvfaq.htm#a4. Accessed December 21, 2015.

American Association for the Study of Liver Diseases; and Infectious Diseases Society of America. *Recommendations for Testing, Managing and Treating Hepatitis C.* http://www.hcvguidelines.org/sites/default/files/full_report.pdf. Accessed December 21, 2015.

7. C. Approximately 15% to 25% of persons clear the hepatitis C virus without treatment; the reasons for this are not understood.

Centers for Disease Control and Prevention. Viral hepatitis: hepatitis C information. http://www.cdc.gov/hepatitis/hcv/hcvfaq.htm#a4. Accessed December 21, 2015.

8. D. The reasons listed in the question put patients at high risk, and imaging is reasonable.

Katz PO, Gerson LB, Vela MF. Diagnosis and management of gastroesophageal reflux disease. *Am J Gastroenterol.* 2013;108:308–328. http://gi.org/guideline/diagnosis-and-managemen-of-gastroesophageal-reflux-disease/. Accessed December 21, 2015.

9. B. Only about one-fourth of patients with gastroesophageal reflux disease (GERD) are able to discontinue routine medication and remain symptom free. It is important to provide anticipatory guidance to patients about the chance of stopping their medications.

Katz PO, Gerson LB, Vela MF. Diagnosis and management of gastroesophageal reflux disease. *Am J Gastroenterol.* 2013;108:308–328. http://gi.org/guideline/diagnosis-and-managemen-of-gastroesophageal-reflux-disease/. Accessed December 21, 2015.

10. C. There are many combinations of medications for the treatment of *H. pylori* eradication, but the combination of omeprazole, amoxicillin, and clarithromycin is considered a first-line regimen.

Chey WD; Practice Parameters Committee of the American College of Gastroenterology. Management of *Helicobacter pylori* infection. *Am J Gastroenterol.* 2007;102:1808–1825. http://gi.org/guideline/management-of-helicobacter-pylori-infection/. Accessed December 21, 2015.

11. A. This student's serology is most consistent with vaccination and not prior infection. Like all healthcare workers, the student should have been vaccinated against hepatitis B virus (HBV), which induces anti-HBs antibody and is thought to be protective.

Centers for Disease Control and Prevention, National Center for HIV/AIDS, STD and TB Prevention. Interpretation of the hepatitis B panel. http://nmhealth.org/publication/view/help/468/. Accessed December 21, 2015.

12. D. The student has been previously vaccinated. A serum antibody level for hepatitis B virus (HBV) is indicated to determine whether there is an adequate immune response.

Centers for Disease Control and Prevention. *Hepatitis B and Healthcare Personnel. CDC Answers Frequently Asked Questions About How to Protect Healthcare Personnel.* http://www.immunize.org/catg.d/p2109.pdf. Accessed December 21, 2015.

13. A. The clinical presentation of this patient likely suggests gastroesophageal reflux disease (GERD). An 8-week course of a proton pump inhibitor (PPI) is the therapy of choice for symptom relief. There are no major differences in the efficacy among PPIs.

Katz PO, Gerson LB, Vela MF. Diagnosis and management of gastroesophageal reflux disease. *Am J Gastroenterol.* 2013;108:308–328. http://gi.org/guideline/diagnosis-and-managemen-of-gastroesophageal-reflux-disease/. Accessed December 21, 2015.

14. A. Conservative management for possible irritable bowel syndrome is reasonable as initial treatment. Additional treatment strategies can be explored at follow-up.

Ford AC, Moayyedi P, Lacy BD, et al. American College of Gastroenterology monograph on the management of irritable bowel syndrome and chronic idiopathic constipation. *Am J Gastroenterol.* 2014;109:S2–S26.

15. C. This dyspepsia can be related to aging. If this continues to be bothersome, the NP should realize that medications to relieve symptoms may not be as effective as they are in a younger patient and that, because of the physiologic aspects of aging, elderly adults may be at high risk for adverse effects.

Wooten JM. Pharmacotherapy considerations in elderly adults. *South Med J.* 2012;105:437–445.

16. B. Upper endoscopy is not required in the presence of typical gastroesophageal reflux disease (GERD) symptoms. Endoscopy is the recommended diagnostic test in the presence of alarm symptoms and for screening of patients at high risk for complications.

Katz PO, Gerson LB, Vela MF. Diagnosis and management of gastroesophageal reflux disease. *Am J Gastroenterol.* 2013;108:308–328. http://gi.org/guideline/diagnosis-and-managemen-of-gastroesophageal-reflux-disease/. Accessed December 21, 2015.

17. C. The location of abdominal pain helps guide the initial evaluation. Associated signs and symptoms are predictive of certain causes of abdominal pain and can help narrow the diagnosis. Symptoms of peptic ulcer disease include concurrent, episodic gnawing or burning pain; pain relieved by food; and nighttime awakening with pain.

Cartwright SL, Knudson MP. Evaluation of acute abdominal pain in adults. *Am Fam Physician.* 2008;77:971–978. http://www.aafp.org/afp/2008/0401/p971.html. Accessed December 21, 2015.

18. B. The anatomic location of the pain and the demographics of this patient (female, age 43) help narrow down the cause of abdominal pain. Symptoms of cholecystitis include nausea and vomiting and often occur after a large or fatty meal.

Cartwright SL, Knudson MP. Evaluation of acute abdominal pain in adults.

Am Fam Physician. 2008;77:971–978. http://www.aafp.org/afp/2008/0401/p971.html. Accessed December 21, 2015.

19. A. Factors associated with diverticulosis include alterations in colonic motility, colonic wall resistance, and dietary issues that cause increased intraluminal pressure and weakness of the bowel wall. There is also a genetic susceptibility to diverticular disease.

Wilkins T, Embry K, George R. Diagnosis and management of acute diverticulitis. *Am Fam Physician.* 2013;87:612–620. http://www.aafp.org/afp/2013/0501/p612.html. Accessed December 21, 2015.

20. D. Hepatitis C virus (HCV) disease progresses in stages, with the progression from inflammation to fibrosis to cirrhosis. The best method of grading and staging liver disease is by biopsy.

American Association for the Study of Liver Diseases; and Infectious Diseases Society of America. *Recommendations for Testing, Managing and Treating Hepatitis C.* http://www.hcvguidelines.org/sites/default/files/full_report.pdf. Accessed December 21, 2015.

21. D. In general, fever is more suggestive of inflammatory diarrhea and would warrant further workup.

Barr W, Smith A. Acute diarrhea in adults. *Am Fam Physician.* 2014;89:180–189. http://www.aafp.org/afp/2014/0201/p180.html. Accessed December 21, 2015.

22. A. Differentiation of a flare and superimposed infection in patients with diarrhea who have a history of inflammatory bowel disease is essential so that correct therapy can be instituted.

Barr W, Smith A. Acute diarrhea in adults. *Am Fam Physician.* 2014;89:180–189. http://www.aafp.org/afp/2014/0201/p180.html. Accessed December 21, 2015.

23. D. No studies have demonstrated a higher test yield with multiple samples.

Barr W, Smith A. Acute diarrhea in adults. *Am Fam Physician.* 2014;89:180–189. http://www.aafp.org/afp/2014/0201/p180.html. Accessed December 21, 2015.

24. C. Patients with mild-moderate *Clostridium difficile* infection (CDI) symptoms should be treated with metronidazole 500 mg orally three times daily for 10 days.

Surawicz CM, Brandt LJ, Binion DG, et al. Guidelines for diagnosis, treatment and prevention of *Clostridium difficile* infections. *Am J Gastroenterol.* 2013;108:478–498. http://gi.org/guideline/diagnosis-and-management-of-c-difficile-associated-diarrhea-and-colitis/. Accessed December 21, 2015.

25. D. Loperamide can be given in all the situations listed in the question. This medication may reduce the diarrhea by about 1 day. The combination of loperamide/simethicone is faster and may provide more complete relief of acute nonspecific diarrhea and gas-related discomfort than loperamide alone.

Barr W, Smith A. Acute diarrhea in adults. *Am Fam Physician.* 2014;89:180–189. http://www.aafp.org/afp/2014/0201/p180.html. Accessed December 21, 2015.

26. C. Although the avoidance of dairy is commonly suggested, there are no supporting data for this recommendation.

Barr W, Smith A. Acute diarrhea in adults. *Am Fam Physician.* 2014;89:180–189. http://www.aafp.org/afp/2014/0201/p180.html. Accessed December 21, 2015.

27. B. Prevalence estimates of irritable bowel syndrome (IBS) in North America range from 5% to 10%, with peak prevalence in those from 20 to 39 years of age. IBS affects 1.5 times more women than men.

Wilkins T, Pepitone C, Alex B, Schade RR. Diagnosis and management of IBS in adults. *Am Fam Physician.* 2012;86:5.

28. C. Abdominal pain is the most common symptom in patients with irritable bowel syndrome (IBS) and is described as a cramping sensation. Pain that is progressive or that awakens the patient from sleep is not characteristic of IBS.

Wilkins T, Pepitone C, Alex B, Schade RR. Diagnosis and management of IBS in adults. *Am Fam Physician.* 2012;86:5.

29. A. A systematic review including more than 4000 patients showed that 4% of those with diarrhea-predominant or mixed presentation irritable bowel syndrome (IBS) had biopsy-proven celiac disease. Although routine lab work and stool testing are low yield, the NP should consider routine testing for celiac disease in these patients.

Wilkins T, Pepitone C, Alex B, Schade RR. Diagnosis and management of IBS in adults. *Am Fam Physician.* 2012;86:5.

30. D. All of the listed symptoms are red alarm symptoms for irritable bowel syndrome (IBS) and should prompt an investigation for other diseases. The diagnostic study of choice for the evaluation is colonoscopy with biopsy.

Wilkins T, Pepitone C, Alex B, Schade RR. Diagnosis and management of IBS in adults. *Am Fam Physician.* 2012;86:5.

31. B. Patients with irritable bowel syndrome (IBS) who exercise have fewer IBS symptoms when compared with patients who do not exercise.

Wilkins T, Pepitone C, Alex B, Schade RR. Diagnosis and management of IBS in adults. *Am Fam Physician.* 2012;86:5.

32. A. Alosetron improves global IBS symptoms and abdominal pain.

Wilkins T, Pepitone C, Alex B, Schade RR. Diagnosis and management of IBS in adults. *Am Fam Physician.* 2012;86:5.

33. D. None of these patients are at increased risk for celiac disease, and none should be tested.

Rubion-Taplia A, Hill ID, Kelly CP, Calderwood AH, Murray JA. ACG clinical guidelines: diagnosis and management of celiac disease. *Am J Gastroenterol.* 2013;108:656.

34. B. IgA anti-tissue transglutaminase antibody is the preferred single test for detection of celiac disease (CD) in individuals older than the age of 2 years. When a high probability of CD exists, the possibility of IgA deficiency is considered, and total IgA should be measured.

Rubion-Taplia A, Hill ID, Kelly CP, Calderwood AH, Murray JA. ACG clinical guidelines: diagnosis and management of celiac disease. *Am J Gastroenterol.* 2013;108:656.

35. C. The treatment for celiac disease is primarily a gluten-free diet, which requires significant patient education, motivation, and follow-up.

Rubion-Taplia A, Hill ID, Kelly CP, Calderwood AH, Murray JA. ACG clinical guidelines: diagnosis and management of celiac disease. *Am J Gastroenterol.* 2013;108:656.

36. A. A gluten-free diet entails strict avoidance of all products containing the proteins from wheat, barley, and rye. Although the term "gluten-free" implies complete elimination of all sources of gluten, this is not possible as a result of

contamination of foods with trace amounts of gluten. Therefore, the term "gluten-free" indicates a diet that contains gluten at such a low level as to be considered harmless. The exact level below which gluten is harmless is not known, but a recent review suggests less than 10 mg per day is unlikely to cause damage in most patients.

Rubion-Taplia A, Hill ID, Kelly CP, Calderwood AH, Murray JA. ACG clinical guidelines: diagnosis and management of celiac disease. *Am J Gastroenterol*. 2013;108:656.

37. A. The diagnosis of drug-induced liver injury (DILI) requires an awareness of potential liver injury from various culprit drugs. An elevation of alanine aminotransferase (ALT) or alkaline phosphatase (AP) > 2 times the upper limit of normal is indicative of apparent liver injury.

Thanavaro J. An overview of drug induced liver injury. *J Nurse Practitioners*. 2011;7:819–826.

38. A. The length of medication use and the drug dosage are the major factors in the development of drug-induced liver injury (DILI). Long duration use of a drug at a high dose is more likely to induce DILI.

Thanavaro J. An overview of drug induced liver injury. *J Nurse Practitioners*. 2011;7:819–826.

39. D. Discovery of the culprit agent and early drug discontinuation is the primary treatment for drug-induced liver injury (DILI) and is essential for the recovery of liver damage. It is not uncommon that liver enzyme elevations may last several months before returning to normal.

Thanavaro J. An overview of drug induced liver injury. *J Nurse Practitioners*. 2011;7:819–826.

40. B. Untreated celiac disease can result in serious consequences, including malignancy and autoimmune disease; early diagnosis and management are crucial to preventing these potential sequelae.

AGA Institute. AGA Institute medical position statement on the diagnosis and management of celiac disease. *Gastroenterology*. 2006;131:1977.

Chapter 5: Common Hematologic Disorders in Primary Care

1. Mr. Frederick is a 66-year-old African American male with a history of HTN and chronic kidney disease who presents with increased edema. His medications are furosemide 10 mg once daily and lisinopril 5 mg once daily. After the physical examination, which lab studies do you anticipate ordering for Mr. Frederick?
   a. Complete blood count
   b. Comprehensive metabolic panel
   c. Glomerular filtration rate
   d. All of the above

2. For Mr. Frederick, what abnormalities do you anticipate in his complete blood count?
   a. Low RBC, low Hgb, low Hct, normal MCV, normal MCHC
   b. Low RBC, low Hgb, low Hct, low MCV, low MCHC
   c. Low RBC, low Hgb, low Hct, elevated MCV, elevated MCHC
   d. None of the above

3. What additional lab studies would you anticipate for Mr. Frederick?
   a. GFR, 24-hour urine
   b. Reticulocytes, RDW, peripheral blood smear
   c. Serum iron, ferritin, and TIBC
   d. All of the above

4. What medication may be used to treat anemia of chronic disease caused by renal failure?
   a. Lisinopril
   b. Furosemide
   c. Erythropoietin alpha
   d. None of the above

5. Anticipated physical changes associated with anemia include which of the following?
   a. Arrhythmias
   b. Extracardiac sounds
   c. Crackling or rales on lung examination
   d. All of the above

6. Mrs. Williams is a 58-year-old white female who presents with c/o fatigue, coolness, numbness, and tingling in her lower extremities and intermittent dizziness when changing positions. Given only this information, which of the following conditions might Mrs. Williams be experiencing?
   a. Thyroid disorders
   b. Anemia
   c. Autoimmune disease
   d. All of the above

7. With this information about Mrs. Williams, you suspect that anemia is the probable cause of her symptoms. Her differential diagnoses should include which of the following conditions?
   a. Anemia of folate deficiency
   b. Anemia of vitamin B$_{12}$ deficiency
   c. Iron-deficiency anemia
   d. All of the above

8. Mrs. Williams is diagnosed with anemia related to a vitamin deficiency. To differentiate which deficiency she is experiencing, which tests do you anticipate need to be completed?
   a. CBC, Schilling test, CMP
   b. CBC, CMP, TIBC
   c. CBC, LFT, ferritin
   d. CBC, ferritin, TIBC

9. Mrs. Williams has been diagnosed with anemia of vitamin B_{12} deficiency. What do you expect her labs to show?
   - a. Decreased RBC, Hgb, Hct; Schilling test positive *(circled)*
   - b. Increased RBC, decreased Hgb, decreased Hct, Schilling test positive
   - c. Normal RBC, Hgb, Hct; Schilling test positive
   - d. Normal Hgb, normal Hct, decreased RBC, Schilling test positive

10. When teaching Mrs. Williams about her anemia, which of the following do you tell her are risk factors for vitamin B_{12}–deficiency anemia?
    - a. Fair-skinned, fair-eyed women of northern European descent
    - b. Low PO intake of vitamin B_{12}–containing foods
    - c. Malabsorption of vitamin B_{12} related to gastric disorders
    - d. All of the above *(circled)*

11. All patients with vitamin B_{12} deficiency can be safely managed on oral vitamin B_{12}.
    - a. True
    - b. False *(circled)*

12. Recommended interventions for vitamin B_{12}–deficiency anemia in a patient with a history of partial gastrectomy should include:
    - a. Vitamin B_{12} PO
    - b. Vitamin B_{12} PR
    - c. Vitamin B_{12} injection *(circled)* *(handwritten: or intranasal)*
    - d. Both B and C

13. Mr. Jones is a 60-year-old male who reports he was recently attempting to donate blood when he was told to follow up with his healthcare provider for further evaluation. He said he was told he had "poor blood." When queried about his health history and medications, Mr. Jones reports he takes aspirin daily for DJD but is otherwise healthy. Which of the following tests will your baseline evaluation include?
    - a. CBC, Schilling test, CMP, ferritin
    - b. CBC, CMP, ferritin, TIBC *(circled)*
    - c. CBC, LFT, ferritin, CMP
    - d. CBC, ferritin, TIBC, Hgb electrophoresis

14. Mrs. Albrecht is a 65-year-old female who presents with complaints of fatigue. PMH significant for ETOH use of four martinis per week for the past 35 years, tobacco use, and diabetes. You know that her history puts her at risk of anemia for which of the following reasons? *(handwritten: ETOH likely Folate)*
    - a. Anemia of folate deficiency *(circled)*
    - b. Anemia of vitamin B_{12} deficiency
    - c. Iron-deficiency anemia
    - d. Anemia caused by blood loss

15. You are aware that Mrs. Albrecht's anemia may also occur simultaneously with other forms of anemia such as which of the following?
    - a. Anemia of folate deficiency
    - b. Anemia of vitamin B_{12} deficiency
    - c. Iron-deficiency anemia
    - d. Both B and C *(circled)*

16. Lab results for a patient with iron-deficiency anemia could be expected to appear as which of the following?
    - a. Decreased Hgb, Hct, MCV, ferritin; increased RDW, TIBC *(circled)*
    - b. Decreased Hgb, Hct, MCV, RDW; increased ferritin, TIBC
    - c. Decreased Hgb, Hct; normal MCV, RDW; increased ferritin, TIBC
    - d. Decreased Hgb, Hct, MCV; increased RDW, ferritin, TIBC

17. When working up a patient for iron-deficiency anemia, you must realize that the lab results may show either a microcytic or a normocytic anemia.
    - a. True *(circled)*
    - b. False

18. Lab results for a patient with folic acid–deficiency anemia would include a hemoglobin electrophoresis.
    - a. True
    - b. False *(circled)* *(handwritten: hemoglobin electrophoresis blood test to detect different types of hemoglobin.)*

19. For your patient with iron-deficiency anemia, patient teaching should include which of the following pieces of information?
    - a. Take your iron tablets on an empty stomach.
    - b. Anticipate dark-colored stools.
    - c. You will not feel better immediately.
    - d. All of the above *(circled)*

20. Common classifications for anemia include:
    - a. Microcytic, macrocytic, normocytic *(circled)*
    - b. Normocytic, hypercytic, hypocytic
    - c. Microcytic, macrocytic, hypocytic
    - d. None of the above

21. Common lab results for a normocytic anemia include which of the following? *(handwritten: anemia where mcv is WNL)*
    - a. Normal retic count, normal MCV *(circled)*
    - b. Low retic count, normal MCV
    - c. High retic count, normal MCV
    - d. None of the above

22. Laboratory results for thalassemia may be similar to laboratory results for which other condition? *(handwritten: until a hemoglobin electrophoresis is completed to diagnose/differentiate)*
    - a. Folate-deficiency anemia
    - b. Iron-deficiency anemia *(circled)*
    - c. Vitamin B_{12}–deficiency anemia
    - d. None of the above

23. In perimenopausal women, anemia may be related to which of the following conditions?
    - a. Dysfunctional uterine bleeding
    - b. Thyroid disease
    - c. PCOS
    - d. All of the above *(circled)*

24. Your patient was just diagnosed with alpha thalassemia minor. What does this tell you?
    - a. She inherited this condition from both parents.
    - b. She inherited this condition from one parent. *(circled)*
    - c. She can expect to have ongoing symptoms of the disorder.
    - d. None of the above

25. Your patient was just diagnosed with beta thalassemia major. What does this tell you?
    a. He inherited this condition from both parents.
    b. He inherited this condition from one parent.
    c. He can expect to have minimal or no symptoms of the disorder.
    d. None of the above

Iron overload can be Fatal

26. Why is it important to differentiate between iron deficiency and alpha thalassemia?
    a. Iron supplementation is contraindicated in alpha thalassemia.
    b. Folate would need to be added to an alpha thalassemia plan of care.
    c. A higher iron dose and folate dose would be needed for alpha thalassemia.
    d. None of the above

27. What are the risk factors for alpha thalassemia?
    a. A familial history of thalassemia
    b. Frequent bleeding episodes
    c. Asian descent
    d. Both A and C

28. What is another name for beta thalassemia major?
    a. Van Cool's anemia
    b. Cool anemia
    c. Cooley's anemia → *Found by Thomas cooley*
    d. None of the above

29. Alpha thalassemias are commonly seen in persons who can trace their descent to which areas?
    a. Southeast Asia, Malaysia, southern China
    b. Mediterranean region, Africa, Southeast Asia
    c. Southeast Asia, Africa, Malaysia
    d. Northern China, Malaysia, Africa

30. Beta thalassemias are commonly seen in persons who can trace their descent to which areas?
    a. Southeast Asia, Malaysia, southern China
    b. Mediterranean region, Africa, Southeast Asia
    c. Southeast Asia, Africa, Malaysia
    d. Northern China, Malaysia, Africa

31. Beta thalassemia major is commonly diagnosed by:
    a. CBC, CMP, and TIBC
    b. Early childhood
    c. CBC, CMP, Schilling test
    d. None of the above

32. You anticipate that your adult patient with sickle cell anemia will:
    a. Have asplenia
    b. Be aware of which medications are most effective for pain
    c. Need careful monitoring for sequelae of the disease
    d. All of the above

33. Your patient has been diagnosed with sickle cell disease. What does this tell you?
    a. She inherited this disease from both parents.
    b. She inherited this disease from one parent.
    c. She can expect to have minimal or no symptoms of the disorder.
    d. None of the above

34. When teaching your patient about living with sickle disease, you emphasize the importance of avoiding which of the following situations?
    a. Extreme heat or cold, dehydration, air travel in unpressurized cabins
    b. Dehydration, vitamin K–containing foods, air travel in pressurized cabins
    c. Air travel in unpressurized cabins, dental procedures
    d. All of the above

35. Which of the following is a serious complication from sickle cell disease?
    a. Cerebrovascular accident
    b. Acute chest syndrome
    c. Pulmonary hypertension
    d. All of the above

36. What does it mean when a person with sickle cell trait has a child with a person who also is diagnosed with sickle cell trait? *Sickle Cell is Autosomal recessive*
    a. They can pass the disease to their children.
    b. Their children will have either the disease or the trait.
    c. There is no risk to the children because the parents have only the trait.
    d. All of the above

37. Which of the following are signs and symptoms of a severe complication of sickle cell disease?
    a. Chest pain, shortness of breath
    b. Joint pain in multiple joints
    c. Abnormal Hgb S values on CBC
    d. All of the above

38. Which medication is commonly used to reduce or prevent complications of sickle cell disease?
    a. Hydrochlorothiazide
    b. Hydroxyurea
    c. Hydroxyzine
    d. Hydrolysis

39. Sickle cell screening in the United States is:
    a. Part of mandatory newborn screening
    b. Offered and recommended for persons at risk prior to conception
    c. Recommended for young children in at-risk groups
    d. All of the above

40. Which of the following is an important immunization for persons with sickle cell disease?
- a. Pneumococcus
- b. Meningococcus
- c. Influenza
- d. All of the above

Chapter 5: Answers and Rationales

1. D. Labs to assess for anemia, potential causes of anemia, and sequelae of disease would be anticipated.

Kidney Disease: Improving Global Outcomes (KDIGO) Anemia Work Group. KDIGO clinical practice guideline for anemia in chronic kidney disease. *Kidney Int Suppl.* 2012;2(4):279–335. http://www.kdigo.org/clinical_practice_guidelines/pdf/KDIGO-Anemia%20GL.pdf. Accessed September 16, 2015.

Kidney Disease: Improving Global Outcomes (KDIGO) Anemia Work Group. KDIGO 2012 clinical practice guideline for the evaluation and management of chronic kidney disease. *Kidney Int Suppl.* 2013;3(1):1–150. http://www.kdigo.org/clinical_practice_guidelines/pdf/CKD/KDIGO_2012_CKD_GL.pdf. Accessed September 16, 2015.

World Health Organization. *Haemoglobin concentrations for the diagnosis of anaemia and assessment of severity.* Vitamin and Mineral Nutrition Information System. Geneva: World Health Organization; 2011. http://www.who.int/vmnis/indicators/haemoglobin.pdf. Accessed September 16, 2015.

2. A. Anemia of chronic disease is a normocytic, normochromic anemia.

Kidney Disease: Improving Global Outcomes (KDIGO) Anemia Work Group. KDIGO clinical practice guideline for anemia in chronic kidney disease. *Kidney Int Suppl.* 2012;2(4):279–335. http://www.kdigo.org/clinical_practice_guidelines/pdf/KDIGO-Anemia%20GL.pdf. Accessed September 16, 2015.

Kidney Disease: Improving Global Outcomes (KDIGO) Anemia Work Group. KDIGO 2012 clinical practice guideline for the evaluation and management of chronic kidney disease. *Kidney Int Suppl.* 2013;3(1):1–150. http://www.kdigo.org/clinical_practice_guidelines/pdf/CKD/KDIGO_2012_CKD_GL.pdf. Accessed September 16, 2015.

World Health Organization. *Haemoglobin concentrations for the diagnosis of anaemia and assessment of severity.* Vitamin and Mineral Nutrition Information System. Geneva: World Health Organization; 2011. http://www.who.int/vmnis/indicators/haemoglobin.pdf. Accessed September 16, 2015.

3. D. Labs to assess for anemia, potential causes of anemia, and sequelae of disease would be anticipated.

Kidney Disease: Improving Global Outcomes (KDIGO) Anemia Work Group. KDIGO clinical practice guideline for anemia in chronic kidney disease. *Kidney Int Suppl.* 2012;2(4):279–335. http://www.kdigo.org/clinical_practice_guidelines/pdf/KDIGO-Anemia%20GL.pdf. Accessed September 16, 2015.

Kidney Disease: Improving Global Outcomes (KDIGO) Anemia Work Group. KDIGO 2012 clinical practice guideline for the evaluation and management of chronic kidney disease. *Kidney Int Suppl.* 2013;3(1):1–150. http://www.kdigo.org/clinical_practice_guidelines/pdf/CKD/KDIGO_2012_CKD_GL.pdf. Accessed September 16, 2015.

4. C. Erythropoietin alpha is used to stimulate red blood cell production and maturation in patients with chronic kidney disease.

Kidney Disease: Improving Global Outcomes (KDIGO) Anemia Work Group. KDIGO clinical practice guideline for anemia in chronic kidney disease. *Kidney Int Suppl.* 2012;2(4):279–335. http://www.kdigo.org/clinical_practice_guidelines/pdf/KDIGO-Anemia%20GL.pdf. Accessed September 16, 2015.

Kidney Disease: Improving Global Outcomes (KDIGO) Anemia Work Group. KDIGO 2012 clinical practice guideline for the evaluation and management of chronic kidney disease. *Kidney Int Suppl.* 2013;3(1):1–150. http://www.kdigo.org/clinical_practice_guidelines/pdf/CKD/KDIGO_2012_CKD_GL.pdf. Accessed September 16, 2015.

5. D. Congestive heart failure and arrhythmias are associated with anemia.

Kidney Disease: Improving Global Outcomes (KDIGO) Anemia Work Group. KDIGO clinical practice guideline for anemia in chronic kidney disease. *Kidney Int Suppl.* 2012;2(4):279–335. http://www.kdigo.org/clinical_practice_guidelines/pdf/KDIGO-Anemia%20GL.pdf. Accessed September 16, 2015.

Kidney Disease: Improving Global Outcomes (KDIGO) Anemia Work Group. KDIGO 2012 clinical practice guideline for the evaluation and management of chronic kidney disease. *Kidney Int Suppl.* 2013;3(1):1–150. http://www.kdigo.org/clinical_practice_guidelines/pdf/CKD/KDIGO_2012_CKD_GL.pdf. Accessed September 16, 2015.

6. D. In a female patient with symptoms of fatigue, numbness, and tingling, you should consider thyroid disorders, vitamin-deficiency anemia, and autoimmune disease. A physical examination also is required to rule out any neurologic or cardiovascular basis for her complaints.

Johnson-Wimbley TD, Graham DY. Diagnosis and management of iron deficiency anemia in the 21st century. *Therap Adv Gastroenterol.* May 2011;4(3):177–184. http://www.ncbi.nlm.nih.gov/pmc/articles/PMC3105608/.

Short MW, Domagalski JE. Iron deficiency anemia: evaluation and management. *Am Fam Physician.* 2013;87(2):98–104.

7. D. When considering vitamin deficiency causes for anemia, folate, vitamin B_{12}, and coexisting iron-deficiency anemia should be evaluated for.

Johnson-Wimbley TD, Graham DY. Diagnosis and management of iron deficiency anemia in the 21st century. *Therap Adv Gastroenterol*. May 2011;4(3):177–184. http://www.ncbi.nlm.nih.gov/pmc/articles/PMC3105608/.

Short MW, Domagalski JE. Iron deficiency anemia: evaluation and management. *Am Fam Physician*. 2013;87(2):98–104.

8. A. The Schilling test differentiates folate-deficiency anemia from vitamin B_{12}–deficiency anemia.

Johnson-Wimbley TD, Graham DY. Diagnosis and management of iron deficiency anemia in the 21st century. *Therap Adv Gastroenterol*. May 2011;4(3):177–184. http://www.ncbi.nlm.nih.gov/pmc/articles/PMC3105608/.

Short MW, Domagalski JE. Iron deficiency anemia: evaluation and management. *Am Fam Physician*. 2013;87(2):98–104.

9. A. The Schilling test helps differentiate vitamin B_{12}–deficiency anemia from other forms of anemia.

Johnson-Wimbley TD, Graham DY. Diagnosis and management of iron deficiency anemia in the 21st century. *Therap Adv Gastroenterol*. May 2011;4(3):177–184. http://www.ncbi.nlm.nih.gov/pmc/articles/PMC3105608/.

Short MW, Domagalski JE. Iron deficiency anemia: evaluation and management. *Am Fam Physician*. 2013;87(2):98–104.

10. D. All of the listed items are risk factors for vitamin B_{12}–deficiency anemia.

Johnson-Wimbley TD, Graham DY. Diagnosis and management of iron deficiency anemia in the 21st century. *Therap Adv Gastroenterol*. May 2011;4(3):177–184. http://www.ncbi.nlm.nih.gov/pmc/articles/PMC3105608/.

Short MW, Domagalski JE. Iron deficiency anemia: evaluation and management. *Am Fam Physician*. 2013;87(2):98–104.

11. B. Some patients may not be able to derive benefit from oral vitamin B_{12} and may require intranasal or injectable vitamin B_{12}.

Johnson-Wimbley TD, Graham DY. Diagnosis and management of iron deficiency anemia in the 21st century. *Therap Adv Gastroenterol*. May 2011;4(3):177–184. http://www.ncbi.nlm.nih.gov/pmc/articles/PMC3105608/.

Short MW, Domagalski JE. Iron deficiency anemia: evaluation and management. *Am Fam Physician*. 2013;87(2):98–104.

12. C. Vitamin B_{12} may be delivered PO, intranasally, or via injection. In the case of a patient with partial gastrectomy, injection or intranasal would be preferred.

Johnson-Wimbley TD, Graham DY. Diagnosis and management of iron deficiency anemia in the 21st century. *Therap Adv Gastroenterol*. May 2011;4(3):177–184. http://www.ncbi.nlm.nih.gov/pmc/articles/PMC3105608/.

Short MW, Domagalski JE. Iron deficiency anemia: evaluation and management. *Am Fam Physician*. 2013;87(2):98–104.

13. B. Lab testing to differentiate iron-deficiency anemia should include complete blood count (CBC), comprehensive metabolic panel (CMP), ferritin, and total iron-binding capacity (TIBC) as baseline testing.

Johnson-Wimbley TD, Graham DY. Diagnosis and management of iron deficiency anemia in the 21st century. *Therap Adv Gastroenterol*. May 2011;4(3):177–184. http://www.ncbi.nlm.nih.gov/pmc/articles/PMC3105608/.

Short MW, Domagalski JE. Iron deficiency anemia: evaluation and management. *Am Fam Physician*. 2013;87(2):98–104.

14. A. A history of alcohol (ETOH) abuse is associated with folate deficiency.

Johnson-Wimbley TD, Graham DY. Diagnosis and management of iron deficiency anemia in the 21st century. *Therap Adv Gastroenterol*. May 2011;4(3):177–184. http://www.ncbi.nlm.nih.gov/pmc/articles/PMC3105608/.

Short MW, Domagalski JE. Iron deficiency anemia: evaluation and management. *Am Fam Physician*. 2013;87(2):98–104.

15. D. Anemia of folate deficiency often occurs concurrently with anemia of vitamin B_{12} deficiency and iron-deficiency anemia.

Johnson-Wimbley TD, Graham DY. Diagnosis and management of iron deficiency anemia in the 21st century. *Therap Adv Gastroenterol*. May 2011;4(3):177–184. http://www.ncbi.nlm.nih.gov/pmc/articles/PMC3105608/.

Short MW, Domagalski JE. Iron deficiency anemia: evaluation and management. *Am Fam Physician*. 2013;87(2):98–104.

16. A. Iron-deficiency anemia lab results will vary based upon the stage of disease and any comorbid anemias, but it is associated with a decrease in hemoglobin (Hgb), hematocrit (Hct), mean corpuscular volume (MCV), and ferritin with an increase in red cell distribution width (RDW) and total iron-binding capacity (TIBC).

Johnson-Wimbley TD, Graham DY. Diagnosis and management of iron deficiency anemia in the 21st century. *Therap Adv Gastroenterol*. May 2011;4(3):177–184. http://www.ncbi.nlm.nih.gov/pmc/articles/PMC3105608/.

Short MW, Domagalski JE. Iron deficiency anemia: evaluation and management. *Am Fam Physician*. 2013;87(2):98–104.

17. A. Depending upon the stage of compensation in iron-deficiency anemia, the labs may appear as either microcytic or normocytic.

Johnson-Wimbley TD, Graham DY. Diagnosis and management of iron deficiency anemia in the 21st century. *Therap Adv Gastroenterol*. May 2011;4(3):177–184. http://www.ncbi.nlm.nih.gov/pmc/articles/PMC3105608/.

Short MW, Domagalski JE. Iron deficiency anemia: evaluation and management. *Am Fam Physician*. 2013;87(2):98–104.

18. B. Hemoglobin electrophoresis is not used to differentiate folic acid–deficiency anemia.

Johnson-Wimbley TD, Graham DY. Diagnosis and management of iron deficiency anemia in the 21st century. *Therap*

Adv Gastroenterol. May 2011;4(3):177–184. http://www.ncbi.nlm.nih.gov/pmc/articles/PMC3105608/.

Short MW, Domagalski JE. Iron deficiency anemia: evaluation and management. *Am Fam Physician.* 2013;87(2):98–104.

19. D. Instructing patients on what to anticipate from oral iron therapy is an important intervention in the management of iron-deficiency anemia.

Johnson-Wimbley TD, Graham DY. Diagnosis and management of iron deficiency anemia in the 21st century. *Therap Adv Gastroenterol.* May 2011;4(3):177–184. http://www.ncbi.nlm.nih.gov/pmc/articles/PMC3105608/.

Short MW, Domagalski JE. Iron deficiency anemia: evaluation and management. *Am Fam Physician.* 2013;87(2):98–104.

20. A. Anemia is generally divided into microcytic, macrocytic, and normocytic categories.

Johnson-Wimbley TD, Graham DY. Diagnosis and management of iron deficiency anemia in the 21st century. *Therap Adv Gastroenterol.* May 2011;4(3):177–184. http://www.ncbi.nlm.nih.gov/pmc/articles/PMC3105608/.

Short MW, Domagalski JE. Iron deficiency anemia: evaluation and management. *Am Fam Physician.* 2013;87(2):98–104.

21. A. The definition of normocytic anemia is anemia with a mean corpuscular volume (MCV) in the normal range.

Johnson-Wimbley TD, Graham DY. Diagnosis and management of iron deficiency anemia in the 21st century. *Therap Adv Gastroenterol.* May 2011;4(3):177–184. http://www.ncbi.nlm.nih.gov/pmc/articles/PMC3105608/.

Short MW, Domagalski JE. Iron deficiency anemia: evaluation and management. *Am Fam Physician.* 2013;87(2):98–104.

22. B. Baseline laboratory results for thalassemia may initially appear similar to iron-deficiency anemia until further testing with hemoglobin electrophoresis is conducted.

Johnson-Wimbley TD, Graham DY. Diagnosis and management of iron deficiency anemia in the 21st century. *Therap Adv Gastroenterol.* May 2011;4(3):177–184. http://www.ncbi.nlm.nih.gov/pmc/articles/PMC3105608/.

Short MW, Domagalski JE. Iron deficiency anemia: evaluation and management. *Am Fam Physician.* 2013;87(2):98–104.

23. D. Perimenopausal women are at risk for iron-deficiency anemia (IDA) related to hormonal disease states.

Johnson-Wimbley TD, Graham DY. Diagnosis and management of iron deficiency anemia in the 21st century. *Therap Adv Gastroenterol.* May 2011;4(3):177–184. http://www.ncbi.nlm.nih.gov/pmc/articles/PMC3105608/.

Short MW, Domagalski JE. Iron deficiency anemia: evaluation and management. *Am Fam Physician.* 2013;87(2):98–104.

24. B. Autosomal recessive traits allow for inheritance of no disease, inheritance of disease in a carrier state, or disease expression. In the case of alpha thalassemia minor, this patient has inherited one altered alpha chain.

Northern California Comprehensive Thalassemia Center. Genetics of thalassemia. http://thalassemia.com/genetics-inheritance.aspx#gsc.tab=0. Accessed January 4, 2016.

25. A. Autosomal recessive traits allow for inheritance of no disease, inheritance of the disease in a carrier state, or disease expression. In the case of beta thalassemia major, both parents must pass on one altered beta chain for the patient to have this severe form of the disease.

Piel FB, Weatherall DJ. The α-thalassemias. *N Engl J Med.* 2014;371(20):1908–1916.

26. A. Iron supplementation is contraindicated in alpha thalassemia because iron overload can prove fatal for patients with alpha thalassemia.

Piel FB, Weatherall DJ. The α-thalassemias. *N Engl J Med.* 2014;371(20):1908–1916.

27. D. Alpha thalassemia is an inherited condition common in patients of Asian descent.

Northern California Comprehensive Thalassemia Center. Genetics of thalassemia. http://thalassemia.com/genetics-inheritance.aspx#gsc.tab=0. Accessed January 4, 2016.

Piel FB, Weatherall DJ. The α-thalassemias. *N Engl J Med.* 2014;371(20):1908–1916.

28. C. Beta thalassemia major was first described by Detroit pediatrician Thomas Cooley in 1925 and is often referred to as Cooley's anemia.

Northern California Comprehensive Thalassemia Center. Genetics of thalassemia. http://thalassemia.com/genetics-inheritance.aspx#gsc.tab=0. Accessed January 4, 2016.

Piel FB, Weatherall DJ. The α-thalassemias. *N Engl J Med.* 2014;371(20):1908–1916.

29. A. Alpha thalassemia is common in Southeast Asian, Malaysian, and southern Chinese populations.

Northern California Comprehensive Thalassemia Center. Genetics of thalassemia. http://thalassemia.com/genetics-inheritance.aspx#gsc.tab=0. Accessed January 4, 2016.

Piel FB, Weatherall DJ. The α-thalassemias. *N Engl J Med.* 2014;371(20):1908–1916.

30. B. Beta thalassemias are common in persons of Mediterranean, African, and Southeast Asian descent.

Northern California Comprehensive Thalassemia Center. Genetics of thalassemia. http://thalassemia.com/genetics-inheritance.aspx#gsc.tab=0. Accessed January 4, 2016.

Piel FB, Weatherall DJ. The α-thalassemias. *N Engl J Med.* 2014;371(20):1908–1916.

31. B. Beta thalassemia major is normally diagnosed in early childhood.

Northern California Comprehensive Thalassemia Center. Genetics of thalassemia. http://thalassemia.com/genetics-inheritance.aspx#gsc.tab=0. Accessed January 4, 2016.

Piel FB, Weatherall DJ. The α-thalassemias. *N Engl J Med.* 2014;371(20):1908–1916.

32. D. According to the National Heart, Lung, and Blood Institute, asplenia is commonly experienced by the age of adulthood in patients with sickle cell disease. Persons with sickle cell disease require ongoing lifetime monitoring for complications of sickle cell disease. By adulthood, they have experienced multiple pain crises.

National Heart, Lung, and Blood Institute. What causes sickle cell disease? 2015. http://www.nhlbi.nih.gov/health/health-topics/topics/sca/causes. Accessed January 4, 2016.

33. A. According to the National Heart, Lung, and Blood Institute, sickle cell disease is an autosomal recessive condition.

National Heart, Lung, and Blood Institute. What causes sickle cell disease? 2015. http://www.nhlbi.nih.gov/health/health-topics/topics/sca/causes. Accessed January 4, 2016.

34. A. According to the National Heart, Lung, and Blood Institute, avoidance of extreme conditions is imperative to prevent sickling and vaso-occlusive crises.

National Heart, Lung, and Blood Institute. What are the signs and symptoms of sickle cell disease? 2015. http://www.nhlbi.nih.gov/health/health-topics/topics/sca/signs. Accessed January 4, 2016.

35. D. According to the National Heart, Lung, and Blood Institute, serious complications of sickle cell disease can be life threatening if not diagnosed and treated effectively.

National Heart, Lung, and Blood Institute. What are the signs and symptoms of sickle cell disease? 2015. http://www.nhlbi.nih.gov/health/health-topics/topics/sca/signs. Accessed January 4, 2016.

36. A. Sickle cell disease is an autosomal recessive trait.

National Heart, Lung, and Blood Institute. What is sickle cell disease? 2015. http://www.nhlbi.nih.gov/health/health-topics/topics/sca. Accessed January 4, 2016.

37. A. Acute chest syndrome is a life-threatening complication of sickle cell disease that requires immediate emergency intervention.

National Heart, Lung, and Blood Institute. What are the signs and symptoms of sickle cell disease? 2015. http://www.nhlbi.nih.gov/health/health-topics/topics/sca/signs. Accessed January 4, 2016.

38. ~~A.~~ *B.* According to the National Heart, Lung, and Blood Institute, hydroxyurea is used to reduce or prevent complications of sickle cell disease.

National Heart, Lung, and Blood Institute. How is sickle cell disease treated? 2015. http://www.nhlbi.nih.gov/health/health-topics/topics/sca/treatment. Accessed January 4, 2016.

39. A. According to the National Heart, Lung, and Blood Institute, screening is recommended.

National Heart, Lung, and Blood Institute. How is sickle cell disease treated? 2015. http://www.nhlbi.nih.gov/health/health-topics/topics/sca/diagnosis. Accessed January 4, 2016.

40. D. The National Heart, Lung, and Blood Institute recommends all of the vaccinations listed for persons with sickle cell disease.

National Heart, Lung, and Blood Institute. How is sickle cell disease treated? 2015. http://www.nhlbi.nih.gov/health/health-topics/topics/sca/treatment. Accessed January 4, 2016.

Chapter 6: Common Endocrine Disorders in Primary Care

1. Cecil is a 14-year-old male who was recently diagnosed with diabetes mellitus type 1 (DM1). His mother is anxious and asks why her son got this disease. You tell her that DM1 is caused by:
   a. Obesity
   b. Inactivity
   c. Poor diet
   d. Autoimmune response

2. James is a 17-year-old male with DM1. You anticipate his treatment regimen may include:
   a. 1–2 basal injections daily *Any of these*
   b. Prandial insulin before each meal
   c. Continuous subcutaneous insulin infusion
   d. All of the above

3. Ronald is a 55-year-old male with newly diagnosed diabetes mellitus type 2 (DM2). His HgbA1C is currently 7.4%. You anticipate his initial treatment regimen will include:
   a. Lifestyle modification
   b. Weight loss as appropriate
   c. Monotherapy with an agent such as metformin
   d. All of the above

4. If Ronald's HgbA1C is not at goal within 3 months, you anticipate starting him on insulin.
   a. True   *If ∅ improvement c̄ monothera[py]*
   b. False   *initiate a second oral agent*

5. Patients who use an insulin pump for management of diabetes should be taught to:
   a. Self-monitor blood glucose at least two times daily
   b. Be alert for hypoglycemia
   c. Self-monitor blood glucose prior to any bolus of insulin
   d. All of the above

6. Glucose monitoring for adolescent patients with DM1 should be anticipated to be done:
   a. Morning and evening
   b. With each meal and prior to activity
   c. More frequently during times of growth and menstruation
   d. All of the above

7. You anticipate that managing DM1 in teenage female clients will be more challenging than in male teens because of:
   a. Dietary changes
   b. Growth
   c. Menstruation
   d. Potential for pregnancy

8. Glucose monitoring for well managed, nonpregnant adult patients should be anticipated to be:
   a. Individualized for each patient
   b. Performed at an increased frequency with illness
   c. Done when symptoms of blood glucose changes are present
   d. Both B and C
   e. All of the above

9. A diagnosis of DM is recommended to be made utilizing which of the following laboratory tests?
   a. Hemoglobin A1C
   b. Fasting plasma glucose (FPG)
   c. Oral glucose tolerance test (OGTT)
   d. Both B and C
   e. Both A and C
   f. All of the above

10. When assessing a patient whom you suspect may have DM1, in addition to FPB or OGTT, what tests do you anticipate ordering in the primary care setting?
    a. Autoantibodies, CMP, UA
    b. Autoantibodies, ABGs, CBC
    c. CMP, ABGs, CBC
    d. None of the above

11. Terri is a 53-year-old Native American female patient with DM2. She is obese, is on monotherapy, has no comorbidities, and denies any complaints of hypoglycemia. She comes to you today for discussion of her current HgbA1C. You tell her:
    a. Your HgbA1C is 6.0%. Keep up the good work.
    b. Your HgbA1C is 8.0%. Great job!
    c. Your HgbA1C is 6.5%. You need to make some modifications to reduce this number.
    d. Your HgbA1C is 6.0%. That is too low; you need to eat more carbohydrates.

12. A hemoglobin A1C of 12 is approximately equivalent to an average blood sugar of:
    a. 298
    b. 175
    c. 200
    d. 325

13. Recommendations for annual screening in diabetic patients include:
    a. Dilated eye exam
    b. Serum creatinine and urinalysis
    c. Neurologic examination
    d. All of the above

14. Risk factors for DM2 include:
    a. Sedentary lifestyle, overweight, Hispanic
    b. Hispanic, Asian/Pacific Islander, underweight
    c. Family history of DM2, Hispanic, active lifestyle
    d. None of the above

15. Treatment for DM2 in adolescents would be expected to include:
    a. Weight loss, diet instruction, insulin
    b. Diet instruction, weight loss, oral medication
    c. Oral medication, insulin
    d. All of the above

16. Treatment for DM2 in adults would be expected to include:
    a. Weight loss, diet instruction, insulin
    b. Diet instruction, weight loss, oral medication
    c. Oral medication, diet instruction, and possibly insulin
    d. None of the above

17. According to the Centers for Disease Control and Prevention (CDC), _____ people have DM in the United States.
    a. Over 29 million
    b. 1 in 3
    c. Over 86 million
    d. Both B and C

18. In persons ages 20 years and older in the United States, _____ American Indians and Alaskan Natives are estimated to have diabetes.
    a. 15.9%
    b. 13.2%
    c. 12.8%
    d. 9%

19. You are contemplating beginning metformin for your patient. You want to teach about side effects of the medication. A serious side effect to caution your patient about is:
    a. Lactic acidosis → rare but serious S/E
    b. Weight loss
    c. Anorexia   } normal S/E but not life threatening
    d. All of the above

20. Which agent would you anticipate beginning in a 32-year-old Hispanic female, BMI 30, with 3 children, nonpregnant, who presents with an HgbA1C of 7.4%?
    a. Thiazolidinediones
    b. Long-acting insulin
    c. Metformin — started as initial tx
    d. Sulfonylureas

21. In some patients the HgbA1C result may be less reliable than in other patients. What clinical conditions would cause you to reconsider the accuracy of the HgbA1C result?
    a. Anemia, thalassemia, and iron deficiency
    b. HTN, thalassemia
    c. Renal failure, HTN
    d. All of the above

22. The AACE recommends aggressive comorbidity management to reduce CVD in patients with DM. In an adult patient with DM and HTN, what are the preferred target measurements in an otherwise healthy adult?
    a. HgbA1C less than 7% and BP less than 120/80
    b. HgbA1C less than 7.5% and BP less than 130/80
    c. HgbA1C less than 8% and BP less than 140/90
    d. HgbA1C less than 9% and BP less than 140/90

23. What medications would you suggest for a nonpregnant adult patient newly diagnosed with HTN, DM, and an HgbA1C of 7%?
    a. Metoprolol, sulfonylurea
    b. Lisinopril, metformin
    c. Metoprolol, metformin
    d. Diltiazem, sulfonylurea

24. Diabetic neuropathy may include:
    a. Loss of sensation in feet, alterations in sensation of feet, increased peripheral pulse amplitude in feet
    b. Loss of sensation in feet, heart rate variability, decreased peripheral pulse amplitude
    c. Loss of sensation in feet, decreased peripheral pulse amplitude, fungal infection of feet/nails
    d. All of the above

25. What is the single best screening test for primary thyroid dysfunction?
    a. Serum thyrotropin (TSH)
    b. T3
    c. T4
    d. TPOAb

26. Mrs. Armbruster is a 40-year-old female who presents to you with c/o weight gain, dry skin, and dysmenorrhea. You are suspicious of a possible thyroid condition and find the following factors in her history merit further screening for possible hypothyroidism:
    a. Her father had Hashimoto's disease
    b. She takes lithium and vitamin B$_{12}$ injections
    c. Her mother had uterine fibroids
    d. Both A and B
    e. All of the above

27. Primary treatment for hypothyroidism includes:
    a. Levothyroxine
    b. Desiccated thyroid
    c. Iodine
    d. All of the above

28. In the management of your patient with primary hypothyroidism, your medication teaching should include:
    a. Take your medication on an empty stomach with a full glass of water.
    b. Do not take with calcium or multivitamins.
    c. Avoid taking with iron.
    d. All of the above

29. Lab recommendations for monitoring persons with hypothyroidism include:
    a. TSH 4–8 weeks after initiation of medication and/or changes in therapy
    b. T4 4–8 weeks after initiation of medication and/or changes in therapy
    c. TSH every 6–12 months once TSH is stable
    d. T4 every 6–12 months once T4 is stable
    e. Both A and C
    f. Both B and D

30. Mrs. Hill is a 38-year-old female with new onset of rapid irregular heart rate, anxiety and agitation, and noted protrusion of her eyes. You know that Mrs. Hill may be at risk for hyperthyroidism based upon the following history:
    a. Family history of Graves' disease
    b. Personal history of rheumatoid arthritis
    c. Female under age 40
    d. All of the above

31. After diagnosing Mrs. Hill with Graves' disease, you discuss her options for treatment with her. You explain that her treatment may include:
    a. Radioactive iodine ablation
    b. Surgery
    c. Anti-thyroid medications
    d. Beta blockers
    e. All of the above

32. Following initial treatment for Graves' disease, you advise your patient that:
    a. Laboratory testing will be necessary to monitor for treatment response.
    b. Levothyroxine may be needed.
    c. Additional treatments may be necessary.
    d. All of the above

33. On examination of a 45-year-old female patient, you palpate a fixed thyroid nodule. You order the initial test(s):
    a. Ultrasound
    b. Fine-needle aspiration biopsy (FNAB)
    c. Laboratory testing for TSH, T4, T3
    d. Both A and C
    e. All of the above

34. When preparing Mr. Jones for an ultrasound-guided FNAB, you instruct him:
    a. NPO after midnight
    b. You will be awake during the procedure with a local anesthetic agent applied.
    c. A fine-gauge needle will be inserted to remove cells for pathology.
    d. Both B and C
    e. All of the above

35. Mr. Jones's FNAB revealed cells that are suspicious for malignancy. You discuss the plan of care with Mr. Jones and inform him that the next step would be:
a. Surgery
b. Radioactive iodine treatment
c. Anti-thyroid medication
d. A wait-and-see approach

36. Mrs. Watson is a 52-year-old female who is preparing to undergo radioactive iodine ablation (RAI) treatment. You instruct her that for the 3–7 days following RAI treatment she should plan to:
a. Not kiss or hug her 2-year-old grandson
b. Avoid grocery shopping
c. Increase her intake of fluids
d. All of the above

37. Thyroid cancer risk factors include which of the following?
a. Radiation exposure in childhood
b. Family history of thyroid cancer
c. Over the age of 40 years
d. Both A and B
e. All of the above

38. The most common type of thyroid cancer is: *70–80% of Thyroid Cancers*
a. Papillary
b. Follicular
c. Medullary
d. Anaplastic

39. Mr. Jones is diagnosed with papillary thyroid cancer stage 1 and is asking about his prognosis. You tell him that the 5-year survival rate for his type of cancer is estimated at:
a. 100%
b. 71%
c. 28%
d. 7%

40. You are performing a routine thyroid examination on your 30-year-old female patient. You palpate a nodule and remember that:
a. Nonpalpable nodules are usually cancerous.
b. Hard nodules are usually benign.
c. Fluctuant nodules are usually benign.
d. Palpation is not effective in diagnosing benign versus cancerous nodules.

Chapter 6: Answers and Rationales

1. D. The CDC implicates an autoimmune response in the cause of DM1.

Centers for Disease Control and Prevention. Basics about diabetes. 2015. http://www.cdc.gov/diabetes/basics/diabetes.html. Accessed January 8, 2016.

2. D. According to the American Association of Clinical Endocrinologists (AACE), persons with DM1 will be managed using either a combination of 1–2 basal injections daily along with prandial insulin before each meal or a continuous subcutaneous insulin infusion.

American Association of Clinical Endocrinologists. AACE/ACE comprehensive diabetes management algorithm. *Endocr Pract.* 2015;21(4):e1–e10. https://www.aace.com/files/aace_algorithm.pdf. Accessed September 22, 2015.

American Association of Clinical Endocrinologists. Clinical practice guidelines. 2016. https://www.aace.com/publications/guidelines. Accessed January 8, 2016.

3. D. According to the AACE, a newly diagnosed DM2 patient with an HgbA1C of less than 7.5% would begin lifestyle modifications, weight loss as appropriate, and monotherapy with an oral agent.

American Association of Clinical Endocrinologists. AACE/ACE comprehensive diabetes management algorithm. *Endocr Pract.* 2015;21(4):e1–e10. https://www.aace.com/files/aace_algorithm.pdf. Accessed September 22, 2015.

American Association of Clinical Endocrinologists. Clinical practice guidelines. 2016. https://www.aace.com/publications/guidelines. Accessed January 8, 2016.

4. B. According to the AACE, if not at goal at 3 months, a patient who entered treatment with HgbA1C at 7.4% would be given a second oral agent to add to his current monotherapy regimen.

American Association of Clinical Endocrinologists. AACE/ACE comprehensive diabetes management algorithm. *Endocr Pract.* 2015;21(4):e1–e10. https://www.aace.com/files/aace_algorithm.pdf. Accessed September 22, 2015.

American Association of Clinical Endocrinologists. Clinical practice guidelines. 2016. https://www.aace.com/publications/guidelines. Accessed January 8, 2016.

5. D. According to the AACE, persons managed with continuous subcutaneous insulin infusion should be prepared to self-monitor blood glucose frequently and be alert for signs or symptoms of hypoglycemia.

American Association of Clinical Endocrinologists. AACE/ACE comprehensive diabetes management algorithm. *Endocr Pract.* 2015;21(4):e1–e10. https://www.aace.com/files/aace_algorithm.pdf. Accessed September 22, 2015.

American Association of Clinical Endocrinologists. Clinical practice guidelines. 2016. https://www.aace.com/publications/guidelines. Accessed January 8, 2016.

6. D. According to the AACE, glucose monitoring for adolescents will need to be more frequent to anticipate changes in insulin needs during activity and with increased metabolic demands such as growth and menstruation.

American Association of Clinical Endocrinologists. AACE/ACE comprehensive diabetes management algorithm. *Endocr Pract.* 2015;21(4):e1–e10. https://www.aace.com/files/aace_algorithm.pdf. Accessed September 22, 2015.

American Association of Clinical Endocrinologists. Clinical practice guidelines. 2016. https://www.aace.com/publications/guidelines. Accessed January 8, 2016.

7. C. According to the AACE, glucose monitoring for adolescents will need to be more frequent to anticipate changes in insulin needs during activity and with increased metabolic demands such as growth and menstruation.

American Association of Clinical Endocrinologists. AACE/ACE comprehensive diabetes management algorithm. *Endocr Pract.* 2015;21(4):e1–e10. https://www.aace.com/files/aace_algorithm.pdf. Accessed September 22, 2015.

American Association of Clinical Endocrinologists. Clinical practice guidelines. 2016. https://www.aace.com/publications/guidelines. Accessed January 8, 2016.

8. E. According to the AACE, glucose monitoring for stable, nonpregnant adult patients should be introduced at diagnosis, individualized based on patient needs, increased with illness related to blood sugar changes, and performed with any symptoms of hypo- or hyperglycemia.

American Association of Clinical Endocrinologists. AACE/ACE comprehensive diabetes management algorithm. *Endocr Pract.* 2015;21(4):e1–e10. https://www.aace.com/files/aace_algorithm.pdf. Accessed September 22, 2015.

American Association of Clinical Endocrinologists. Clinical practice guidelines. 2016. https://www.aace.com/publications/guidelines. Accessed January 8, 2016.

9. D. According to the AACE, the HgbA1C should be used as an additional diagnostic tool but not the primary diagnostic criterion for initial diagnosis of DM. The HgbA1C is not recommended to assist with diagnosis of gestational DM or DM1.

American Association of Clinical Endocrinologists. AACE/ACE comprehensive diabetes management algorithm. *Endocr Pract.* 2015;21(4):e1–e10. https://www.aace.com/files/aace_algorithm.pdf. Accessed September 22, 2015.

American Association of Clinical Endocrinologists. Clinical practice guidelines. 2016. https://www.aace.com/publications/guidelines. Accessed January 8, 2016.

10. A. Assessment for autoantibodies, renal function, and ketosis should be anticipated. Additionally, in an emergency/inpatient setting, ABGs would also be done to assess for ketoacidosis.

American Association of Clinical Endocrinologists. AACE/ACE comprehensive diabetes management algorithm. *Endocr Pract.* 2015;21(4):e1–e10. https://www.aace.com/files/aace_algorithm.pdf. Accessed September 22, 2015.

American Association of Clinical Endocrinologists. Clinical practice guidelines. 2016. https://www.aace.com/publications/guidelines. Accessed January 8, 2016.

11. A. An HgbA1C of less than or equal to 6.5% is the goal recommended by the AACE.

American Association of Clinical Endocrinologists. AACE/ACE comprehensive diabetes management algorithm. *Endocr Pract.* 2015;21(4):e1–e10. https://www.aace.com/files/aace_algorithm.pdf. Accessed September 22, 2015.

American Association of Clinical Endocrinologists. Clinical practice guidelines. 2016. https://www.aace.com/publications/guidelines. Accessed January 8, 2016.

12. A. According to the National Institute of Diabetes and Digestive and Kidney Diseases, an HgbA1C of 12% is equivalent to an average blood sugar of 298 mg/dL.

National Institute of Diabetes and Digestive and Kidney Diseases. The A1C test and diabetes: can the A1C test result in a different diagnosis than the glucose tests? 2014. http://www.niddk.nih.gov/health-information/health-topics/diagnostic-tests/a1c-test-diabetes/Pages/index.aspx#9. Accessed January 8, 2016.

13. D. According to the AACE, annual evaluations for diabetic patients should include evaluations of renal function and neurologic function and a dilated eye examination.

American Association of Clinical Endocrinologists. AACE/ACE comprehensive diabetes management algorithm. *Endocr Pract.* 2015;21(4):e1–e10. https://www.aace.com/files/aace_algorithm.pdf. Accessed September 22, 2015.

American Association of Clinical Endocrinologists. Clinical practice guidelines. 2016. https://www.aace.com/publications/guidelines. Accessed January 8, 2016.

14. A. According to AACE, overweight persons with a sedentary lifestyle, especially from an at-risk racial or ethnic group, are at a higher risk of the development of DM2.

American Association of Clinical Endocrinologists. Clinical practice guidelines. 2016. https://www.aace.com/publications/guidelines. Accessed January 8, 2016.

15. B. According to the AACE, DM2 is growing more common in adolescents. As with older patients with DM2, dietary teaching, weight loss, and oral medications would be anticipated treatments.

American Association of Clinical Endocrinologists. Clinical practice guidelines. 2016. https://www.aace.com/publications/guidelines. Accessed January 8, 2016.

16. C. According to the AACE, adults with DM2 would be started on oral therapy initially if their HgbA1C is < 9%, but may require insulin if their HgbA1C is > 9% or is not well managed after a period of time on oral medications.

American Association of Clinical Endocrinologists. AACE/ACE comprehensive diabetes management algorithm. *Endocr Pract.* 2015;21(4):e1–e10. https://www.aace.com/files/aace_algorithm.pdf. Accessed September 22, 2015.

American Association of Clinical Endocrinologists. Clinical practice guidelines. 2016. https://www.aace.com/publications/guidelines. Accessed January 8, 2016.

17. A. According to the CDC, more than 29 million Americans currently have diabetes, over 86 million have pre-diabetes, and 1 in 3 adults will develop diabetes in their lifetime.

Centers for Disease Control and Prevention. Diabetes in the United States: a snapshot. 2014. http://www.cdc.gov/diabetes/pubs/statsreport14/diabetes-infographic.pdf. Accessed January 8, 2016.

18. A. According to the CDC, American Indians and Alaskan Natives are estimated to have diabetes at a rate of 15.9%, compared to non-Hispanic blacks at 13.2%, Hispanics 12.8%, Asian Americans 9%, and white non-Hispanics 7.6%.

Centers for Disease Control and Prevention. National Diabetes Statistics Report, 2014. 2014. http://www.cdc.gov/diabetes/pubs/statsreport14/national-diabetes-report-web.pdf. Accessed January 8, 2016.

19. A. According to the National Institutes of Health, lactic acidosis is a rare but serious side effect of metformin and can be potentially life threatening. The other side effects listed—weight loss, anorexia, and others including bloating, gas, and diarrhea—while troubling, are not normally serious or life threatening.

National Library of Medicine. Metformin. 2016. https://www.nlm.nih.gov/medlineplus/druginfo/meds/a696005.html. Accessed January 8, 2016.

20. C. According to the AACE, adults with DM2 would be started on an oral monotherapy such as metformin initially if their HgbA1C is < 7.5%. The additional benefit of slight weight loss in the case of metformin is also beneficial in this young obese patient.

American Association of Clinical Endocrinologists. AACE/ACE comprehensive diabetes management algorithm. *Endocr Pract.* 2015;21(4):e1–e10. https://www.aace.com/files/aace_algorithm.pdf. Accessed September 22, 2015.

American Association of Clinical Endocrinologists. Clinical practice guidelines. 2016. https://www.aace.com/publications/guidelines. Accessed January 8, 2016.

21. A. According to the AACE, hemoglobinopathies, iron deficiency, hemolytic anemia, and thalassemia can cause the HgbA1C to be misleading.

American Association of Clinical Endocrinologists. AACE/ACE comprehensive diabetes management algorithm. *Endocr Pract.* 2015;21(4):e1–e10. https://www.aace.com/files/aace_algorithm.pdf. Accessed September 22, 2015.

American Association of Clinical Endocrinologists. Clinical practice guidelines. 2016. https://www.aace.com/publications/guidelines. Accessed January 8, 2016.

22. B. The AACE recommends that in an otherwise healthy adult an HgbA1c of less than 7.5% and BP less than 130/80 are desired. A more intensive goal should be considered in patients who can safely achieve them, while a less aggressive goal may be necessary for patients with significant comorbidities.

American Association of Clinical Endocrinologists. AACE/ACE comprehensive diabetes management algorithm. *Endocr Pract.* 2015;21(4):e1–e10. https://www.aace.com/files/aace_algorithm.pdf. Accessed September 22, 2015.

American Association of Clinical Endocrinologists. Clinical practice guidelines. 2016. https://www.aace.com/publications/guidelines. Accessed January 8, 2016.

23. B. According to the AACE, a first-line oral monotherapy treatment for DM should be selected. An angiotensin-converting enzyme (ACE) inhibitor would be preferred as a first-line treatment for HTN in this DM patient related to its additive benefit of slowing progression of nephropathy and retinopathy.

American Association of Clinical Endocrinologists. AACE/ACE comprehensive diabetes management algorithm. *Endocr Pract.* 2015;21(4):e1–e10. https://www.aace.com/files/aace_algorithm.pdf. Accessed September 22, 2015.

American Association of Clinical Endocrinologists. Clinical practice guidelines. 2016. https://www.aace.com/publications/guidelines. Accessed January 8, 2016.

24. B. According to the AACE, diabetic neuropathy evaluations should include foot inspection, assessment for peripheral vascular compromise, and assessment for cardiovascular autonomic neuropathy.

American Association of Clinical Endocrinologists. AACE/ACE comprehensive diabetes management algorithm. *Endocr Pract.* 2015;21(4):e1–e10. https://www.aace.com/files/aace_algorithm.pdf. Accessed September 22, 2015.

American Association of Clinical Endocrinologists. Clinical practice guidelines. 2016. https://www.aace.com/publications/guidelines. Accessed January 8, 2016.

25. A. Serum thyrotropin, also known as TSH, is considered the best screening test for primary thyroid dysfunction by the AACE and the American Thyroid Association (ATA).

Garber JR, Cobin RH, Gharib H; American Association of Clinical Endocrinologists and American Thyroid Association Taskforce on Hypothyroidism in Adults. Clinical practice guidelines for hypothyroidism in adults: cosponsored by the American Association of Clinical Endocrinologists and the American Thyroid Association. *Thyroid.* 2012;22(12):1200–1235. doi:10.1089/thy.2012.0205.

26. D. The AACE and ATA joint guidelines list a first-degree family history of autoimmune thyroiditis, a personal history of pernicious anemia, and use of certain medications such as lithium as reasons to screen for hypothyroidism.

Garber JR, Cobin RH, Gharib H; American Association of Clinical Endocrinologists and American Thyroid Association Taskforce on Hypothyroidism in Adults. Clinical practice guidelines for hypothyroidism in adults: cosponsored by the American Association of Clinical Endocrinologists and the American Thyroid Association. *Thyroid.* 2012;22(12):1200–1235. doi:10.1089/thy.2012.0205.

27. A. The AACE and ATA joint guidelines list levothyroxine as the primary treatment medication for hypothyroidism.

Garber JR, Cobin RH, Gharib H; American Association of Clinical Endocrinologists and American Thyroid Association Taskforce on Hypothyroidism in Adults. Clinical practice guidelines for hypothyroidism in adults: cosponsored by the American Association of Clinical Endocrinologists and the American Thyroid Association. *Thyroid*. 2012;22(12):1200–1235. doi:10.1089/thy.2012.0205.

28. D. The AACE and ATA joint guidelines state that levothyroxine should be taken alone, on an empty stomach, with a full glass of water to allow for full absorption and efficacy of levothyroxine.

Garber JR, Cobin RH, Gharib H; American Association of Clinical Endocrinologists and American Thyroid Association Taskforce on Hypothyroidism in Adults. Clinical practice guidelines for hypothyroidism in adults: cosponsored by the American Association of Clinical Endocrinologists and the American Thyroid Association. *Thyroid*. 2012;22(12):1200–1235. doi:10.1089/thy.2012.0205.

29. E. The AACE and ATA joint guidelines state that TSH levels should be monitored 4–8 weeks after the initiation of treatment, 4–8 weeks after medication changes, and every 6–12 months once the TSH is stable.

Garber JR, Cobin RH, Gharib H; American Association of Clinical Endocrinologists and American Thyroid Association Taskforce on Hypothyroidism in Adults. Clinical practice guidelines for hypothyroidism in adults: cosponsored by the American Association of Clinical Endocrinologists and the American Thyroid Association. *Thyroid*. 2012;22(12):1200–1235. doi:10.1089/thy.2012.0205.

30. D. The AACE and ATA joint guidelines state risk factors for Graves' disease include family history of the disease, personal history of autoimmune disease, and female gender under the age of 40.

Bahn RS, Burch HB, Cooper DS, et al. Hyperthyroidism and other causes of thyrotoxicosis: management guidelines of the American Thyroid Association and American Association of Clinical Endocrinologists. *Endocr Pract*. 2011;17(3). https://www.aace.com/files/hyperguidelinesapril2013.pdf. Accessed September 24, 2015.

31. E. The AACE and ATA joint guidelines include the following treatment recommendations for Graves' disease: surgical removal of all or part of the thyroid gland, radioactive iodine ablation of the thyroid, anti-thyroid medications to treat the cause of Graves' disease, and beta blockers not to treat the cause of Graves' disease but to treat the symptoms of Graves' while awaiting treatment response.

Bahn RS, Burch HB, Cooper DS, et al. Hyperthyroidism and other causes of thyrotoxicosis: management guidelines of the American Thyroid Association and American Association

of Clinical Endocrinologists. *Endocr Pract*. 2011;17(3). https://www.aace.com/files/hyperguidelinesapril2013.pdf. Accessed September 24, 2015.

32. D. The AACE and ATA joint guidelines note that treatment for Graves' disease will need to be individualized by patient and may need readjustment or additional treatments to achieve the desired response. Additionally, thyroid replacement may be necessary following ablation treatments and/or surgery.

Bahn RS, Burch HB, Cooper DS, et al. Hyperthyroidism and other causes of thyrotoxicosis: management guidelines of the American Thyroid Association and American Association of Clinical Endocrinologists. *Endocr Pract*. 2011;17(3). https://www.aace.com/files/hyperguidelinesapril2013.pdf. Accessed September 24, 2015.

33. D. The AACE, Associazione Meidici Endorinologi (EAM), and European Thyroid Association (ETA) Medical Guidelines for the Diagnosis and Management of Thyroid Nodules recommend initial evaluation of a thyroid nodule to include laboratory evaluation of thyroid hormone levels as well as ultrasound. An FNAB may be recommended following ultrasound and laboratory tests if further suspicion for malignancy exists.

Bahn RS, Burch HB, Cooper DS, et al. Hyperthyroidism and other causes of thyrotoxicosis: management guidelines of the American Thyroid Association and American Association of Clinical Endocrinologists. *Endocr Pract*. 2011;17(3). https://www.aace.com/files/hyperguidelinesapril2013.pdf. Accessed September 24, 2015.

Gharib H, Papini E, Paschke R, et al. American Association of Clinical Endocrinologists, Associazione Medici Endocrinologi, and European Thyroid Association medical guidelines for clinical practice for the diagnosis and management of thyroid nodules. https://www.aace.com/files/thyroid-guidelines.pdf. Accessed January 9, 2016.

34. D. The American Thyroid Association recommends that an ultrasound-guided FNAB, which is a minimally invasive procedure, may be performed with or without a local anesthetic agent, will not require the patient to be NPO after midnight, and will use a fine-gauge needle to remove cells for pathology.

American Thyroid Association. Thyroid nodules. 2016. http://www.thyroid.org/thyroid-nodules/. Accessed January 9, 2016.

35. A. The American Association of Clinical Endocrinologists, Associazione Medici Endocrinologi, and European Thyroid Association Medical Guidelines for Clinical Practice for the Diagnosis and Management of Thyroid Nodules recommend surgical removal of thyroid tissue suspicious for malignancy.

Gharib H, Papini E, Paschke R, et al. American Association of Clinical Endocrinologists, Associazione Medici

Endocrinologi, and European Thyroid Association medical guidelines for clinical practice for the diagnosis and management of thyroid nodules. https://www.aace.com/files/thyroid-guidelines.pdf. Accessed January 9, 2016.

36. D. The American Thyroid Association recommends avoiding close contact with other persons, especially children and pregnant women, in the 3–7 days following treatment with RAI. The amount of time needed for increased distance is relative to the dosing amount of the RAI. Patients should be instructed to increase fluids, avoid sharing food or utensils, do laundry and dishes separately, and sleep alone for 3–7 days following treatment to avoid exposing others to RAI and to aid in flushing the RAI out of the body.

American Thyroid Association. Radioactive iodine. 2016. http://www.thyroid.org/radioactive-iodine/. Accessed January 9, 2016.

EndocrineWeb. Radioactive iodine for hyperthyroidism: the most common hyperthyroid treatment in the US. 2014. http://www.endocrineweb.com/conditions/hyperthyroidism/radioactive-iodine-hyperthyroidism. Accessed January 9, 2016.

37. E. The American Thyroid Association and the Centers for Disease Control and Prevention (CDC) note that while most cases of thyroid cancer are in patients without readily identifiable risk patterns, a history of radiation exposure in childhood, family history of thyroid cancer, and being over the age of 40 years increase the likelihood of thyroid cancer.

American Thyroid Association. Thyroid cancer. 2016. http://www.thyroid.org/cancer-of-the-thyroid/. Accessed January 9, 2016.

Centers for Disease Control and Prevention. Thyroid cancer and the environment. 2014. http://ephtracking.cdc.gov/showCancerThyroidEnv.action. Accessed January 9, 2016.

38. A. The American Thyroid Association states that papillary thyroid cancer comprises 70–80% of all thyroid cancers diagnosed.

American Thyroid Association. Thyroid cancer. 2016. http://www.thyroid.org/cancer-of-the-thyroid/. Accessed January 9, 2016.

39. A. The American Cancer Society estimates the 5-year survival rate of Stage 1 papillary thyroid cancer at near 100%. Conversely, anaplastic thyroid cancer is considered Stage IV at diagnosis and is estimated to have a 5-year survival rate of approximately 7%.

American Cancer Society. Thyroid cancer survival by type and stage. 2015. http://www.cancer.org/cancer/thyroidcancer/detailedguide/thyroid-cancer-survival-rates. Accessed January 9, 2016.

40. D. The AACE, EAM, and ETA Medical Guidelines for Clinical Practice for the Diagnosis and Management of Thyroid Nodules state that clinical presentation of a nodule is not diagnostic, because both benign and malignant pathology can cause thyroid nodules. Further diagnostics are required to evaluate the thyroid nodule found on clinical examination.

Gharib H, Papini E, Paschke R, et al. American Association of Clinical Endocrinologists, Associazione Medici Endocrinologi, and European Thyroid Association medical guidelines for clinical practice for the diagnosis and management of thyroid nodules. https://www.aace.com/files/thyroid-guidelines.pdf. Accessed January 9, 2016.

Chapter 7: Common Women's Health Disorders in Primary Care

1. Which statement is incorrect regarding the use of intrauterine devices (IUDs)?
   a. The IUD is a safe and highly effective means of contraception.
   b. The effectiveness of IUDs is heavily dependent on user compliance.
   c. Three IUDs are available in the United States.
   d. Failure rates within the first year after insertion are less than 1%.

2. Which statement is consistent with key recommendations for IUDs?
   a. Adolescents should not be offered an IUD.
   b. Women who are at high risk for sexually transmitted infections (STIs) should not receive an IUD.
   c. If a woman with an IUD becomes pregnant, the IUD should be removed.
   d. Prophylactic antibiotics should be routinely administered for all women prior to IUD insertion.

3. Which of the following are potential side effects of IUDs?
   a. Headaches and nausea
   b. Hair loss and breast tenderness
   c. Depression and decreased libido
   d. All of the above

4. According to the Centers for Disease Control and Prevention, which suggestion is inconsistent with recommendations for establishing and maintaining rapport when providing contraceptive services?
   a. Explain how personal information will be used and ensure privacy and confidentiality.
   b. Demonstrate expertise, trustworthiness, and accessibility.
   c. Ask open-ended questions and listen without judgment.
   d. None of the above

5. Which condition requires additional considerations when prescribing estrogen-containing contraceptives?
   a. Breast cancer
   b. Hypotension
   c. Age younger than 30 years old
   d. Alcohol use

6. What recommendation is inaccurate for a woman who has missed a dose of an oral contraceptive?
    a. If the woman is on a combined oral contraceptive and has missed only 1 pill less than 48 hours ago, she should take the missed pill as soon as possible. The remaining pills should be taken at the usual time each day. No backup method is required.
    b. If the woman is on combined oral contraceptive and has missed 2 or more pills and the last pill was taken greater than 48 hours ago, she should take the most recently missed pill as soon as possible. The remaining pills should be taken at the usual time each day. A backup method is required for 7 consecutive days.
    c. If the woman is on a progestin-only pill, once a pill is missed the women must use a backup method for the next month and consider Plan B if she has had recent unprotected sex.
    d. If the woman is using a combined vaginal ring and has delayed insertion of a new ring for less than 48 hours, she should insert the ring as soon as possible and keep the ring in until the regularly scheduled removal day. Backup contraception should be used for 7 days.

7. According to CDC guidelines, what is the recommended treatment for gonococcal infections of the cervix, urethra, and rectum?
    a. Ceftriaxone 250 mg PO in a single dose
    b. Azithromycin 1 g orally in a single dose
    c. Ceftriaxone 250 mg IM in a single dose plus azithromycin 1 g orally in a single dose
    d. Cefazolin 250 mg IM in a single dose plus azithromycin 1 g orally in a single dose

8. Which statement is inconsistent with screening guidelines for gonococcal infections?
    a. Annual screening for *Neisseria gonorrhoeae* infection is recommended for all women older than 30 years.
    b. Annual screening is recommended for all sexually active women younger than 25 years.
    c. Annual screening is recommended for all sexually active women older than 25 years who are at increased risk for infection.
    d. Increased risk for infection for gonorrhea infection includes anyone with a new sex partner or more than one sex partner.

9. Which statement is incorrect regarding the symptoms of gonorrhea in women?
    a. Most women with gonorrhea have no symptoms, or only mild symptoms.
    b. Gonorrhea can cause a burning sensation during urination.
    c. Gonorrhea will not alter menstrual cycles.
    d. Women with gonorrhea may have increased vaginal discharge.

10. What are the potential complications of gonorrhea in women?
    a. Pelvic inflammatory disease (PID)
    b. Increased risk of ectopic pregnancy
    c. Infertility
    d. All of the above

11. Gonorrhea can be diagnosed using all of the following methods *except*:
    a. Blood work
    b. Endocervical or vagina specimens
    c. Rectal swab specimens
    d. Urine specimen

12. Which STI is most prevalent in the United States?
    a. Chlamydia
    b. Gonorrhea
    c. Syphilis
    d. Genital herpes

13. Your patient is being treated for chlamydia today. She asks when she can resume sex. What instructions should be given to the patient?
    a. You should not have sex again until you and your partner have completed treatment.
    b. If you are prescribed a single dose of medication, you should wait 7 days after the medication before having sex.
    c. If you are prescribed medication for 7 days, you should wait 7 days after completing the medication before having sex.
    d. All of the above

14. Which statement regarding expedited partner therapy (EPT) is inconsistent with CDC guidelines?
    a. EPT is the clinical practice of treating the sex partner of a patient diagnosed with HIV.
    b. EPT is the clinical practice of treating the sex partner of patients diagnosed with chlamydia.
    c. EPT involves a clinical assessment of the patient and treatment of both the patient and their partner if an STI is identified.
    d. The CDC has recommended EPT as a useful option to help facilitate partner management.

15. Which one of the following is not a recommended treatment regimen for patients with chlamydia?
    a. Erythromycin base 500 mg four times daily orally for 7 days
    b. Azithromycin 1 g orally as a single dose
    c. Doxycycline 100 mg orally twice a day for 7 days
    d. Levofloxacin 750 mg orally daily for 3 days

16. Casey is a 24-year-old female who reports she has not had a menstrual period for over 3 months. She states that she began menses at age 12 years old and had 5-day menstrual periods monthly since that time. What would you assess to determine the cause of her secondary amenorrhea?
    a. Pregnancy testing
    b. BMI
    c. Endocrine issues
    d. All of the above

CDC Recommends ✓
Levaquin 500mg QD X 7D

17. Ruby is a 28-year-old marathon runner who reports to you today with concerns about recurrent stress fractures in her lower extremities and recent cessation of her menstrual periods. You consider that the cause of her amenorrhea may be related to:
    a. Functional hypothalamic amenorrhea
    b. Thyroid dysfunction
    c. Anorexia nervosa
    d. All of the above

18. Shaunette is a 17-year-old female who presents to you along with her mother for concerns over her lack of menses. She states she is not sexually active, denies exercising to excess, and denies any recent illness. Her examination is unremarkable with the exception of erosion of enamel from teeth, thin hair, and cachectic appearance with a BMI of 17.5. You suspect:
    a. Functional hypothalamic amenorrhea
    b. Thyroid dysfunction
    c. Eating disorder
    d. All of the above

19. Jeanette is a 35-year-old female who presents to your office with c/o nausea, dizziness, and "feeling tired." She is G0P0 and reports she is "a little late" for her menstrual period but that is "not that unusual." States she is sexually active and uses condoms for birth control and STI prevention. You anticipate ordering which of the following diagnostic tests:
    a. Urinalysis
    b. Serum hCG test
    c. Thyroid panel
    d. CBC

20. Delilah is a 30-year-old female who presents with c/o dysuria, urgency, and burning on urination. Your differential diagnoses for Delilah would include:
    a. Uncomplicated UTI
    b. Vaginal infection
    c. STI
    d. All of the above

21. For a nonpregnant female patient with an uncomplicated UTI, what treatment regimen would you anticipate?
    a. Trimethoprim-sulfamethoxazole DS for 3 days
    b. Norfloxacin for 10 days
    c. Ciprofloxacin for 7 days
    d. Trimethoprim-sulfamethoxazole DS for 5 days

    [handwritten: → as initial tx]

22. Chauntay returns to the clinic today with c/o dysuria and urgency. You review her record and note she is a 26-year-old nonpregnant female who has been treated for UTI two times in the past 3 months. Your next step is:
    a. UA with C&S
    b. Begin trimethoprim-sulfamethoxazole DS for 3 days
    c. Begin ciprofloxacin for 3 days
    d. Begin phenazopyridine until symptoms resolve

23. Nonpharmacologic treatment for prevention of UTI should include:
    a. Postcoital voiding
    b. Increased fluids
    c. Showering as opposed to bathing
    d. All of the above

24. The most common causative bacteria in UTI in premenopausal nonpregnant females is:
    a. E. coli
    b. Coliform
    c. S. saprophyticus
    d. S. aureus

25. Concerning symptoms in a female patient with suspected UTI include which of the following?
    a. High fever
    b. Flank pain
    c. Nausea and vomiting
    d. All of the above

26. Prophylactic or intermittent antimicrobial therapy may be useful in female patients with recurrent UTI.
    a. True
    b. False

27. Mrs. Brownlee is a 50-year-old female who presents today with c/o dysfunctional uterine bleeding, night sweats, sleep disturbance, and irritability. You assess that she is probably experiencing:
    a. Perimenopause
    b. Menopause
    c. Uterine infection
    d. Cystitis

    [handwritten: menopause – defined as an abscence of menstruation >1 yr]

28. Common changes occurring in menopause include:
    a. Vaginal dryness
    b. Hot flashes
    c. Sleep disturbance
    d. All of the above

29. The average age of menopause is:
    a. 41
    b. 43
    c. 51
    d. 53

30. Evaluation of dysfunctional uterine bleeding in a 50-year-old female should first include:
    a. Uterine biopsy
    b. Hormone therapy
    c. Hysterectomy
    d. Uterine ablation

    [handwritten: → done to R/o uterine pathology prior to starting HRT]

31. Health risks after menopause include:
    a. Cardiovascular disease
    b. Stroke
    c. Bone thinning
    d. All of the above

32. Which medication increases the risk of endometrial cancer in postmenopausal women?
    a. Progesterone
    b. Estrogen
    c. Combined estrogen–progesterone compounds
    d. Calcium

33. Which of the following medications is associated with an increased risk of stroke and deep vein thrombosis (DVT)?
    a. Progesterone
    b. Vitamin D
    c. Combined estrogen–progesterone compounds
    d. Calcium

34. Screening recommendations for menopausal women include:
    a. DEXA scanning
    b. Mammography
    c. Cholesterol monitoring
    d. All of the above

35. Health maintenance activities for postmenopausal women include:
    a. Balanced diet
    b. Weight-bearing exercise
    c. Mammography screening
    d. All of the above

36. Vitamin supplementation for postmenopausal women includes:
    a. Vitamin D and calcium
    b. Vitamin B and vitamin D
    c. Calcium and vitamin B
    d. Vitamin C and vitamin B

Chapter 7: Answers and Rationales

1. B. Once the IUD is inserted, the patient only has to check the string to ensure that the IUD is still in place. Compliance is not a concern with IUDs.

   Hardeman J, Weiss BD. Intrauterine devices: an update. *Am Fam Physician*. 2014:89;445–450. http://www.aafp.org/afp/2014/0315/p445.html. Accessed January 9, 2016.

2. C. The risk of ectopic pregnancy is higher in women who become pregnant with an IUD in place in comparison with women who do not have an IUD. Ectopic pregnancies are less common in this population. Once ectopic pregnancy is excluded, the IUD should be removed.

   Hardeman J, Weiss BD. Intrauterine devices: an update. *Am Fam Physician*. 2014:89;445–450. http://www.aafp.org/afp/2014/0315/p445.html. Accessed January 9, 2016.

3. D. Side effects of the 2 levonorgestrel-releasing IUDs (LNG-IUD) are similar to those of other progestin-based contraceptives and include all of the side effects listed.

Hardeman J, Weiss BD. Intrauterine devices: an update. *Am Fam Physician*. 2014:89;445–450. http://www.aafp.org/afp/2014/0315/p445.html. Accessed January 9, 2016.

4. D. All answers listed are recommended for establishing and maintaining rapport when providing contraceptive services.

   Klein DA, Arnold JJ, Reese ES. Provision of contraception: key recommendations from the CDC. *Am Fam Physician*. 2015:91;625–633. http://www.aafp.org/afp/2015/0501/p625.html. Accessed January 9, 2016.

5. A. The presence of breast cancer is an unacceptable health risk (Category 4) for prescribing estrogen-containing contraceptives. The risk becomes a category 3 (proven risks usually outweigh its advantages) if the woman has been in complete remission for 5 years.

   Klein DA, Arnold JJ, Reese ES. Provision of contraception: key recommendations from the CDC. *Am Fam Physician*. 2015:91;625–633. http://www.aafp.org/afp/2015/0501/p625.html. Accessed January 9, 2016.

6. C. If the missed pill is more than 3 hours past the recommended dose (i.e., > 27 hours since previous dose), the woman should take 1 pill as soon as possible and take the remaining pills at the usual time each day. Backup contraception should be used for 2 consecutive days, and the woman should consider if she had recent unprotected intercourse.

   Klein DA, Arnold JJ, Reese ES. Provision of contraception: key recommendations from the CDC. *Am Fam Physician*. 2015:91;625–633. http://www.aafp.org/afp/2015/0501/p625.html. Accessed January 9, 2016.

7. C. As dual therapy, ceftriaxone and azithromycin should be administered together on the same day, preferably simultaneously and under direct observation.

   Centers for Disease Control and Prevention. 2015 Sexually transmitted diseases treatment guidelines. http://www.cdc.gov/std/tg2015/default.htm. Accessed September 25, 2015.

8. A. Annual screening is recommended for all sexually active women younger than 25 years and all sexually active women older than 25 years who are at increased risk for infection.

   Centers for Disease Control and Prevention. 2015 Sexually transmitted diseases treatment guidelines. http://www.cdc.gov/std/tg2015/default.htm. Accessed September 25, 2015.

9. C. Women with gonorrhea may experience vaginal bleeding between periods.

   Centers for Disease Control and Prevention. Gonorrhea— CDC fact sheet. 2015. http://www.cdc.gov/std/gonorrhea/stdfact-gonorrhea-detailed.htm. Accessed January 9, 2016.

10. D. Untreated gonorrhea can cause serious and permanent health problems in both men and women.

    Centers for Disease Control and Prevention. Gonorrhea— CDC fact sheet. 2015. http://www.cdc.gov/std/gonorrhea/stdfact-gonorrhea-detailed.htm. Accessed January 9, 2016.

11. A. Gonorrhea cannot be diagnosed with a blood sample. The nucleic acid amplification test (NAAT) is now considered the test of choice by the CDC because it is very sensitive.

Association of Public Health Laboratories, Centers for Disease Control and Prevention. Laboratory diagnostic testing for *Chlamydia trachomatis* and *Neisseria gonorrhoeae*. 2009. http://www.aphl.org/aphlprograms/infectious/std/Documents/ID_2009Jan_CTGCLab-Guidelines-Meeting-Report.pdf. Accessed January 9, 2016.

12. A. Chlamydia has the highest number of reported cases of all STIs, with 1,401,906 cases reported in 2013. Many cases of chlamydia, gonorrhea, and syphilis continue to go undiagnosed and unreported.

Centers for Disease Control and Prevention. 2013 sexually transmitted disease surveillance: chlamydia. 2014. http://www.cdc.gov/std/stats13/chlamydia.htm. Accessed January 9, 2016.

13. D. It is important that both the patient and her partner are treated and that they are clear about when it's safe to resume sex.

Centers for Disease Control and Prevention. Chlamydia—CDC fact sheet (detailed). 2015. http://www.cdc.gov/std/chlamydia/stdfact-chlamydia-detailed.htm. Accessed January 9, 2016.

14. A. EPT is not recommended for the treatment of a sex partner with HIV.

Centers for Disease Control and Prevention. Sexually transmitted diseases—expedited partner therapy. 2015. http://www.cdc.gov/std/ept/. Accessed January 9, 2016.

15. D. The CDC currently recommends that levofloxacin be prescribed at the 500 mg dose and given daily for 7 days.

Centers for Disease Control and Prevention. 2015 Sexually transmitted treatment guidelines: chlamydial infections. 2015. http://www.cdc.gov/std/tg2015/chlamydia.htm. Accessed January 9, 2016.

16. D. Secondary amenorrhea is cessation of menses following normal menarche. It can be caused by pregnancy, endocrine issues and low BMI.

Gordon CM. Functional hypothalamic amenorrhea. *N Engl J Med*. 2010;363:365–371. doi:10.1056/NEJMcp0912024.

Klein DA, Poth MA. Amenorrhea: an approach to diagnosis and management. *Am Fam Phys*. 2013;87(11):781–788.

17. A. Functional hypothalamic amenorrhea can be brought on by high levels of prolonged physical or emotional stress.

Gordon CM. Functional hypothalamic amenorrhea. *N Engl J Med*. 2010;363:365–371. doi:10.1056/NEJMcp0912024.

Klein DA, Poth MA. Amenorrhea: an approach to diagnosis and management. *Am Fam Phys*. 2013;87(11):781–788.

18. C. According to the American Psychiatric Association (APA), Shaunette is displaying symptoms of an eating disorder.

American Psychiatric Association. *Practice Guideline for the Treatment of Patients with Eating Disorders*. 3rd ed. Washington, DC: American Psychiatric Association; 2006.

Gordon CM. Functional hypothalamic amenorrhea. *N Engl J Med*. 2010;363:365–371. doi:10.1056/NEJMcp0912024.

Klein DA, Poth MA. Amenorrhea: an approach to diagnosis and management. *Am Fam Phys*. 2013;87(11):781–788.

US Department of Agriculture, US Department of Health and Human Services. *Dietary Guidelines for Americans, 2010*. 7th ed. Washington, DC: US Government Printing Office; 2010.

19. B. A female of childbearing years with delayed menstruation and signs or symptoms consistent with pregnancy should be tested for pregnancy. Because of the relative early stage of the suspected pregnancy a serum hCG test would be appropriate.

Gordon CM. Functional hypothalamic amenorrhea. *N Engl J Med*. 2010;363:365–371. doi:10.1056/NEJMcp0912024.

Klein DA, Poth MA. Amenorrhea: an approach to diagnosis and management. *Am Fam Phys*. 2013;87(11):781–788.

20. D. Differentials to consider for urinary irritation should include vaginal infection, STI, and UTI.

American College of Obstetricians and Gynecologists. *Treatment of Urinary Tract Infections in Nonpregnant Women*. Washington, DC: American College of Obstetricians and Gynecologists; 2008. (ACOG Practice Bulletin no. 91). http://www.guideline.gov/content.aspx?id=12628. Accessed September 25, 2015.

21. D. According to American College of Obstetricians and Gynecologists, Trimethoprim-sulfamethoxazole DS may be used for initial treatment of uncomplicated UTI in a nonpregnant female.

American College of Obstetricians and Gynecologists. *Treatment of Urinary Tract Infections in Nonpregnant Women*. Washington, DC: American College of Obstetricians and Gynecologists; 2008. (ACOG Practice Bulletin no. 91). http://www.guideline.gov/content.aspx?id=12628. Accessed September 25, 2015.

22. A. It is important in the case of recurrent UTI in premenopausal women to determine if the recurrence is related to re-infection or treatment failure related to resistant microbes. The urinalysis (UA) with culture and sensitivity (C&S) will determine the infectious agent, thereby targeting treatment more effectively.

American College of Obstetricians and Gynecologists. *Treatment of Urinary Tract Infections in Nonpregnant Women*. Washington, DC: American College of Obstetricians and Gynecologists; 2008. (ACOG Practice Bulletin no. 91). http://www.guideline.gov/content.aspx?id=12628. Accessed September 25, 2015.

23. D. American College of Obstetricians and Gynecologists (ACOG) recommends hygienic measures to reduce risk factors for UTI.

American College of Obstetricians and Gynecologists. *Treatment of Urinary Tract Infections in Nonpregnant Women.* Washington, DC: American College of Obstetricians and Gynecologists; 2008. (ACOG Practice Bulletin no. 91). http://www.guideline.gov/content.aspx?id=12628. Accessed September 25, 2015.

24. A. The most common isolate in premenopausal nonpregnant females with UTI is *E. coli.*

American College of Obstetricians and Gynecologists. *Treatment of Urinary Tract Infections in Nonpregnant Women.* Washington, DC: American College of Obstetricians and Gynecologists; 2008. (ACOG Practice Bulletin no. 91). http://www.guideline.gov/content.aspx?id=12628. Accessed September 25, 2015.

25. D. Pyelonephritis must be considered in patients with UTI and systemic and higher renal symptoms.

American College of Obstetricians and Gynecologists. *Treatment of Urinary Tract Infections in Nonpregnant Women.* Washington, DC: American College of Obstetricians and Gynecologists; 2008. (ACOG Practice Bulletin no. 91). http://www.guideline.gov/content.aspx?id=12628. Accessed September 25, 2015.

26. A. ACOG recommends either intermittent or prophylactic antimicrobial use in recurrent UTI.

American College of Obstetricians and Gynecologists. *Treatment of Urinary Tract Infections in Nonpregnant Women.* Washington, DC: American College of Obstetricians and Gynecologists; 2008. (ACOG Practice Bulletin no. 91). http://www.guideline.gov/content.aspx?id=12628. Accessed September 25, 2015.

27. A. ACOG defines menopause as the absence of menstruation for greater than 1 year. Perimenopause is the time period of hormonal changes that occurs for up to 10 years prior to cessation of menstruation.

American College of Obstetricians and Gynecologists. Perimenopausal bleeding and bleeding after menopause. 2011. http://www.acog.org/Patients/FAQs/Perimenopausal-Bleeding-and-Bleeding-After-Menopause. Accessed January 9, 2016.

Goodman NF, Cobin RH, Ginzburg SB, et al. American Association of Clinical Endocrinologists. American Association of Clinical Endocrinologists Medical Guidelines for Clinical Practice for the diagnosis and treatment of menopause: executive summary of recommendations. *Endocr Pract.* 2011;17(6):949–954.

28. D. ACOG states that common changes occurring in menopause and perimenopause include vasomotor disturbances, vulvovaginal atrophy, and sleep disturbance.

American College of Obstetricians and Gynecologists. The menopause years. 2015. http://www.acog.org/Patients/FAQs/The-Menopause-Years. Accessed January 9, 2016.

Goodman NF, Cobin RH, Ginzburg SB, et al. American Association of Clinical Endocrinologists. American Association of Clinical Endocrinologists Medical Guidelines for Clinical Practice for the diagnosis and treatment of menopause: executive summary of recommendations. *Endocr Pract.* 2011;17(6):949–954.

29. C. ACOG states that 51 is the average age of menopause.

American College of Obstetricians and Gynecologists. Perimenopausal bleeding and bleeding after menopause. 2011. http://www.acog.org/Patients/FAQs/Perimenopausal-Bleeding-and-Bleeding-After-Menopause. Accessed January 9, 2016.

Goodman NF, Cobin RH, Ginzburg SB, et al. American Association of Clinical Endocrinologists. American Association of Clinical Endocrinologists Medical Guidelines for Clinical Practice for the diagnosis and treatment of menopause: executive summary of recommendations. *Endocr Pract.* 2011;17(6):949–954.

30. A. ACOG states that evaluation of the uterus and endometrium should be done prior to initiation of hormonal therapy or treatment initiation in dysfunctional uterine bleeding to rule out uterine pathology.

American College of Obstetricians and Gynecologists. Perimenopausal bleeding and bleeding after menopause. 2011. http://www.acog.org/Patients/FAQs/Perimenopausal-Bleeding-and-Bleeding-After-Menopause. Accessed January 9, 2016.

Goodman NF, Cobin RH, Ginzburg SB, et al. American Association of Clinical Endocrinologists. American Association of Clinical Endocrinologists Medical Guidelines for Clinical Practice for the diagnosis and treatment of menopause: executive summary of recommendations. *Endocr Pract.* 2011;17(6):949–954.

31. D. ACOG discusses health risks faced by menopausal women.

American College of Obstetricians and Gynecologists. Perimenopausal bleeding and bleeding after menopause. 2011. http://www.acog.org/Patients/FAQs/Perimenopausal-Bleeding-and-Bleeding-After-Menopause. Accessed January 9, 2016.

Goodman NF, Cobin RH, Ginzburg SB, et al. American Association of Clinical Endocrinologists. American Association of Clinical Endocrinologists Medical Guidelines for Clinical Practice for the diagnosis and treatment of menopause: executive summary of recommendations. *Endocr Pract.* 2011;17(6):949–954.

32. B. ACOG states that women with an intact uterus at menopause should not be given estrogen-only medications, because they are associated with an increased risk of endometrial cancer.

American College of Obstetricians and Gynecologists. The menopause years. 2015. http://www.acog.org/Patients/FAQs/The-Menopause-Years. Accessed January 9, 2016.

Goodman NF, Cobin RH, Ginzburg SB, et al. American Association of Clinical Endocrinologists. American Association of Clinical Endocrinologists Medical Guidelines for Clinical Practice for the diagnosis and treatment of menopause: executive summary of recommendations. *Endocr Pract.* 2011;17(6):949–954.

33. C. ACOG states that combined estrogen–progesterone compounds increase the risk of stroke and DVT.

American College of Obstetricians and Gynecologists. The menopause years. 2015. http://www.acog.org/Patients/FAQs/The-Menopause-Years. Accessed January 9, 2016.

Goodman NF, Cobin RH, Ginzburg SB, et al. American Association of Clinical Endocrinologists. American Association of Clinical Endocrinologists Medical Guidelines for Clinical Practice for the diagnosis and treatment of menopause: executive summary of recommendations. *Endocr Pract.* 2011;17(6):949–954.

34. D. ACOG recommends routine screening for breast cancer, cardiovascular disease, and osteoporosis.

American College of Obstetricians and Gynecologists. The menopause years. 2015. http://www.acog.org/Patients/FAQs/The-Menopause-Years. Accessed January 9, 2016.

Goodman NF, Cobin RH, Ginzburg SB, et al. American Association of Clinical Endocrinologists. American Association of Clinical Endocrinologists Medical Guidelines for Clinical Practice for the diagnosis and treatment of menopause: executive summary of recommendations. *Endocr Pract.* 2011;17(6):949–954.

35. D. ACOG recommends routine health maintenance to help manage symptoms of menopause and prevent health conditions that increase in women after menopause.

American College of Obstetricians and Gynecologists. The menopause years. 2015. http://www.acog.org/Patients/FAQs/The-Menopause-Years. Accessed January 9, 2016.

Goodman NF, Cobin RH, Ginzburg SB, et al. American Association of Clinical Endocrinologists. American Association of Clinical Endocrinologists Medical Guidelines for Clinical Practice for the diagnosis and treatment of menopause: executive summary of recommendations. *Endocr Pract.* 2011;17(6):949–954.

36. A. ACOG states that postmenopausal women should include vitamin D and calcium in their diet for bone health.

American College of Obstetricians and Gynecologists. The menopause years. 2015. http://www.acog.org/Patients/FAQs/The-Menopause-Years. Accessed January 9, 2016.

Goodman NF, Cobin RH, Ginzburg SB, et al. American Association of Clinical Endocrinologists. American Association of Clinical Endocrinologists Medical Guidelines for Clinical Practice for the diagnosis and treatment of menopause: executive summary of recommendations. *Endocr Pract.* 2011;17(6):949–954.

Chapter 8: Common Men's Health Disorders in Primary Care

1. Which statement is accurate regarding prostate cancer?
   a. Men with localized disease frequently are symptomatic.
   b. There is no consensus regarding the optimal treatment for the patient with clinically localized disease.
   c. Approximately 50% of men with prostate cancer have localized disease.
   d. The incidence rate of prostate cancer is higher among black men, and this incidence has significantly increased from 2002–2011.

2. Which of the following is the most commonly used tumor grading system for prostate cancer?
   a. Karnofsky score
   b. Apache II score
   c. Gleason score
   d. Nottingham grade system

3. Which statement is not consistent with the new prostate-specific antigen (PSA) screening guideline from the American Urological Association?
   a. The target range for "routine" PSA screening has been expanded to ages 55 to 69.
   b. No screening is recommended for men younger than 40.
   c. No screening is recommended for men older than 70 or with life expectancy shorter than 15 years.
   d. Every other year screening is recommended.

4. What does the US Preventive Services Task Force recommend for screening for testicular cancer?
   a. All adolescent and adult males should be taught self-testicular examinations.
   b. All adolescent and adult males should have screening PSA testing for testicular cancer.
   c. Screening by self-examination or clinical examination is unlikely to offer meaningful health benefits.
   d. None of the above

5. Management of testicular cancer may consists of:
   a. Surgery
   b. Radiation
   c. Chemotherapy
   d. All of the above

6. Which of the following causes of scrotal swelling requires urgent surgical repair?
   a. Epididymitis
   b. Testicular torsion
   c. Henoch-Schonlein purpura vasculitis
   d. Varicocele

7. Which of the following is a modifiable risk factor associated with erectile dysfunction (ED)?
   a. Hypertension
   b. Diabetes
   c. Heart disease
   d. All of the above

8. Which category of medications may be considered for the management of erectile dysfunction?
   a. Tricyclic antidepressants
   b. Phosphodiesterase type 5 (PDE 5) inhibitors *Sildenafil, Vardenafil etc.*
   c. Selective serotonin reuptake inhibitors
   d. Angiotensin-converting enzyme inhibitors

9. Which statement is not consistent with the Princeton Consensus Panel regarding the management of erectile dysfunction in patients with cardiovascular disease?
   a. Patients at high risk should not receive treatment for sexual dysfunction until their cardiac condition has stabilized.
   b. Patients with unstable angina and uncontrolled hypertension are at high risk.
   c. The majority of patients treated for erectile dysfunction are in the high-risk category for cardiovascular disease. *majority are actually low risk*
   d. Patients whose risk is indeterminate should undergo further evaluation by a cardiologist before receiving drug therapy for sexual dysfunction.

10. Which statement accurately describes recommended approaches to the discussion of treatment options for erectile dysfunction?
    a. The spouse should not be present during the discussion of treatment options.
    b. Psychotherapy is rarely helpful alone or in combination with medical and surgical options.
    c. If one oral agent is ineffective, surgical options should be offered.
    d. The choice of treatment should ideally be made jointly by the provider, the patient, and the patient's partner.

11. Your patient with erectile dysfunction presents today to discuss how to take his new medication vardenafil. Which statement is incorrect regarding this medication?
    a. Side effects related to peripheral vasodilation include nasal congestion, headache, and dyspepsia.
    b. Concomitant use of this medication with organic nitrates or nitrites is contraindicated.
    c. The patient should take his medication approximately 60 minutes prior to sexual intercourse.
    d. This medication should be stored in the refrigerator to prevent disintegration of the drug.

12. Which statement accurately describes the initial diagnosis and evaluation of erectile dysfunction?
    a. Extensive lab evaluation for comorbid diseases is recommended.
    b. A complete medical, sexual, and psychosocial history is recommended.
    c. Medications rarely contribute to erectile dysfunction.
    d. Penile duplex ultrasonography is a useful diagnostic tool.

13. According to the updated American Urological Association (AUA) clinical guidelines, which of the following statements about recommendations for the diagnosis of lower urinary tract symptoms (LUTS) secondary to benign prostatic hyperplasia (BPH) is not correct?
    a. Men with suspected LUTS should be asked about a relevant medical history and complete the AUA symptom index.
    b. Physical examination should include a digital rectal examination.
    c. Laboratory tests should include prostate-specific antigen testing and urinalysis.
    d. Serum creatinine level should be measured routinely in the initial evaluation of men with LUTS secondary to BPH.

14. Which statement is true regarding overactive bladder (OAB) in men?
    a. OAB is common in men, and it significantly affects quality of life. *≈ 30%*
    b. OAB is not common in men, and it does not significantly affect quality of life.
    c. OAB is more common in women than in men.
    d. OAB is common in men, but most men are not troubled by it.

15. Your patient is a 70-year-old white man with LUTS secondary to BPH. According to the updated AUA clinical guidelines, which of the following statements would most likely apply to his treatment?
    a. If the AUA symptom index score is less than 8, he can be treated with watchful waiting.
    b. Persistent, bothersome LUTS after basic management should be treated by the nurse practitioner.
    c. Alpha-adrenergic blockers have not been linked to intraoperative floppy iris syndrome in patients with cataract.
    d. 5-Alpha-reductase inhibitors alone are the first treatment of choice of LUTS secondary to BPH with predominant bladder outlet obstruction (BOO) symptoms.

16. Which symptom would be a concern about the possible diagnosis of prostate cancer in a male over 50 years of age?
    a. Hesitancy, dribbling, and urgency
    b. Decreased force of urinary stream
    c. Pain and feeling of a full bladder
    d. Rapid onset of obstructive symptoms of urinary output

17. A young male client presents with a complaint of a feeling of fullness in the scrotum. Physical exam reveals a round, soft, bluish discolored, nontender, nonadherent testicular mass resembling a "bag of worms"; there is no variation in size with respiration or Valsalva maneuver. The mass transilluminates and is located anterior to the testes. The most likely diagnosis is:
    a. Varicocele
    b. Hernia
    c. Tumor
    d. Spermatocele

18. In the male, sexually transmitted disease can present as:
    a. Epididymitis
    b. Prostatitis
    c. Urethritis
    d. All of the above

19. Which statement is inaccurate regarding genital herpes?
    a. Genital herpes is a sexually transmitted illness caused by two types of viruses.
    b. About 1 out of every 6 people between the ages of 14 and 49 years has genital herpes.
    c. Herpes can only be spread by having vaginal sex with someone who has the disease.
    d. Genital herpes can be cured with antibiotics.

20. Which statement is accurate regarding the symptoms of genital herpes?
    a. Sores are generally limited to blisters on the mouth.
    b. Blisters associated with genital herpes are rarely painful.
    c. Repeat outbreaks of genital herpes are common.
    d. The number of outbreaks tends to increase over a period of years.

21. Which statement is inaccurate regarding strategies to reduce the risk of contracting genital herpes?
    a. The only way to avoid sexually transmitted diseases is to avoid vaginal, anal, and oral sex.
    b. The use of latex condoms may not fully protect people from getting genital herpes.
    c. Women who are pregnant cannot contract genital herpes, so condoms are unnecessary during pregnancy.
    d. Being in a long-term mutually monogamous relationship with a partner who has been tested and has negative STI test results can lower your risk of getting genital herpes.

22. Which statement is inaccurate regarding human immunodeficiency virus (HIV) transmission? *Preseminal + Vaginal + human milk*
    a. Blood, semen, and rectal fluids from an HIV-infected person are the only fluids that can transmit HIV.
    b. In the United States, HIV is spread mainly by having sex or sharing injection drug equipment such as needles with someone who has HIV.
    c. Anal sex is the highest risk behavior.
    d. HIV is not spread through saliva.

23. Which statement is not consistent with HIV screening guidelines?
    a. Screening for HIV infection should be performed routinely for all patients ages 10–75 years.
    b. All patients initiating treatment for TB should be screened routinely for HIV.
    c. All patients seeking treatment for STIs should be screened routinely for HIV during each visit for a new complaint.
    d. Persons at high risk for HIV infection should be screened for HIV at least annually.

24. Which statement is correct regarding HIV antibody testing?
    a. Enzyme-linked immunosorbent assays (ELISA) tests can detect HIV antibodies about 3 weeks after exposure.
    b. Only a blood sample can be used to detect HIV antibodies.
    c. Rapid HIV testing can provide results within 12 hours.
    d. A Western blot test is not needed to confirm ELISA or rapid HIV test results.

25. Which statement is inaccurate regarding inguinal hernias?
    a. The history and physical examination is usually sufficient to make the diagnosis.
    b. Inguinal hernias have a 9:1 male predominance with a higher incidence among men 40 to 59 years of age.
    c. Symptomatic patients often present with groin pain.
    d. Surgical repair is recommended for all inguinal hernias.

26. In which clinical situations would imaging with magnetic resonance be helpful to diagnose a hernia?
    a. Suspected sports hernia
    b. Recurrent hernia
    c. Possible hydrocele
    d. Activity-related groin pain with no identifiable hernia on exam

27. Which statement is inaccurate regarding the use of alpha-adrenergic medications for BPH?
    a. Alpha blockers are appropriate and effective treatment options for patients with moderate to severe lower urinary tract symptoms (LUTS) due to BPH.
    b. Alfuzosin, doxazosin, tamsulosin, and terazosin all appear to have equal clinical effectiveness.
    c. The older, less costly, generic alpha blockers require dose titration and blood pressure monitoring.
    d. The most common adverse event associated with alpha blockers is dry mouth.

28. Which statement is inaccurate regarding the use of 5-alpha reductase inhibitor (5-ARI) drugs for BPH?
    a. 5-ARIs should not be used in men with LUTS secondary to BPH without prostatic enlargement.
    b. 5-ARIs should not be used in refractory hematuria presumably due to prostatic bleeding. *(Finasteride has been proven to help e this)*
    c. 5-ARIs may prevent progression of LUTS secondary to BPH.
    d. 5 ARIs may reduce the risk of urinary retention and future prostate-related surgery.

29. The preferred method of diagnosing epididymitis is by:
    a. Gram stain of the urethral secretions demonstrating > 5 WBC per oil-immersion field *helps dx gonococcal inf*
    b. Culture of the urethral secretions demonstrating the presence of nitrites ≥ 10 WBC per high-power field
    c. Complete blood count demonstrating an elevated WBC > 10,000
    d. None of the above

30. Your 40-year-old patient comes in because of scrotal swelling and is concerned that he has epididymitis. He wants some basic information before he agrees to any diagnostic testing. Which statement is incorrect regarding the treatment of epididymitis?

a. Over-the-counter nonsteroidal agents can help with the discomfort.

b. A cold gel pack may help pain and swelling.

c. Antibiotics will always be prescribed.

d. A jock strap should be worn to support the scrotum.

31. Which statement is incorrect regarding the etiology of epididymitis?

a. In men younger than about 39 years of age, the cause is usually *Chlamydia trachomatis* or *Neisseria gonorrhoeae*.

b. In men older than 39 years of age, the causes are usually coliforms, which are bacteria (e.g., *Escherichia coli*) that live in the intestines.

c. Chemical epididymitis is an inflammation caused by the retrograde (backward) flow of urine when exercising or having sex with a full bladder.

d. Epididymitis is never viral in origin. *(mumps is a viral cause)*

32. A 17-year-old male presents to the practice with scrotal pain, swelling, and inflammation of the epididymis that started 3 weeks ago. Which statement is incorrect regarding treatment?

a. No treatment should be given until urine cultures are back.

b. Goals of treatment include improvement of signs and symptoms and prevention of transmission to others.

c. Treatment goals include decreasing potential complications such as infertility and chronic pain.

d. The recommended drug therapy includes ceftriaxone 250 mg IM in a single dose and doxycycline 100 mg twice daily for 10 days.

33. The prevalence of reduced libido is estimated to be 5–15% in men. Which of the following may be an etiological factor for low libido?

a. Alcoholism and depression

b. Prescription and recreational drugs

c. Relationship problems and psychosocial factors

d. All of the above

34. Which statement is inaccurate regarding the treatment for premature ejaculation?

a. Seeking psychological assistance or couples therapy may be helpful.

b. Behavioral methods include the start-and-stop method and the squeeze method.

c. Selective serotonin reuptake inhibitors help delay ejaculation.

d. Premature ejaculation rarely goes away without treatment.

35. Which of the following symptoms is not initially expected in adult men who have testosterone deficiency?

a. Decreased vigor

b. Decreased muscle mass and body hair

c. Decreased libido

d. Depressed mood

36. Population screening for male hypogonadism is not recommended. The Endocrine Society suggests screening only in situations in which prevalence is high. Which type of patient would not fall into this high-prevalence group?

a. Patients on long-term steroids

b. Patients with end-stage-renal disease on hemodialysis

c. Patients with type 1 DM *only Type II are high*

d. Men with osteoporosis or low-trauma fracture *risk*

37. Which of the following lab tests is usually the most important single test in the evaluation of male hypogonadism?

a. Serum total testosterone concentration

b. Serum free testosterone concentration

c. Serum luteinizing hormone (LH) and follicle-stimulating hormone (FSH)

d. Semen analysis

38. Which statement is inaccurate regarding abnormal serum free testosterone (SHBG) levels?

a. Obesity decreases SHBG levels.

b. Liver disease and hypothyroidism slightly increase SHBG levels.

c. Insulin resistance increases SHGB levels.

d. Although serum total testosterone concentration falls slightly with increasing age, SHBG falls to a greater degree.

39. At what time of the day should testosterone levels be drawn?

a. Ideally between 8:00 and 10:00 a.m. in a fasting patient.

b. Ideally between 4:00 and 6:00 p.m. in a fasting patient.

c. Ideally before 8:00 a.m. in a non-fasting patient.

d. The timing of blood draws is not clinically significant.

40. Which statement is inaccurate regarding testosterone treatment for erectile dysfunction?

a. Testosterone treatment for ED can cause acne, an enlarged prostate, and gynecomastia.

b. Testosterone treatment can increase the risk of heart disease and sleep apnea symptoms.

c. Women and children need to avoid touching any unwashed area where testosterone gel has been applied, because the medication can be transferred through skin contact.

d. A goal testosterone level for men taking testosterone treatment is 800–900 ng/dL.

recommend repletion 400-700

Chapter 8: Answers and Rationales

1. B. There are several commonly accepted initial interventions including active surveillance, radiotherapy, and radical prostatectomy. A discussion of the benefits and harms of each intervention should be offered to the patient.

Centers for Disease Control and Prevention. Prostate cancer trends. 2015. http://www.cdc.gov/cancer/prostate/statistics/trends.htm. Accessed January 9, 2016.

Thompson I, Thrasher JB, Aus G, et al. Guideline for the management of clinically localized prostate cancer: 2007 update. *J Urol.* 2007;177(6):2106–2131.

2. C. The most commonly used tumor grading system is the Gleason score. This system assigns a grade for each prostate cancer from 1 (least aggressive) to 5 (most aggressive) based on the degree of architectural differentiation of the tumor.

Thompson I, Thrasher JB, Aus G, et al. Guideline for the management of clinically localized prostate cancer: 2007 update. *J Urol.* 2007;177(6):2106–2131.

3. A. Compared to the 2009 best practice policy document, the guidelines narrow the age range in which informed decision making around PSA screening should be offered to men at average risk for prostate cancer to ages 55 to 69.

Carter HB, Albertsen PC, Barry MJ, et al. Early detection of prostate cancer: AUA guideline. *J Urol.* 190(2):419–426. http://dx.doi.org/10.1016/j.juro.2013.04.119.

4. C. Screening by self-examination or clinician examination is unlikely to offer meaningful health benefits, given the very low incidence and high cure rate of even advanced testicular cancer. Potential harms of screening include false-positive results, anxiety, and harms from diagnostic tests or procedures.

US Preventive Services Task Force. Clinical summary: testicular cancer: screening, April 2011. 2011. http://www.uspreventiveservicestaskforce.org/Page/Document/ClinicalSummaryFinal/testicular-cancer-screening. Accessed January 9, 2016.

5. D. There are different types of treatments for patients with testicular cancer. Treatment options depend on the stage of the cancer and how well it is expected to respond to the treatment.

Testicular Cancer Society. Understanding testicular cancer. 2002–2016. http://www.testicularcancersociety.org/understanding_testicular_cancer.html?gclid=Cj0KEQjw0tCuBRDIjJ_Mlb6zzpQBEiQAyjCoBndmwDJmp2FmEjG50Shmd52hkRrLf1N7vfZpxriDfVEaAs_L8P8HAQ. Accessed January 9, 2016.

6. B. Timely diagnosis and treatment of testicular torsion is key to preserving testicular function. If repaired within 6 hours of symptom onset, the salvage rate of the testicle is as high as 80% to 100%.

Crawford P, Crop JA. Evaluation of scrotal masses. *Am Fam Physician.* 2014;89;723–727.

7. D. Risk factors and disease processes that affect the function of the arterial or venous systems are expected to have a negative impact on erectile function. Because the risk of developing ED is increased in the presence of diabetes, heart disease, and hypertension, it is logical to conclude that optimal management of these diseases may prevent the development of ED.

American Urological Association. The management of erectile dysfunction. 2005. http://www.auanet.org/education/guidelines/erectile-dysfunction.cfm. Accessed January 9, 2016.

8. B. Oral phosphodiesterase type 5 inhibitors, unless contraindicated, should be offered as a first line of therapy for erectile dysfunction.

American Urological Association. The management of erectile dysfunction. 2005. http://www.auanet.org/education/guidelines/erectile-dysfunction.cfm. Accessed January 9, 2016.

9. C. The majority of patients treated for ED are actually in the low-risk category for cardiovascular disease.

Nehra A, Jackson G, Miner M, et al. The Princeton III consensus recommendations for the management of erectile dysfunction and cardiovascular disease. *Mayo Clin Proc.* 2012;87(8):766–778. http://www.ncbi.nlm.nih.gov/pmc/articles/PMC3498391/. Accessed September 25, 2015.

10. D. The patient's partner should always be included in the decision-making process for treatment.

American Urological Association. The management of erectile dysfunction. 2005. http://www.auanet.org/education/guidelines/erectile-dysfunction.cfm. Accessed January 9, 2016.

11. D. Refrigeration is not needed for this medication.

American Urological Association. The management of erectile dysfunction. 2005. http://www.auanet.org/education/guidelines/erectile-dysfunction.cfm. Accessed January 9, 2016.

12. B. The initial evaluation should take into account not only medical information but also the sexual and psychosocial history. Often, this information is adequate to determine an etiological base for ED.

Heidelbaugh JJ. Management of erectile dysfunction. *Am Fam Physician.* 2010;81:305–312.

13. D. Baseline renal insufficiency appears to be no more common in men with BPH than in men of the same age group in the general population, and serum creatinine levels provide no additional helpful information in the diagnostic evaluation of BPH.

American Urological Association. American Urological Association guideline: management of benign prostatic hyperplasia (BPH). 2010. https://www.auanet.org/common/pdf/education/clinical-guidance/Benign-Prostatic-Hyperplasia.pdf. Accessed January 9, 2016.

14. A. About 30% of all men have OAB symptoms, but it is believed that many cases go untreated because men may feel embarrassed about having symptoms and don't discuss it with their healthcare provider. Quality of life is impacted due to its common set of symptoms that can include frequent urination, a constant urge to go, leakage, and nighttime urination.

American Urological Association. American Urological Association guideline: management of benign prostatic hyperplasia (BPH). 2010. https://www.auanet.org/common/pdf/education/clinical-guidance/Benign-Prostatic-Hyperplasia.pdf. Accessed January 9, 2016.

15. A. An AUA symptom index score less than 8 is not causing considerable symptoms or quality of life issues, thus it is appropriate to watch the patient and reevaluate at least annually.

American Urological Association. American Urological Association guideline: management of benign prostatic hyperplasia (BPH). 2010. https://www.auanet.org/common/pdf/education/clinical-guidance/Benign-Prostatic-Hyperplasia.pdf. Accessed January 9, 2016.

16. D. An enlarged prostate, which can occur due to prostate cancer, can cause urinary tract obstruction by obstructing the urethra.

Kim ED. Urinary tract obstruction. 2014. http://emedicine.medscape.com/article/438890-overview#a8. Accessed January 9, 2016.

17. A. A varicocele is a dilation of the pampiniform venous plexus along the spermatic cord. Patients may be asymptomatic or may complain of a dull, dragging discomfort on the affected side. Palpation reveals the classic "bag of worms" along the spermatic cord. The mass disappears when the patient lies down and reappears when the patient stands.

Crawford P, Crop JA. Evaluation of scrotal masses. *Am Fam Physician*. 2014:89;723–727.

18. D. Sexually transmitted illnesses can involve the epididymis, the prostate, and the urethra.

Centers for Disease Control and Prevention. Sexually transmitted diseases (STDs): treatment. 2015. http://www.cdc.gov/std/treatment/. Accessed January 9, 2016.

19. D. There is no cure for herpes. Antiviral medications can help prevent or shorten outbreaks.

Centers for Disease Control and Prevention. Genital herpes—CDC fact sheet. http://www.cdc.gov/std/herpes/stdfact-herpes-detailed.htm. Accessed September 25, 2015.

20. C. Repeat outbreaks of genital herpes are common, especially during the first year after infection. Repeat outbreaks are usually shorter and less severe than the first outbreak.

Centers for Disease Control and Prevention. Genital herpes—CDC fact sheet. http://www.cdc.gov/std/herpes/stdfact-herpes-detailed.htm. Accessed September 25, 2015.

21. C. Women who are pregnant can contract genital herpes. It is important to avoid getting herpes during pregnancy because it can sometimes lead to miscarriage and is a risk factor for premature birth. Infection can be passed from the mother to the child and can potentially cause neonatal herpes.

Centers for Disease Control and Prevention. Genital herpes—CDC fact sheet. http://www.cdc.gov/std/herpes/stdfact-herpes-detailed.htm. Accessed September 25, 2015.

22. A. HIV can be spread by other fluids, including preseminal fluid, vaginal fluids, and human milk.

Centers for Disease Control and Prevention. HIV Transmission. 2015. http://www.cdc.gov/hiv/basics/transmission.html. Accessed January 9, 2016.

23. A. Routine screening for HIV infection should be performed for all patients ages 12–64.

Branson BM, Hunter Handsfield H, Lampe MA, et al. Revised recommendations for HIV testing of adults, adolescents, and pregnant women in health-care setting. *MMWR*. 2006;55(RR14):1–17. http://www.cdc.gov/mmwr/preview/mmwrhtml/rr5514a1.htm. Accessed January 9, 2016.

24. A. ELISA testing can detect HIV antibodies quickly after exposure.

Centers for Disease Control and Prevention. HIV/AIDS: laboratory tests. 2015. http://www.cdc.gov/hiv/testing/laboratorytests.html. Accessed January 9, 2016.

25. D. In the past, surgical repair was recommended because of the risk for incarceration or strangulation. Recent studies have shown that small, minimally symptomatic, first occurrence hernias do not require repair, but patients should be followed carefully. Symptoms of incarceration and strangulation require prompt evaluation.

Leblanc KE, Leblanc LL, Leblanc, KA. Inguinal hernias: diagnosis and management. *Am Fam Physician*. 2013:87; 844–848.

26. D. Activity-related groin pain with a normal physical examination may occur with inguinal hernias. Magnetic resonance imaging may be useful in differentiating inguinal and femoral hernias with a high sensitivity and specificity.

Leblanc KE, Leblanc LL, Leblanc, KA. Inguinal hernias: diagnosis and management. *Am Fam Physician*. 2013:87; 844–848.

27. D. The most common side effect of alpha blockers is dizziness, which occurs in approximately 14% of patients.

American Urological Association. American Urological Association guideline: management of benign prostatic hyperplasia (BPH). 2010. https://www.auanet.org/common/pdf/education/clinical-guidance/Benign-Prostatic-Hyperplasia.pdf. Accessed January 9, 2016.

28. B. One of the early intraprostatic effects of finasteride has been the suppression of vascular endothelial growth factor (VEGF). Initially, anecdotally and then in long-term follow-up studies, it was noted that men with prostate-related bleeding (e.g., all other causes of hematuria had been excluded) responded to finasteride therapy with a reduction or cessation of such bleeding and a reduced likelihood of recurrent bleeding. A prospective study verified these observations.

American Urological Association. American Urological Association guideline: management of benign prostatic hyperplasia (BPH). 2010. https://www.auanet.org/common/pdf/education/clinical-guidance/Benign-Prostatic-Hyperplasia.pdf. Accessed January 9, 2016.

29. A. Gram stain is the preferred rapid diagnostic test for evaluating urethritis, because it is highly sensitive and specific for documenting both urethritis and the presence or absence of gonococcal infection.

Centers for Disease Control and Prevention. Epididymitis. 2011. http://www.cdc.gov/std/treatment/2010/epididymitis.htm. Accessed January 9, 2016.

30. C. Antibiotics are only prescribed if a bacterial infection is causing epididymitis.

Davis CP. Epididymitis. 2015. http://www.emedicinehealth.com/testicle_infection_epididymitis/article_em.htm. Accessed January 9, 2016.

31. D. A viral cause of epididymitis is the mumps.

Davis CP. Epididymitis. 2015. http://www.emedicinehealth.com/testicle_infection_epididymitis/article_em.htm. Accessed January 9, 2016.

32. A. Empiric therapy is indicated before laboratory test results are available to help prevent the transmission to others and to decrease potential complications.

Centers for Disease Control and Prevention. Epididymitis. 2011. http://www.cdc.gov/std/treatment/2010/epididymitis.htm. Accessed January 9, 2016.

33. D. All of the above are possible causes of reduced libido.

Cunningham GR. Treatment of male sexual dysfunction. 2015. http://www.uptodate.com/contents/treatment-of-male-sexual-dysfunction. Accessed January 9, 2016.

34. D. Premature ejaculation often goes away without treatment but should be treated if it happens frequently.

Familydoctor.org. Premature ejaculation: treatment. 2014. http://familydoctor.org/familydoctor/en/diseases-conditions/premature-ejaculation/treatment.html. Accessed January 9, 2016.

35. B. Decreased muscle mass and body hair are less common and do not occur for a year or many years.

Bhasin S, Cunningham GR, Hayes FJ, et al. Testosterone therapy in men with androgen deficiency syndromes: an endocrine society clinical practice guideline. *J Clin Endocrinol Metab.* 2010;95:2536.

36. C. Patients with type 2 DM fall into a high-risk category for hypogonadism.

Bhasin S, Cunningham GR, Hayes FJ, et al. Testosterone therapy in men with androgen deficiency syndromes: an endocrine society clinical practice guideline. *J Clin Endocrinol Metab.* 2010;95:2536.

37. A. Serum total testosterone concentration is the best test, because a low value usually indicates hypogonadism.

Bhasin S, Cunningham GR, Hayes FJ, et al. Testosterone therapy in men with androgen deficiency syndromes: an endocrine society clinical practice guideline. *J Clin Endocrinol Metab.* 2010;95:2536.

38. C. Insulin resistance decreases SHBG concentrations.

Bhasin S, Cunningham GR, Hayes FJ, et al. Testosterone therapy in men with androgen deficiency syndromes: an endocrine society clinical practice guideline. *J Clin Endocrinol Metab.* 2010;95:2536.

39. A. Interpretation of serum testosterone levels should take into consideration the diurnal fluctuation of testosterone, which reaches a maximum level at about 8:00 in the morning and a minimum level at about 8:00 pm. It's easier to appreciate a normal from a subnormal level when the normal is higher, so a lab draw between 8:00 and 10:00 a.m. is recommended. Because food decreases testosterone levels, patients should have their levels drawn in a fasting state.

Bhasin S, Cunningham GR, Hayes FJ, et al. Testosterone therapy in men with androgen deficiency syndromes: an endocrine society clinical practice guideline. *J Clin Endocrinol Metab.* 2010;95:2536.

40. D. The Endocrine Society guidelines recommend repletion to 400–700 ng/dL.

Bhasin S, Cunningham GR, Hayes FJ, et al. Testosterone therapy in men with androgen deficiency syndromes: an endocrine society clinical practice guideline. *J Clin Endocrinol Metab.* 2010;95:2536.

Chapter 9: Common Musculoskeletal Disorders in Primary Care

1. It is estimated that _____ adults in the United States will experience low back pain (LBP) at some point in their lives.
   a. 1 in 4
   b. 80% of
   c. 50% of
   d. 1 in 3

2. John is a 25-year-old male who presents to you for treatment after "pulling" his back at work today. Management of uncomplicated acute LBP should include:
   a. Ibuprofen and walking
   b. Acetaminophen and yoga
   c. Naproxen and bed rest
   d. All of the above

3. Adjuvant treatments of LBP may include:
   a. Heat, physical therapy
   b. Cold, aggressive stretching
   c. Sleep modification, aggressive stretching
   d. Aqua therapy, aggressive stretching

4. Your patient asks about treating with a chiropractor. Your best response should be that chiropractic care:
   a. Is recommended for some patients with acute low back pain
   b. Is strongly recommended for all patients with acute low back pain
   c. Is not recommended for patients with acute low back pain
   d. None of the above

5. Imaging studies recommended for a patient with uncomplicated acute low back pain would include:
   a. CT
   b. MRI
   c. X-ray
   d. None of the above

6. A patient presents to your clinic with new complaints of LBP. Your initial evaluation should include:
  a. Focused history and physical exam
  b. Attention to neurologic involvement
  c. Identification of red flags
  d. All of the above

7. Sam is a 25-year-old male who presents following a motor vehicle accident with c/o low back pain, difficulty urinating, numbness in his buttocks and thighs and sudden onset of sexual dysfunction. Signs and symptoms that merit emergent referral include:
  a. Difficulty urinating
  b. Numbness in buttocks and thighs
  c. Sexual dysfunction
  d. All of the above

8. Differential diagnoses in low back pain should include:
  a. Back sprain, tumor, fracture
  b. Renal stones, pancreatitis, aortic aneurysm
  c. Systemic illness, ankylosing spondylitis
  d. All of the above

9. Sarah is a 25-year-old female who reports a recent motor vehicle accident and comes to you with complaints of neck pain and numbness into her right shoulder. When ordering imaging for Sarah, you know that:
  a. If the CT is negative, you may order an MRI too.
  b. You are concerned about imaging for fracture and ligamentous injury.
  c. You should follow imaging guidelines.
  d. All of the above

[handwritten note: Recommend non-contrast CT, MRI if indicated]

10. Cervical radiculopathy should be considered in patients who present with:
  a. Scapular winging, deltoid weakness, breast pain
  b. Deltoid weakness, dental pain, nausea
  c. Chest or deep breast pain, headache
  d. Both A and C
  e. All of the above

11. For patients with complaints of radiculopathy, differential diagnosis would include:
  a. Cerebrovascular accident (CVA)
  b. Myocardial infarction (MI)
  c. Malignancy
  d. Trauma
  e. All of the above

12. Imaging recommendations for neck pain may include:
  a. CT
  b. CT with myelogram
  c. MRI
  d. All of the above

13. John presents to your clinic with complaints of low back pain. You administer an Oswestry Disability Index and your patient scores 38%. You interpret this to mean:
  a. John is completely disabled.
  b. John's back pain is moderately interfering with his ability to manage everyday life.
  c. John feels able to complete all activities of daily living without increased pain or disability.
  d. None of the above

14. Suzette is an 18-year-old female patient who presents to your clinic with complaints of knee pain following a soccer game. Your differential diagnoses will include:
  a. ACL
  b. MCL
  c. Meniscal injury
  d. Both A and C
  e. All of the above

15. Suzette tells you that as she was running to kick a soccer ball, she planted her foot and her "knee just kept going," causing her to twist the knee and fall to the ground. She states she heard a loud "pop" and she could not bear weight on the knee. You anticipate performing what examinations to arrive at your diagnosis?
  a. Full knee exam with ballottement positive and Lachman's positive
  b. Full knee exam with McMurray's positive and ballottement positive
  c. Full knee exam with Valgus stress positive and Varus stress negative
  d. Full knee exam with Apley's negative and Valgus stress positive

16. Suzette asks you if she needs "an X-ray or something." Your best response is:
  a. The examination is positive for an ACL tear.
  b. An X-ray will be done to rule out fracture.
  c. An MRI will be done in anticipation of surgery.
  d. Both B and C
  e. All of the above

17. You are aware when evaluating Suzette that patients with a finding of an ACL tear often have:
  a. Meniscal tear
  b. Articular cartilage injury
  c. Other ligamentous tears
  d. All of the above

18. When evaluating a patient for a suspected meniscal tear, you anticipate a positive finding on:
  a. X-ray
  b. McMurray's
  c. Posterior drawers
  d. All of the above

19. Concerning history and physical exam findings for complaints of knee pain may include:
   a. Locking, giving away
   b. Locking, antalgia
   c. Severe pain, unable to bear weight
   d. Both A and C
   e. All of the above

20. In a young sexually active patient with complaints of unilateral knee pain, your differentials should include:
   a. Malignancy
   b. Sprains and strains
   c. Fracture
   d. *N. gonorrhoeae* infection
   e. Both B and D
   f. All of the above

21. Your patient presents with c/o stiffness and pain in her left knee. She requests a knee brace. You discuss with her that bracing:
   a. May be used postoperatively
   b. Is not recommended as treatment for pain in the absence of injury
   c. Should be utilized as part of an ongoing program of rehabilitation
   d. All of the above

22. Your 58-year-old male patient reports pain in bilateral knees, worsened with standing or walking and stiff after sitting for a period of time. He has no history of cardiovascular disease, peptic ulcer disease (PUD), or renal or liver disease. You anticipate your plan of care may include:
   a. Patellar taping, exercise, NSAIDs
   b. Exercise, weight loss, heat
   c. Wedge insoles, acetaminophen
   d. All of the above

23. Nonmodifiable risk factors for arthritis include:
   a. Age, gender
   b. Inheritance, obesity
   c. Obesity, gender
   d. All of the above

24. Modifiable risk factors for arthritis include:
   a. Obesity, joint injuries
   b. Infection, occupational risks
   c. Crutch use, diet
   d. Both A and B
   e. All of the above

25. It is estimated that _____ adults in the United States have arthritis.
   a. 80% of
   b. 1 of every 5
   c. 68% of
   d. 1 of every 4

26. Mrs. Jones reports she has been having pain in her hip for the past 3 weeks. When exploring her history further, you know it

will be important to narrow her complaints in an effort to make a definitive diagnosis. Hip pain etiologies can be broken into:
   a. Anterior, lateral, posterior
   b. Anterior, posterior, caudal
   c. Caudal, cephalo, posterior
   d. Dorsal, anterior, caudal

27. Mrs. Jones's history and physical narrow her complaints to the anterior hip. This tells you that the likely cause of her pain is:
   a. Intra-articular surfaces, hip flexor strain, stress fracture, iliopsoas bursitis
   b. Trochanteric bursitis, gluteus medius injury, iliotibial band syndrome
   c. Lumbosacral spine arthropathy, spinal disc disease, spinal stenosis
   d. Spinal disc disease, hip flexor strain, trochanteric bursitis

28. Mr. Robinson is a 45-year-old male who presents today with c/o pain in bilateral wrists, hands, and knees; sensation of fever intermittently; and warm joints. What is your differential diagnosis for Mr. Robinson?
   a. Osteoarthritis
   b. Rheumatoid arthritis
   c. Psoriatic arthritis
   d. All of the above

29. James comes to you today with complaints of severe shoulder and knee pain. He states the pain feels like his bones and joints are breaking. When queried about recent activities, he states he returned 1 week ago from a vacation to the Caribbean, where he went parasailing and water skiing. You assess that his differential diagnosis should include:
   a. Dengue
   b. Chikungunya
   c. Sprains
   d. Tendinitis
   e. All of the above

30. Thomas is a 19-year-old cross-country athlete who reports that while running in a wooded uneven terrain he "twisted" his left ankle. He states he is unsure if he "rolled it in or out," but he now has severe pain and seems unable to bear weight. On examination you notice pain with palpation of medial malleolus, decreased range of motion, and an inability to bear weight. You assess your need for imaging based upon:
   a. Ohio Ankle Rules
   b. Orlando Ankle Rules
   c. Ottawa Ankle Rules — *malleolar pain + unable to bear weight indicates imaging*
   d. None of the above

31. Upon further evaluation of Thomas's injury, the lateral ankle is grossly swollen and exquisitely painful with severe laxity on stress maneuvers. His X-ray is negative for fracture. You rate this as a Grade _____ sprain.
   a. I
   b. II
   c. III
   d. IV

32. NSAIDs are commonly used in the care of orthopedic injuries and complaints. Caution should be used, however, in some specific populations such as patients with:
   a. Cardiovascular disease
   b. Gastrointestinal disease
   c. Chronic kidney disease
   d. All of the above

33. Robert is a 58-year-old male who presents to you with complaints of hip pain unrelieved by NSAIDs. He requests an opioid pain reliever. You tell him that opioid pain relievers are never used in chronic orthopedic pain.
   a. True
   b. False

34. The physical examination of Robert's hip pain would include:
   a. FABER test
   b. FADIR test
   c. Ober test
   d. All of the above

35. Rosemarie is a 60-year-old female who works on an assembly line. She reports that several months ago she started having numbness in her hand along her thumb and index finger. She states it worsens overnight and sometimes awakens her. Her differential diagnosis should include:
   a. Carpal tunnel syndrome
   b. Medial epicondylitis
   c. Lateral epicondylitis
   d. None of the above

36. When exploring Rosemarie's past medical history, you make note of:
   a. Breast cancer
   b. Hypothyroidism
   c. Osteoporosis
   d. Osteoarthritis

37. Evaluations that can be done in your office to assess for carpal tunnel syndrome include:
   a. Phalen's
   b. Finkelstein's
   c. Tinel's
   d. Both A and C
   e. All of the above

38. Carpal tunnel syndrome is diagnosed by:
   a. X-ray
   b. ANA titers
   c. Electrodiagnostic studies
   d. CT scan

39. Justin presents to your office with a complaint of elbow pain. Justin states he has recently started playing golf at least 3 times a week. You anticipate his pain on palpation to be located in the region of his:
   a. Preolecranon
   b. Medial epicondyle *"golfers elbow"*
   c. Lateral epicondyle
   d. Antecubital fossa

40. Janet presents to your office with a complaint of elbow pain. Janet reports she plays tennis at least 4 times a week. You anticipate her pain on palpation to be located in the region of her:
   a. Preolecranon
   b. Medial epicondyle
   c. Lateral epicondyle *"tennis elbow"*
   d. Antecubital fossa

Chapter 9: Answers and Rationales

1. B. The National Institute of Neurological Disorders and Stroke estimates that 80% of adults will experience low back pain at some point in their lives.

   National Institute of Neurological Disorders and Stroke. Low back pain fact sheet. 2015. http://www.ninds.nih.gov/disorders/backpain/detail_backpain.htm. Accessed January 9, 2016.

2. A. The American College of Occupational and Environmental Medicine (ACOEM), the American College of Physicians, and the American Pain Society recommend aerobic activity and nonsteroidal anti-inflammatory drugs (NSAIDs) for treatment of acute low back pain.

   American College of Occupational and Environmental Medicine (ACOEM). *Occupational Medicine Practice Guidelines: Evaluation and Management of Health Problems and Functional Recovery in Workers.* 3rd ed. Elk Grove Village, IL: American College of Occupational and Environmental Medicine; 2011:333–796.

3. A. The ACOEM, American College of Physicians, and American Pain Society list heat and a structured therapy program for treatment of acute low back pain.

   American College of Occupational and Environmental Medicine (ACOEM). *Occupational Medicine Practice Guidelines: Evaluation and Management of Health Problems and Functional Recovery in Workers.* 3rd ed. Elk Grove Village, IL: American College of Occupational and Environmental Medicine; 2011:333–796.

4. A. The ACOEM recommends chiropractic treatment for some patients with acute low back pain based on the Clinical Prediction Rule.

   American College of Occupational and Environmental Medicine (ACOEM). *Occupational Medicine Practice Guidelines: Evaluation and Management of Health Problems and Functional Recovery in Workers.* 3rd ed. Elk Grove Village, IL: American College of Occupational and Environmental Medicine; 2011:333–796.

5. D. The ACOEM, American College of Physicians, and American Pain Society do not recommend imaging studies for acute low back pain in the absence of red flags.

   American College of Occupational and Environmental Medicine (ACOEM). *Occupational Medicine Practice Guidelines:*

Evaluation and Management of Health Problems and Functional Recovery in Workers. 3rd ed. Elk Grove Village, IL: American College of Occupational and Environmental Medicine; 2011:333–796.

6. D. According to the American College of Physicians and the American Pain Society, a focused history and physical examination should be conducted to allow the clinician to stratify patients into one of three categories: nonspecific low back pain, back pain potentially associated with radiculopathy or spinal stenosis, or back pain potentially associated with another specific spinal cause.

Chou R, Qaseem A, Snow V, et al; Clinical Efficacy Assessment Subcommittee of the American College of Physicians; American College of Physicians; American Pain Society Low Back Pain Guidelines Panel. Diagnosis and treatment of low back pain: a joint clinical practice guideline from the American College of Physicians and the American Pain Society. *Ann Intern Med.* 2007;147(7):479–491. http://annals.org/article.aspx?articleid=736814. Accessed January 9, 2016.

7. D. According to the ACOEM, the American College of Physicians, and the American Pain Society, symptoms of cauda equina syndrome require emergent referral for imaging and decompression.

American College of Occupational and Environmental Medicine (ACOEM). *Occupational Medicine Practice Guidelines: Evaluation and Management of Health Problems and Functional Recovery in Workers.* 3rd ed. Elk Grove Village, IL: American College of Occupational and Environmental Medicine; 2011:333–796.

8. D. According to the American College of Physicians and the American Pain Society, the differential diagnoses should include systemic illness, serious back complaints, and common low back syndromes.

Chou R, Qaseem A, Snow V, et al; Clinical Efficacy Assessment Subcommittee of the American College of Physicians; American College of Physicians; American Pain Society Low Back Pain Guidelines Panel. Diagnosis and treatment of low back pain: a joint clinical practice guideline from the American College of Physicians and the American Pain Society. *Ann Intern Med.* 2007;147(7):479–491. http://annals.org/article.aspx?articleid=736814. Accessed January 9, 2016.

9. D. The American College of Radiology recommends imaging of suspected C-spine injury with non-contrast CT and MRI as indicated by NEXUS criteria.

Daffner RH, Weissman BN, Appel M, et al; Expert Panel on Musculoskeletal Imaging. ACR Appropriateness Criteria: stress (fatigue/insufficiency) fracture, including sacrum, excluding other vertebrae. Reston, VA: American College of Radiology; 2011.

10. D. According to the North American Spine Society, atypical presentations of radiculopathy should be considered when evaluating the diagnoses listed.

North American Spine Society. *Diagnosis and Treatment of Cervical Radiculopathy from Degenerative Disorders.* Burr Ridge, IL: North American Spine Society; 2010. https://www.spine.org/Documents/ResearchClinicalCare/Guidelines/CervicalRadiculopathy.pdf. Accessed January 9, 2016.

11. E. According to the North American Spine Society, complaints that resemble radiculopathy should be considered with attention to red flags and life-threatening etiologies.

North American Spine Society. *Diagnosis and Treatment of Cervical Radiculopathy from Degenerative Disorders.* Burr Ridge, IL: North American Spine Society; 2010. https://www.spine.org/Documents/ResearchClinicalCare/Guidelines/CervicalRadiculopathy.pdf. Accessed January 9, 2016.

12. D. The American College of Radiology recommends imaging of suspected C-spine injury with CT and MRI as indicated by NEXUS criteria.

Rubin DA, Weissman BN, Appel M, et al; Expert Panel on Musculoskeletal Imaging. *ACR Appropriateness Criteria: Chronic Wrist Pain.* Reston, VA: American College of Radiology; 2012.

13. B. The Oswestry Disability Index score of 38% demonstrates that John rates his low back pain as moderately interfering with his ability to manage everyday life.

Fairbank JCT, Pynsent PB. The Oswestry Disability Index. *Spine.* 2000;25(22):2940–2953. http://www.rehab.msu.edu/_files/_docs/Oswestry_Low_Back_Disability.pdf. Accessed January 9, 2016.

14. E. According to the American Academy of Orthopaedic Surgeons (AAOS), the differentials stated should be considered during evaluation of a knee injury in an athlete.

American Academy of Orthopaedic Surgeons (AAOS). *American Academy of Orthopaedic Surgeons Clinical Practice Guideline on Management of Anterior Cruciate Ligament Injuries.* Rosemont, IL: American Academy of Orthopaedic Surgeons; 2014.

15. A. According to the American Academy of Family Physicians (AAFP) and AAOS, a Lachman's is the most accurate examination technique to identify ACL tear. An effusion would be anticipated in this clinical presentation.

American Academy of Orthopaedic Surgeons (AAOS). Anterior cruciate ligament (ACL) injuries. 2014. http://orthoinfo.aaos.org/topic.cfm?topic=A00549. Accessed January 9, 2016.

Cimino F, Volk BS, Setter D. Anterior cruciate ligament injury: diagnosis, management, and prevention. *Am Fam Physician.* 2010;82(8):917–922. http://www.aafp.org/afp/2010/1015/p917.html. Accessed January 9, 2016.

16. E. According to the AAFP and AAOS, a Lachman's is the most accurate examination technique to identify ACL tear; however, an X-ray can be done to rule out fracture and an MRI would be advisable in this young patient to identify possible meniscal tear or cartilage injury and in anticipation of probable surgical repair.

American Academy of Orthopaedic Surgeons (AAOS). Anterior cruciate ligament (ACL) injuries. 2014. http://orthoinfo.aaos.org/topic.cfm?topic=A00549. Accessed January 9, 2016.

Cimino F, Volk BS, Setter D. Anterior cruciate ligament injury: diagnosis, management, and prevention. *Am Fam Physician.* 2010;82(8):917–922. http://www.aafp.org/afp/2010/1015/p917.html. Accessed January 9, 2016.

17. D. According to the AAFP and AAOS, in the case of an ACL tear, up to 50% will present with injury to meniscus, articular cartilage, and/or other ligaments.

American Academy of Orthopaedic Surgeons (AAOS). Anterior cruciate ligament (ACL) injuries. 2014. http://orthoinfo.aaos.org/topic.cfm?topic=A00549. Accessed January 9, 2016.

Cimino F, Volk BS, Setter D. Anterior cruciate ligament injury: diagnosis, management, and prevention. *Am Fam Physician.* 2010;82(8):917–922. http://www.aafp.org/afp/2010/1015/p917.html. Accessed January 9, 2016.

18. B. A positive McMurray's would be anticipated in meniscal tear.

Ebell MH. Evaluating the patient with a knee injury. *Am Fam Physician.* 2005;71(6):1169–1172. http://www.aafp.org/afp/2005/0315/p1169.html. Accessed January 9, 2016 .

19. D. According to the AAOS, examination findings of locking, giving away, severe pain, or inability to bear weight are concerning and require further evaluation.

American Academy of Orthopaedic Surgeons (AAOS). *American Academy of Orthopaedic Surgeons Clinical Practice Guideline on Management of Anterior Cruciate Ligament Injuries.* Rosemont, IL: American Academy of Orthopaedic Surgeons; 2014.

20. F. According to the AAFP, the AAOS, and the Centers for Disease Control and Prevention (CDC), differentials covering injury, infection, and malignancy should be considered.

American Academy of Orthopaedic Surgeons (AAOS). Anterior cruciate ligament (ACL) injuries. 2014. http://orthoinfo.aaos.org/topic.cfm?topic=A00549. Accessed January 9, 2016.

Cimino F, Volk BS, Setter D. Anterior cruciate ligament injury: diagnosis, management, and prevention. *Am Fam Physician.* 2010;82(8):917–922. http://www.aafp.org/afp/2010/1015/p917.html. Accessed January 9, 2016.

Centers for Disease Control and Prevention. Gonorrhea—STD fact sheet. 2015. http://www.cdc.gov/std/Gonorrhea/STDFact-gonorrhea.htm. Accessed January 9, 2016.

21. D. According to the AAOS, bracing is not routinely done for prophylaxis and should be initiated as part of a rehabilitation program.

American Academy of Orthopaedic Surgeons (AAOS). Anterior cruciate ligament (ACL) injuries. 2014. http://orthoinfo.aaos.org/topic.cfm?topic=A00549. Accessed January 9, 2016.

22. D. According to the American Academy of Rheumatology, a treatment plan for osteoarthritis should include the modalities stated.

Hochberg MC, Altman RD, April KT, et al. American College of Rheumatology 2012 recommendations for the use of non-pharmacologic and pharmacologic therapies in osteoarthritis of the hand, hip, and knee. *Arthritis Care Res* (Hoboken). 2012;64(4):465–474.

23. A. The CDC lists age, gender, and inheritance of certain genetic conditions as nonmodifiable risk factors for arthritis.

Centers for Disease Control and Prevention. Arthritis: risk factors. 2015. http://www.cdc.gov/arthritis/basics/risk_factors.htm. Accessed January 9, 2016.

24. D. The CDC lists obesity, joint injuries, infection, and participation in certain occupations as modifiable risk factors for arthritis.

Centers for Disease Control and Prevention. Arthritis: risk factors. 2015. http://www.cdc.gov/arthritis/basics/risk_factors.htm. Accessed January 9, 2016.

25. B. The CDC states 1 in 5 adults in the United States has a form of arthritis.

Centers for Disease Control and Prevention. Arthritis: risk factors. 2015. http://www.cdc.gov/arthritis/basics/risk_factors.htm. Accessed January 9, 2016.

26. A. The American College of Rheumatology divides the regions of hip pain as anterior, lateral, and posterior hip pain.

Hochberg MC, Altman RD, April KT, et al. American College of Rheumatology 2012 recommendations for the use of non-pharmacologic and pharmacologic therapies in osteoarthritis of the hand, hip, and knee. *Arthritis Care Res* (Hoboken). 2012;64(4):465–474.

27. A. The American College of Rheumatology lists the referral regions for anterior hip pain.

Hochberg MC, Altman RD, April KT, et al. American College of Rheumatology 2012 recommendations for the use of non-pharmacologic and pharmacologic therapies in osteoarthritis of the hand, hip, and knee. *Arthritis Care Res* (Hoboken). 2012;64(4):465–474.

28. D. In considering causes of joint pain without trauma, osteoarthritis, rheumatoid arthritis and psoriatic arthritis would be considered during the differential diagnosis process.

Hochberg MC, Altman RD, April KT, et al. American College of Rheumatology 2012 recommendations for the use of non-pharmacologic and pharmacologic therapies in osteoarthritis of the hand, hip, and knee. *Arthritis Care Res* (Hoboken). 2012;64(4):465–474.

29. E. The CDC reports that dengue and chikungunya are infectious diseases characterized by severe joint pain and fever that are transmissible in the Caribbean. Tendinitis and sprains would also be possible based upon the activities James reports.

Centers for Disease Control and Prevention. Chikungunya virus: symptoms, diagnosis, & treatment. 2015. http://www.cdc.gov/chikungunya/symptoms/index.html. Accessed January 9, 2016.

Centers for Disease Control and Prevention. Dengue. 2015. http://www.cdc.gov/dengue/. Accessed January 9, 2016.

Centers for Disease Control and Prevention. Malaria. 2015. http://www.cdc.gov/malaria/. Accessed January 9, 2016.

30. C. According to the Ottawa Ankle Rules Criteria, imaging would be appropriate based upon malleolar pain and an inability to bear weight.

Tiemstra JD. Update on acute ankle sprains. *Am Fam Physician.* 2012;85(12):1170–1176. http://www.aafp.org/afp/2012/0615/p1170.html. Accessed January 9, 2016.

31. C. AAFP notes that ankle sprains are graded as a I, II, or III for no rupture, partial rupture, or full rupture of the tendon. It is difficult to differentiate amount of rupture utilizing only stress maneuvers. Clinical evaluation of bruising, swelling, and pain is also considered when grading sprains and determining plan of care.

Tiemstra JD. Update on acute ankle sprains. *Am Fam Physician.* 2012;85(12):1170–1176. http://www.aafp.org/afp/2012/0615/p1170.html. Accessed January 9, 2016.

32. D. The American College of Rheumatology notes that NSAIDs are not suitable for specific populations.

Hochberg MC, Altman RD, April KT, et al. American College of Rheumatology 2012 recommendations for the use of non-pharmacologic and pharmacologic therapies in osteoarthritis of the hand, hip, and knee. *Arthritis Care Res* (Hoboken). 2012;64(4):465–474.

33. B. The American College of Rheumatology recommends opioid pain relief for certain patients who do not benefit fully from NSAIDs.

Hochberg MC, Altman RD, April KT, et al. American College of Rheumatology 2012 recommendations for the use of non-pharmacologic and pharmacologic therapies in osteoarthritis of the hand, hip, and knee. *Arthritis Care Res* (Hoboken). 2012;64(4):465–474.

34. D. The American College of Rheumatology recommends a full physical examination of the hip for patients with pain.

Hochberg MC, Altman RD, April KT, et al. American College of Rheumatology 2012 recommendations for the use of non-pharmacologic and pharmacologic therapies in osteoarthritis of the hand, hip, and knee. *Arthritis Care Res* (Hoboken). 2012;64(4):465–474.

35. A. The ACOEM describes the signs and symptoms of carpal tunnel syndrome.

Carpal tunnel syndrome. In: Hegmann KT, ed. *Occupational Medicine Practice Guidelines: Evaluation and Management of Common Health Problems and Functional Recovery in Workers.* 3rd ed. Elk Grove Village, IL: American College of Occupational and Environmental Medicine; 2011:1–73.

36. B. A history of DM, hypothyroidism, rheumatoid arthritis, and recent pregnancy can place one at risk for developing carpal tunnel syndrome.

Carpal tunnel syndrome. In: Hegmann KT, ed. *Occupational Medicine Practice Guidelines: Evaluation and Management of Common Health Problems and Functional Recovery in Workers.* 3rd ed. Elk Grove Village, IL: American College of Occupational and Environmental Medicine; 2011:1–73.

37. D. The ACOEM describes Phalen's and Tinel's for the evaluation of carpal tunnel syndrome.

Carpal tunnel syndrome. In: Hegmann KT, ed. *Occupational Medicine Practice Guidelines: Evaluation and Management of Common Health Problems and Functional Recovery in Workers.* 3rd ed. Elk Grove Village, IL: American College of Occupational and Environmental Medicine; 2011:1–73.

38. C. Electrodiagnostic studies are used for confirmatory diagnosis of carpal tunnel syndrome.

Carpal tunnel syndrome. In: Hegmann KT, ed. *Occupational Medicine Practice Guidelines: Evaluation and Management of Common Health Problems and Functional Recovery in Workers.* 3rd ed. Elk Grove Village, IL: American College of Occupational and Environmental Medicine; 2011:1–73.

39. B. The American Academy of Orthopedic Surgeons provides anticipated examination findings for medial epicondylitis, sometimes known as "golfer's elbow."

Amin NH, Kumar NS, Schickendantz MS. Medial epicondylitis: evaluation and management. *J Am Acad Orthop Surg.* 2015;23:348–355.

40. C. The AAFP provides anticipated examination findings for lateral epicondylitis, also known as "tennis elbow."

Johnson GW, Cadwallader K, Scheffel SB, et al. Treatment of lateral epicondylitis. *Am Fam Physician.* 2007;76(6):843–848. http://www.aafp.org/afp/2007/0915/p843.html. Accessed January 10, 2016.

Chapter 10: Common Neurologic Disorders in Primary Care

1. A 72-year-old woman reports 2 weeks of episodic dizziness. She states the "room seems to spins in circles" when she gets in and out of bed. It also occurs when she looks up toward the ceiling. The episodes typically last less than 2 minutes. She denies any hearing problems or tinnitus. On exam, a Dix-Hallpike maneuver produces rotary nystagmus. The most probable diagnosis is:
   a. Benign positional vertigo
   b. Acute labyrinthitis
   c. Meniere's syndrome
   d. Brainstem ischemia

2. A 30-year-old patient presents with a 5-week history of recurrent headaches that awaken him during the night. The pain is severe, lasts about 1 hour, and is located behind his left eye. Additional symptoms include lacrimation and nasal

discharge. His physical exam is within normal limits. The most likely diagnosis is:

a. Common migraine
b. Classic migraine
c. Cluster headache → *characterized by episodes of severe head pain, and associated autonomic symptoms*
d. Increased intracranial pressure (ICP)

3. A 22-year-old woman presents with a 3-year history of recurrent, unilateral, pulsating headaches with vomiting and photophobia. The headaches, which generally last 3 hours, can be aborted by resting in a dark room. She can usually tell that she is going to get a headache. She explains, "I see little squiggles before my eyes for about 15 minutes." This presentation is most consistent with:

a. Tension-type headache
b. Migraine without aura
c. Migraine with aura
d. Cluster headache

4. Prophylactic treatment for migraine headaches includes:

a. Propranolol (Inderal)
b. Ergotamine (Cafergot)
c. Prednisone
d. Enalapril (Vasotec)

Prophylaxis meds good: BB's, TCA, CCB, NSAID, Anti-epileptic

5. You are examining a 55-year-old woman who has a history of angina and migraine headache. Which of the following represents the best choice for abortive migraine therapy for this patient?

a. Verapamil (Calan)
b. Ergotamine (Cafergot)
c. Ibuprofen (Motrin)
d. Sumatriptan (Imitrex)

avoid Cardiovascular drugs in cardiac patients

6. With appropriately prescribed headache prophylactic therapy, the patient should be informed to expect:

a. Virtual resolution of headaches
b. No fewer but less severe headaches
c. Fewer and less severe headaches
d. That lifelong therapy is advised

7. An 18-year-old college freshman is brought to the student health center with a chief complaint of headache, fever, and neck pain. On physical examination, he has positive Kernig and Brudzinski signs. The most likely diagnosis is:

a. Encephalitis
b. Meningitis
c. Subarachnoid hemorrhage
d. Epidural hematoma

8. Which of the following is most consistent with findings in patients with Parkinson's disease?

a. Rigid posture with monocular vision loss
b. Mask-like facies and altered cognitive function
c. Excessive arm swinging with ambulation and flexed posture
d. Tremor at rest with bradykinesia

9. Treatment options to control motor symptoms of Parkinson's disease include all of the following *except*:

a. Levodopa-carbidopa
b. Selegiline (Eldepryl)
c. Apomorphine (Apokyn)
d. Nortriptyline (Pamelor) → *Can help c̄ depression but not motor.*

10. When caring for a patient with a recent transient ischemic attack (TIA), you consider that: → *Aspirin*

a. Long-term antiplatelet therapy is indicated.
b. This person has a relatively low risk of future stroke.
c. Women present with this disorder more often than men.
d. Rehabilitation will be needed to minimize the effects of the resulting neurologic insult.

11. Patients should be instructed that the symptoms of TIA include:

a. Weakness or numbness of the hand, tongue, cheek, face, or extremities
b. Trouble speaking normally or at all
c. Trouble seeing clearly with one or both eyes
d. All of the above

12. The nurse practitioner understands that the most common form of facial paralysis in the adult client is:

a. Facial nerve fasciitis
b. Trigeminal neuralgia
c. Bell's palsy
d. Herpes zoster

13. A 76-year-old woman consults you because of leg discomfort. Her legs are comfortable during the day, but in the evening she develops an uncomfortable creepy-crawly sensation that keeps her awake for hours. The feeling is temporarily relieved by movement; she will awaken, pace around, and sometimes run water on her legs to achieve relief. Which of the following is the best initial treatment for her condition?

a. Zolpidem 5 mg PO at bedtime
b. Trazodone 50 mg PO at bedtime
c. Stretching exercises of the legs
d. Pramipexole 0.125 mg PO in the evening

14. Your patient is complaining of extreme fatigue and states he is always sleepy. You decide to use the Epworth Sleepiness Questionnaire to screen him for a sleep disorder. This tool asks patients to determine the likelihood of them dozing off or falling asleep during all of the following situations *except*:

a. Sitting and reading
b. In a car stopped for a few minutes
c. Sex
d. Watching TV

15. Which statement is incorrect regarding signs and symptoms of multiple sclerosis?

a. Signs and symptoms of multiple sclerosis depend on where the nerves are demyelinated.
b. Visual changes, numbness, and tingling or weakness are common early symptoms.

c. Muscle spasticity and painful involuntary muscle contractions are common symptoms.

d. Men are more likely to develop multiple sclerosis and frequently have incontinence.

16. Which statement is accurate regarding lab and diagnostic testing for evaluating multiple sclerosis?

a. MRI of the brain can be useful in making the diagnosis of multiple sclerosis earlier and with more confidence.

b. The purpose of lab data is to exclude other diseases.

c. The diagnosis can be made without cerebrospinal fluid or evoked potential testing.

d. All of the above

17. Your patient comes in with a complaint of tremor. She states that it has an abrupt onset and resolves without treatment. Her description of the tremor characteristics is unclear. It sometimes occurs at rest and sometimes with activity. She is unclear how long it lasts. On examination you are able to eliminate the tremor with distraction. What type of tremor syndrome do you suspect?

a. Cerebellar tremor

b. Essential tremor

c. Psychogenic tremor → deals c stress

d. Parkinsonian tremor

18. Your patient presents with episodic vertigo and is concerned about hearing loss. Which of the following etiologies of dizziness would you suspect?

a. Presyncope due to orthostatic hypotension

b. Vestibular migraine

c. Meniere's disease

d. Disequilibrium due to neuropathy

19. Which statement is inaccurate regarding psychiatric causes of lightheadedness?

a. Questions about anxiety and depression should be included in the patient history, because psychiatric causes of lightheadedness are common.

b. Patients with depression and alcohol intoxication may have dizziness.

c. Hyperventilation syndrome is an important cause of lightheadedness.

d. Patients with panic disorder rarely experience dizziness.

20. Which statement is accurate regarding dizziness associated with vestibular neuritis? → usual occurs. post-viral

a. Patients with vestibular neuritis have mild vertigo and some hearing loss.

b. Patients with vestibular neuritis have intense vertigo that often begins acutely after an upper respiratory or flulike illness.

c. Vestibular neuritis is often related to head trauma.

d. Drugs such as meclizine and promethazine should be avoided in patients with vestibular neuritis.

21. Patient education is an important component of vertigo treatment. Which statement is inaccurate regarding treatment for symptoms?

a. Antihistamines and anti-nausea medications may help alleviate symptoms.

b. Staying still and not moving your head may help alleviate symptoms.

c. Canalith repositioning may help alleviate symptoms in patients with BPPV.

d. Sedative medications may help relieve symptoms.

22. Appropriate treatment for Meniere's disease would include:

a. Hydration

b. Meclizine

c. Diuresis   diuretic and sodium are restriction are tx strategies

d. Corticosteroids

23. Which statement is inaccurate regarding the association between seizures and diabetes mellitus?

a. Approximately 25% of all diabetic patients experience different types of seizures.

b. Diabetic patients who have had diabetic ketoacidosis (DKA) have seizures more frequently.

c. The cause of seizures in diabetics is due to abnormal blood sugars.

d. Many non-ketotic diabetic patients are resistant to frequently used antiepileptic drugs for partial seizures.

24. Causes of a provoked seizure may include:

a. Newly diagnosed brain lesion

b. Medication use

c. Central nervous system infection

d. All of the above

25. Which one of the following patients does not require immediate neuroimaging following a seizure?

a. A patient with new-onset focal seizures

b. A young adult with known alcoholism

c. A patient with new-onset seizure over the age of 40

d. A patient over 50 with seizure associated with a fall

26. Which of the following is essential in the diagnostic evaluation of the patient with possible epilepsy?

a. Electrocardiogram

b. Electroencephalography (EEG)

c. Lumbar puncture

d. Brain magnetic resonance imaging (MRI)

27. Which statement is accurate regarding the initiation of anti-epileptic drug (AED) therapy?

a. AED therapy should generally be started after 2 or more unprovoked seizures.

b. AED therapy should be started with 1 provoked seizure.

c. About 50% of patients with newly diagnosed epilepsy will become seizure free with the first medication prescribed.

d. Drug therapy must be individualized and take into account drug effectiveness for seizure type, potential side effects, patient lifestyle, and cost.

after having 1st Seizure a pt is >50% likely to have a Repeat

28. Which statement is true regarding driving for patients with seizures?

    a. All patients with seizures will have to surrender their driving license.

    b. The laws governing when a person with seizures can drive vary from state to state.

    c. All healthcare providers must report patients with seizures to the department of motor vehicles.

    d. Patients can drive immediately after they start AED therapy.

29. Which statement is inaccurate regarding the diagnosis of Parkinson's disease?

    a. The diagnosis is clinical and relies on the presence of cardinal features.

    b. Cardinal features include bradykinesia, rigidity, tremor, and postural instability.

    c. Symptom onset is usually rapid with full-blown symptoms occurring over several months.

    d. A sustained response to therapy with levodopa helps confirm the diagnosis.

30. Which statement is inaccurate regarding the prognosis for Parkinson's disease?

    a. It is not possible to estimate exactly how quickly or slowly the disease will progress.

    b. Risk factors for a more rapid decline in motor function include older age at diagnosis.

    c. The incidence of dementia increases with patient age and duration of the disease.

    d. Parkinson's disease may progress more slowly in patients who do not have tremor.

[handwritten in margin: Pt's who do not have a tremor generally have faster progression]

31. Which statement is accurate regarding nonmotor symptoms of Parkinson's disease?

    a. Fatigue may occur in the early stages of the disease.

    b. Autonomic dysfunction occurs early in the disease and may include urinary frequency, diarrhea, and hypertension.

    c. Depression and psychosis occur in a small percentage of patients with Parkinson's disease.

    d. All of the above

[handwritten in margin: fatigue occurs in 1/3]

32. Which mnemonic can help in the evaluation of syncope?

    a. SNOOP

    b. POUND

    c. CHESS *[handwritten: → CHF Hematocrit >30%, ECG abnormal,]*

    d. CHAD *[handwritten: Shortness of breath, Systolic BP<90]*

33. Which of the following is not a type of neurally mediated syncope?

    a. Vasovagal syncope

    b. Cardiac syncope

    c. Carotid sinus syncope

    d. Situational syncope

34. Which diagnostic test would be appropriate for the evaluation of neurally mediated syncope or orthostatic syncope?

    a. Tilt-table testing

    b. Echocardiogram

    c. Exercise stress testing

    d. Electrophysiologic study

35. Cerebrovascular syncope can occur in the setting of an occlusive disease when preferential blood flow is diverted from the brain to the arm during activity. This is commonly referred to as:

    a. Carotid sinus syndrome

    b. Subclavian steal syndrome

    c. Lown-Ganong-Levine syndrome

    d. Aicardi syndrome

36. Modifiable risk factors for both TIA and stroke include all of the following *except*:

    a. Cigarette smoking

    b. Diabetes

    c. Hypertension

    d. Family history

37. The clinical diagnosis of TIA may be difficult, because the patient's signs and symptoms frequently are resolved by the time of the evaluation. The diagnosis depends on all of the following *except*:

    a. Careful history including onset, duration, and resolution of symptoms

    b. Detailed neurologic examination

    c. Detailed cardiovascular examination

    d. EEG

38. Which imaging modality should be ordered for the evaluation of patients with suspected acute cerebral infarction?

    a. Noncontrast brain computed tomography (CT)

    b. Magnetic resonance imaging (MRI)

    c. Cerebral perfusion study

    d. Conventional angiography

39. Sleep disorders are common in older adults. Serious health consequences can result from inadequate rest including:

    a. Depression

    b. Memory difficulties

    c. Increased risk for falls

    d. All of the above

40. Nonpharmacologic management of chronic insomnia includes all of the following *except*:

    a. Avoiding exercise during the 4 hours before bedtime

    b. Setting aside time to relax before bed

    c. Taking naps to help with daytime sleepiness

    d. Keeping the bedroom at a comfortable temperature and as dark as possible

41. Which statement is not accurate regarding tremors?

    a. A rest tremor occurs in a body part that is relaxed and completely supported by gravity.

    b. A rest tremor may worsen with mental stress and improve with voluntary movement.

    c. The most common pathologic tremor is related to medications that exacerbate the tremor.

    d. The first step in the evaluation of tremor is to categorize the tremor based on triggers and frequency of anatomic distribution of the movement disorder.

[handwritten: 50% of cases]

Chapter 10: Answers and Rationales

1. A. The Dix-Hallpike maneuver tests for canalithiasis of the posterior semicircular canal, which is the most common cause of benign paroxysmal positional vertigo (BPPV).

Post RE, Dickerson LM. Dizziness: a diagnostic approach. *Am Fam Physician.* 2010;82:361–368.

2. C. Cluster headaches are characterized by brief episodes of severe head pain with associated autonomic symptoms.

Hainer BI, Matheson EM. Approach to acute headache in adults. *Am Fam Physician.* 2013;87: 682–687.

3. C. This patient's symptoms are congruent with the diagnostic criteria for migraine with aura. An aura may consist of reversible visual symptoms, sensory symptoms, or dysphasic speech disturbance.

Lipton RB, Bigal ME, Steiner TJ, et al. American Academy of Neurology: classification of primary headaches. *Neurology.* 2004;63:429.

4. A. A number of medications can be used for prevention of migraines. Categories of medication for prophylaxis include beta-adrenergic blockers, tricyclic antidepressants, calcium-channel blockers, antiepileptic drugs, and nonsteroidal anti-inflammatory drugs (NSAIDs). Propranolol is a beta-adrenergic blocker.

Moloney MF, Cranwell-Bruce LA. Pharmacological management of migraine headaches. *Nurse Pract.* 2010;35:23.

5. C. Triptans and ergot alkaloids are contraindicated in patients with known cardiovascular disease because they work by causing vasoconstriction. Calcium channel blockers (Verapamil) are not effective for aborting migraines.

Moloney MF, Cranwell-Bruce LA. Pharmacological management of migraine headaches. *Nurse Pract.* 2010;35:23.

6. C. Complete resolution of migraines is not possible. Patients should be instructed that the goal of therapy is to reduce the number and severity of their headaches.

Gilmore B, Magdalena M. Treatment of acute migraine headache. *Am Fam Physician.* 2011;83:271–280.

7. B. The classic triad of meningitis is fever, neck stiffness, and altered mental status. Other symptoms suggestive of meningitis include positive Kernig and Brudzinski signs.

Bhimra A. Acute community-acquired bacterial meningitis in adults: an evidence-based review. *Cleve Clin J Med.* 2012; 79:393–400.

8. D. Features that increase the likelihood of Parkinson's disease include those associated with bradykinesia including micrographia, a shuffling walk, difficulties performing motor tasks, and tremor at rest.

Gazewood JD, Richards DR, Clebak K. Parkinson disease: an update. *Am Fam Physician.* 2013;87:267–272.

9. D. Nortriptyline can be used in Parkinson's disease to help with depression, but it does not have any effect on motor symptoms.

Gazewood JD, Richards DR, Clebak K. Parkinson disease: an update. *Am Fam Physician.* 2013;87:267–272.

10. A. Patients with large-vessel atherosclerosis and small-vessel disease with TIA should receive aspirin. Patients with atrial fibrillation with or without a cerebrovascular ischemic event should be treated with long-term anticoagulation—either with warfarin (Coumadin) or one of the novel agents such as dabigatran (Pradaxa), rivaroxaban (Xarelto), or apixaban (Eliquis).

Sonni S, Thaler DE. Transient ischemic attack: omen and opportunity. *Cleve Clin J Med.* 2013;80:566–575.

11. D. Patients should know the symptoms of TIA so they can receive appropriate care. Symptoms of TIA are the same as stroke except TIA symptoms go away quickly. The mnemonic FAST (F = face is uneven, A = arm is weak, S = speech is strange, T = time to call an ambulance) can help patients remember the signs of stroke.

American Stroke Association. TIA (transient ischemic attack). 2012. http://www.strokeassociation.org/STROKEORG/AboutStroke/TypesofStroke/TIA/TIA-Transient-Ischemic-Attack_UCM_310942_Article.jsp. Accessed January 10, 2016.

12. C. Bell's palsy is a form of temporary facial paralysis due to damage to the 7th cranial nerve.

National Institute of Neurological Disorders and Stroke. Bell's Palsy fact sheet. 2015. http://www.ninds.nih.gov/disorders/bells/detail_bells.htm. Accessed January 10, 2016.

13. D. These symptoms are suggestive of restless legs syndrome; pramipexole is a treatment option for restless legs syndrome.

Aurora RN, Kristo DA, Bista SR, et al. The treatment of restless legs syndrome and periodic limb movement disorder in adults: an update for 2012: practice parameters with an evidence-based systemic review and meta-analyses: an American Academy of Sleep Medicine clinical guideline. 2012 http://www.aasmnet.org/resources/practiceparameters/treatmentrls.pdf. Accessed January 10, 2016.

14. C. Sleepiness associated with sex is not evaluated with the Epworth Sleepiness Questionnaire.

Johns MW. Sleepiness in different situations measured by the Epworth Sleepiness Scale. *Sleep.* 1994;17:703–710. https://web.stanford.edu/~dement/epworth.html. Accessed January 10, 2016.

15. D. The incidence of multiple sclerosis is higher in women than men and both incontinence and urinary retention may occur.

Maloni HW. Multiple sclerosis: managing patients in primary care. *Nurse Pract.* 2013;38:24–35.

16. D. Lab and diagnostic testing includes a wide variety of supportive and confirmatory tests in the evaluation of multiple sclerosis.

Maloni HW. Multiple sclerosis: managing patients in primary care. *Nurse Pract.* 2013;38:24–35.

17. C. The clinical features of tremor provide important diagnostic clues. The characteristics of this patient's tremor are consistent with a psychogenic tremor. Frequently, it is associated with a stressful life event. The incidence of psychogenic tremor is unknown.

Crawford P, Zimmerman EE. Differentiation and diagnosis of tremor. *Am Fam Physician*. 2011;83:697–702.

18. C. Hearing loss and duration of symptoms help to narrow the differential diagnosis in patients with vertigo. Meniere's disease is due to increased endolymphatic fluid in the inner ear and affects hearing.

Post RE, Dickerson LM. Dizziness: a diagnostic approach. *Am Fam Physician*. 2010;82:361–368.

19. D. One in 4 patients with dizziness meets the criteria for panic disorder.

Yardley L, Owen N, Nazareth I, et al. Panic disorder with agoraphobia associated with dizziness. *J Nerv Ment Dis*. 2001;189:321–327.

20. B. Vestibular neuritis is believed to be a viral or postviral inflammatory disorder affecting the vestibular portion of the 8th cranial nerve.

Shaia WT, Meyers AD. Dizziness evaluation. 2015. http://emedicine.medscape.com/article/1831429-overview#a3. Accessed January 10, 2016.

21. B. Staying still can make it harder to cope with vertigo. Balance rehabilitation can help the brain to adjust its responses to changes in the vestibular system.

Vestibular Disorders Association. Benign Paroxysmal Positional Vertigo. http://vestibular.org/understanding-vestibular-disorders/types-vestibular-disorders/benign-paroxysmal-positional-vertigo.

22. C. The cause of Meniere's disease is not well understood but appears to be related to abnormal volume or composition of fluid in the inner ear. A diuretic and sodium restriction are recommended treatment strategies.

Kerber KA, Baloh RW. The evaluation of a patient with dizziness. *Neurol Clin Prac*. 2011;1:24–33. http://cp.neurology.org/content/1/1/24.full. Accessed January 10, 2016.

23. C. The pathogenesis of seizures in diabetic patients is not completely understood, but the literature suggests that it is likely multifactorial including immune abnormalities, microvascular lesions in the brain, metabolic factors, and gene mutation.

Yun C, Xuefeng W. Association between seizures and diabetes mellitus: a comprehensive review of the literature. *Curr Diabetes Rev*. 2013;9:350–354.

24. D. Provoked seizures are caused by various underlying diseases.

Wilden JA, Cohen-Gadol AA. Evaluation of first nonfebrile seizure. *Am Fam Physician*. 2012;86:334–340.

25. B. Recommendations for imaging after a first seizure depend on age, seizure type, and associated risk factors. Immediate neuroimaging is indicated when a serious structural brain lesion is suspected and should be considered for patients with focal seizures and for those over the age of 40.

Harden CL, Huff JS, Schwartz TH, et al. Reassessment: neuro imaging in the emergency patient presenting with seizure (an evidence-based review). Report of the Therapeutics and Technology Assessment Subcommittee of the American Academy of Neurology. *Neurology*. 2007;69:1772–1780.

26. B. Electroencephalography should be ordered in all patients with suspected seizure of unknown etiology to detect focal lesions not visible with neuroimaging. It also facilitates the diagnosis of particular epilepsy syndromes.

Wilden JA, Cohen-Gadol AA. Evaluation of first nonfebrile seizure. *Am Fam Physician*. 2012;86:334–340.

27. B. AED therapy is indicated after the first occurrence of seizure, because it is implied that the patient has a more than 50% risk for repeated seizures.

Fountain NB, Van Ness PC, Swain-Eng R, et al. Quality improvement in neurology: AAN epilepsy quality measures: Report of the Quality Measurement and Reporting Subcommittee of the American Academy of Neurology. *Neurology*. 2011;76:76–94.

28. B. Every state regulates driver's license eligibility of persons with epilepsy. The most common requirement is that they be seizure free for a specific period of time and submit a healthcare provider's evaluation of their ability to drive safely. Nurse practitioners should use the state driving laws database to determine requirements for their patients.

Epilepsy Foundation. State driving laws database. https://www.epilepsy.com/driving-laws. Accessed January 10, 2016.

29. C. Symptoms of Parkinson's disease are gradual and progressive.

Gazewood JD, Richards DR, Clebak K. Parkinson disease: an update. *Am Fam Physician*. 2013;87:267–272.

30. D. Patients with Parkinson's disease who do not have tremor are more likely to have a quicker progression of symptoms.

American Academy of Neurology. AAN guideline for patients and their families: diagnosis and prognosis of new onset Parkinson disease, initiation of treatment for Parkinson disease (2002), neuroprotective and alternative therapies for Parkinson disease. http://tools.aan.com/professionals/practice/guidelines/Diagnosis_Prognosis_PD_Sum.pdf. Accessed January 10, 2016.

31. A. Fatigue is present in one-third of patients at diagnosis and is associated with severity.

Gazewood JD, Richards DR, Clebak K. Parkinson disease: an update. *Am Fam Physician*. 2013;87:267–272.

32. C. CHESS is the mnemonic from the San Francisco Syncope Rule, which helps healthcare providers evaluate the short-term risk of syncope. C = congestive heart failure, H = hematocrit > 30%, E = ECG abnormalities, S = shortness of breath, and S = systolic BP < 90 mm Hg.

Quinn J, McDermott D, Stiell I, et al. Derivation of the San Francisco Syncope Rule to predict patients with short-term serious outcomes. *Ann Emerg Med.* 2004;43:224–232.

33. B. Cardiac arrhythmias can cause syncope, but the etiology is a drop in cardiac output, not a neurally mediated reflex. Cardiac arrhythmia–related syncope includes sinus node dysfunction, AV conduction, paroxysmal supraventricular tachycardia, ventricular tachycardia, Wolff-Parkinson-White syndrome, and inherited syndromes.

Thanavaro JL. Evaluation and management of syncope. *Clin Schol Rev.* 2009;2:65–77.

34. A. A tilt-table test promotes venous pooling in the lower extremities and provokes a vasovagal response. In neurally mediated syncope, the tilt-table test will cause symptoms similar to the patient's symptoms prior to syncope. In orthostatic syncope, a positive tilt-table test will uncover symptomatic hypotension without bradycardia.

Baron-Esquivias G, Martinez-Rubio A. Tilt table test: state of the art. *Indian Pacing Electrophysiol J.* 2003;3:239–252.

35. B. Patients with atherosclerotic occlusive plaques in the subclavian artery may develop either vertebrobasilar symptoms or exercise-induced arm pain due to subclavian artery occlusive disease.

Bayat I. Subclavian steal syndrome: treatment and management. 2015. http://emedicine.medscape.com/article/462036-treatment. Accessed January 10, 2016.

36. D. Family history of stroke increases the risk of stroke by 30%. This association is stronger with large-vessel and small-vessel stroke but not cardioembolic stroke.

Sonni S, Thaler DE. Transient ischemic attack: omen and opportunity. *Cleve Clin J Med.* 2013;80:566–575.

37. D. An EEG is not valuable in the workup of TIA symptoms. An ECG is indicated to evaluate for arrhythmias, especially atrial fibrillation.

Sonni S, Thaler DE. Transient ischemic attack: omen and opportunity. *Cleve Clin J Med.* 2013;80:566–575.

38. A. Noncontrast brain CT is considered the first-line imaging for patients with acute stroke. Noncontrast head CT is broadly available and quick. Imaging is done to look for other causes of new focal neurologic deficits besides ischemic disease and to evaluate any contraindications (intracranial hemorrhage) to therapy.

Sonni S, Thaler DE. Transient ischemic attack: omen and opportunity. *Cleve Clin J Med.* 2013;80:566–575.

39. D. There are many adverse consequences of sleep abnormalities including those listed above. Sleep is also important in the prevention of cardiovascular problems, diabetes, obesity, and fatigue.

Rajki M. Sleep problems in older adults: serious health consequences can result from inadequate rest. *Adv NPs PAs.* 2011;2(12):16–22.

40. C. Taking naps will make it harder to sleep during the night. Daytime napping should be avoided.

Harsora P, Kessmann J. Nonpharmacologic management of chronic insomnia. *Am Fam Physician.* 2009;79:125–130.

41. C. The most common pathologic tremor is essential tremor, which is familial in about 50% of cases.

Crawford P, Zimmerman EE. Differentiation and diagnosis of tremor. *Am Fam Physician.* 2011;83:697–702.

Chapter 11: Common Psychiatric Disorders in Primary Care

1. The PHQ-9 is best used to evaluate:
   a. Bipolar disorders
   b. Anxiety disorders
   c. Depression
   d. Mood disorders

2. The CAGE AID questionnaire is best used to evaluate:
   a. Bipolar disorders
   b. Alcohol and drug use
   c. Tobacco and alcohol use
   d. Depression

3. The MDQ13 is best used to screen for:
   a. Bipolar disorders
   b. Anxiety disorders
   c. Obsessive compulsive disorder
   d. Depression

4. The GAD 7 is best used to screen for:
   a. Bipolar disorders → generalized Anxiety Disorder
   b. Anxiety disorders
   c. Depression
   d. Alcohol and drug abuse

5. The Patient Stress Questionnaire is best used in:
   a. Primary care settings
   b. Acute care settings
   c. Urgent care settings
   d. All settings

6. The AUDIT is best used to screen for:
   a. Alcohol abuse disorders
   b. Anxiety disorders
   c. Abuse and neglect
   d. None of the above

7. Which tool is used to screen for suicide risk?
   a. C-SSRS
   b. SAFE-T   *Pg 568*
   c. SBQ-R
   d. All of the above

8. Sam is a 23-year-old male who presents with c/o difficulty in social situations and "worrying too much." He states he is unable to apply for a job, because he is afraid he will be rejected;

he is unable to go for interviews, because he worries so much he will fail that he does not try. He states people have always told him he "is a worrier," but he feels it is getting in the way of him leading a normal life. He states he often refuses going out with friends because of worry and feels he is going to be "alone forever" if he "can't get this under control." He states the past year has been very stressful since graduating from college. He reports when queried that he often has difficulty sleeping because he is thinking about "something over and over." Sam's differential diagnoses should include:

a. BAD
b. GAD
c. PUD
d. Both A and B
e. All of the above

9. First-line treatment for generalized anxiety may include:
   a. Antidepressants and cognitive behavioral therapy
   b. Antidepressants and anti-anxiolytics
   c. Benzodiazepines
   d. All of the above
   e. Both A and B

10. Serious side effects of antidepressants to consider when prescribing should include:
    a. Increased risk of suicide in young adults and adolescents
    b. Cardiovascular disease
    c. Respiratory depression
    d. Risk of addiction

11. A serious side effect of escitalopram to consider when prescribing is:
    a. Increased risk of suicidal ideation
    b. ST wave changes
    c. Increased risk of cerebrovascular accident
    d. QT prolongation risk

12. When prescribing duloxetine for your patient, you consider that this medication:
    a. Requires cautious dose adjustment because of rapid onset
    b. Requires frequent dosing adjustment
    c. Requires careful monitoring related to side effect profile
    d. Lowers seizure threshold

Contraind un Seizure pts (handwritten annotation)

13. Venlafaxine should be used cautiously in patients with:
    a. Hyperthyroidism, glaucoma
    b. CHF, recent MI
    c. HTN, glaucoma
    d. All of the above

14. Paroxetine should be avoided with:
    a. Thiazide diuretics
    b. Swiss cheese
    c. White wine
    d. Linezolid

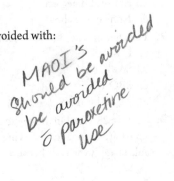

MAOI's should be avoided / be avoided c̄ paroxetine use (handwritten annotation)

15. It is not uncommon for comorbid conditions to accompany generalized anxiety disorder. Examples of these include:
    a. Phobias, panic disorders, depression
    b. Panic disorders, substance abuse, migraines
    c. Depression, migraines, eating disorders
    d. Eating disorders, panic disorders, phobias

16. Cognitive behavioral therapy is used to treat:
    a. Depression
    b. Anxiety disorders
    c. Bipolar disorder
    d. All of the above

17. Schizophrenia typically begins to manifest:
    a. In the 20s
    b. In the middle ages
    c. Later in life
    d. In childhood

18. Bessie reports she is hearing voices that are troubling and telling her that people are "out to get" her. When you attempt to challenge the voices, she becomes angry and agitated. You understand that this is because to Bessie:
    a. The hallucinations are very real.
    b. The delusions are very vivid.
    c. Her disorganized thinking cannot allow her to process what you are saying.
    d. All of the above

19. Bessie has been diagnosed with schizophrenia. You understand that this means she may experience:
    a. Hallucinations
    b. Delusions
    c. Disorganized thoughts and behavior
    d. All of the above

20. Depression occurs most frequently in middle-aged women.
    a. True
    b. False

21. Eating disorders can cause long-term harm to:
    a. Bones and teeth
    b. Heart and digestive system
    c. All of the above
    d. None of the above

22. Susan comes to you for a physical examination to establish a new patient relationship. You notice that she is an attractive female with a normal BMI. You are concerned that Susan may have an eating disorder because:
    a. Her ENT exam is abnormal with erosions noted to lower teeth.
    b. She reports a 24-hour diet recall of 1800 kcal yesterday.
    c. You are not concerned because her weight is normal.
    d. None of the above

23. Janet comes to you accompanied by her mother. Janet's mother reports that Janet regularly eats cloth. When planning care for Janet, you explain to Janet and her mother that:
    a. Pica is the routine ingestion of nonfood items.
    b. Rumination disorder is the practice of eating cloth or dirt.
    c. There is no harm to Janet's behavior so it should be ignored.
    d. None of the above

24. Your female patient has been taking buspirone for the past 6 months. She reports that she recently found out she is pregnant and is quite anxious about the impact the medication may have on her baby. You explain to her that the medication is a pregnancy category:
    a. A—there is no risk to the developing fetus.
    b. B—animal studies have not shown a risk to the fetus.
    c. C—animal studies have shown a risk to the fetus.
    d. D—positive evidence of fetal risk based on human studies.
    e. X—fetal and animal studies have demonstrated a definite risk to the fetus.

25. Farrah was started on buspirone 2 days ago and she is calling your office to ask why she is not feeling better yet. You explain that:
    a. It takes up to 2 weeks to become fully effective.
    b. She probably needs a dose adjustment.
    c. She should feel better by tomorrow.
    d. None of the above

26. All of the following are benzodiazepines except:
    a. Acetazolamide
    b. Chlordiazepoxide
    c. Diazepam
    d. Lorazepam

27. James was diagnosed with bipolar disorder. He said he once knew someone who was manic-depressive and asks if he has the same thing. Your best response is:
    a. Bipolar disorder is a broad diagnosis with multiple subtypes.
    b. If your friend had manic depression, then you have the same thing.
    c. Your can expect a similar disease process as your acquaintance.
    d. None of the above

28. Patients with bipolar disorder can be expected at some time to exhibit the following traits:
    a. Abnormally elevated mood
    b. Depression
    c. Irritability
    d. All of the above

29. According to the DSM-5, bereavement may be a trigger for depression but is not a subtype of depression.
    a. True
    b. False

30. Medical causes to consider when assessing a patient for major depressive disorder include:
    a. Thyroid dysfunction
    b. Bipolar disorder
    c. Anemia
    d. All of the above

31. In addition to pharmacologic interventions for bipolar disorder, you anticipate that your patient will also need the following (*circle all that apply*):
    a. Cognitive behavioral therapy
    b. Family-focused therapy
    c. Social rhythm therapy
    d. Psychoeducation

32. The 2014 National Survey on Drug Use and Health reports that two-thirds of persons over the age of _____ have used alcohol in the preceding 12 months.
    a. 10 years
    b. 12 years
    c. 14 years
    d. 16 years

33. According to SAMHSA's 2014 Behavioral Health Barometer, men are _____ more likely to have illicit drug dependence than women.
    a. 10 times
    b. 5 times
    c. 3 times
    d. 2 times

34. According to SAMHSA, each year approximately _____ people under 21 years of age die as a result of underage drinking.
    a. 1000
    b. 2500
    c. 5000
    d. 7500

35. According to the Centers for Disease Control and Prevention (CDC), alcohol use causes _____ deaths each year.
    a. 15,000
    b. 39,000
    c. 57,000
    d. 88,000

36. Zachary is exhibiting agitation, anxiety, and obsessive thoughts and behaviors. He reports the need to repetitively perform certain tasks prior to leaving for work each morning. Zachary is exhibiting symptoms of:
    a. Generalized anxiety disorder
    b. Obsessive compulsive disorder
    c. Bipolar disorder
    d. Major depressive disorder

37. In the United States, 0.6 ounces of alcohol can be found in:
    a. 16 ounces of beer
    b. 12 ounces of malt liquor
    c. 5 ounces of wine
    d. 2 ounces of 80-proof liquor

38. Characteristics of post-traumatic stress disorder (PTSD) include:
    a. Recurrent upsetting dreams
    b. Flashbacks
    c. Distressing memories
    d. Intense psychological distress
    e. All of the above

39. According to the National Survey on Drug Use and Health (NSDUH) from 2014, _____% of adults over the age of 18 experienced a major depressive episode in that calendar year.
    a. 2.2
    b. 4.4
    c. 6.6
    d. 8.8

40. According to SAMHSA, _____ million or _____ of persons in the United States experience an anxiety disorder in any given year.
    a. 20 million, 9%
    b. 40 million, 18%
    c. 60 million, 24%
    d. 80 million, 36%

Chapter 11: Answers and Rationales

1. C. According to the Substance Abuse and Mental Health Services Administration (SAMHSA), the PHQ-9 is the most common screening tool for depression.

    SAMHSA-HRSA Center for Integrated Health Solutions. Screening tools. http://www.integration.samhsa.gov/clinical-practice/screening-tools. Accessed January 10, 2016.

2. B. According to SAMHSA, the CAGE AID tool is best used to screen for alcohol and drug abuse.

    SAMHSA-HRSA Center for Integrated Health Solutions. Screening tools. http://www.integration.samhsa.gov/clinical-practice/screening-tools. Accessed January 10, 2016.

3. A. According to SAMHSA, the Mood Disorders Questionnaire (MDQ13) is designed to evaluate bipolar disorders.

    SAMHSA-HRSA Center for Integrated Health Solutions. Screening tools. http://www.integration.samhsa.gov/clinical-practice/screening-tools. Accessed January 10, 2016.

4. B. The Generalized Anxiety Disorders (GAD) 7 is best used to identify whether a complete assessment for anxiety is warranted.

SAMHSA-HRSA Center for Integrated Health Solutions. Screening tools. http://www.integration.samhsa.gov/clinical-practice/screening-tools. Accessed January 10, 2016.

5. A. According to SAMHSA, the Patient Stress Questionnaire is a tool used in primary care settings.

    SAMHSA-HRSA Center for Integrated Health Solutions. Screening tools. http://www.integration.samhsa.gov/clinical-practice/screening-tools. Accessed January 10, 2016.

6. A. According to SAMHSA, the AUDIT is a 10-item screening questionnaire to identify alcohol use disorders.

    SAMHSA-HRSA Center for Integrated Health Solutions. Screening tools. http://www.integration.samhsa.gov/clinical-practice/screening-tools. Accessed January 10, 2016.

7. D. According to SAMHSA, the Columbia-Suicide Severity Rating Scale (C-SSRS), the Suicide Assessment Five-Step Evaluation and Triage (SAFE-T), and the Suicide Behaviors Questionnaire (SBQ-R) are all used to evaluate for suicide risk.

    SAMHSA-HRSA Center for Integrated Health Solutions. Screening tools. http://www.integration.samhsa.gov/clinical-practice/screening-tools. Accessed January 10, 2016.

8. D. According to the DSM-5, generalized anxiety disorder (GAD) is characterized by excessive worrying. Repetitive thoughts can also be associated with mania experienced in GAD, but symptoms of peptic ulcer disease (PUD) are not stated in this case.

    American Psychiatric Association. *Diagnostic and Statistical Manual of Mental Disorders (DSM-5)*. 5th ed. Washington, DC: American Psychiatric Association; 2013.

9. E. Antidepressants, anti-anxiolytics, and cognitive behavioral therapy are considered first-line therapies for generalized anxiety disorder. Benzodiazepines may be used limitedly for a short timeframe but are not a good choice long term related to the risk of addiction.

    Mayo Clinic. Generalized anxiety disorder. 2014. http://www.mayoclinic.org/diseases-conditions/generalized-anxiety-disorder/basics/treatment/con-20024562. Accessed January 10, 2016.

10. A. Careful monitoring for suicidal ideation in young adults and adolescents should be anticipated when using antidepressants.

    Mayo Clinic. Generalized anxiety disorder. 2014. http://www.mayoclinic.org/diseases-conditions/generalized-anxiety-disorder/basics/treatment/con-20024562. Accessed January 10, 2016.

11. D. Escitalopram should be avoided in patients with a history of dysrhythmia related to the risk of the life-threatening side effect of QT prolongation.

    Mayo Clinic. Generalized anxiety disorder. 2014. http://www.mayoclinic.org/diseases-conditions/

generalized-anxiety-disorder/basics/treatment/con-20024562. Accessed January 10, 2016.

12. D. Duloxetine should not be used in seizure-sensitive persons related to its side effect of lowering the seizure threshold.

Mayo Clinic. Generalized anxiety disorder. 2014. http://www.mayoclinic.org/diseases-conditions/generalized-anxiety-disorder/basics/treatment/con-20024562. Accessed January 10, 2016.

13. D. Prescribing considerations for venlafaxine would include caution when using in patients with the conditions listed.

Mayo Clinic. Generalized anxiety disorder. 2014. http://www.mayoclinic.org/diseases-conditions/generalized-anxiety-disorder/basics/treatment/con-20024562. Accessed January 10, 2016.

14. D. Monoamine oxidase (MAO) inhibitors should be avoided within 14 days of paroxetine use.

Drugs.com. Paroxetine. 2016. http://www.drugs.com/paroxetine.html. Accessed January 10, 2016.

15. A. It is common for patients with generalized anxiety disorder to exhibit symptoms of other mental health disorders.

Mayo Clinic. Generalized anxiety disorder. 2014. http://www.mayoclinic.org/diseases-conditions/generalized-anxiety-disorder/basics/treatment/con-20024562. Accessed January 10, 2016.

16. D. Cognitive behavioral therapy alone or in combination with medications and adjuvant treatment may be used to treat multiple mental health issues.

Mayo Clinic. Cognitive behavioral therapy. 2013. http://www.mayoclinic.org/tests-procedures/cognitive-behavioral-therapy/basics/why-its-done/prc-20013594. Accessed January 10, 2016.

17. A. Common age of onset for schizophrenia is in the 20s.

Mayo Clinic. Schizophrenia. 2014. http://www.mayoclinic.org/diseases-conditions/schizophrenia/basics/symptoms/con-20021077. Accessed January 10, 2016.

18. A. Hearing or seeing things that are not real is defined as hallucinations.

Mayo Clinic. Schizophrenia. 2014. http://www.mayoclinic.org/diseases-conditions/schizophrenia/basics/symptoms/con-20021077. Accessed January 10, 2016.

19. D. Disorganized thinking, hallucinations, and delusions are all characteristics of schizophrenia.

Mayo Clinic. Schizophrenia. 2014. http://www.mayoclinic.org/diseases-conditions/schizophrenia/basics/symptoms/con-20021077. Accessed January 10, 2016.

20. A. Depression occurs twice as frequently in women as opposed to men and is most common in females between the ages of 40 and 59 years.

Mayo Clinic. Depression in women: understanding the gender gap. 2013. http://www.mayoclinic.org/diseases-conditions/depression/in-depth/depression/art-20047725. Accessed January 10, 2016.

21. C. Eating disorders can have an impact on multiple body systems by either mechanical or chemical irritation as well as malnutrition.

Mayo Clinic. Eating disorders. 2015. http://www.mayoclinic.org/diseases-conditions/eating-disorders/basics/definition/con-20033575. Accessed January 10, 2016.

22. A. Patients with bulimia nervosa can be normal to slightly overweight, will frequently distort or hide the actual amount of food consumed, and will often show signs of purge behaviors such as dental erosions.

Mayo Clinic. Eating disorders. 2015. http://www.mayoclinic.org/diseases-conditions/eating-disorders/basics/definition/con-20033575. Accessed January 10, 2016.

23. A. Pica is the ingestion of nonfood items that can have serious medical consequences.

Mayo Clinic. Eating disorders. 2015. http://www.mayoclinic.org/diseases-conditions/eating-disorders/basics/definition/con-20033575. Accessed January 10, 2016.

24. B. Buspirone is a pregnancy category B.

Drugs.com. FDA pregnancy categories. 2016. http://www.drugs.com/pregnancy-categories.html. Accessed January 10, 2016.

25. A. Buspirone may take 1 to 2 weeks before the patient recognizes its effects.

Mayo Clinic. Buspirone (oral route). 2016. http://www.mayoclinic.org/drugs-supplements/buspirone-oral-route/proper-use/drg-20062457. Accessed January 10, 2016.

26. A. According to the Physicians' Drug Reference (PDR), acetazolamide is a carbonic anhydrase inhibitor and not a benzodiazepine.

Mayo Clinic. Drugs and supplements. http://www.mayoclinic.org/drugs-supplements/. Accessed January 10, 2016.

Physicians' Drug Reference (PDR). http://www.pdr.net/drug-summary/diamox?druglabelid=649. Accessed January 19, 2016.

27. A. SAMHSA and the *Diagnostic and Statistical Manual of Mental Disorders 5th Edition* (DSM-5) categorize bipolar disorder into several subtypes.

Substance Abuse and Mental Health Services Administration. Mental disorders. 2015. http://www.samhsa.gov/disorders/mental. Accessed January 10, 2016.

28. D. According to SAMHSA and the DSM-5, bipolar disorder is characterized by alternating periods of manic episodes and depressive episodes.

Substance Abuse and Mental Health Services Administration. Mental disorders. 2015. http://www.samhsa.gov/disorders/mental. Accessed January 10, 2016.

29. A. The DSM-5 does not view bereavement as a subtype of depression or as a reason to exclude major depressive disorder as a diagnosis but rather as a potential trigger for major depressive disorder.

American Psychiatric Association. *Diagnostic and Statistical Manual of Mental Disorders (DSM-5)*. 5th ed. Washington, DC: American Psychiatric Association; 2013.

30. D. The American Psychiatric Association Practice Guideline for the Treatment of Patients with Major Depressive Disorder lists depressive symptoms of lethargy, malaise, inability to complete activities of daily living (ADLs), and disinterest in normal activities as symptoms of major depressive disorder.

Gelenberg AJ, Freeman MP, Markowitz JC, et al. *Practice Guideline for the Treatment of Patients with Major Depressive Disorder*. 3rd ed. 2010. https://psychiatryonline.org/pb/assets/raw/sitewide/practice_guidelines/guidelines/mdd.pdf. Accessed January 10, 2016.

31. A, B, C, D. SAMHSA and the Health Resources Services Administration (HRSA) Standards for Bipolar Excellence (STABLE): A Performance Measurement and Quality Improvement Project identify that therapies in addition to medication are necessary to assist patients with bipolar disorder.

National Coordinating Council. STABLE resource toolkit. http://www.integration.samhsa.gov/images/res/STABLE_toolkit.pdf. Accessed October 28, 2015.

32. B. According to the SAMHSA, two-thirds of persons over the age of 12 years have used alcohol in the preceding 12 months.

Substance Abuse and Mental Health Services Administration. Alcohol, tobacco, and other drugs. 2015. http://www.samhsa.gov/atod. Accessed January 10, 2016.

33. D. Men reported 3.8% illicit drug dependence compared to 1.9% of women.

Substance Abuse and Mental Health Services Administration. Alcohol, tobacco, and other drugs. 2015. http://www.samhsa.gov/atod. Accessed January 10, 2016.

34. C. According to SAMHSA, underage drinking claims the lives of approximately 5000 persons annually.

Substance Abuse and Mental Health Services Administration. Alcohol, tobacco, and other drugs. 2015. http://www.samhsa.gov/atod. Accessed January 10, 2016.

35. D. According to the CDC, alcohol use causes the death of 88,000 persons in the United States each year.

Centers for Disease Control and Prevention. Fact sheets—alcohol use and your health. http://www.cdc.gov/alcohol/fact-sheets/alcohol-use.htm. Accessed January 10, 2016.

36. B. The SAMHSA and HRSA STABLE Resource Toolkit identifies the symptoms exhibited by Zachary as consistent with bipolar disorder.

National Coordinating Council. STABLE resource toolkit. http://www.integration.samhsa.gov/images/res/STABLE_toolkit.pdf. Accessed October 28, 2015.

37. C. According to the CDC, 0.6 ounces of pure alcohol is equivalent to 12 ounces of beer, 8 ounces of malt liquor, 5 ounces of wine, or 1.5 ounces of 80-proof liquor.

Centers for Disease Control and Prevention. Fact sheets—alcohol use and your health. http://www.cdc.gov/alcohol/fact-sheets/alcohol-use.htm. Accessed January 10, 2016.

38. E. According to SAMHSA, a patient with PTSD may experience some or all of the symptoms listed.

Substance Abuse and Mental Health Services Administration. Mental disorders. 2015. http://www.samhsa.gov/disorders/mental. Accessed January 10, 2016.

39. C. According to SAMHSA, major depressive disorder was experienced by 6.6% of adults over the age of 18 years in 2014.

Substance Abuse and Mental Health Services Administration. Population data/NSDUH. 2015. http://www.samhsa.gov/data/population-data-nsduh. Accessed January 10, 2016.

40. B. SAMHSA estimates that 18% of persons, equivalent to 40 million, in the United States experience an anxiety disorder in any given year.

Substance Abuse and Mental Health Services Administration. Mental disorders. 2015. http://www.samhsa.gov/disorders/mental. Accessed January 10, 2016.

Chapter 12: Common Dermatologic Disorders in Primary Care

1. Josiah comes to your clinic today with complaints of a red, itchy rash with blistering in a linear pattern. Your working diagnosis for Josiah is:
   a. Rhus dermatitis → *Poison IVY*
   b. Scabies
   c. Pediculosis
   d. Atopic dermatitis

2. Jamie is a nurse who presents to you with complaints of reddened dry skin and itching along her hands on both the palmar and dorsal surfaces. Her differentials should include:
   a. Latex allergy
   b. Contact dermatitis
   c. Scabies
   d. Both A and B
   e. Both A and C
   f. All of the above

3. Rhus dermatitis can be spread from person to person via contact with the vesicles.
   a. True
   b. False

4. When explaining to Jamie why she developed contact dermatitis on the area covered by her latex gloves, you know this skin reaction can be related to:
   a. Exposure to a chemical or irritant
   b. A type I hypersensitivity reaction
   c. A type IV hypersensitivity reaction
   d. All of the above

5. Sonya is diagnosed with contact dermatitis caused by a nickel allergy. Your plan of care may include which topical agents?
   a. Antihistamines
   b. Corticosteroids
   c. Nickel-blocking agents
   d. Both A and B
   e. Both A and C
   f. All of the above

6. David is diagnosed with contact dermatitis caused by rhus exposure. Your plan of care may include which agents?
   a. Oral antihistamines
   b. Topical and oral corticosteroids
   c. Rhus-blocking agents
   d. Both A and B
   e. Both A and C
   f. All of the above

7. Eczema is estimated to affect _____ persons in the United States.
   a. 31.6 million
   b. 25.4 million
   c. 17.8 million
   d. 15.4 million

8. Sam presents with a lichenified red pruritic rash to his volar antecubital fossa and popliteal fossa region. Sam reports he has had some irritation in these areas since childhood that comes and goes. You know that the probable working diagnosis for Sam is:
   a. Atopic dermatitis
   b. Contact dermatitis
   c. Scabies
   d. Psoriasis

9. Sam asks you what atopic dermatitis is. Your best response is:
   a. A type of eczema
   b. An inherited condition
   c. Allergy related
   d. All of the above

10. When teaching Sam about living with his atopic dermatitis, you tell him that he needs to:
   a. Avoid tight clothing, take warm showers, immediately moisturize after showering

   b. Avoid loose clothing, take warm showers, avoid heavy moisturizers
   c. Take warm showers, apply moisturizers frequently, avoid touching other persons until skin is clear
   d. None of the above

11. Sam asks if there are other types of eczema. Your best response is:
   a. Yes, such as dyshidrotic and nummular
   b. Yes, such as anatropic and dyshidrotic
   c. Yes, such as nummular and anatropic
   d. No, there are no other forms of eczema

12. In addition to moisturizers and careful skin care, other treatments used for eczema include:
   a. Topical corticosteroids
   b. Topical calcineurin inhibitors
   c. Phototherapy
   d. All of the above

13. Charlotte comes to you today with complaints of a "bite" to her lower leg. Charlotte denies that she has been in dark basements or cleaning out unused closets. She states she works as a physical education teacher. Upon examination you note a fluctuant, red, swollen, painful, pus-filled area. You assess that Charlotte is at risk for:
   a. Methicillin-resistant *Staphylococcus aureus* (MRSA)
   b. Brown recluse spider bite
   c. Hymenoptera insect bite
   d. None of the above

14. You have been asked to speak with a group of coaches about MRSA. You discuss with them how they can help prevent the spread of MRSA as follows:
   a. Athletes should be instructed to seek care from a healthcare provider and keep all wounds fully covered.
   b. Athletes should be advised to avoid whirlpools, swimming pools, and shared equipment.
   c. Coaches should be advised to clean all surfaces using approved products.
   d. All of the above

15. In an adult patient with CA-MRSA, you anticipate treatment may include:
   a. Incision and drainage
   b. Antibiotic therapy
   c. Instructions on hygiene
   d. All of the above

16. In the case of a patient with CA-MRSA who has repeated infections or close family members with CA-MRSA, you would recommend:
   a. Nasal decolonization only
   b. Skin decolonization only
   c. Both nasal and skin decolonization
   d. Nasal decolonization, skin decolonization, and oral antibiotics

17. In the absence of active infection, culture following decolonization is not recommended.
    a. True
    b. False

18. Psoriasis is a contagious skin disease.
    a. True
    b. False

19. Jennifer presents to your clinic with complaints of recent onset of joint pain. During examination you note reddened skin plaques that the patient states she has had "forever." Your working diagnosis is:
    a. Rheumatoid arthritis
    b. Eczema
    c. Osteoarthritis
    d. Psoriatic arthritis

20. Jolynn is a 24 year-old female who presents with c/o waking up at night "itching" and has noticed "bumps" on her skin. Upon examination, you notice a raised linear papular rash on the webspace of bilateral hands and on her buttock. The working diagnosis is:
    a. Pediculosis pubis
    b. Sarcoptes scabiei
    c. Cimex lectularius
    d. Demodex folliculorum

21. Jolynn reports she is sexually active. She asks about what her treatment should include. You tell her that:
    a. She and her sexual partner will need treatment.
    b. She should plan to clean all linens in hot water.
    c. She will need a prescription to treat her scabies infection.
    d. All of the above

22. Differential diagnoses for a patient with symptoms of scabies should include:
    a. Pediculosis pubis
    b. Contact dermatitis
    c. Norwegian scabies
    d. All of the above

23. You are seeing a patient in follow-up from the urgent care center. He states he was diagnosed with Norwegian scabies. He asks you what the difference is between Norwegian scabies and "regular" scabies. Your best reply is:
    a. Norwegian scabies is more commonly seen in patients with immune compromise.
    b. Norwegian scabies is highly contagious.
    c. Norwegian scabies is less easily transmitted.
    d. Both A and B
    e. Both A and C

24. Joshua is a nurse at an extended care facility. He was recently diagnosed with scabies. You recommend that he:
    a. Not return to work until he has been effectively treated
    b. Not return to work until 5 days after the itching stops
    c. Not return to work until 2 months after the itching stops
    d. Not return to work caring for patients

25. As of 2012, there were _____ cases of melanoma skin cancer in the United States.
    a. 25,843
    b. 38,952
    c. 57,895
    d. 67,753

26. Persons with dark skin may get other types of skin cancer but do not get melanoma.
    a. True
    b. False

27. Risk factors for skin cancer include:
    a. Fair skin, light hair, green or brown eyes
    b. Blond or red hair, skin that tans profusely and rarely burns, fluorescent light exposure
    c. Skin that freckles, blue or green eyes, history of sunburns early in life
    d. Family history of skin cancer, brown hair, skin that tans easily

28. The ABCDE of skin cancer stands for:
    a. Asymmetry, border, color, diameter, erythema
    b. Asymmetry, border, change, diameter, ecchymosis
    c. Asymmetry, border, color, diameter, evolving
    d. None of the above

29. Sunscreen should be at least:
    a. SPF 45
    b. SPF 30
    c. SPF 25
    d. SPF 15

30. Sunglasses should:
    a. Wrap around and have UVA protection
    b. Wrap around and have UVB protection
    c. Wrap around and have UVA, UVB, and UVC protection
    d. Wrap around and have UVA and UVB protection

31. Malignant melanoma is diagnosed via the use of:
    a. Punch biopsy
    b. Shave biopsy
    c. Excisional biopsy
    d. Fine-needle aspiration

32. The most common type of skin cancer is:
    a. Basal cell
    b. Squamous cell
    c. Malignant melanoma
    d. Actinic keratosis

33. A raised, rough, scaly, wart-like patch would be most suspicious for:
    a. Molluscum contagiosum
    b. Squamous cell carcinoma
    c. Basal cell carcinoma
    d. Malignant melanoma

34. A translucent, shiny, pearly bump with raised edge and lowered center would be most suspicious for:
    a. Molluscum contagiosum
    b. Squamous cell carcinoma

c. Basal cell carcinoma
d. Malignant melanoma

35. Treatment of most basal cell carcinomas typically includes:
    a. Removal of the lesion
    b. Oral chemotherapy
    c. Intravenous chemotherapy
    d. External beam radiation
    e. All of the above

36. Treatment of squamous cell carcinoma typically includes:
    a. Removal of the lesion
    b. Oral chemotherapy
    c. Intravenous chemotherapy
    d. External beam radiation
    e. All of the above

37. Treatment of malignant melanoma is dependent upon staging of disease but may include:
    a. Full excision of the lesion and all borders
    b. Chemotherapy
    c. Radiation
    d. Immunotherapy
    e. All of the above

38. Staging of malignant melanoma includes examination of the lesion for:
    a. Thickness
    b. Mitotic rate
    c. Ulceration
    d. All of the above

39. Targeted therapy for malignant melanoma includes:
    a. BRAF inhibitors
    b. MEK inhibitors
    c. C-KIT modifiers
    d. Both A and B
    e. All of the above

40. The 5-year survival rate for a person diagnosed with Stage IV malignant melanoma is approximately:
    a. 5–10%
    b. 10–15%
    c. 15–20%
    d. 20–25%

Chapter 12: Answers and Rationales

1. A. The American Academy of Family Practice provides the clinical picture of rhus dermatitis, commonly known as poison ivy.

   Usatine RP, Riojas M. Diagnosis and management of contact dermatitis. http://www.aafp.org/afp/2010/0801/p249.pdf. Accessed January 10, 2016.

2. D. According to the American Academy of Dermatology, contact dermatitis and latex allergy can coexist in the case of a presentation with glove use.

Eichenfield LF, Tom WL, Chamlin SL, et al. Guidelines of care for the management of atopic dermatitis. *J Am Acad Dermatol.* 2014;70(2):338–351.

3. B. Rhus dermatitis is spread via contact with the oil from the leaves on the plant, which may remain on surfaces for up to 5 years, but is not spread via blister fluid.

   Centers for Disease Control and Prevention. NIOSH fast facts: protecting yourself from poisonous plants. http://www.cdc.gov/niosh/docs/2010-118/pdfs/2010-118.pdf.

4. D. The Centers for Disease Control and Prevention (CDC) states that a chemical irritant or a Type I or Type IV hypersensitivity response can be responsible for this skin reaction.

   Centers for Disease Control and Prevention. Frequently asked questions—contact dermatitis and latex allergy. 2013. http://www.cdc.gov/OralHealth/infectioncontrol/faq/latex.htm. Accessed January 10, 2016.

5. B. According to the American Academy of Family Practice, topical corticosteroids would be recommended to treat this nickel allergy.

   Usatine RP, Riojas M. Diagnosis and management of contact dermatitis. http://www.aafp.org/afp/2010/0801/p249.pdf. Accessed January 10, 2016.

6. F. The American Academy of Family Practice provides the treatment modality for uncomplicated rhus dermatitis, commonly known as poison ivy.

   Usatine RP, Riojas M. Diagnosis and management of contact dermatitis. http://www.aafp.org/afp/2010/0801/p249.pdf. Accessed January 10, 2016.

7. A. According to the National Eczema Association, approximately 31.6 million persons in the United States have eczema.

   National Eczema Association. Atopic dermatitis. https://nationaleczema.org/eczema/types-of-eczema/atopic-dermatitis-2/. Accessed January 10, 2016.

8. A. According to the National Eczema Association, chronic atopic dermatitis has the clinical presentation of a lichenified region of itching and redness, primarily at the areas where the elbows and knees bend.

   National Eczema Association. Atopic dermatitis. https://nationaleczema.org/eczema/types-of-eczema/atopic-dermatitis-2/. Accessed January 10, 2016.

9. D. According to the National Eczema Association, atopic dermatitis is an allergy-mediated, inherited condition that is a form of eczema.

   National Eczema Association. Atopic dermatitis. https://nationaleczema.org/eczema/types-of-eczema/atopic-dermatitis-2/. Accessed January 10, 2016.

10. A. According to the National Eczema Association, care of the skin in a patient with eczema is very important to reduce the itch-scratch cycle and provide for good skin hygiene.

    National Eczema Association. Treatment. https://nationaleczema.org/eczema/treatment/. Accessed January 10, 2016.

11. A. According to the National Eczema Association, atopic dermatitis, dyshidrotic, and nummular are all types of eczema.

National Eczema Association. Atopic dermatitis. https://nationaleczema.org/eczema/types-of-eczema/atopic-dermatitis-2/. Accessed January 10, 2016.

12. D. The National Eczema Association lists all of the above as well as psychodermatology, immunosuppressants, and alternative therapies to treat eczema.

National Eczema Association. Treatment. https://national eczema.org/eczema/treatment/. Accessed January 10, 2016.

13. A. The Infectious Diseases Society of America (IDSA) provides the clinical picture of MRSA.

Centers for Disease Control and Prevention. General information about MRSA in the community. 2013. http://www.cdc.gov/mrsa/community/index.html. Accessed January 10, 2016.

Liu C, Bayer A, Cosgrove SE, et al; Infectious Diseases Society of America. Clinical practice guidelines by the Infectious Diseases Society of America for the treatment of methicillin-resistant *Staphylococcus aureus* infections in adults and children. *Clin Infect Dis.* 2011;52(3):e18–55.

14. D. The CDC provides the plan of care and teaching protocol for coaches and care providers of persons affected by community-acquired MRSA (CA-MRSA).

Centers for Disease Control and Prevention. MRSA information for coaches, athletic directors, and team healthcare providers. 2013. http://www.cdc.gov/mrsa/community/team-hc-providers/index.html. Accessed January 10, 2016.

15. D. IDSA recommends treatment that may include hygiene measures, incision and drainage, and probable antibiotic use.

Liu C, Bayer A, Cosgrove SE, et al; Infectious Diseases Society of America. Clinical practice guidelines by the Infectious Diseases Society of America for the treatment of methicillin-resistant *Staphylococcus aureus* infections in adults and children. *Clin Infect Dis.* 2011;52(3):e18–55. http://cid.oxfordjournals.org/content/52/3/e18.full. Accessed January 10, 2016.

16. C. IDSA recommends treatment of CA-MRSA in close household contacts and in persons with repeated infections should include nasal and skin decolonization.

Liu C, Bayer A, Cosgrove SE, et al; Infectious Diseases Society of America. Clinical practice guidelines by the Infectious Diseases Society of America for the treatment of methicillin-resistant *Staphylococcus aureus* infections in adults and children. *Clin Infect Dis.* 2011;52(3):e18–55. http://cid.oxfordjournals.org/content/52/3/e18.full. Accessed January 10, 2016.

17. A. IDSA does not recommend routine cultures following decolonization treatment.

Liu C, Bayer A, Cosgrove SE, et al; Infectious Diseases Society of America. Clinical practice guidelines by the Infectious Diseases Society of America for the treatment of methicillin-resistant *Staphylococcus aureus* infections in adults and children.

Clin Infect Dis. 2011;52(3):e18–55. http://cid.oxfordjournals.org/content/52/3/e18.full. Accessed January 10, 2016.

18. B. The CDC recognizes psoriasis as an autoimmune skin disease.

Centers for Disease Control and Prevention. Psoriasis. 2015. http://www.cdc.gov/psoriasis/index.htm. Accessed January 10, 2016.

19. D. The CDC provides a clinical picture of psoriatic arthritics, which is characterized by psoriatic plaques and joint inflammation.

Centers for Disease Control and Prevention. Psoriasis. 2015. http://www.cdc.gov/psoriasis/index.htm. Accessed January 10, 2016.

20. B. According to the CDC, this clinical picture is of scabies.

Centers for Disease Control and Prevention. What is crusted (Norwegian) scabies? http://www.cdc.gov/parasites/scabies/gen_info/faqs.html#crusted. Accessed January 10, 2016.

21. D. According to the CDC, her treatment should include treatment of sexual partners and close contacts, cleansing of linens in hot water, and a prescription medication for the elimination of the scabies mite.

Centers for Disease Control and Prevention. What is crusted (Norwegian) scabies? http://www.cdc.gov/parasites/scabies/gen_info/faqs.html#crusted. Accessed January 10, 2016.

22. D. According to the CDC, differential diagnoses for scabies could include all of the above.

Centers for Disease Control and Prevention. What is crusted (Norwegian) scabies? http://www.cdc.gov/parasites/scabies/gen_info/faqs.html#crusted. Accessed January 10, 2016.

23. D. According to the CDC, Norwegian scabies is highly contagious and more common in immunosuppressed individuals.

Centers for Disease Control and Prevention. What is crusted (Norwegian) scabies? http://www.cdc.gov/parasites/scabies/gen_info/faqs.html#crusted. Accessed January 10, 2016.

24. A. According to the CDC, any person who works with close skin-to-skin contact such as caregivers in childhood centers, laundries, or extended care/hospital facilities should refrain from work until fully cleared following effective treatment for scabies.

Centers for Disease Control and Prevention. What is crusted (Norwegian) scabies? http://www.cdc.gov/parasites/scabies/gen_info/faqs.html#crusted. Accessed January 10, 2016.

25. D. The CDC estimates that in 2012, the most recent year for which statistics are available, 67,753 people were diagnosed with melanoma skin cancer.

Centers for Disease Control and Prevention. Skin cancer statistics. 2015. http://www.cdc.gov/cancer/skin/statistics/index.htm. Accessed January 10, 2016.

26. B. According to the CDC, while lighter skinned individuals are at a higher risk of skin cancer, melanoma can occur in all races and skin types.

Centers for Disease Control and Prevention. What are the risk factors for skin cancer? 2014. http://www.cdc.gov/cancer/skin/basic_info/risk_factors.htm. Accessed January 10, 2016.

27. C. According to the CDC, lighter skinned, fair-eyed individuals with family history of cancer and history of early sunburns have a higher risk of skin cancer.

Centers for Disease Control and Prevention. What are the risk factors for skin cancer? 2014. http://www.cdc.gov/cancer/skin/basic_info/risk_factors.htm. Accessed January 10, 2016.

28. C. The CDC provides the evaluation mnemonic to assist in the diagnosis of skin cancer for the evaluation of suspicious lesions.

Centers for Disease Control and Prevention. What are the risk factors for skin cancer? 2014. http://www.cdc.gov/cancer/skin/basic_info/risk_factors.htm. Accessed January 10, 2016.

29. D. The CDC recommends a sunscreen of at least SPF 15 that protects against UVA and UVB waves.

Centers for Disease Control and Prevention. What can I do to reduce my risk of skin cancer? 2014. http://www.cdc.gov/cancer/skin/basic_info/prevention.htm. Accessed January 10, 2016.

30. D. The CDC recommends eye protection that guards against UVA and UVB waves and wraps around to protect the eye.

Centers for Disease Control and Prevention. What can I do to reduce my risk of skin cancer? 2014. http://www.cdc.gov/cancer/skin/basic_info/prevention.htm. Accessed January 10, 2016.

31. C. According to the American Cancer Society, malignant melanoma should be removed using a wide excisional margin technique to allow for appropriate staging of melanoma skin cancer.

American Cancer Society. How is melanoma skin cancer diagnosed? 2015. http://www.cancer.org/cancer/skincancer-melanoma/detailedguide/melanoma-skin-cancer-diagnosed. Accessed January 10, 2016.

32. A. According to the American Cancer Society, basal cell carcinoma is the most common form of skin cancer.

American Cancer Society. What are basal and squamous cell skin cancers? 2015. http://www.cancer.org/cancer/skincancer-basalandsquamouscell/detailedguide/skin-cancer-basal-and-squamous-cell-what-is-basal-and-squamous-cell. Accessed January 10, 2016.

33. B. The American Cancer Society provides a clinical picture of squamous cell carcinoma.

American Cancer Society. What are basal and squamous cell skin cancers? 2015. http://www.cancer.org/cancer/skincancer-basalandsquamouscell/detailedguide/skin-cancer-basal-and-squamous-cell-what-is-basal-and-squamous-cell. Accessed January 10, 2016.

34. C. The American Cancer Society provides a clinical picture of basal cell carcinoma.

American Cancer Society. What are basal and squamous cell skin cancers? 2015. http://www.cancer.org/cancer/skincancer-basalandsquamouscell/detailedguide/skin-cancer-basal-and-squamous-cell-what-is-basal-and-squamous-cell. Accessed January 10, 2016.

35. A. According to the American Cancer Society, most cases of basal cell carcinoma are effectively treated with removal of the lesion.

American Cancer Society. What are basal and squamous cell skin cancers? 2015. http://www.cancer.org/cancer/skincancer-basalandsquamouscell/detailedguide/skin-cancer-basal-and-squamous-cell-what-is-basal-and-squamous-cell. Accessed January 10, 2016.

36. A. According to the American Cancer Society, most cases of squamous cell carcinoma are effectively treated with removal of the lesion.

American Cancer Society. What are basal and squamous cell skin cancers? 2015. http://www.cancer.org/cancer/skincancer-basalandsquamouscell/detailedguide/skin-cancer-basal-and-squamous-cell-what-is-basal-and-squamous-cell. Accessed January 10, 2016.

37. E. According to the American Cancer Society, most cases of malignant melanoma may require treatment beyond lesion removal.

American Cancer Society. How is melanoma skin cancer treated? 2015. http://www.cancer.org/cancer/skincancer-melanoma/detailedguide/melanoma-skin-cancer-treating-general-info. Accessed January 10, 2016.

38. D. According to the American Cancer Society, examination of the malignant melanoma lesion will allow for examination of the characteristics of the lesion to enable appropriate staging and determination of treatment recommendations.

American Cancer Society. How is melanoma skin cancer treated? 2015. http://www.cancer.org/cancer/skincancer-melanoma/overviewguide/melanoma-skin-cancer-overview-staging. Accessed January 10, 2016.

39. E. According to the American Cancer Society, targeted therapy for malignant melanoma is directed at blocking particular proteins and gene expressions to arrest the spread of the melanoma.

American Cancer Society. Targeted therapy for melanoma skin cancer. 2015. http://www.cancer.org/cancer/skincancer-melanoma/detailedguide/melanoma-skin-cancer-treating-targeted-therapy. Accessed January 10, 2016.

40. C. According to the American Cancer Society, the 5-year survival rate for malignant melanoma is 15–20%.

American Cancer Society. What are the survival rates for melanoma skin cancer, by stage? 2015. http://www.cancer.org/cancer/skincancer-melanoma/detailedguide/melanoma-skin-cancer-survival-rates. Accessed January 10, 2016.

Chapter 13: Common Geriatric Issues in Primary Care

1. A variety of screening tools are available to evaluate cognitive assessment. Which statement is <u>inaccurate</u> regarding the mini-mental-status exam (MMSE)?
   a. The MMSE has been the most widely used cognitive test for dementia in US clinical practice.
   b. The maximal score on the MMSE is 30 points.
   c. The test has good sensitivity and specificity in a large hospitalized sample but is not sensitive for mild dementia.
   d. Scores are rarely influenced by demographic variables of patients screened.

2. Initial labs to consider in the evaluation of altered cognitive function include all of the following *except*:
   a. CBC and CMP
   b. Syphilis serology
   c. Thyroid panel and vitamin B_{12}
   d. Genetic testing

3. Which statement is <u>accurate</u> regarding imaging for patients with cognitive decline?
   a. All patients with early cognitive decline should get a computed tomography (CT) scan of the brain, with and without contrast.
   b. Magnetic resonance imaging (MRI) is helpful in distinguishing between different types of dementia.
   c. MRI is reasonable for patients with cognitive decline to rule out normal pressure hydrocephalus, subdural hematoma, and cerebrovascular disease.
   d. Positron emission tomography (PET) scanning is the most reliable method of diagnosing the cause of cognitive decline.

4. What tasks are involved in the Mini-Cog test?
   a. Clock drawing task and an uncued recall of three unrelated words
   b. Stating date including year, season, date, day, and month
   c. Serial 7s, beginning with 100 and counting backward
   d. An interview to evaluate impairment in 6 domains

5. According to the Cocoa PHSS, which of the following statements is <u>inaccurate</u> regarding the differentiation of delirium from dementia?
   a. In dementia, patients are usually alert; in delirium, there is decreased consciousness or patients are hyperalert.
   b. In dementia, psychomotor function is usually agitated or lethargic; in delirium, psychomotor function is usually normal.
   c. The onset of dementia is chronic; the onset of delirium is acute or subacute.
   d. In dementia, speech is aphasic and anomic, and word finding is a problem; in delirium the speech is slow and incoherent.

6. Which statement is <u>inaccurate</u> regarding strategies to prevent mild cognitive impairment (MCI) or dementia?
   a. Statin medications and vitamin E may delay or prevent dementia.
   b. Smoking and depression are linked to an increased risk for MCI and dementia; smoking cessation strategies and treatment of depression are recommended.
   c. Regular physical activity may be an important strategy for reducing risk of MCI and dementia.
   d. Cognitive activities such as mental exercises may reduce risk.

7. Which statement is true regarding of the Saint Louis University Mental Status (SLUMS) tool?
   a. It is less sensitive than the MMSE for early cognitive changes.
   b. The tool includes assessment in 14 cognitive domains.
   c. The 5-item delayed recall in the SLUMS tool has been shown to be an excellent discriminator of normal cognition versus mild cognitive changes.
   d. The SLUMS tool quantifies dementia in mild, moderate, severe, profound, and terminal stages.

8. Which statement is <u>inaccurate</u> regarding the importance of evaluating functional activities in older adults with dementia?
   a. Patients with dementia will experience a decline in functional ability over time.
   b. The majority of care costs in patients with dementia are related to functional disability.
   c. Compromised functional ability is unsafe for patients with dementia and is anxiety producing for their families.
   d. There are no good tools to help evaluate instrumental activities of daily living.

9. Which of the following medications would be appropriate for the initial treatment of dementia?
   a. Donepezil
   b. Cyclobenzaprine
   c. Metoclopramide
   d. Thorazine

10. Why are cholinesterase inhibitors used in the treatment of Alzheimer's disease (AD)?
    a. Patients with AD have reduced cerebral production of choline acetyl transferase.
    b. This decrease in choline acetyl transferase leads to a decrease in acetylcholine synthesis.
    c. Reduced acetylcholine synthesis results in impaired cortical cholinergic function.
    d. All of the above

11. Which statement is <u>inaccurate</u> regarding older adult drivers?
    a. Fatal crash rates increase starting at ages 70–74 and are highest among drivers who are 85 or older.

b. Most older drivers were not wearing seat belts at the time of a fatal crash.

c. Older drivers tend to avoid driving during bad weather and at night.

d. Older drivers are less likely to drink and drive than other adult drivers.

12. Which statement is accurate regarding the association between motor vehicle crashes or adverse driving events in the older population?

a. There may be a modest increase in total crash risk and at-fault risk for older adults with cardiac disease.

b. Patients with insulin-dependent diabetes should not need driving restrictions as long as they demonstrate satisfactory control of their diabetes and recognize the warning symptoms of hypoglycemia.

c. Patients with musculoskeletal problems such as diminished cervical range of motion or a slowed walking pace have been associated with an increased crash risk.

d. All of the above

13. Which medications are considered inappropriate to use in older adults according to the Beers criteria?

a. Tertiary tricyclic antidepressants

b. Long-acting sulfonylureas

c. Skeletal muscle relaxants

d. All of the above

14. Why are antispasmodic agents such as belladonna, dicyclomine, and propantheline not recommended for use in older adults?

a. These drugs may cause orthostatic hypotension.

b. These drugs are highly anticholinergic, and effectiveness is uncertain.

c. These drugs have a high potential for pulmonary toxicity, and safer alternatives are available.

d. These drugs may induce heart failure in older adults.

15. Hearing loss is highly prevalent in older patients, and part of the assessment of hearing loss includes the tuning fork exam. Which statement is correct regarding findings associated with tuning fork tests?

a. No lateralization on the Weber test and air conduction greater than bone conduction laterally on a Rinne test indicate no hearing loss.

b. Lateralization to sound to one side and bone conduction greater than air conduction on the side of lateralization indicate a sensorineural hearing loss.

c. Lateralization to sound to one side and air conduction greater than bone conduction on the side of lateralization indicate a conductive hearing loss.

d. No lateralization on the Weber test and bone conduction greater than air conduction on a Rinne test indicate sensorineural hearing loss.

16. While many older adults could benefit from hearing aids, fewer than 15% of Americans older than the age of 50 with hearing loss actually use this assistive device. Reasons for low usage include all of the following *except*:

a. Cost

b. Appearance

c. Comfort

d. Good performance in different environments

17. Causes of conductive hearing loss include all of the following *except*:

a. Cerumen impaction

b. Middle-ear infections

c. Presbycusis → *age related hearing loss*

d. Perforations of the tympanic membrane

18. Causes of age-related hearing loss include all of the following *except*:

a. Medications

b. Noise trauma

c. Acoustic neuroma

d. Otis media with effusion

19. Which statement is incorrect regarding behavioral therapies for urinary incontinence?

a. Bladder training and pelvic muscle exercises are only effective for stress incontinence.

b. Behavioral therapy should be the first-line therapy for older patients with urinary incontinence.

c. Behavioral therapy and pelvic muscle exercises can be used together to help with urinary incontinence.

d. Bladder training involves frequent voluntary voiding to keep bladder volume low and central nervous system and pelvic mechanisms to suppress urgency.

20. Which of the following is the most reliable clinical assessment for confirming stress incontinence?

a. Incontinence Questions Tool

b. Three-day voiding diary

c. Cough stress test

d. Post-void residual urine measurement

21. Why is it important to assess how urinary incontinence affects quality of life?

a. A description of how quality of life is impacted by incontinence helps uncover comorbidities that may need to be treated.

b. A urologic referral is recommended for any patient who has significant symptom burden.

c. The severity of urinary incontinence symptoms and their effect on quality of life determine the aggressiveness of treatment.

d. All of the above

22. Which signs or symptoms are indications for a urologic referral?

a. Marked prostate enlargement

b. Pelvic pain associated with incontinence

c. Incontinence with new-onset neurologic symptoms

d. All of the above

23. Which statement is not consistent with the updated definition of geriatric failure to thrive?
   a. Weight loss of more than 5%
   b. Decreased appetite and poor nutrition
   c. Physical activity and dehydration
   d. Associated with dehydration, immune dysfunction, and low cholesterol

24. A comprehensive initial assessment for patients suspected of having failure to thrive should include:
   a. Evaluation of impaired physical and cognitive function
   b. Evaluation of malnutrition
   c. Evaluation of depression
   d. All of the above

25. For the initial evaluation of geriatric failure to thrive, which of the following is not recommended?
   a. Complete blood count
   b. Urine culture
   c. Thyroid panel
   d. Chemistry panel

26. Which statement is inaccurate regarding nutrition for older adults?
   a. Recommended dietary allowances (RDAs) of vitamins and minerals for older patients are not significantly different from those recommended for middle-age adults.
   b. Recommendations for calcium and vitamin D intake increase for both men and women older than 70 years.
   c. Ten to 15% of total calories should come from fat for patients over 70 years of age.
   d. Protein requirements are influenced by activity levels, medications, protein content of the diet, and health status.

27. Which statement is true regarding the Mini Nutritional Assessment (MNA) tool?
   a. This tool includes a malnutrition indicator score, and patients receiving less than 8 points are malnourished.
   b. Body mass index (BMI) is not measured on this tool, because it is an inadequate predictor of malnutrition.
   c. This tool asks family and other care providers to provide their assessment of the nutritional status of the patient.
   d. Mobility is not a component of this assessment tool.

28. Which statement is inaccurate regarding sarcopenia?
   a. Sarcopenia is defined as a decline in walking speed or grip strength associated with low muscle mass.
   b. Sarcopenia was originally defined as having muscle mass greater than 2 standard deviations below the mean for healthy young adults assessed by a variety of imaging techniques.
   c. Progressive resistance training (PRT) is not helpful in improving strength and physical functioning to combat sarcopenia in geriatric patients.
   d. Sarcopenia represents a major cause of falls and functional deterioration in older persons.

PRT us an effective strategy to improve physical function

29. According to the AD8 dementia screening interview, which of the following changes (over the last several years) may indicate progressive cognitive problems?
   a. Problems making decisions
   b. Repeating the same things over and over
   c. Less interest in hobbies and activities
   d. All of the above

30. The strongest modifiable risk factors for falls in older persons include all of the following *except*:
   a. Balance impairment
   b. Gait impairment
   c. Cognitive impairment
   d. Muscle weakness

31. Which statement is not accurate regarding falls in older patients?
   a. All patients who are older than 65 should be asked annually about whether they have fallen and if they are having difficulty with walking or balance.
   b. A gait and balance evaluation should be performed in every person who reports a single fall.
   c. The Get Up and Go test is the most time-efficient method of assessing for fall risk.
   d. There is good evidence from randomized control trials to direct providers in determining the most effective strategies for fall prevention.

32. What information should be included on the fall-prevention prescription?
   a. Referrals for physical therapy, podiatry, and ophthalmology if indicated
   b. Type of exercise recommended
   c. Recommendations for calcium and Vitamin D
   d. All of the above

33. Which statement is inaccurate regarding fall prevention?
   a. Reducing medication use can decrease falls in elderly patients.
   b. Vitamin D supplementation of at least 800 international units should be given to older persons with proven vitamin D deficiency.
   c. Treatment for osteoporosis should include 1200 mg of calcium daily and bisphosphonates indefinitely to reduce fractures from falls.
   d. All patients should receive a home safety checklist.

Bisphosphonate x 5 yrs only

34. Why is maintaining a driver's license so important to older adults?
   a. Driving represents a person's freedom, independence, and self-sufficiency.
   b. Driving enables a person to get food, clothing, and health care.
   c. Driving helps a person to participate in society and maintain emotional and spiritual needs.
   d. All of the above

35. What agency is responsible for licensing drivers?
  a. National Highway Traffic Safety Administration (NHTSA)
  b. Individual states
  c. Individual counties
  d. Healthcare providers

36. Which statement is inaccurate regarding the NP's initial approach for beginning a conversation related to discouraging or preventing a senior patient from driving?
  a. Refrain from discussing this issue with adult children who will likely have a bias and will want their parent to stop driving.
  b. Contact the state's department of motor vehicles to inquire about regulations regarding licensure and operation.
  c. Complete physical exam with particular attention to the assessment of driving-related skills (ADRS).
  d. Discuss known accidents or near accidents and explore patient's perceptions of the seriousness of these incidents.

37. Giving bad news such as discussing a life-threatening illness or discussing a poor prognosis can be challenging for the nurse practitioner. Which statement is not accurate regarding the SPIKES model for having difficult conversations?
  a. The setup (S) is important, so find a private space to prepare yourself for difficult questions and the emotions that may arise during the planned conversation.
  b. Begin by giving the facts and avoid exploring the perceptions (P) of the patient and family.
  c. Invite (I) the patient and family to tell you how much information they want and then give them the facts (K = knowledge).
  d. Empathize (E) by acknowledging their feelings and then summarize and strategize.

38. Which statement is true regarding pain control at end of life?
  a. Both pharmacologic and nonpharmacologic strategies should be considered to treat pain in the elderly at the end of life; palliative sedation may be a valid palliative care option.
  b. The sequential use of analgesic drugs according to the World Health Organization (WHO) ladder is an inexpensive and effective method for relieving pain.
  c. All opioids are considered effective, but there are no well designed specific studies in the elderly population.
  d. All of the above

39. Which tool may be helpful in determining prognosis in terminally ill patients?
  a. APACHE II score
  b. Gleason score
  c. PaP score
  d. IPSS score

40. Which statement is not accurate regarding referral of patients to hospice care?
  a. Hospice is recommended for any terminally ill patient who chooses a palliative care approach.
  b. Hospice care is built on the concept that the dying patient has physical, social, and spiritual aspects of suffering.
  c. Hospice is a philosophy, not a place. It can be provided in the patient home, nursing home, or hospital setting.
  d. Recommending and referring to hospice care by nurse practitioners has been approved by state legislation.

Chapter 13: Answers and Rationales

1. D. Scores on the MMSE may be influenced by age, education, language, and motor and visual impairments.

Fried W, Schmidt R, Stronegger WJ, et al. Mini mental state examination: influence of sociodemographic, environmental and behavioral factors and vascular risk factors. *J Clin Epidemiol.* 1996;49:73.

2. D. The value of genetic testing for making a diagnosis remains uncertain. It is suggested that formal genetic counseling be recommended if genetic testing is considered.

Mayeux AU, Saunders R, Shea S, et al. Utility of the apolipoprotein E genotype in the diagnosis of Alzheimer's disease. Alzheimer's Disease Centers Consortium on Apolipoprotein E and Alzheimer's Disease. *N Engl J Med.* 1998;338:506–511.

3. C. Structural neuroimaging with either a noncontrast head CT or MRI is the routine initial evaluation of all patients with dementia.

American College of Radiology. ACR appropriateness criteria for dementia and movement disorders. http://www.acr.org/Quality-Safety/Appropriateness-Criteria. Accessed January 10, 2016.

4. A. The Mini-Cog test involves clock drawing and recalling three words. It has the advantage of high sensitivity for predicting dementia status in a short testing time relative to the MMSE, it is easy to administer, and the diagnostic value is not altered by the subject's education or language.

Bonson S, Scanlan J, Brush M, et al. The mini-cog: a cognitive "vital signs" measure for dementia screening in multilingual elderly. *Int J Geriatri Psychiatry.* 2000;15:1021.

5. B. In dementia, psychomotor function is usually normal, and psychomotor function becomes agitated or lethargic in the patient with delirium.

St. Louis University. Geriatric mnemonics and screening tools. http://aging.slu.edu/uploads/pdf/Saint-Louis-University-Geriatric-Evaluation_2013.pdf. Accessed January 10, 2016.

6. A. Rationale: There are no proven strategies to prevent MCI or dementia. The use of statin drugs and vitamin E has failed to delay or prevent dementia in large clinical trials.

Daviglus ML, Bell CC, Berrettini W, et al. National Institutes of Health State-of-the-Science Conference Statement: preventing Alzheimer's disease and cognitive decline. *NIH Consens State Sci Statements.* 2010;27(4):1–27.

7. C. The SLUMS tool has better sensitivity than the MMSE for early cognitive changes and discriminates between normal cognition and mild cognitive changes. It is available for general use with no fee. It is widely used by the Veterans Administration system.

Segal-Gidan F. Cognitive screening tools. *Clin Rev.* 2013; 23:12–18.

Saint Louis University. VAMC SLUMS examination. http://medschool.slu.edu/agingsuccessfully/pdfsurveys/slumsexam_05.pdf. Accessed January 10, 2016.

8. D. The Functional Activities Questionnaire (FAQ) measures instrumental activities of daily living and demonstrates good sensitivity (85%) and high reliability (exceeding 0.80).

Utility of the Functional Activities Questionnaire for Distinguishing Mild Cognitive Impairment from Very Mild Alzheimer's Disease. http://www.ncbi.nlm.nih.gov/pmc/articles/PMC2997338/.

9. A. Donepezil is a cholinesterase inhibitor, which is a drug category that is recommended as a first-line choice for the treatment of dementia.

MedlinePlus. Donezepil. 2014. http://www.nlm.nih.gov/medlineplus/druginfo/meds/a697032.html. Accessed January 11, 2016.

10. D. Three cholinesterase inhibitors are currently approved for use in AD.

Press D, Alexander M. Cholinesterase inhibitors in the treatment of dementia. 2015. http://www.uptodate.com/contents/cholinesterase-inhibitors-in-the-treatment-of-dementia. Accessed January 10, 2016.

11. B. More than 79% of older drivers were wearing seat belts at the time of a fatal crash.

Centers for Disease Control and Prevention. Injury prevention & control: motor vehicle safety. 2015. http://www.cdc.gov/motorvehiclesafety/older_adult_drivers/. Accessed January 10, 2016.

12. D. Many medical conditions may impact the safety of the older driver. Nurse practitioners should consult the *Physician's Guide to Assessing and Counseling Older Drivers* for assistance with determining crash risk for their patients.

American Medical Association, National Highway Traffic Safety Administration. *Physician's Guide to Assessing and Counseling Older Drivers.* http://www.nhtsa.gov/people/injury/olddrive/OlderDriversBook/pages/Contents.html. Accessed January 10, 2016.

13. D. Overuse and misuse of drugs used in older adults is common. Several "drugs-to-avoid" lists are available to identify medications that may cause a wide variety of side effects in the elderly. The Beers criteria provide a helpful tool for identifying these drugs and potential problems, and NPs should consult this list before prescribing to older adults.

The American Geriatrics Society 2012 Updated Beers Criteria Update Expert Panel. American Geriatrics Society updated Beers criteria for potentially inappropriate medication use in older adults. *J Am Geriatr Soc.* 2012;60:616–631. http://www.americangeriatrics.org/files/documents/beers/2012AGS BeersCriteriaCitations.pdf. Accessed January 10, 2016.

14. B. Anticholinergic drugs may cause blurred vision, constipation, drowsiness, sedation, memory impairment, and difficulty with urination.

The American Geriatrics Society 2012 Updated Beers Criteria Update Expert Panel. American Geriatrics Society updated Beers criteria for potentially inappropriate medication use in older adults. *J Am Geriatr Soc.* 2012;60:616–631. http://www.americangeriatrics.org/files/documents/beers/2012AGS BeersCriteriaCitations.pdf. Accessed January 10, 2016.

15. A. Normal findings on a tuning fork exam include no sound lateralization on the Weber test and air conduction greater than bone conduction. This finding is consistent with no hearing loss but can also indicate sensorineural hearing loss bilaterally.

Genther DJ, Lin FR. Managing hearing impairment in older adults. In: Williams BA, Chang A, eds. *Current Diagnosis & Treatment: Geriatrics.* 2nd ed. New York: McGraw-Hill; 2014: 460–466.

16. D. Performance may be variable for patients with hearing aids, but there is ongoing work on improving amplification of sounds.

Neumann SI, Wolfe J. New and notable in hearing aids. 2013. http://www.listeningandspokenlanguage.org/Parent GuideHA.aspx. Accessed January 10, 2016.

17. C. Presbycusis is age-related hearing loss and results in sensorineural hearing loss.

Walling AD, Dickson GM. Hearing loss in older adults. *Am Fam Physician.* 2012;85:1150–1156.

18. D. Otitis media with effusion is caused by infection and is not more prevalent in the older population.

Walling AD, Dickson GM. Hearing loss in older adults. *Am Fam Physician.* 2012;85:1150–1156.

19. A. Bladder training and pelvic muscle exercises are effective for stress, urge, and mixed incontinence.

Hersh L, Salzman B. Clinical management of urinary incontinence in women. *Am Fam Physician.* 2013;87:634–640.

20. C. The cough test is easy to perform and has good specificity and sensitivity for stress incontinence. Confirmatory urodynamic evaluation is required, because the results may be inconclusive.

Khandelwal C, Kistler C. Diagnosis of urinary incontinence. *Am Fam Physician.* 2013;87:543–550.

21. C. Urinary incontinence is not a normal result of aging, and patients with incontinence may experience depression and limited social and sexual function. Providers should evaluate how incontinence is affecting quality of life and choose appropriate therapies based on the overall impact incontinence is having on the patient's lifestyle.

Khandelwal C, Kistler C. Diagnosis of urinary incontinence. *Am Fam Physician*. 2013;87:543–550.

22. D. All of the above will require a more extensive workup and require a urologic referral. All patients with an unclear etiology for urinary incontinence after the initial assessment should also be referred to a specialist for further evaluation.

Khandelwal C, Kistler C. Diagnosis of urinary incontinence. *Am Fam Physician*. 2013;87:543–550.

23. C. Geriatric failure to thrive is often associated with dehydration, not physical activity; physical inactivity occurs with this syndrome.

Robertson RG, Montagnini M. Geriatric failure to thrive. *Am Fam Physician*. 2004;70:343–350.

24. D. A comprehensive initial assessment should include information about physical and psychological health, functional ability, and socioeconomic factors.

Robertson RG, Montagnini M. Geriatric failure to thrive. *Am Fam Physician*. 2004;70:343–350.

25. B. A urinalysis, not a culture, is recommended for the initial workup.

Robertson RG, Montagnini M. Geriatric failure to thrive. *Am Fam Physician*. 2004;70:343–350.

26. C. Current recommendations suggest that 25–30% of total calories should come from fat; some fat in the diet is required for fat-soluble vitamins.

Yukawa, M. Defining adequate nutrition for older adults In: Williams BA, Chang A, eds. *Current Diagnosis & Treatment: Geriatrics*. 2nd ed. 2014. New York: McGraw-Hill; 2014: 494–500.

27. A. The MNA is the most well validated nutritional screening tool for the elderly and enables a patient to be categorized as normal (adequate nutrition), borderline (at risk of malnutrition), or undernutrition. A score between 8 and 11 points indicates risk for malnutrition and a score less than 8 indicates a malnourished patient. The original MNA was developed on the basis of a study comparing a population of frail elderly and healthy elderly in Toulouse, France.

Guigoz Y, Vellas B, Garry PJ. Mini nutritional assessment: a practical assessment tool for grading the nutritional state of elderly patients. In: Vellas BJ, Guigoz Y, Garry PJ, Albarede JL, eds. *The Mini Nutritional Assessment: MNA. Nutrition in the Elderly*. 1997:15–60. http://www.cabdirect.org/abstracts/19971409869.html;jsessionid=522FF0C20132 F44ADC02ACAC9E954E35. Revised MNA available at: http://www.mna-elderly.com/. Accessed January 10, 2016.

28. C. More than 100 randomized controlled trials showed PRT to be an effective strategy for improving physical functioning in older people. PRT involves exercising against an increasing external load.

Liu CJ, Latham NK. Progressive resistance strength training for improving physical function in older adults. *Cochrane Database Syst Rev* 2009;3:CD002759.

29. D. The AD8 is a brief instrument to help discriminate between signs of normal aging and mild dementia.

Galvin JE, Roe CM, Powlishta KK, ET AL. The AD8: a brief informant interview to detect dementia. *Neurology*. 2005; 65(4):559–564. http://www.alz.org/documents_custom/ad8 .pdf. Accessed January 10, 2016.

30. C. Rationale: Cognitive impairment is a risk factor for falls in older persons, but it is not modifiable.

Panel on Prevention of Falls in Older Persons, American Geriatrics Society, British Geriatrics Society. Summary of the updated American Geriatrics Society/British Geriatrics Society clinical practice guideline for prevention of falls in older persons. *J Am Geriatr Soc*. 2011;59:148–157.

31. D. Multifactorial interventions are most effective, but there is conflicting evidence about which interventions to recommend.

Panel on Prevention of Falls in Older Persons, American Geriatrics Society, British Geriatrics Society. Summary of the updated American Geriatrics Society/British Geriatrics Society clinical practice guideline for prevention of falls in older persons. *J Am Geriatr Soc*. 2011;59:148–157.

32. D. Nurse practitioners may not intervene with fall prevention because of a perception that it is not an acute problem. A fall-prevention prescription can simplify the multifactorial interventions that should be explored.

Moncada LVV. Management of falls in older persons: a prescription for prevention. *Am Fam Physician*. 2011;84: 1267–1276.

33. C. A dose of 1200 mg of daily calcium is recommended as a treatment for osteoporosis, but bisphosphonate therapy is recommended for up to 5 years.

Favus MJ. Bisphosphonates for osteoporosis. *N Engl J Med*. 2010;363:2027–2035.

34. D. Driving is considered an essential component of maintaining a person's lifestyle, and making a decision to remove the ability of a patient to drive is a difficult decision for the nurse practitioner.

Novak J, McGee C, Curry K. Older adults and driving: NP role in assessment and management. *Am J Nurse Pract*. 2012;16:26–32.

35. B. Although the NHTSA makes recommendations for safe driving, individual states are responsible for licensing drivers, monitoring licensed drivers, and enforcing state driving laws.

Novak J, McGee C, Curry K. Older adults and driving: NP role in assessment and management. *Am J Nurse Pract*. 2012;16:26–32.

36. A. Adult children should be included in fact finding, because they are the most likely people who have witnessed the patient's driving skills. Legitimate reasons that can prompt adult children to request driving restrictions may include close calls, actual accidents, and signs of dementia or sensory loss.

Novak J, McGee C, Curry K. Older adults and driving: NP role in assessment and management. *Am J Nurse Pract.* 2012; 16:26–32.

37. B. Exploring patient and family perceptions is an important component of building trust. NPs should always ask what the patient and family already know or what they think is going on.

Baile WF, Buckman R, Lenzi R, et al. SPIKES—a six step protocol for delivering bad news: application to the patient with cancer. *Oncologist.* 2000;5:302–311. http://hiv.ubccpd .ca/files/2012/09/Summary-on-Breaking-Bad-News.pdf. Accessed January 10, 2016.

38. D. There are many treatment strategies for pain management at end of life. The WHO ladder is a helpful tool to help determine titration of medications.

Dalacorte RR, Rigo JC, Dalacorte A. Pain management in the elderly at the end of life. *N Am J Med Sci.* 2011;3:348–354.

39. C. The palliative prognosis score divides patients into three specific risk classes based on the following six predictive factors of death: dyspnea, anorexia, Karnofsky Performance Status (KPS), Clinical Prediction of Survival (CPS), total white blood count (WBC), and lymphocyte percentage. The PaP score is a simple instrument that permits a more accurate quantification of expected survival and is suitable for use in clinical practice.

Maltoni M, Nanni O, Pirovano M, et al. Successful validation of the palliative prognostic score in terminally ill cancer patients. Italian Multicenter Study Group on Palliative Care. *J Pain Symptom Manage.* 1999;17(4):240–247.

40. D. Nurse practitioners have demonstrated safe and responsible care and have expert knowledge that allows them to provide high-level assessments of patients' needs and recognize when hospice care is needed by their patients. To date nurse practitioners are authorized to be Part B Medicare providers, but they are unable to order hospice care for their patients. Instead, they must find a physician to sign orders at an additional cost for these services when needed.

American Association of Nurse Practitioners. Fact sheet: ordering home health care S227 and HR2267. 2012. http:// www.aanp.org/component/content/article/68-articles/331- ordering-home-health-care. Accessed January 10, 2016.

ndex